Diagnostic Cerebral Angiography

Second Edition

Diagnostic Cerebral Angiography

Second Edition

Anne G. Osborn, M.D., F.A.C.R.
Professor of Radiology
William H. and Patricia N. Child Presidential Endowed Chair
  Honoring Pioneering Utah Women in Medicine
University of Utah School of Medicine
Salt Lake City, Utah
and
Nycomed Amersham Visiting Professor in Diagnostic Imaging
Armed Forces Institute of Pathology
Washington, D.C.

With a chapter on technical aspects of cerebral angiography by
John M. Jacobs, M.D.
Clinical Associate Professor of Radiology
University of Utah School of Medicine
Salt Lake City, Utah

Illustrated by
Julian Maack, M.F.A., C.M.I
Director, Department of Medical Illustration
University of Utah School of Medicine
Salt Lake City, Utah

Computer images and layout by
Lisa-Antoinette Quillman, B.F.A.
Graphic Artist, Department of Radiology
University of Utah School of Medicine
Salt Lake City, Utah

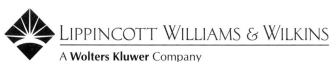

LIPPINCOTT WILLIAMS & WILKINS
A **Wolters Kluwer** Company
Philadelphia · Baltimore · New York · London
Buenos Aires · Hong Kong · Sydney · Tokyo

Acquisitions Editor: Joyce-Rachel John
Developmental Editor: Delois Patterson
Manufacturing Manager: Dennis Teston
Production Manager: Cassie Moore
Cover Designer: Wanda Kossack
Indexer: Ann Cassar
Compositor: Lippincott Williams & Wilkins Desktop Division
Printer: Kingsport Press

Printed in the United States of America

9 8 7 6 5 4 3 2 1

Library of Congress Cataloging-in-Publication Data

Osborn, Anne G., 1943–
    Diagnostic cerebral angiography / Anne G. Osborne; with a chapter on technical aspects of cerebral angiography by John M. Jacobs; illustrated by Julian Maack; computer images and layout by Lisa-Antoinette Quillman. — 2nd ed.
        p.   cm.
    Rev. ed. of: Introduction to cerebral angiography / Anne G. Osborn. c1980.
    Includes bibliographical references and index.
    ISBN 0-397-58404-0
    1. Brain—Blood-vessels—Radiography. 2. Angiography.
I. Jacobs, John M., M.D. II. Osborn, Anne G., 1943–   Introduction to cerebral angiography. III. Title
    [DNLM: 1. Cerebral Angiography. WL 141081da 1999]
RC386.6.A54082 1999
616.8′047572—dc21
DNLM/DLC   98-39295
for Library of Congress   CIP

To my parents,
who, having opened all the doors for their children
now prepare to walk through a very special set of their own.
With great love, much affection, and many thanks.

Contents

Preface

The first edition of this book, published in 1980 as *Introduction to Cerebral Angiography,* has been through sixteen printings. In the nearly two decades since that first publication, the increasing sophistication of noninvasive techniques has radically changed the role of cerebral angiography itself. Though the anatomical foundations of neuroangiography have of course remained unchanged and high quality analog subtraction films can still be useful, the advent of superselective techniques and 1024 x 1024 digital biplane studies has provided us with new, breathtakingly detailed images of the craniocervical vasculature. Thanks to our neuropathology colleagues and advances in decoding the human genome, we also understand a great deal more about the disease processes that affect the brain blood vessels.

So, at last it was time for a radical revision.

Diagnostic Cerebral Angiography is, in essence, really a brand-new book. Only a handful of illustrations (mostly a few of Julian Maack's elegant line drawings) were retained from the first edition and the text has been written entirely from scratch. Almost nothing of the old dowager (the book, not me!) remains.

As is the case with all my books, *Diagnostic Cerebral Angiography* is designed as a teaching text. I have attempted to amalgamate, consolidate, simplify, and illustrate the pathology, epidemiology, and (of course) imaging findings for just about every major disease (and many important minor ones) that affects the craniocerebral vessels. For easy review, key information is summarized and highlighted in the special boxes that accompany each chapter. The references were updated and the text changed to reflect new information available within three months of publication.

So what isn't in here? That will become obvious as you read. As this book focuses on cerebral angiography (the conventional kind), noninvasive studies are used very sparingly and only to illustrate special points. I have chosen to focus on the diagnostic aspect of cerebral angiography, so the interventional cases are also limited.

Finally, the closing chapter by John Jacobs is a very straightforward and nicely illustrated "how-to" section that presents the basic techniques of performing a cerebral angiogram.

I hope you'll enjoy the second go-'round.

Anne G. Osborn
Salt Lake City, Utah

Acknowledgments

No one really writes a book alone, even a "single author" text such as this one. So a number of thanks are due. To our neuroradiology section, so ably led by Ric Harnsberger, for the commitment to quality and education that forms the foundation of all that we do. To our incomparable Chief of Medical Illustrations, Julian Maack, whose elegant line drawings have graced our texts and journal articles for more than twenty years. To Lisa Quillman, whose technical know-how and artist's eye were essential in designing the computerized figures. To Roland, Vangee, the file room personnel and all the technicians whose day-to-day diligence helps make us productive. And finally, to my beloved husband and eternal companion Ron. Your patience, forbearance, and unfailing good cheer throughout the whole intense creative process kept me sane and whole. I love you.

Anne G. Osborn

SECTION I

Normal Gross and Angiographic Anatomy of the Craniocervical Vasculature

CHAPTER 1

The Aortic Arch and Great Vessels

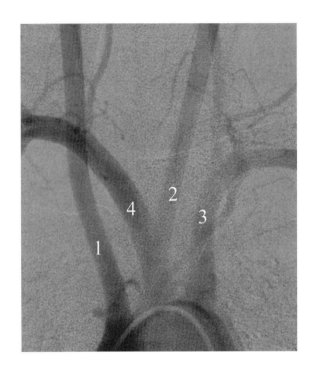

Cerebral angiography begins at the aortic arch. Understanding the normal anatomy, common variants, and important anomalies of the aortic arch is a prerequisite for safe, efficient catheterization of the craniocervical vessels. Atheromatous lesions of the aortic arch are also an independent risk factor for arterial embolism and ischemic stroke. Therefore, the discussion of cerebral angiography begins with the normal development, gross anatomy, and imaging of the aortic arch and great vessels.

AORTIC ARCH

Normal Development

Introduction

Normal development of the human aortic arch and great vessels involves the formation and selective regression of paired vascular arches that connect the embryonic aortic sac (ventral aorta) with the paired dorsal aortae. Five pairs of arches arise that correspond to pharyngeal arches 1, 2, 3, 4, and 6 (the fifth arch never develops at all or appears briefly and then regresses) (1). Initially developing as undifferentiated plexiform networks, the embryonic vascular arches arise in a craniocaudal sequence and form primitive arterial arcades around the pharyngeal arches (1).

Some segments of the developing fetal craniocerebral vasculature partially regress or disappear completely, whereas others persist as anlage for the definitive aortic arch, great vessels, and their branches. Structures that arise from the first three pairs of arches are bilateral and symmetrical, but those that originate from the fourth and sixth arches develop asymmetrically (1–4) (Table 1-1).

Three to Four Weeks of Fetal Development

The first pair of pharyngeal arches, also called the maxillomandibular arches, appears at about 22 days of fetal development. By day 24 a corresponding pair of vascular arches arises from the aortic sac. The *first aortic arches* are plexiform vessels that connect the embryonic ventral aorta to the paired dorsal aortae (1).

The second pair of pharyngeal arches, the hyoid arches, appears by day 24. The *second aortic arches* appear by day 26 as the first pair regresses.

The *third and fourth aortic arches* appear on day 28; the *sixth arches* form on day 29. By day 29 the first and second arches have largely disappeared (Fig. 1-1). The proximal ends of the second arches, the *hyoid arteries*, persist as stems for the developing *stapedial arteries* and may contribute some components to the definitive external carotid arteries (ECAs) (5) (see Chapter 2).

TABLE 1-1. *Aortic arch and great vessels: normal development*

Embryonic precursor	Primitive artery formed	Regression/remodeling pattern	Becomes
Bulbus cordis	Truncus arteriosus	Aorticopulmonary septum forms	Ascending aorta, pulmonary trunk
Aortic sac	Ventral aorta	Persists	Ascending aorta, brachiocephalic trunk
Dorsal aortae	Carotid arteries (distal)	Right partially regresses (distal to SCA)	Part of RSCA, right distal ICA
		Left persists	Left distal ICAs, descending aorta
Cervical plexi	Cervical intersegmental arteries	C1–6 (proximal segments regress)	Vertebral arteries
		C7	Subclavian arteries
Dorsal plexi	Longitudinal neural arteries	Midline fusion	Basilar artery
Aortic arches			
I	Mandibular arteries	Involute	± distal ECA
II	Hyoid arteries	Mostly involute	Caroticotympanic arteries
	Stapedial arteries	Partially involute	Distal segments persist as middle meningeal artery, internal maxillary branches of ECA
III	Carotid arteries (proximal)	Persists	CCAs, proximal ICAs, ECA (*de novo* sprout)
IV	Right and left primitive aortic arches	Asymmetric remodeling	Right → proximal SCA Left → definitive aortic arch
VI	Ductus arteriosus	Asymmetric remodeling Right partial Left persists	Right pulmonary arteries Left pulmonary arteries Ductus arteriosus

SCA, subclavian; ECA, external carotid artery; CCA, common carotid artery; ICA, internal carotid artery, C, cervical intersegmental artery.

During early fetal development, intracranial blood flow is derived primarily from the *primitive carotid arteries.* The proximal aspects of these vessels, the future common carotid arteries (CCAs), arise from the ventral aorta and third arches. The distal segments, the future internal carotid arteries (ICAs), represent cephalad continuations of the paired dorsal aortae (Fig. 1-1).

Each distal ICA divides into a cranial division (that will give rise to the future anterior cerebral artery) and a caudal division (the precursor of the posterior communicating artery) (5,6).

Five Weeks of Fetal Development

By day 35 the third, fourth, and sixth arches are well developed (Fig. 1-2A). The dorsal aortic segments between the third and fourth arches regress. The *internal carotid arteries* are now supplied entirely by the ventral aorta and third aortic arches (Fig. 1-2B). A new

source of blood flow to the hindbrain develops from two vascular plexi that lie dorsal to the third and fourth arches. These plexiform vessels, the paired *longitudinal neural arteries,* eventually fuse in the midline and become the definitive basilar artery.

The longitudinal neural arteries are initially supplied from below by the cervical intersegmental arteries. However, four transient connections between each longitudinal neural artery and its corresponding carotid artery also develop. The most prominent and cephalad of these primitive anastomoses is the *trigeminal artery* (3,5,6). Other embryonic anastomoses between the carotid and hindbrain circulations are the *primitive otic, hypoglossal, and proatlantal intersegmental arteries* (Fig. 1-2).

Development of the *external carotid arteries* (ECAs) is less clear and more speculative (5). The ECAs probably sprout *de novo* from the aortic sac or ventral end of the third arches (common carotid arteries). Remnants of the first and second arches may contribute some distal ECA branches (see Chapter 2).

Six Weeks of Fetal Development

The caudal divisions of the primitive internal carotid arteries, which will become the definitive *posterior communicating arteries*, anastomose with the paired longitudinal neural arteries (Fig. 1-3). As these cranial anastomoses are established, the transient connections between the longitudinal neural arteries and the ICAs involute. If these embryonic anastomoses fail to regress, so-called persistent carotid–basilar anastomoses such as a primitive trigeminal artery result (6,7) (see Chapter 3).

At this stage, connections between the seven cervical intersegmental arteries also begin to coalesce and form the definitive *vertebral arteries*. The proximal connections between the first six cervical intersegmental arteries and the dorsal aortae regress. The seventh intersegmental arteries enlarge and will become the definitive *subclavian arteries*. The *pulmonary arteries* initially sprout from the fourth arch but become secondarily reconnected to the sixth arches (7) (Fig. 1-3).

Seven Weeks of Fetal Development

The fourth and sixth arches undergo asymmetric remodeling to supply blood to the upper extremities, dorsal aorta, and lungs (1). The left fourth aortic arch and the dorsal aorta become the definitive aortic arch and the most cranial portion of the descending aorta (Fig. 1-4). The right dorsal aorta remains connected to the right fourth arch but gradually loses its connections with both the midline descending aorta and the right sixth arch (Figs. 1-3 and 1-4).

Both seventh cervical segmental arteries, arising from their respective fourth arches, enlarge into the developing limb buds and form the proximal *subclavian arteries*. The right fourth dorsal aortic segment distal to the seventh cervical segmental artery and the subclavian artery then involutes. The definitive right subclavian artery (RSCA) thus receives its blood supply from the brachiocephalic artery, which is itself a remnant of the embryonic third and fourth arches (1,3,7) (Fig. 1-4).

The *basilar artery* forms as the paired longitudinal neural arteries coalesce across the midline (Figs. 1-3 and 1-4). In turn, the developing basilar artery anastomoses inferiorly with the vertebral arteries that have been formed by coalescence of the longitudinal anastomoses between the cervical intersegmental arteries.

Eight Weeks of Fetal Development

By 8 weeks the developing aortic arch and great vessels approach their definitive configuration. The *external and internal carotid arteries* now arise from a common trunk that represents remnants of the ventral aorta and third aortic arches (Fig. 1-5). The ductus arteriosus remains open and connects the pulmonary trunk to the proximal descending aorta (Table 1-1).

Gross Anatomy

The thoracic aorta has four major segments: (a) the ascending aorta, (b) the transverse aorta, (c) the aortic isthmus, and (d) the descending aorta.

Ascending Aorta

The ascending aorta is about 5 cm in length. From its origin at the base of the left ventricle, the aorta ascends obliquely behind the sternum (see Fig. 1-27). The *right* and *left coronary arteries* originate from the anterior and left posterior sinuses.

Transverse Aorta

The transverse aorta consists primarily of the aortic arch. The arch lies in the superior mediastinum, beginning at the level of the second right sternocostal articulation. The aorta then curves backward and to the left over the left pulmonary hilum (see Fig. 1-27). The aortic arch thus has two curvatures: one that is convex upward and another that is convex forward and curving to the left. The major branches that arise from the transverse aorta are the *brachiocephalic trunk,* the *left common carotid artery* (LCCA), and the *left subclavian artery* (LSCA).

Aortic Isthmus

The fetal aorta narrows just distal to the left subclavian artery (LCSA). This normally narrowed area between the LSCA and site of the ductus arteriosus is called the aortic isthmus. The aorta just beyond the ductus may have a fusiform enlargement called the aortic spindle. These features may persist into adulthood and should not be mistaken for disease (7) (see below).

Descending Aorta

The descending thoracic aorta begins at the left of the fourth thoracic vertebra and extends inferiorly to the diaphragm (7).

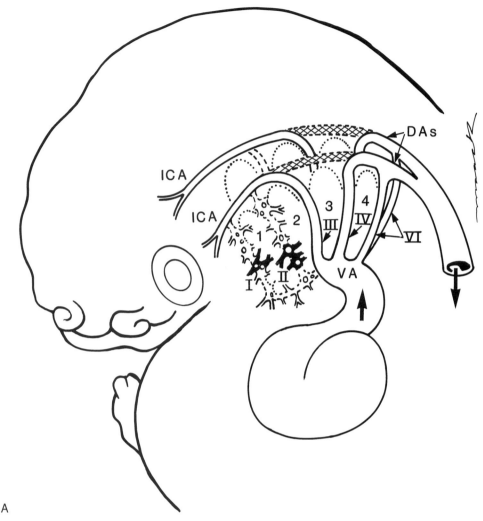

A

FIG. 1-1. A: Oblique three-dimensional anatomic sketch depicts the craniocerebral vasculature at approximately 4 gestational weeks (6 to 8 mm crown-rump stage). The relationship between the embryonic pharyngeal pouches (1–4) and the developing aortic arches (I–VI) is shown. The third, fourth, and sixth arches (*solid lines*) have appeared. The plexiform first and second arches have regressed (*dotted lines*) except for some small remnants (*solid black areas*) that may persist as part of the future distal external carotid arteries. The primitive internal carotid arteries (ICAs) are formed from cephalad continuation of the dorsal aortae (DAs), whereas the common carotid arteries are derived from the ventral aorta (VA) and third arches. The dorsal aortic segments between the third and fourth arches, indicated by the cross-hatched areas, are still patent at this stage but will eventually regress completely.

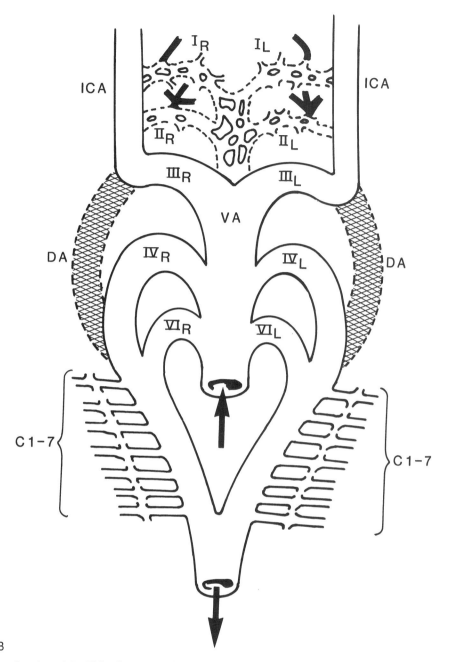

B

FIG. 1-1. *Continued.* **B:** This diagrammatic sketch (anteroposterior view) depicts the developing aortic arches (I–VI) and craniocervical vasculature at approximately 4 gestational weeks. The plexiform first and second arches (*dotted lines*) have largely regressed, except for small remnants (*solid black areas*) that are annexed later by the future external carotid arteries (see Fig. 2-2). The third and fourth arches are prominent; the sixth arches are beginning to develop. The dorsal aortic (DA) segments between the third and fourth arches (indicated by the cross-hatched areas) are still present but will soon regress. Cephalad continuation of the right and left dorsal aortic segments from their junction with the third arches forms the primitive internal carotid arteries (ICAs); their more proximal segments (i.e., the future common carotid arteries) are formed by the ventral aorta (VA) and third arches. The seven cervical intersegmental arteries are also depicted (C1–7). Their mid-segments are beginning to coalesce and will eventually form the definitive vertebral arteries. Direction of blood flow is indicated by the large black arrows.

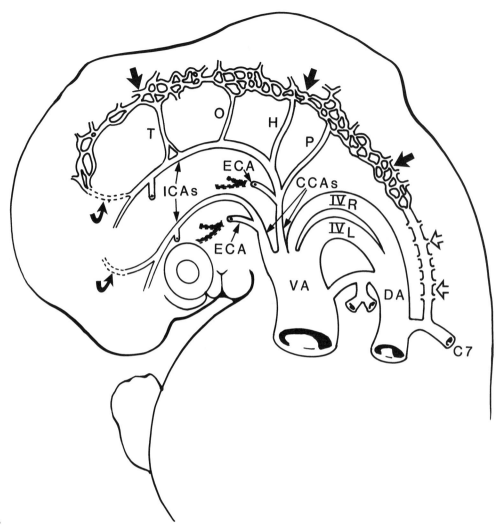

A

FIG. 1-2. A: Three-dimensional sketch at approximately 5 gestational weeks. Development of the paired plexiform longitudinal neural arteries (*solid black arrows*) is depicted. The vertebral arteries (*open arrows*) form as longitudinal anastomoses between the seven cervical intersegmental arteries. The proximal connections between the C1–6 arteries and the dorsal aorta (DA) are regressing. For simplification, only one set of longitudinal neural and cervical intersegmental arteries is shown. These vessels are the precursors of the vertebrobasilar circulation. Initially, the longitudinal neural arteries are supplied from below via the cervical intersegmental arteries. At this stage several temporary connections between the developing vertebrobasilar circulation and the carotid arteries also form. From cephalad to caudad, these arteries are the trigeminal (T), otic (O), hypoglossal (H), and proatlantal intersegmental arteries (P) (this vessel forms slightly later). These transient anastomoses regress as the caudal divisions of the primitive internal carotid arteries (ICAs) anastomose with the cranial ends of the longitudinal neural arteries and form the future posterior communicating arteries (*dotted lines with curved arrows*). Persistence of the transient embryonic interconnections is abnormal and results in a so-called primitive carotid–basilar anastomosis (see Chapters 3 and 4). Sprouting of the external carotid arteries (ECAs) from the proximal common carotid arteries (CCAs) is also depicted. These vessels will annex first and second arch remnants (*solid black areas*). VA, ventral aorta.

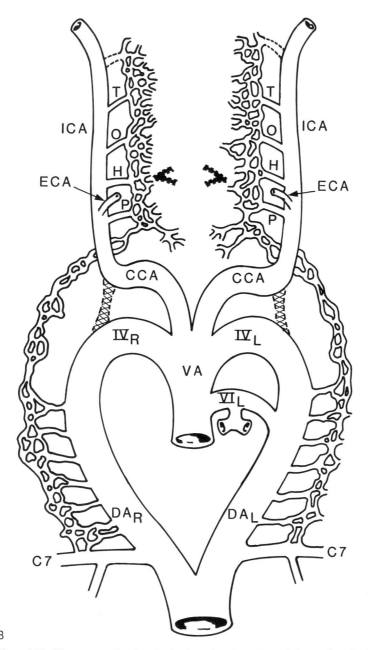

B

FIG. 1-2. *Continued.* **B:** Diagrammatic sketch depicts development of the embryologic craniocervical vasculature at approximately 35 gestational days. Both dorsal aortic segments that previously connected the third and fourth arches, indicated by the small cross-hatched areas, have regressed. The primitive internal carotid arteries (ICAs) now receive blood supply through the ventral aorta (VA) and common carotid arteries (CCAs), the former third arches. The external carotid arteries (ECAs) sprout from the CCAs. The fourth arches are both still prominent. The right sixth arch has involuted as the left sixth arch is forming the ductus arteriosus and pulmonary arteries. The vertebral arteries are formed as plexiform longitudinal anastomoses between the cervical intersegmental arteries. The seventh cervical segments (C7) are enlarging and will become the subclavian arteries. Connections between the proximal six segments and the dorsal aortae (DA) are starting to regress and eventually will disappear completely (see Fig. 1-3). Transient anastomoses between the paired plexiform longitudinal neural arteries are also depicted. From top down, these are the trigeminal (T), otic (O), hypoglossal (H), and proatlantal intersegmental arteries (P). The position of the future posterior communicating artery is indicated by the dotted lines.

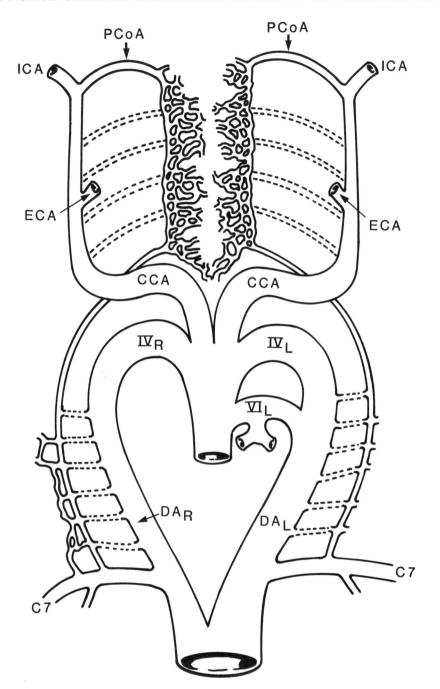

FIG. 1-3. Diagrammatic sketch of the fetal craniocervical vasculature at approximately 6 gestational weeks. The external carotid arteries (ECAs) arise from the common carotid arteries (CCAs). The caudal divisions of the ICAs, the future posterior communicating arteries (PCoAs; *arrows*), now join the cephalad aspects of the plexiform longitudinal neural arteries. The vertebral arteries arise from the enlarging seventh cervical intersegmental arteries (C7) and supply the caudal end of the longitudinal neural arteries. The temporary connections between the carotid arteries and plexiform longitudinal arteries have regressed, as have the connections between the first six cervical segments and the aortic arches (*dotted lines*). DA, dorsal aorta. Roman numerals indicate embryonic aortic arches.

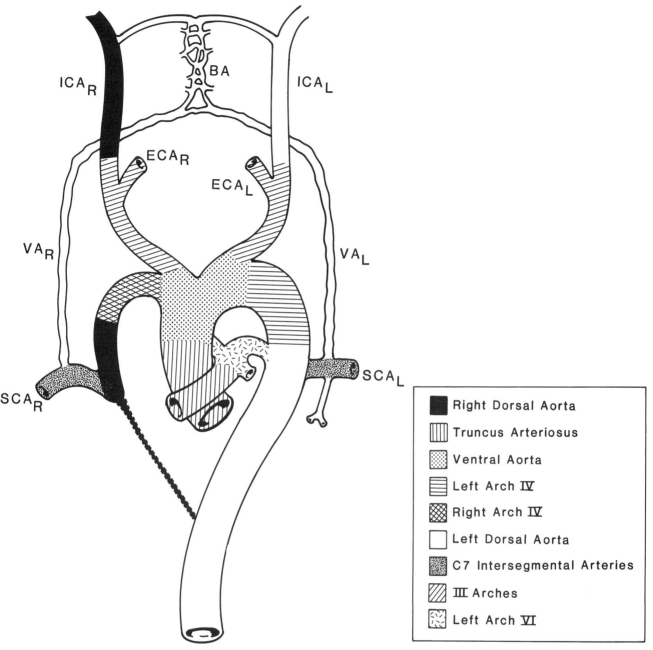

FIG. 1-4. Diagrammatic sketch of the craniocerebral vasculature at 7 weeks of development. The arch and great vessels are approaching their definitive form. Origins of these vessels from their embryonic precursors are depicted schematically. The fourth and sixth aortic arches are undergoing asymmetric remodeling to supply blood to the upper extremities, dorsal aorta, and lungs. The right sixth arch has involuted (leaving only part of the right pulmonary artery). The right dorsal aorta distal to the origin of the subclavian artery (SCA) is regressing (*dotted lines*) but remains connected to the right fourth arch. The right third and fourth arches are forming the brachiocephalic trunk; the left fourth arch becomes the definitive aortic arch. The left dorsal aorta becomes the proximal descending aorta. The first six cervical intersegmental arteries have become the definitive vertebral arteries (VAs); the C7 arteries have enlarged to become part of the developing subclavian arteries (SCAs). The longitudinal neural arteries are fusing across the midline to form the definitive basilar artery (BA).

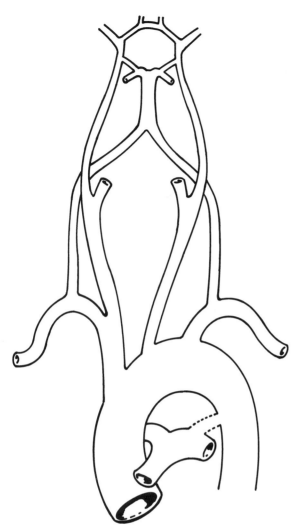

FIG. 1-5. This anatomic sketch depicts the craniocerebral vasculature at 8 weeks of fetal development. The definitive arch and great vessels have formed and are approaching their final configuration. The pulmonary trunk remains connected to the descending aorta via the ductus arteriosus (*dotted lines*).

Relationships

The aortic arch is anatomically related to a number of important structures, the most important of which are discussed below (7).

Anterior

The left vagus nerve (cranial nerve X [CN X]) and cervical sympathetic branches lie in front of the aortic arch.

Posterior

The trachea, left recurrent laryngeal nerve, esophagus, thoracic duct, and vertebral column lie behind the arch.

Superior

The great vessels, i.e., the brachiocephalic trunk and left common carotid and left subclavian arteries, are the most important structures that lie immediately above the aortic arch. The left brachiocephalic vein is also superior to the arch.

Inferior

The pulmonary bifurcation, ligamentum arteriosum, and left recurrent laryngeal nerve all lie below the arch.

Branches

The human aorta usually gives origin to three major branches that arise from the superior aspect of the arch (Fig. 1-6). In normal order of origin they are the brachio-

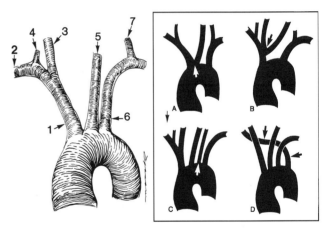

FIG. 1-6. Diagrammatic sketch of the normal aortic arch and its most common branching pattern is shown on the left.

1, Brachiocephalic trunk (innominate artery)
2, Right subclavian artery
3, Right common carotid artery
4, Right vertebral artery
5, Left common carotid artery
6, Left subclavian artery
7, Left vertebral artery

Diagrammatic sketches of frequently encountered aortic arch variants and common anomalies are shown on the right. **A:** Common origin of the innominate and left common carotid arteries from the arch (*arrow*). **B:** Origin of the left common carotid artery (*arrow*) from the innominate artery (brachiocephalic trunk). In this arrangement only two great vessels arise from the arch. **C:** Origin of the left vertebral artery (*arrow*) directly from the aortic arch. In this arrangement four great vessels arise from the arch. **D:** An aberrant right subclavian artery (*arrows*) arises directly from the arch as the fourth and last great vessel.

cephalic trunk (also called the innominate artery), left common carotid artery, and left subclavian artery (see box below).

Brachiocephalic Artery

The brachiocephalic trunk is the first and largest branch that arises from the aortic arch convexity. The brachiocephalic artery ascends posterolateral to the trachea. At the level of the sternoclavicular joint, the brachiocephalic trunk bifurcates into its two terminal branches, the *right subclavian artery* and the *right common carotid artery* (RCCA) (Fig. 1-7).

Left Common Carotid Artery

The left common carotid artery arises from the aortic arch apex just distal to the brachiocephalic artery origin. It initially ascends in front of the trachea, then passes posterolaterally and ascends along its left side. At about the upper border of the thyroid cartilage, the LCCA bifurcates into the *left internal and external carotid arteries* (Fig. 1-8).

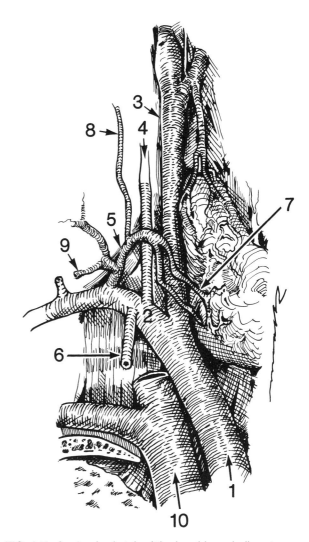

FIG. 1-7. Anatomic sketch of the brachiocephalic artery and its major branches.

1, Brachiocephalic (innominate) artery
2, Right subclavian artery
3, Right common carotid artery
4, Right vertebral artery
5, Thyrocervical trunk
6, Internal thoracic artery
7, Inferior thyroid artery
8, Ascending cervical artery
9, Transverse cervical artery
10, Brachiocephalic vein

Aortic Arch: Normal Anatomy and Variants

Normal development
 Left fourth embryonic arch
Key relationships
 Anterior: CN X (vagus nerve)
 Posterior: Trachea, esophagus, left recurrent laryngeal nerve
 Superior: Great vessels, left brachiocephalic vein
 Inferior: Pulmonary trunk and bifurcation, left recurrent laryngeal nerve
Branches
 Brachiocephalic artery
 Left common carotid artery
 Left subclavian artery
Common variants
 Brachiocephalic trunk and LCCA share common origin (25% to 30%)
 LCCA arises from brachiocephalic trunk (7%)
 LCCA and LSCA form a left-sided brachiocephalic trunk (1% to 2%)
 Left vertebral artery (LVA) arises directly from arch (0.5%)
Anomalies
 Left arch with aberrant right subclavian artery (0.4% to 2%)
 Right arch with aberrant left subclavian artery (most common type of right arch; frequent cause of symptomatic vascular ring)
 Right arch with mirror-image branching (occurs without ring but invariably associated with cyanotic congenital heart disease)
 Double aortic arch (DAA)

CN, cranial nerve; IV, fourth embryonic vascular arch; LCCA, left common carotid artery; LSCA, left subclavian artery.

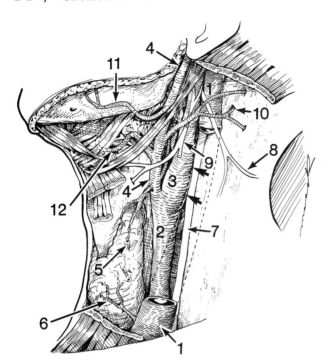

FIG. 1-8. Anatomic sketch of the left common carotid artery and its adjacent structures (oblique lateral view).

1, Internal jugular vein (cut across and partially removed to show carotid artery)
2, Common carotid artery
3, Internal carotid artery (*arrows on bulb*)
4, External carotid artery
5, Superior thyroid artery
6, Inferior thyroid artery (from thyrocervical trunk)
7, Vagus nerve (CN X)
8, Accessory nerve (CN XI)
9, Glossopharyngeal nerve (CN IX)
10, Occipital artery
11, Facial artery
12, Lingual artery

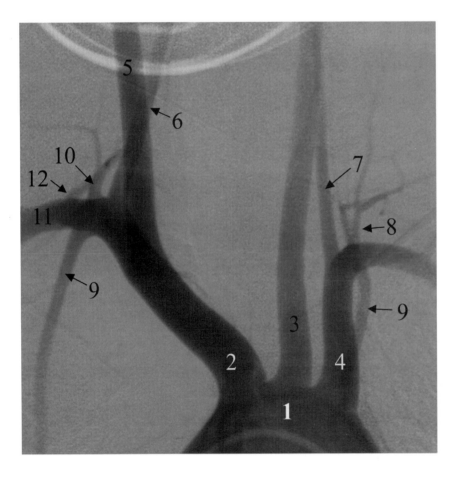

FIG. 1-9. Normal aortic arch angiogram in a 26-year-old patient (early arterial phase, shallow left anterior oblique view). The great vessels and some of their proximal branches are easily observed.

1, Aortic arch
2, Brachiocephalic (innominate) artery
3, Left common carotid artery
4, Left subclavian artery
5, Right common carotid artery
6, Right vertebral artery
7, Left vertebral artery
8, Left thyrocervical trunk
9, Right and left internal thoracic (mammary) arteries
10, Right thyrocervical trunk
11, Right subclavian artery
12, Right costocervical trunk

Left Subclavian Artery

The left subclavian artery (LSCA) arises from the aortic arch a few millimeters distal to the LCCA origin (see Fig. 9-1A). The left recurrent laryngeal nerve lies medial to the LSCA in the thorax. The LSCA ascends into the neck, then courses laterally to the medial border of the anterior scalene muscle. It is crossed anteriorly by the left phrenic nerve and thoracic duct.

Normal Angiographic Anatomy

Conventional Angiography

The left anterior oblique (LAO) position is typically used to image the aortic arch. The aortic arch itself and great vessel origins are usually delineated well on this standard projection (Fig. 1-9). The location and branching angles of the great vessels as they arise from the arch vary significantly (Figs. 1-9 and 1-10). Typically the branching angles are not affected by atherosclerosis or

hypertension, nor are they consistently correlated with age (8).

Origins of major branches from the great vessels often overlap each other on a single projection. Multiple views may be necessary to delineate vessel origins not easily seen on the routine LAO projection (Fig. 1-11). Selective catheterization of the proximal arch vessels with high-resolution digital subtraction angiography is often the most effective way to profile vascular origins and delineate individual branching patterns (Fig. 1-12).

Other Imaging Techniques

Although catheter angiography remains the definitive procedure for evaluating the aortic arch and great vessel origins, useful noninvasive adjuncts include routine computed tomography (CT) and CT angiography (CTA), contrast-enhanced magnetic resonance angiography (MRA), cine MR imaging, flow quantification, and echocardiography and color Doppler sonography (9–11).

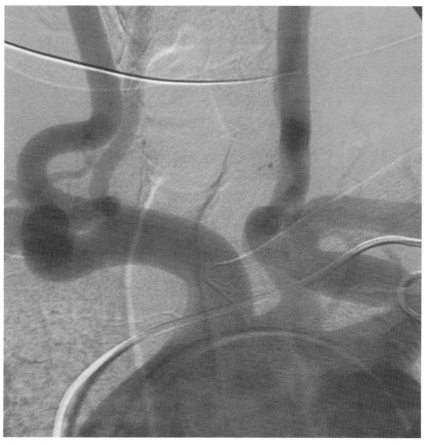

FIG. 1-10. Normal aortic arch angiogram in a 72-year-old patient (mid-arterial phase, shallow left anterior oblique projection). Some tortuosity and ectasia of the great vessels is present, but there is no angiographic evidence of atherosclerosis.

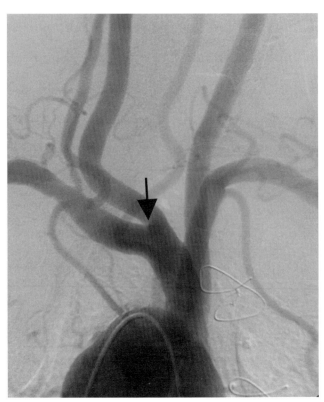

A   B

FIG. 1-11. Aortic arch angiogram (mid-arterial phase) in a 60-year-old patient is shown. On the standard left anterior oblique projection **(A)** the great vessel origins are well visualized, but the brachiocephalic artery bifurcation into the right subclavian and common carotid arteries (*arrow*) is poorly seen because of vessel overlap. In the opposite view **(B)** (i.e., the right anterior oblique projection) the brachiocephalic bifurcation (*arrow*) is profiled, but the great vessel origins are obscured by overlapping vessels.

Normal Variants

The typical order of great vessel origins (i.e., brachiocephalic trunk as the first branch followed by the LCCA and LSCA) is found in approximately two thirds of all cases. Many variations from this pattern occur. The number of great vessels that arise from the aortic arch may be as few as two or as many as six (7,8) (Fig. 1-6).

Common Origin of the Brachiocephalic and Left Common Carotid Arteries

A shared origin of the brachiocephalic trunk and LCCA is the most frequently encountered normal variant in aortic arch branching patterns. Sometimes called a bovine configuration, this arrangment occurs in 27% of all cases (Figs. 1-6A and 1-13). In 7% of cases, the LCCA arises from the proximal brachiocephalic artery instead of the aortic arch (Figs. 1-6B and 1-14). In 1% to 2% of cases, the LCCA and LSCA share a common origin and form a left-sided brachiocephalic trunk (7).

Arch Origin of the Left Vertebral Artery

The left VA arises directly from the aortic arch in 0.5% of cases. In this arrangement there are four (not three) great vessels that originate from the arch (Fig. 1-6C). The LVA is often hypoplastic and usually arises between the LCCA and LSCA (Fig. 1-15). Occasionally the LVA arises distal to the SCA (6).

Miscellaneous Variants

The RCCA and RSCA may arise separately from the aortic arch. In rare instances, the external and internal carotid arteries arise independently from the aortic arch. Anomalies such as aberrant course of the petrous internal carotid artery are common in such cases (see Chapter 3).

"Lumps" and "Bumps"

These are normal anatomic variants that can mimic acute aortic and brachiocephalic vessel injury at aortography. These variants include aortic "spindle," classic or

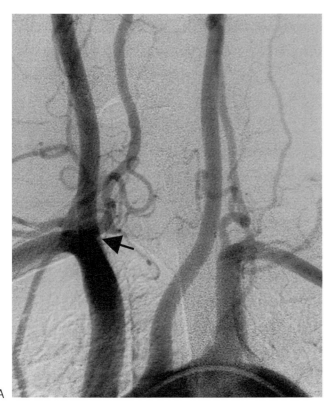
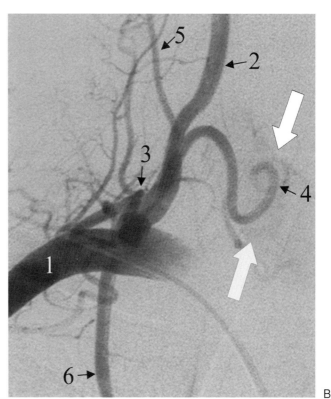

FIG. 1-12. The use of selective arteriography to profile arch vessels and their branches is demonstrated in this case. The standard left anterior oblique projection **(A)** shows the great vessels well, but the right vertebral artery (*arrow*) is obscured by the overlapping right common carotid artery. Selective injection of the right subclavian artery **(B)** shows its major branches. A faint vascular blush in the thyroid gland is indicated by the white arrows.

1, Right subclavian artery
2, Right vertebral artery
3, Thyrocervical trunk
4, Inferior thyroid artery
5, Ascending cervical artery
6, Internal thoracic artery

atypical ductal diverticulae, and infundibulae of the brachiocephalic arteries and adjacent branches (12).

A narrowed segment between the LSCA and the ductus arteriosis, the *aortic isthmus*, is present in newborn infants but usually disappears after 2 months of age. A circumferential bulge just beyond the ductus may persist into adulthood. This variant is called an *aortic spindle*. The junction between the isthmus and spindle is marked by an inferior indentation on aortic arch angiograms and is considered a normal variant (Fig. 1-16).

A *ductus diverticulum* is a focal bulge along the anteromedial aspect of the aortic isthmus. It is present in 33% of infants and 9% of adults and is a normal variant. A classic ductus diverticulum has smooth, uninterrupted margins and gently sloping symmetric shoulders (12).

Anomalies

Embryology

The normal aortic arch represents persistence of the left fourth embryonic vascular arch (see Table 1-1). The most widely used system to explain and classify common arch malformations is based on abnormal development of the fetal aortic arches (6,13–15). Persistence, migration, or interruption of these embryonic arches at abnormal locations explains the subsequent development of various congenital anomalies.

Most arch anomalies consist of errors in laterality (i.e., right aortic arch [RAA]) and/or errors in the level of interruption of the contralateral arch, which in turn determines the presence or absence of aberrant great vessels (14).

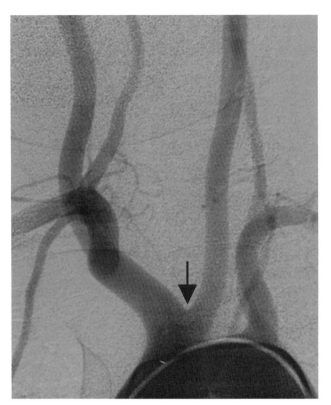

FIG. 1-13. Aortic arch angiogram (arterial phase, LAO view) shows a common origin of the brachiocephalic trunk and left common carotid artery (*arrow*). This normal variant occurs in about one fourth of all cases (see Fig. 1-6A).

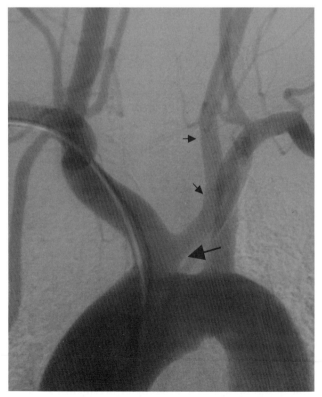

FIG. 1-14. Aortic arch angiogram (arterial phase, LAO view) shows a left common carotid artery (*small arrows*) originating from the brachiocephalic trunk (*large arrow*). In this normal variant there are only two great vessels that arise from the aortic arch.

Aortic arch anomalies are classically divided according to site of the arch (e.g., left, right, or double), location of supraaortic vessels, and position of the descending aorta. Anomalies also may exist with or without additional abnormalities such as stenosis, atresia, coarctation, or diverticulum (14,15).

Some uncommon or atypical malformations are difficult to classify. Newer morphologic approaches to classifying aortic arch anomalies detail each anomaly on the basis of its abnormality of position and caliber (see box below) (14).

Classification of Aortic Arch Anomalies

Position of aorta
   Transverse characteristics (axial plane)
      Side of arch
         Left aortic arch (LAA)
         Right aortic arch (RAA)
         Double aortic arch (DAA)
      Side of descending aorta (relative to arch)
         Ipsilateral
         Midline
         Contralateral
      Site of interruption/involuted segment
         Distal to subclavian artery
         Between common carotid and subclavian
            arteries
         Proximal to common carotid artery
   Vertical characteristics (level of arch in coronal
      plane)
      Below manubrium (normal)
      Manubrial
      Above manubrium
Caliber of aorta
   Size
      Normal
      Abnormal
         Stenotic (coarctation)
         Atretic (interruption)
         Ectatic
   Site of abnormality
      Ascending aorta
      Arch
      Descending aorta
      Great vessels
Number of anomalies
   Solitary
   Multiple
      Position
      Caliber
   Miscellaneous associated abnormalities (e.g.,
      diverticulum)

Data in this box adapted and modified from the concepts in ref. 14.

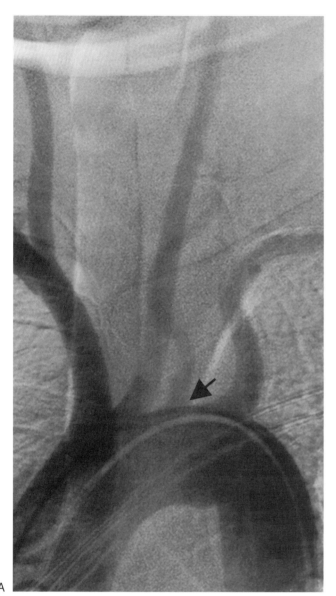 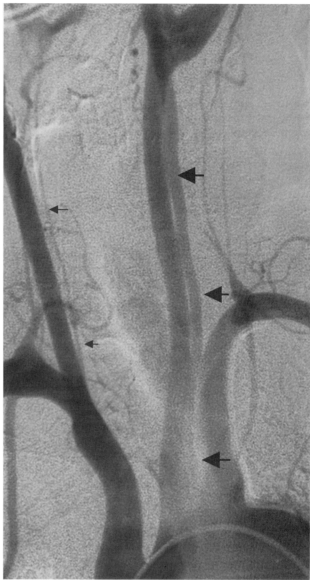

A   B

FIG. 1-15. A: Aortic arch angiogram (early arterial phase, LAO view) shows a large left vertebral artery arising directly from the aortic arch (*arrow*). In this arrangement there are four great vessels that arise from the aortic arch. **B:** Aortic arch angiogram in another patient shows a left vertebral artery that arises directly from the aortic arch (*large arrows*). Only the thyrocervical trunk and internal thoracic (mammary) artery arise from the subclavian artery. The right vertebral artery (*small arrows*) is hypoplastic.

A detailed delineation of complex congenital heart disease with all the possible aortic arch anomalies is beyond the scope of this text. Here we delineate only the most common anomalies and rare but important anomalies that may be encountered when performing cerebral angiography.

Left Aortic Arch with Aberrant Branching Patterns

A left aortic arch with an *aberrant right subclavian artery* (ARSCA) is the most common congenital arch anomaly, with a reported prevalence ranging from 0.4%

to 2% (6,16). This malformation results from persistence of the embryonic right dorsal aorta combined with involution of the arch segment between the RCCA and RSCA.

In this anomaly, the first branch that arises from the arch is the RCCA, followed in sequence by the LCCA and LSCA. The ARSCA arises as the last arch branch and crosses the mediastinum from left to right behind the esophagus (Figs. 1-6D and 1-17) (15).

Occasionally an ARSCA arises from a common trunk with the LSCA. This arrangement, sometimes called a bitruncus arch, forms a relatively uncommon type of vas-

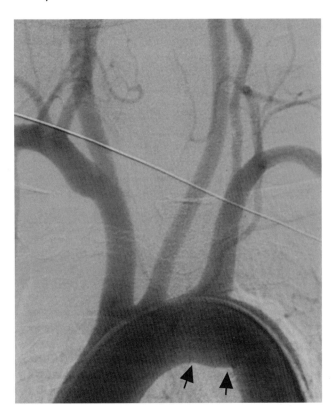

FIG. 1-16. Aortic arch angiogram (arterial phase, LAO view) shows an indentation (*arrows*) along the inferior curve of the aortic arch. This is a relatively common normal variant and should not be mistaken for a dissection.

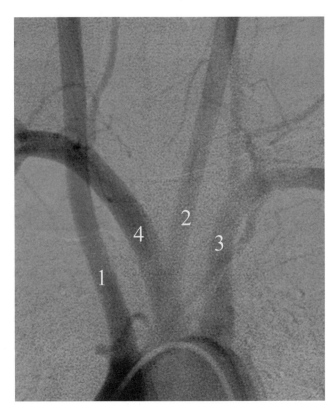

FIG. 1-17. Aortic arch angiogram (arterial phase, LAO view) shows a left arch with an aberrant right subclavian artery (ARSCA). This is the most common congenital arch anomaly, seen in 0.4% to 2% of cases (see also Fig. 1-6D).

1, Right common carotid artery
2, Left common carotid artery
3, Left subclavian artery
4, Aberrant right subclavian artery

cular ring. Here only two great vessels arise from the aortic arch (Fig. 1-18). Compression of the trachea by the bicarotid truncus in front and the bisubclavian truncus behind may cause stridor (17).

Although an ARSCA typically exists as an isolated anomaly and is discovered incidentally, it also may be associated with an aneurysm or a remnant (Kommerell's) diverticulum (Fig. 1-19). Here the aberrant artery arises from a diverticulumlike structure that is thought to represent a persisting segment of the distal embryonic right aortic arch (18,19).

Right Aortic Arch Anomalies

Right aortic arch anomalies represent persistence of the right fourth embryonic arch.

A *right aortic arch with an aberrant left subclavian artery* is the most common type of right aortic arch (20). It is one of the most common causes of a symptom-producing vascular ring (21). In this anomaly, four vessels originate from the right arch (Fig. 1-20). The LCCA is the first branch to arise from the right-sided arch (Fig. 1-

20A), followed by the RCCA (Fig. 1-20A and B) and RSCA (Fig. 1-20C). The aberrant LSCA arises as the last branch and usually originates from a posterior aortic diverticulum at the junction of the right arch and retroesophageal descending aorta (Fig. 1-21A) (20–22).

In the most common form of *right aortic arch with mirror-image branching*, the left side of the hypothetical double aortic arch is interrupted between either the left ductus arteriosus or descending aorta. In this anomaly, a left innominate artery is the first aortic branch. It courses anterior to the trachea and gives rise to both the LCCA and LSCA. The second branch is the RCCA and the third is the RSCA (Fig. 1-21B). The left ductus arteriosus connects the subclavian portion of the innominate artery to the left pulmonary artery.

A right aortic arch with mirror-image branching does not produce a vascular ring. However, this type of RAA is invariably associated with cyanotic congenital heart disease, particularly tetralogy of Fallot, truncus arterio-

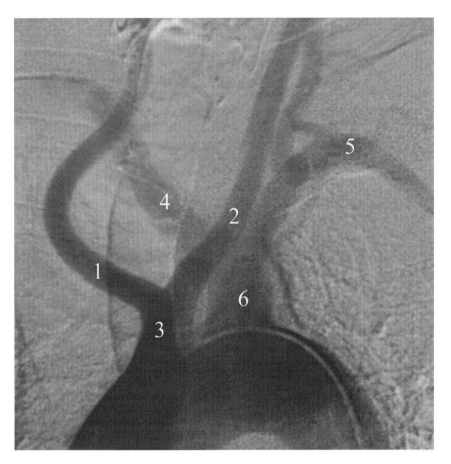

FIG. 1-18. Aortic arch angiogram (early arterial phase, LAO view) shows only two great vessels. Both the right (1) and left (2) common carotid arteries arise together from a single trunk (3). An aberrant right subclavian artery (4) and a normally positioned left subclavian artery (5) also arise from a common trunk (6). This relatively uncommon anomaly is sometimes called a bitruncus arch because only two great vessels arise from the arch itself. This arrangement forms a type of incomplete vascular ring around the trachea, which can be compressed by the bicarotid trunk (3) in front and the subclavian trunk (6) behind.

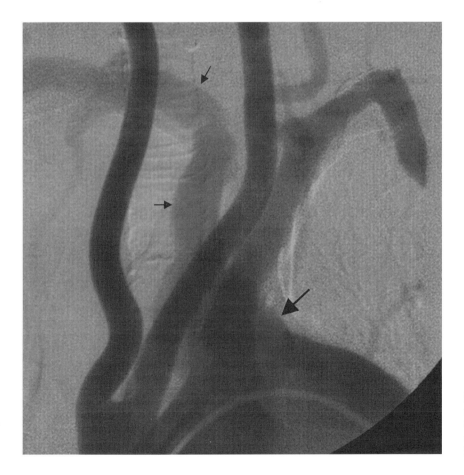

FIG. 1-19. Aortic arch angiogram (early arterial phase, LAO view) shows an aberrant right subclavian artery (*small arrows*) with aneurysmal dilatation at its origin (*large arrow*).

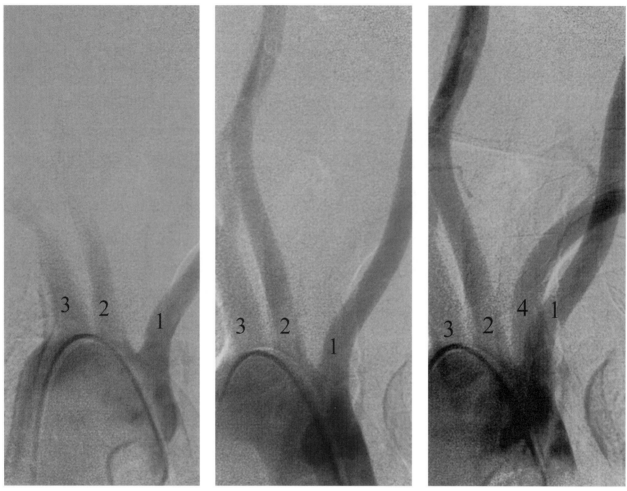

A

B,C

FIG. 1-20. Aortic arch angiogram, anteroposterior view, shows a right aortic arch with an aberrant left subclavian artery. This is a common form of complete vascular ring. Early **(A)** and mid-arterial phase **(B)** frames show that the left common carotid artery (1) is the first branch that arises from the right-sided aortic arch. The right common carotid (2) and subclavian (3) arteries are also seen. **(C)** Late arterial view shows opacification of the left subclavian artery (4), the last vessel that arises from the arch.

sus, and (less commonly) tricuspid atresia (15,17,20, 23).

Double Aortic Arch Anomalies

A double aortic arch (DAA) is one of the most common causes of a symptomatic vascular ring or sling (15,17,20,23–25). Embryologically, a DAA represents persistence of both fourth fetal aortic arches. A *double aortic arch with both arches patent* is the most common form. The ascending aorta divides into right- and left-sided arches. The right is larger than the left in approximately 50% to 75% of cases. The two arches encircle the trachea and esophagus, then join posteriorly to form the descending aorta (which is usually on the left side). A

common carotid and a subclavian artery arises from each arch (Figs. 1-22, 1-23, and 1-24) (15,17,20).

A *double aortic arch with left arch atresia* is less common. In this anomaly the left arch is atretic and persists as a fibrous cord. Subtypes of this malformation are based on the precise site of left arch atresia (15,17,20).

Other Aortic Arch Anomalies

Other rare forms of arch and great vessel anomalies that may produce a symptomatic vascular ring include *left aortic arch with right descending aorta, right aortic arch with left descending aorta* (the so-called circumflex aorta) (Fig. 1-25), *right aortic arch with mirror-image branching and ligamentum arteriosum from the left pul-*

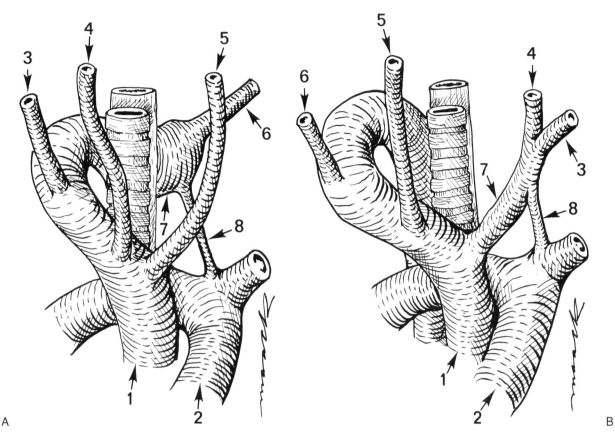

A

B

FIG. 1-21. A: Anatomic diagram depicts the most common type of right aortic arch (RAA), i.e., RAA with aberrant left subclavian artery (ALSCA). The distal aortic arch is retroesophageal and the left ductus arteriosus connects to an aortic diverticulum. The ALSCA arises from the aortic diverticulum. An RAA with an ALSCA does form a true vascular ring but usually does not cause stridor (modified and adapted with permission from ref. 15).

　1, Aorta
　2, Pulmonary trunk
　3, Right subclavian artery
　4, Right common carotid artery
　5, Left common carotid artery
　6, Aberrent left subclavian artery
　7, Aortic diverticulum
　8, Ligamentum arteriosum

B: Anatomic diagram depicts the most common type of right aortic arch (RAA) with mirror-image branching. The aorta descends on the right side. A left innominate artery is the first branch that arises from the arch. No vascular ring is formed, but this type of RAA is almost always associated with cyanotic congenital heart disease (modified and adapted with permission from ref. 15).

　1, Aorta
　2, Pulmonary trunk
　3, Left subclavian artery
　4, Left common carotid artery
　5, Right common carotid artery
　6, Right subclavian artery
　7, Left innominate artery
　8, Ligamentum arteriosum

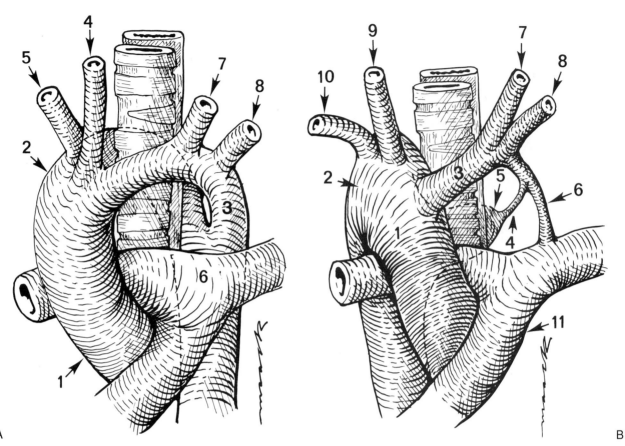

A   B

FIG. 1-22. A: Anteroposterior anatomic diagram depicts a functioning double aortic arch (DAA) with patent right and left arches. The aorta descends on the left. Each arch gives rise to its respective brachiocephalic arteries, i.e., the common carotid and subclavian arteries. Note that in this configuration the left-sided arch tends to be the anterior arch, whereas the right arch is the posterior arch (modified and adapted with permission from ref. 15).

   1, Ascending aorta
   2, Right arch
   3, Left arch
   4, Right common carotid artery
   5, Right subclavian artery
   6, Pulmonary trunk
   7, Left common carotid artery
   8, Left subclavian artery

B: Anteroposterior anatomic diagram depicts a double aortic arch (DAA) with left arch atresia. In the most common type the left arch is atretic distal to the subclavian artery origin. The aorta descends on the right.

   1, Ascending aorta
   2, Right arch
   3, Patent part of left arch
   4, Atretic part of left arch (connects to an aortic diverticulum)
   5, Aortic diverticulum
   6, Left ductus
   7, Left common carotid artery
   8, Left subclavian artery
   9, Right common carotid artery
   10, Left subclavian artery
   11, Pulmonary trunk

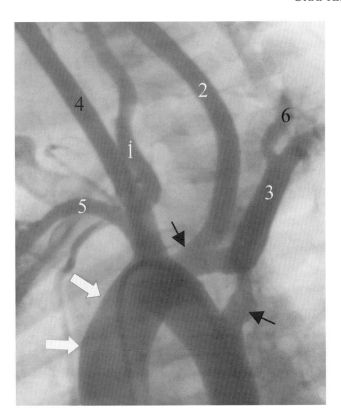

FIG. 1-23. Photographic reversal of a conventional aortic arch angiogram, mid-arterial phase, left anterior oblique view. A true functioning double aortic arch is present. Esophagram (not shown) in this patient with stridor disclosed both a right-sided extrinsic indentation and a posterior indentation. The right-sided arch (*white outlined arrows*) is dominant. There is a smaller left-sided arch (*black arrows*). A focal area of narrowing distal to the left subclavian artery origin is present. The right arch gives origin to the right subclavian (5) and common carotid (4) arteries. The left arch gives origin to the left common carotid (2) and subclavian (3) arteries. The right (1) and left (6) vertebral arteries arise normally from their respective subclavian arteries (case courtesy of Ina Tonkin, M.D.).

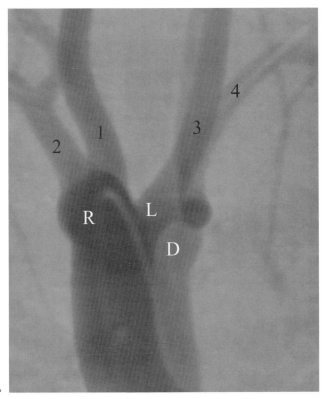

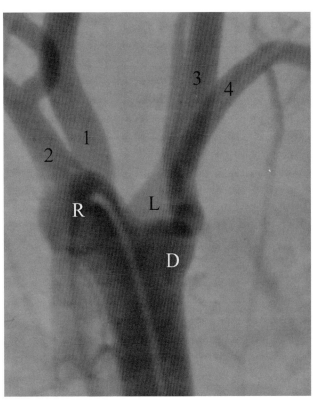

A

B

FIG. 1-24. A magnetic resonance imaging scan (not shown) in this 3-year-old child with stridor showed a true double aortic arch that encircled the trachea and esophagus. An aortic arch angiogram was performed. Early **(A)** and mid-arterial **(B)** phase frames (anteroposterior view) show that the right common (1) and right subclavian (2) arteries arise from the right arch (R). The left common (3) and left subclavian (4) arteries originate from the posterior left-sided arch (L). The two arches join to form a midline descending aorta. A diverticulum (D) is present at the proximal aspect of the descending aorta (case courtesy of Ina Tonkin, M.D.).

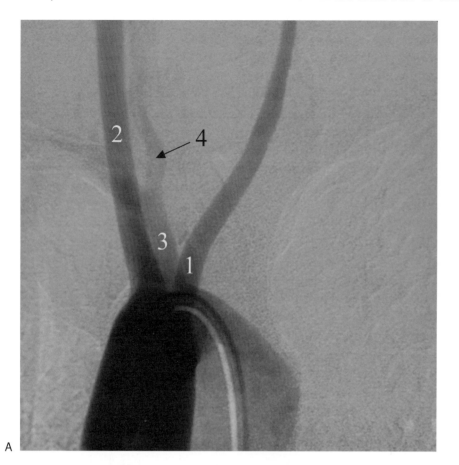

A

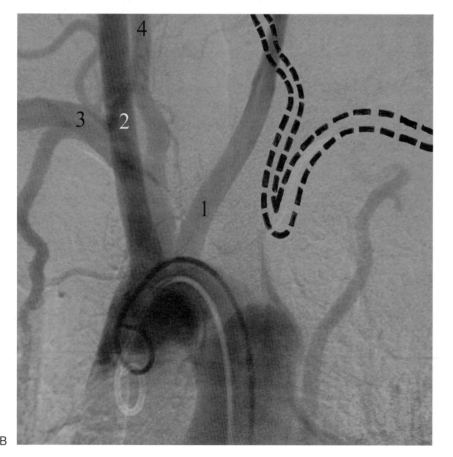

B

FIG. 1-25. A right aortic arch with a left descending aorta, sometimes called a circumflex aorta, is depicted. This case probably represents a double aortic arch with left arch atresia. Early **(A)** and late **(B)** shallow LAO angiograms are shown. The left subclavian artery is occluded but filled on a later phase of the angiogram (subclavian steal) via a large right vertebral artery (4). Its position is indicated (**B,** *dotted lines*). The first arch branch is the left common carotid artery (1). The right common carotid artery (2) is the second branch that arises from the arch, whereas the right subclavian artery (3) is the third great vessel arising from the arch.

monary artery to the aortic diverticulum, and *common origin of the carotid arteries* (so-called bicarotid truncus) with aberrant right subclavian artery (17,20,26,27).

A *cervical aortic arch* may present as a pulsatile neck mass. In this uncommon anomaly the aortic arch lies above the manubrium (Fig. 1-26). A right cervical aortic arch is more common than a left-sided cervical arch. In both instances, branching of the arch vessels is variable and may be aberrant.

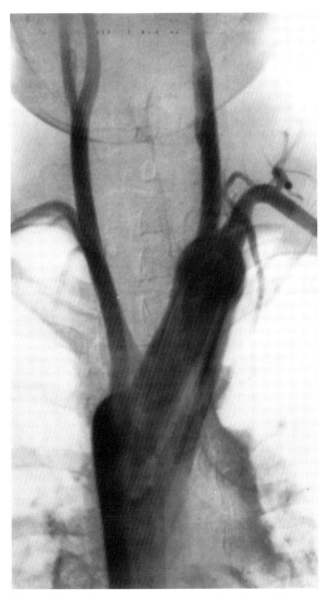

FIG. 1-26. Aortic arch angiogram (arterial phase, left anterior oblique view) in a woman with thoracic outlet syndrome, and a pulsatile supraclavicular mass demonstrate a left cervical aortic arch and right descending thoracic aorta.

GREAT VESSELS AND THEIR BRANCHES

Brachiocephalic Trunk

The two major branches of the brachiocephalic trunk are the right subclavian and the right common carotid arteries (Figs. 1-7 and 1-27).

Right Subclavian Artery

From its origin at the brachiocephalic trunk the right subclavian artery (RSCA) courses superolaterally, ascending approximately 2 cm above the clavicle and passing behind the scalenus anterior muscle. Major branches that arise from the RSCA are the right vertebral and internal thoracic arteries and the thyrocervical and costocervical trunks (see Figs. 1-7, 1-12B, and 1-27).

The *right vertebral artery* (RVA) arises from the posterosuperior aspect of the RSCA and courses superiorly. It enters the foramen transversarium of the C6 transverse process.

The *internal thoracic* (mammary) artery arises inferiorly from the first part of the subclavian artery, opposite the thyrocervical trunk. It descends behind the costal cartilages.

The *thyrocervical trunk* arises from the anterior aspect of the right subclavian artery near the anterior scalene muscle and divides almost immediately into inferior thyroid, suprascapular, and superficial cervical branches. The inferior thyroid artery gives rise to a small but important branch, the *ascending cervical artery*, which anastomoses with the vertebral, ascending pharyngeal, occipital, and deep cervical arteries (see Fig. 1-7).

The *costocervical trunk* arises from the RSCA distal to the thyrocervical trunk and vertebral arteries. It has superior intercostal and deep cervical branches.

Right Common Carotid Artery

The right common carotid artery (RCCA) arises from the brachiocephalic trunk behind the right sternoclavicular joint. It ascends posterolaterally and is separated from the left common carotid artery by the trachea, thyroid gland, larynx, and pharynx. The RCCA courses cephalad in the carotid space accompanied by the internal jugular vein and vagus nerve (CN X). At about the C4 or C5 level the RCCA terminates by dividing into the *right external carotid artery* and the *right internal carotid artery* (Figs. 1-7 and 1-27). These two important vessels are discussed in subsequent chapters.

The common carotid arteries (CCAs) typically do not have named branches, but occasionally the superior thyroid, ascending pharyngeal, or occipital arteries arise from a CCA prior to its bifurcation into the internal and external carotid arteries (22) (see Chapter 2).

There are significant positional variations in the level of the common carotid bifurcation as well as in the rela-

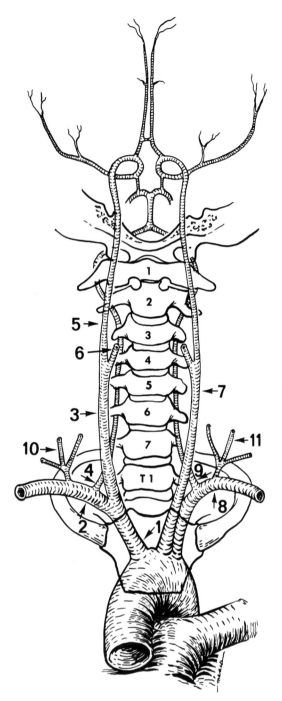

FIG. 1-27. Anatomic sketch of the aortic arch, the great vessels and their major branches (anteroposterior view).

   1, Innominate artery (brachiocephalic trunk)
   2, Right subclavian artery
   3, Right common carotid artery
   4, Right vertebral artery
   5, Right internal carotid artery
   6, Right external carotid artery
   7, Left common carotid artery
   8, Left subclavian artery
   9, Left vertebral artery
   10, Right thyrocervical trunk
   11, Left thyrocervical trunk

tionship between the external and internal carotid arteries. Multiple angiographic projections may be required to profile the bifurcation completely (see Chapter 4).

Left Common Carotid Artery

The left common carotid artery (LCCA) is usually the second major vessel that arises from the aortic arch. At about the upper border of the thyroid cartilage, the LCCA bifurcates into the internal and external carotid arteries (Fig. 1-8).

Left Subclavian Artery

Proximal branches of the left subclavian artery are the left vertebral and internal thoracic arteries and the left thyrocervical and costocervical trunks (Figs. 1-27 and 1-28).

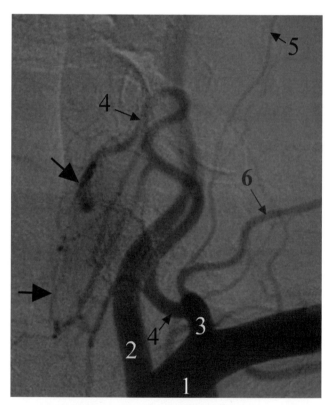

FIG. 1-28. Selective left subclavian angiogram, arterial phase, anteroposterior view. A prominent thyroid blush (*large black arrows*) is present.

   1, Left subclavian artery
   2, Left vertebral artery
   3, Thyrocervical trunk
   4, Inferior thyroid artery
   5, Ascending cervical artery
   6, Transverse cervical artery

Left Vertebral Artery

The left vertebral artery (LVA) arises from the postero-superior aspect of the LSCA near its apex (Figs. 1-6 and 1-28). Occasionally the LVA arises from the proximal LSCA near the arch (Fig. 1-29) or from the arch itself (Fig. 1-15).

From its origin the LVA passes cephalad to enter the foramen transversarium of the C6 vertebral segment (see Fig. 10-1). In approximately 12% of cases the vertebral artery enters the foramen at other levels. The level at which the vertebral artery enters the foramen transversarium is determined by which specific embryonic cervical intersegmental vessel persisted to form the proximal vertebral artery (28).

Left Thyrocervical Trunk

The thyrocervical trunk arises from the apex of the LSCA distal to the LVA origin. Major branches of this vessel include the *inferior thyroid artery* and *ascending cervical artery*. A prominent vascular blush in the thyroid gland is sometimes seen with selective injection of the LSCA (Fig. 1-28).

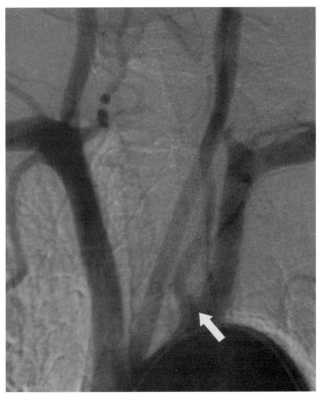

FIG. 1-29. Aortic arch angiogram, arterial phase, left anterior oblique view shows unusually low origin of the left vertebral artery from the subclavian artery (*arrow*).

REFERENCES

1. Larsen WJ. Development of the vasculature. In: *Human embryology*, 2nd ed. New York: Churchill Livingstone, 1997.
2. Padget DH. The development of the cranial arteries in the human embryo. *Contrib Embryol* 1922;32:205–262.
3. Padget DH. Designation of the embryonic intersegmental arteries in reference to the vertebral artery and subclavian stem. *Anat Rec* 1954;1119:349–356.
4. Edwards JE. Anomalies of the derivatives of the aortic arch system. *Med Clin North Am* 1948;32:925–949.
5. Lambiase RE, Haas RA, Carney WI Jr, Rogg J. Anomalous branching of the left common carotid artery with associated atherosclerotic changes: a case report. *AJNR* 1991;12:187–189.
6. Haughton VM, Rosenbaum AE. The normal and anomalous aortic arch and brachiocephalic arteries. In: Newton TH, Potts DG, eds. *Radiology of the skull and brain*. Vol. 2, Book 2. St. Louis: Mosby, 1974: 1145–1163.
7. Williams PL, Warwick R, Dixon M, Bannister LH, eds. *Gray's anatomy*, 38th ed. New York: Churchill Livingstone, 1995:1510–1513.
8. Zamir M, Sinclair P. Origin of the brachiocephalic trunk, left carotid, and left subclavian arteries from the arch of the human aorta. *Invest Radiol* 1991;26:128–133.
9. Ho VB, Kenney JV, Sahn DJ. Contributions of newer MR imaging strategies for congenital heart disease. *Radiographics* 1997;16:43–60.
10. Chung JW, Park JH, Im J-G, et al. Spiral CT angiography of the thoracic aorta. *Radiographics* 1996;16:811–824.
11. Krinsky G, Rofsky N, Flyer M, et al. Gadolinium-enhanced three-dimensional MR angiography of acquired arch vessel disease. *AJR* 1996;167:981–987.
12. Fisher RG, Sanchez-Torres M, Wigham CT, Thomas JW. "Lumps" and "bumps" that mimic acute aortic and brachiocephalic vessel injury. *Radiographics* 1997;17:825–834.
13. Caldemeyer KS, Carrico JB, Mathews VP. The radiology and embryology of anomalous arteries of the head and neck. *AJR* 1998;170: 197–203.
14. Beigelman C, Mowrey-Gerosa I, Gamsu G, Grenier P. New morphologic approach to the classification of anomalies of the aortic arch. *Eur Radiol* 1995;5:435–442.
15. Shuford WH, Sybers RG, eds. *The aortic arch and its malformations*. Springfield, IL: Charles C. Thomas Publisher, 1974.
16. Freed K, Low VHS. The aberrant subclavian artery. *AJR* 1997;166: 481–484.
17. Jaffe RB. Magnetic resonance imaging of vascular rings. *Semin Ultrasound CT MR* 1990;11:206–220.
18. Hogg JP, Dominic AJ, Conselman RL, Hurst JL. Expanding aneurysm of aberrant right subclavian artery. *Clin Imaging* 1997;21:195–199.
19. Salomonowitz E, Edwards JE, Hunter DW, et al. The three types of aortic diverticula. *AJR* 1984;142:673–679.
20. Jaffe RB. Radiographic manifestations of congenital anomalies of the aortic arch. *Radiol Clin North Am* 1991;29:319–334.
21. Pickhardt PJ, Siegel MJ, Gutierrez FR. Vascular rings in symptomatic children: frequency of chest radiographic findings. *Radiology* 1997;203: 423–426.
22. Hopkins KL, Patrick LE, Simoneaux SF, et al. Pediatric great vessel anomalies: initial clinical experience with spiral CT angiography. *Radiology* 1996;200:811–815.
23. Kocis KC, Midgley FM, Ruckman RN. Aortic arch complex anomalies: 20-year experience with symptoms, diagnosis, associated cardiac defects, and surgical repair. *Pediatr Cardiol* 1997;18:127–132.
24. Tonkin ILD, Gold RE, Moser D, Laster RE Jr. Evaluation of vascular ring with digital subtraction angiography. *AJR* 1984;142:1287–1291.
25. Lowe GM, Donaldson JS, Backer CL. Vascular rings: 10-year review of imaging. *Radiographics* 1991;11:637–646.
26. Shuford WH, Sybers RG, Gordon IJ, et al. Circumflex retroesophageal right aortic arch simulating mediastinal tumor or dissecting aneurysm. *AJR* 1986;146:491–496.
27. Moes CAF, Freedom RM. Rare types of aortic arch anomalies. *Pediatr Cardiol* 1993;14:93–101.
28. Gailloud P, Khan HG, Khaw N, et al. The supraisthmic anastomatic arch. *AJR* 1998;170:497–498.

CHAPTER 2

The External Carotid Artery

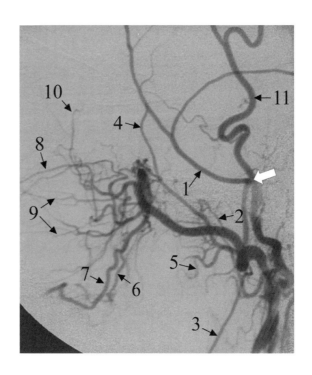

The common carotid arteries (CCAs) terminate by dividing into the external and internal carotid arteries. The external carotid artery (ECA) is the smaller of the two terminal CCA branches. The ECA supplies most head and neck structures (excluding the brain and eye). It also may contribute significant vascular supply to a broad spectrum of intracranial lesions such as vascular malformations and neoplasms.

The ECA has numerous important anastomoses with the internal carotid arteries (ICAs) and the vertebrobasilar system. As selective catheterization of the ECA for interventional procedures becomes increasingly more widespread, understanding normal ECA anatomy and recognizing potentially dangerous anastomotic pathways becomes a necessity.

In this chapter, the embryology of the ECA is first considered briefly. Understanding how the ECA develops from its primitive precursors helps explain the spectrum of anatomic variants and anomalies that may be encountered when catheterizing this vessel. Next, the normal gross and imaging anatomy of the ECA are discussed. Beginning with the ECA trunk and its main branches, the deep branches of the ECA are examined in more detail. The chapter concludes with a brief discussion of basic functional neuroangiography as it is applied to the external carotid system.

EXTERNAL CAROTID ARTERY: MAIN TRUNK

Normal Development

Overview and General Principles

The craniocerebral vasculature develops through hemodynamically induced modeling and remodeling of numerous primitive vascular precursors (see Chapter 1). The embryology of the external carotid artery (ECA) is incompletely understood (1,2). As with most of the cerebral vasculature, the ECA develops through a combination of outgrowths from some vessels, involution of others, and assimilation of preexisting channels that arise from undifferentiated precursor vessels (3).

Main ECA Trunk

The pharyngeal pouches first appear at 3 to 4 gestational weeks. A network of plexiform vessels that surrounds these pouches coalesces to form arc-shaped anastomotic channels that connect the ventral and dorsal aortae. These fenestrated channels are the embryonic *first and second aortic arches* (Fig. 2-1; also see Fig. 1-1A).

At around 4 weeks the first and second aortic arches begin to regress. Other transient channels called the *ventral pharyngeal arteries* (VPAs) grow simultaneously

31

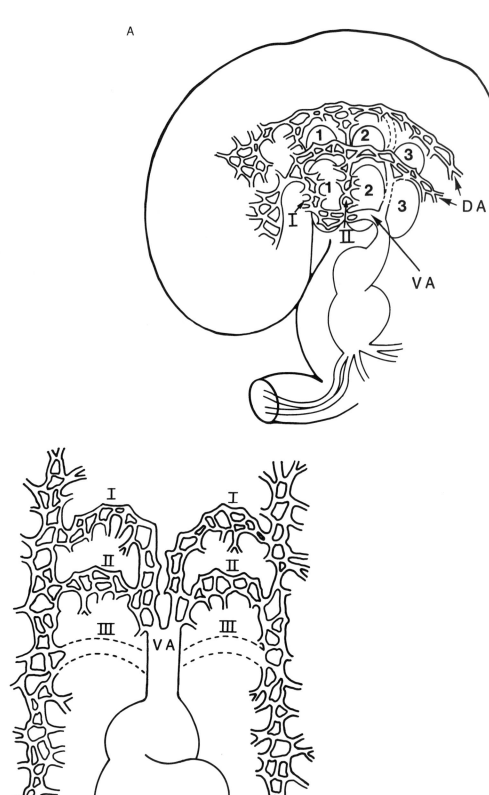

FIG. 2-1. Lateral **(A)** and anteroposterior **(B)** anatomic diagrams depict the fetal vasculature at approximately 3½ gestational weeks (3- to 5-mm stage; compare with Fig. 1-1 at 4 weeks of development). The primitive heart is shown with the aortic sac and ventral aortae (VA). The first three pharyngeal pouches (1–3) have appeared. Plexiform vessels are coalescing around these pouches to form anastomotic channels between the VAs and paired dorsal aortae (DA). These are the first two embryonic aortic arches, designated here as I and II. The third arch (III) has not developed yet, but its future position is indicated by the dotted lines.

from the ventral aorta to supply the pharyngeal pouches (Fig. 2-2). The primitive hyoidostapedial arteries, which develop from first and second arch remnants, then establish anastomoses with the VPAs at their cranial ends.

The definitive external carotid trunks arise as *de novo* outgrowths (sprouts) from the embryonic third aortic arches (4,5). The VPAs regress as the ECAs develop and assimilate their proximal stems (Fig. 2-3; also see Fig. 1-3) (1,6).

Distal ECA Branches

The *first aortic arches* function until the neural tube closes and the pharynx differentiates into pouches. The first arches then regress, although some remnants persist and are annexed later by outgrowths from the second aortic arches.

As the second pharyngeal pouches develop, a plexus of vessels between the first and second pouches on each side forms the *second aortic arches* (Fig. 2-1B). Their proximal aspects coalesce and establish primitive channels called the hyoid arteries. The *hyoid arteries* unite with

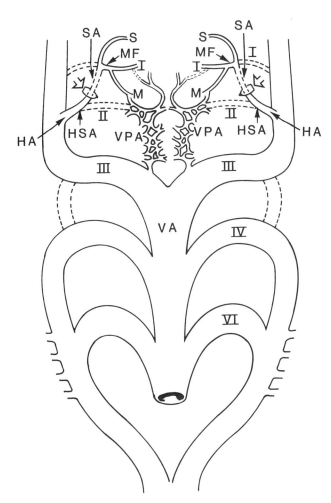

FIG. 2-2. Anteroposterior diagram depicts the fetal cranio-cerebral vasculature at approximately 29 gestational days. The first two aortic arches are beginning to regress (*dotted lines*). Blood supply to their corresponding pharyngeal pouches is now mostly derived from transient channels called the ventral pharyngeal arteries (VPAs) that grow from the ventral aorta (VA) and aortic sac. The proximal aspects of the second arches are coalescing to form the primitive hyoid arteries (HA). Each HA joins with its corresponding stapedial artery (SA), a first arch remnant, to form a trunk that is sometimes called the hyoidostapedial artery (HSA). The HSAs are shown here passing through the developing ring of the stapes (*open arrows*). Each stapedial artery anastomoses with the cranial end of its corresponding VPA, eventually annexing its terminal distribution. Both fully developed stapedial arteries will then have a supraorbital (S) and a maxillofacial division (MF). Each maxillofacial division has two major branches, the infraorbital (I) and maxillary (M) arteries.

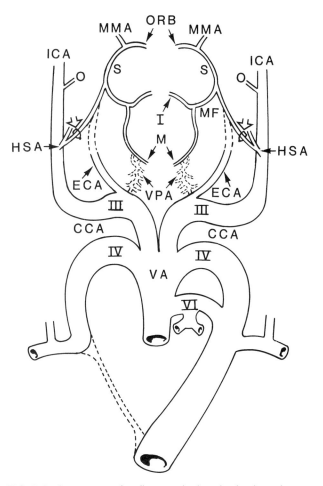

FIG. 2-3. Anteroposterior diagram depicts the fetal craniocerebral circulation at approximately 6 to 7 gestational weeks. The ventral pharyngeal arteries (VPAs, *small dotted lines*) have regressed as the developing ECAs sprout from the third arches and incorporate the VPA stems. The primitive stapedial arteries and their branches are being annexed by the distal ends of the sprouting ECAs (*large dotted lines*). Each HSA, shown here as they pass through the stapes (*open arrows*), will regress, and its distal branches are incorporated as part of the definitive ECAs. The ophthalmic arteries (O) are also shown sprouting from the internal carotid arteries (ICAs). (The paired, plexiform dorsal longitudinal neural arteries are also present at this stage but for simplification are not shown in this diagram; see Fig. 1-3). S, supraorbital division of HSA with extracranial MMA and orbital (ORB) branches; MF, maxillofacial trunk of STA with infraorbital (I) and maxillary (M) branches.

distal plexiform remnants from the first arches to form the *stapedial arteries* (Fig. 2-2).

Each embryonic hyoidostapedial artery (HSA) passes through the developing stapes and then divides into three branches (Fig. 2-3). These three vessels, supra- and infra-orbital branches and a mandibular branch, follow a course that parallels the three divisions of the trigeminal nerve (CN V). The embryonic HSA thus consists of three parts: (a) a main trunk derived from the hyoid artery (a second aortic arch structure), (b) a maxillofacial division with an infraorbital (maxillary) branch and a mandibular branch (partly derived from the first arch), and (c) a supraorbital division (2).

The maxillofacial division of the HSA becomes the definitive *internal maxillary artery* (IMA). It is usually annexed by the ECA trunk as the ECA sprouts from the common carotid artery (Fig. 2-3). The main HSA proximal to the stapes partially regresses and persists as the *caroticotympanic artery*, a branch of the petrous internal carotid artery (Fig. 2-4; also see Fig. 3-19) (2,7).

The supraorbital division of the HSA supplies the intracranial segment of the *middle meningeal artery* (MMA). It also gives off *orbital branches* that are incorporated into the ophthalmic artery (OA; a branch of the internal carotid artery).

The definitive ECAs have highly variable vascular territories (see below). These patterns are determined by whether and to what extent their embryonic precursors are assimilated by the sprouting main ECA trunks (Fig. 2-5). Some vascular territories, especially those supplying the orbit and cranial meninges, are often annexed by branches of the definitive internal carotid arteries (see Chapters 3 and 4), whereas others usually remain part of the external carotid circulation.

Gross Anatomy

The ECA originates from the common carotid artery (CCA) at the mid-cervical level as the smaller of its two terminal branches (8) (Fig. 2-6). The ECA usually arises from the common carotid bifurcation at approximately the C4 vertebral level but may arise as low as T3 or as high as the hyoid bone (9).

Relationships

The main ECA trunk lies in the carotid space and is anatomically related to a number of important structures (Fig. 2-7). The major structures that lie adjacent to the ECA are discussed below.

Anterior

The anterior margin of the sternomastoid lies superficial and lateral to the ECA. At various points the ECA is crossed by the hypoglossal nerve (cranial nerve [CN] XII), the stylohyoid muscle, and the posterior belly of the digastric muscle (8).

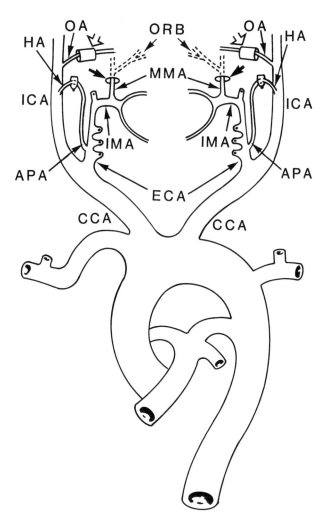

FIG. 2-4. Anteroposterior diagram depicts the fetal circulation at approximately 8 to 10 weeks. The ventral pharyngeal arteries have disappeared. The definitive external carotid arteries (ECAs) have annexed the stapedial artery branches. The maxillofacial branches have become the internal maxillary artery (IMA) and the extracranial segment of the middle meningeal artery (MMA). The MMA passes cephalad through the foramen spinosum (ring indicated by the black arrow). The supraorbital division of the primitive stapedial artery (*dotted lines*) has become the intracranial MMA segment and orbital arteries (ORB). The ORBs supply all orbital structures except the globes. The ophthalmic arteries (OAs) are shown sprouting from the internal carotid arteries (ICAs) and passing through the optic canals (*open arrows*). The OAs supply the globes and will eventually annex most of the ORBs as well. The embryonic hyoid artery (HA), the proximal aspect of the hyoidostapedial trunk, has mostly regressed. A small remnant of the embryonic HA persists as the caroticotympanic artery (a branch of the petrous internal carotid artery segment). It is shown here passing through the ring of the stapes and anastomosing with inferior tympanic branches from the ascending pharyngeal artery (APA).

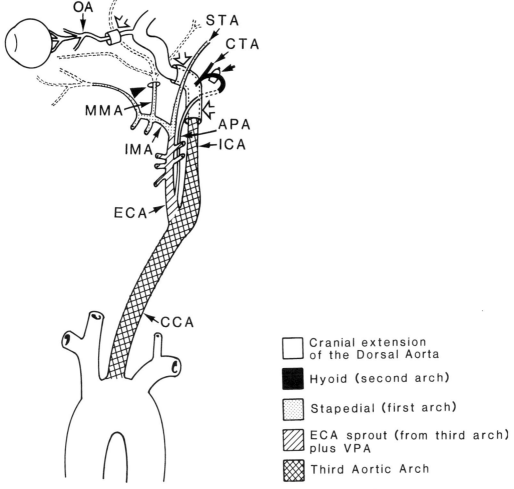

FIG. 2-5. Anatomic diagram turned from anteroposterior to a left anterior oblique (LAO) position depicts the definitive left common carotid artery as well as the external and internal carotid arteries. The embryonic origin of these vessels is also shown. CTA, caroticotympanic artery; small single arrow, stapes; arrowhead, foramen spinosum; double arrows, optic canal; open arrows, carotid canal. Distal ramifications from the IMA, MMA, and orbital branches of the OA are indicated by the dotted lines. There are many potential anastomoses between these vessels. Variations in their vascular territories are also common.

Posterior

The ECA initially lies in front of, and medial to, the internal carotid artery (ICA). As the ECA ascends, it gradually courses posterolaterally, branching to supply the facial structures. The internal jugular vein courses posterolaterally to the ICA and ECA (Fig. 2-7). The small carotid body (glomus caroticum) lies in the carotid bifurcation between the ECA and ICA. The vagus nerve (CN X) courses inferiorly in the carotid sheath between the ICA and internal jugular vein and medial to the ECA (see Figs. 1-8 and 3-3).

Lateral

High deep cervical lymph nodes and the deep lobe of the parotid gland are lateral and slightly posterior to the proximal and distal ECA segments, respectively.

Medial

Initially the pharyngeal wall, superior laryngeal nerve (a branch of CN X), and ascending pharyngeal artery (APA) lie medial to the ECA. At a higher level the ICA crosses behind the ECA trunk and then lies medial to it. These two vessels are separated by the styloid process, the styloglossus and stylopharyngeus muscles, and the glossopharyngeal nerve (CN IX) (8).

Summary

Thus, the ECA:

1. Originates from the CCA bifurcation at about the C4 level.
2. Initially lies *anterior* and *medial* to the ICA, then courses *posterolaterally* as it ascends in the carotid sheath.
3. Lies *in front of* the internal jugular vein.

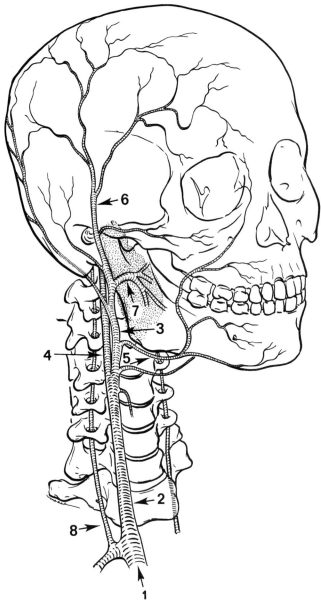

FIG. 2-6. The right common carotid artery, carotid bifurcation, and some of the main external carotid artery (ECA) branches are depicted in this oblique anatomic diagram. The parotid gland is indicated by the stippled area.

1, Brachiocephalic trunk
2, Right common carotid artery
3, Right external carotid artery (main trunk)
4, Right internal carotid artery
5, Facial artery (the lingual and superior thyroid arteries arise more proximally from the ECA and are cut off)
6, Superficial temporal artery
7, Internal maxillary artery
8, Right vertebral artery

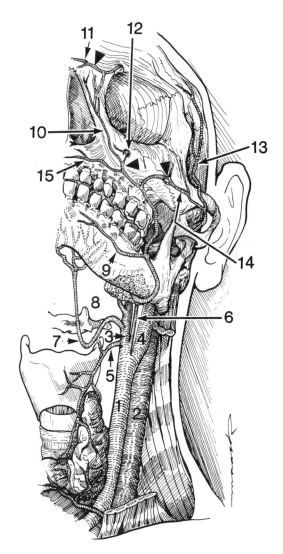

FIG. 2-7. Anteroposterior anatomic sketch shows the left common carotid artery and related structures. The sternomastoid muscle has been partially removed to expose the carotid artery and internal jugular vein. The submandibular gland is indicated by the stippled area. The carotid bifurcation and proximal ECA branches are depicted in detail. Potential anastomoses between branches representing the facial, ophthalmic, internal maxillary, and transverse facial artery pedicles are indicated by the arrowheads (also see Fig. 2-29).

1, Left common carotid artery
2, Left internal jugular vein
3, Left external carotid artery
4, Left internal carotid artery
5, Superior thyroid artery
6, Ascending pharyngeal artery
7, Lingual artery
8, Facial artery
9, Inferior labial branch of the facial artery
10, Angular artery and nasal branches of the facial artery (note anastomosis with branches of the ophthalmic artery)
11, Orbital branches of the ophthalmic artery (an internal carotid artery branch)
12, Infraorbital artery (note anastomosis between this branch of the maxillary artery and the facial artery)
13, Superficial temporal artery
14, Transverse facial artery (note anastomosis with facial artery branches)
15, Superior labial branch of the facial artery

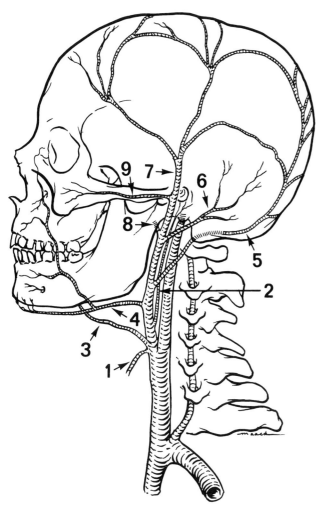

FIG. 2-8. Lateral anatomic diagram depicts the external carotid artery and its major branches:

1, Superior thyroid artery
2, Ascending pharyngeal artery
3, Lingual artery
4, Facial artery
5, Occipital artery
6, Posterior auricular artery
7, Superficial temporal artery;
8, Internal maxillary artery (cut off)
9, Transverse facial artery (a branch of the superficial temporal artery)

4. Is *covered by* the sternomastoid muscle and *crossed by* the hypoglossal nerve.
5. Lies *anterolateral* to the vagus nerve.

Branches

The ECA has eight major branches (Fig. 2-8; see box below). The main ECA trunk rapidly decreases in size as it gives off branches to the tongue, deep face, and neck. It terminates medial to (or within) the parotid gland by

dividing into its two main distal branches, the superficial temporal artery (STA) and the maxillary artery. The ECA branches, territories supplied, and functional hemodynamic balance between adjacent arterial trunks are quite variable (6,10,11).

Superior Thyroid Artery

The superior thyroid artery is typically the first ECA branch. It usually arises from the anterior wall of the ECA, coursing anteroinferiorly and slightly medially toward the apex of the thyroid gland (Fig. 2-7; also see Fig. 1-8). In approximately 20% of cases the superior thyroid artery arises from the carotid bifurcation. Less com-

---

External Carotid Artery: Normal Anatomy and Variations

Normal development
  Proximal trunk from
    Ventral pharyngeal artery
    De novo "sprout" (from embryonic third aortic arch)
  Distal branches from
    Primitive hyoid artery (second arch)
    Primitive stapedial artery (first arch)
Key relationships
  Anteromedial, then posterolateral to ICA
  Anterior to IJV
  Anterolateral to CN X (vagus nerve)
  Terminates medial to (or within) parotid gland
Branches
  Superior thyroid artery
  Ascending pharyngeal artery
  Lingual artery (LA)
  Facial artery (FA)
  Occipital artery (OccA)
  Posterior auricular artery (PAA)
  Superficial temporal artery
  Maxillary artery
Vascular territory
  Most of head and neck (except orbit, brain)
Common variants
  Origins, branching patterns, territories are
    normally quite variable
Anomalies
  "Nonbifurcating" carotid artery (ECA branches
    arise separately from a CCA that does not
    bifurcate)
  Aberrant origin of ECA branches from ICA and VA

ECA, external carotid artery; ICA, internal carotid artery; CCA, common carotid artery; VA, vertebral artery; IJV, internal jugular vein; CN X vagus nerve.

mon origins of this vessel include the common carotid (10%) and lingual (2%) arteries (12,13).

The superior thyroid artery supplies the larynx and most of the upper thyroid gland (Table 2-1). This vessel has extensive anastomoses with its counterpart from the opposite ECA as well as the inferior thyroid artery, a branch of the thyrocervical trunk that supplies the isthmus and inferior poles of the thyroid gland. Both thyroid arteries may anastomose with the lowest thyroid artery, the arteria thyroidea ima. This vessel is an inconstant branch that arises from the brachiocephalic trunk or aortic arch (13).

Ascending Pharyngeal Artery

The ascending pharyngeal artery (APA) is the smallest and first posterior ECA branch. It usually originates from the common carotid bifurcation or proximal ECA (see Figs. 1-8 and 2-8); occasionally the APA arises from a common trunk with the occipital artery (see Fig. 2-14).

The APA ascends behind the ICA and anteromedial to the internal jugular vein. The APA has anteriorly directed *pharyngeal branches* that supply the pharynx and eustachian tube. Posteriorly directed *inferior tympanic* and *muscular branches* supply the tympanic cavity and prevertebral muscles. An important vessel, the *neuromeningeal branch*, supplies the dura and lower cranial nerves (8,13–17).

The APA anastomoses with many other ECA rami such as the middle meningeal, accessory meningeal, dorsal pharyngeal, and ascending palatine arteries. The *inferior tympanic artery* from the APA anastomoses with the caroticotympanic artery, a branch of the petrous internal carotid artery (Figs. 2-4 and 2-5). The APA also has extensive anastomoses with other important ICA branches such as the vidian artery and inferolateral trunk (Table 2-1).

The APA may anastomose with meningeal or cervical branches of the vertebral artery at the C3 level (15–17). The rich anastomotic system between the APA and the carotid and vertebral arteries may serve as an important supply of collateral blood flow. It also poses a potential

TABLE 2-1. *External Carotid Artery: Branches, Territories, and Major Anastomoses*

Branch	Territory supplied	Major anastomoses
Superior thyroid artery	Larynx, upper thyroid	Subclavian artery via inferior thyroid artery
Ascending pharyngeal	Pharynx; middle ear; CNS VII and IX-XII; dura (clivus, petrous ridge, posterior cavernous sinus)	ICA via inferolateral trunk (C4 segment), vidian artery (C2/C3 segment), caroticotympanic artery (C2 segment)
		ECA via occipital artery
		Vertebral artery via musculospinal branches, neuromeningeal branches
		Subclavian artery via ascending cervical artery (C3 segment)
Lingual artery	Tongue, oral cavity, sublingual gland	ECA via facial artery, superior thyroid artery
Facial artery	Face (cheek, lips, palate, submandibular, gland, etc.)	ICA via ophthalmic artery
		ECA via lingual artery, transverse facial artery, (superficial temporal artery)
Occipital artery	Posterior neck, scalp; some dura; CN VII	ECA via ascending pharyngeal artery, superficial temporal artery, posterior auricular artery, superficial temporal artery
		Vertebral artery via musculospinal branches (C1/C2 segments)
		Subclavian artery via ascending cervical artery (C1/C2 segments)
Posterior auricular artery	Scalp; pinna; external auditory canal	ECA via occipital artery, superior temporal artery
Superficial temporal artery	Scalp; ear; parotid gland	ICA via ophthalmic artery
		ECA via facial artery, occipital artery, maxillary artery
Internal maxillary artery	Deep face, nose	ICA via Inferolateral trunk (C4 segment), ophthalmic artery (ethmoid, deep collaterals), vidian artery (C2/C3 segment)
		ECA via superficial temporal artery, facial artery

Only the main anastomoses are shown; most ECA branches also anastomose with their counterparts from the contralateral ECA.

ICA, internal carotid artery; ECA, external carotid artery.

hazard during therapeutic embolization of extracranial vascular lesions (see Fig. 17-15).

Lingual Artery

The lingual artery is the second anterior ECA branch. It initially courses superiorly, medial to the pharyngeal muscles and the hyoglossus muscle. It then loops down and forward before curving upward toward the tongue (see Figs. 2-7 and 1-8). The LA provides the major vascular supply to the tongue and oral cavity (Table 2-1). In 10% to 20% of cases the LA shares a common trunk with the facial artery (8,14,18).

Facial Artery

The facial artery, also called the external maxillary artery, is the third anteriorly directed ECA branch. It originates from the anterior aspect of the ECA just above the lingual artery. In approximately 10% of cases the FA shares a common trunk with the lingual artery (18).

From its origin the FA first ascends, then curves inferolaterally over the submandibular gland and around the mandible. It then passes anteriorly and superiorly across the cheek (see Figs. 1-8, 2-7, and 2-8).

The facial artery terminates near the medial canthus of the eye by becoming the *angular artery*. Here the FA anastomoses with branches of the ophthalmic artery, a branch of the ICA (Fig. 2-7). This anastomosis between orbital branches of the ICA and the ECA is an important potential pathway for collateral blood flow in the event of ICA occlusion (Table 2-1; also see Chapter 17).

The facial artery exists in hemodynamic balance with other ECA arterial pedicles such as the internal maxillary and transverse facial arteries (see Fig. 2-29) (10,17–19). The terminal distribution of the FA is thus quite variable, although it usually supplies most of the face, palate, lip, and cheek. Major branches of the FA include the *ascending palatine artery, submental artery, buccal and masseteric branches, superior and inferior labial arteries,* and a *lateral nasal artery* (Fig. 2-7).

Occipital Artery

The occipital artery (OccA) originates from the posterior aspect of the ECA. It courses posterosuperiorly, passing between the occipital bone and the first cervical vertebra (Fig. 2-8). Its terminal branches supply the musculocutaneous structures of the posterior neck and scalp and also provide meningeal rami to the posterior fossa (see Fig. 2-17B).

Numerous anastomoses are present between muscular branches of the OccA and segmental branches from the vertebral and ascending cervical arteries, scalp rami of other ECA branches, and posterior fossa meningeal branches (Table 2-1). The OccA may arise from, or have sizable direct anastomoses with, the vertebral artery at the C1 or C2 levels (see Figs. 2-16, 2-20, and 17-14) (17,20).

Posterior Auricular Artery

The posterior auricular artery (PAA) is a small branch that arises from the posterior aspect of the ECA just above the occipital artery origin. The PAA also may arise from the OA. The PAA courses posterosuperiorly to supply the scalp, pinna, and external auditory canal (Fig. 2-8). The PAA may give rise to the *stylomastoid artery*, a small but important branch that supplies the chorda tympani. The stylomastoid artery also may arise from the OA itself (see Fig. 2-17). It anastomoses with petrosal branches from the middle meningeal artery (17).

Superficial Temporal Artery

The ECA divides into the maxillary and superficial temporal arteries just inferior to the mandibular condyle. The superficial temporal artery (STA) is the smaller of the two terminal ECA branches. From its origin, the STA runs behind the condyle, passing from deep to superficial as it passes upward and forward (Figs. 2-8 and 2-9) (21).

The STA is essentially a cutaneous artery that supplies the anterior two thirds of the scalp, part of the ear, and the parotid gland (Table 2-1). The *transverse facial artery* arises near (or from) the origin of the STA and courses horizontally forward. Branches of the transverse facial artery anastomose with those of the facial and maxillary arteries to supply the deep face and cheek (Fig. 2-7).

Maxillary Artery

The maxillary artery, sometimes called the internal maxillary artery (IMA), is the larger terminal ECA branch. The IMA arises within the parotid gland behind the neck of the mandible (Fig. 2-6). It runs obliquely forward and medially in the masticator space. The IMA terminates within the pterygopalatine fossa by dividing into branches that supply the deep face and nose (Fig. 2-9). The IMA is in hemodynamic balance with the facial artery (see Fig. 2-29) and is a major source of potential collateral blood flow from the external to internal carotid systems (see above box; see also Chapter 17).

Normal Angiographic Anatomy

The ECA origin and its proximal branches are best delineated using multiple projections of common carotid angiograms (Fig. 2-10). The distal ECA branches are especially well seen when the ICA is occluded at or near the carotid bifurcation (see Fig. 2-16).

Superior Thyroid Artery

Usually the first anterior ECA branch, the superior thyroid artery courses inferomedial to the common carotid

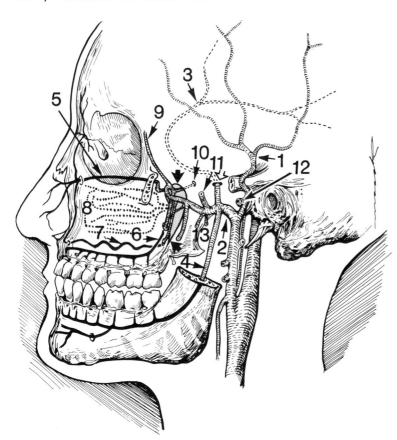

FIG. 2-9. Anatomic sketch depicts the terminal external carotid artery bifurcation. The distal internal maxillary artery divides within the ptery-gopalatine fossa (*large black arrows*).

1, Superficial temporal artery (note prominent "hairpin" turn where the artery loops over the zygoma)
2, Internal maxillary artery (IMA)
3, Middle meningeal artery (foramen spinosum is indicated by the outlined arrow)
4, Inferior alveolar artery
5, Infraorbital artery
6, Superior alveolar artery
7, Greater (descending) palatine artery
8, Sphenopalatine artery and branches (*dotted lines*)
9, Anterior deep temporal artery
10, Artery of the foramen rotundum
11, Middle deep temporal artery (cut off)
12, Transverse facial artery (cut off)
13, Buccal branches of the IMA

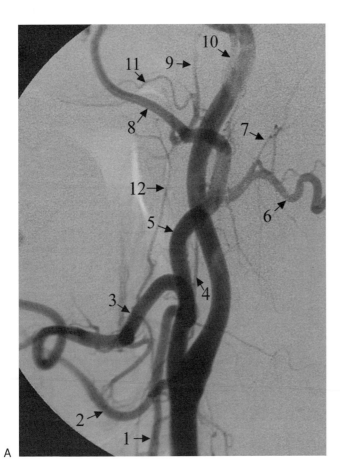

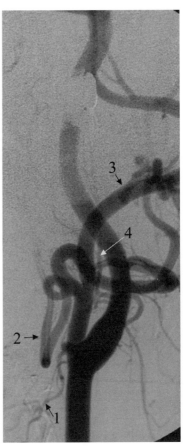

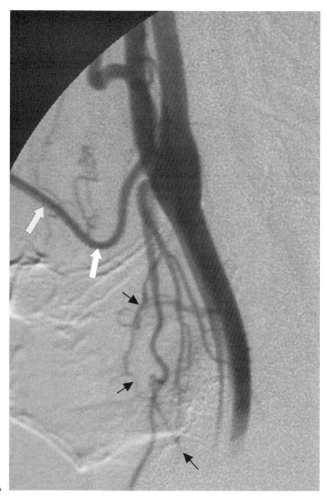
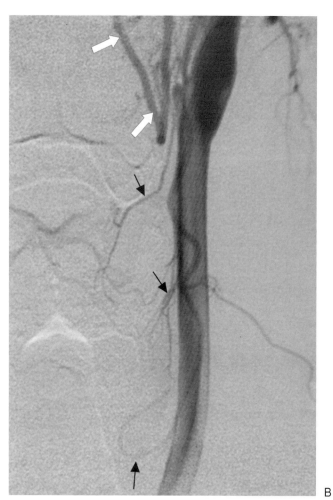

A

B

FIG. 2-11. Lateral **(A)** and anteroposterior **(B)** views of a left common carotid angiogram show the superficial thyroid artery and its numerous branches (*small black arrows*). The lingual artery, with its distinctive U-shaped curve, is indicated by the large white arrows.

FIG. 2-10. Lateral **(A)** and anteroposterior **(B)** views of a left common carotid angiogram show the ECA and its major branches:

1, Superior thyroid artery
2, Lingual artery
3, Facial artery (note anterosuperior course of the distal facial artery, indicated by the arrowheads)
4, Ascending pharyngeal artery
5, Main ECA trunk
6, Occipital artery
7, Posterior auricular artery
8, Maxillary artery
9, Middle meningeal artery
10, Superficial temporal artery
11, Transverse facial artery (superficial temporal artery branch)
12, Ascending palatine artery (facial artery branch)

artery (Fig. 2-11; see also Figs. 1-8 and 2-7). The superior thyroid artery divides almost immediately into fine rami that course toward the thyroid apex. A prominent vascular blush within the thyroid gland itself sometimes is seen.

Ascending Pharyngeal Artery

The ascending pharyngeal artery (APA) is a small vessel that originates from the common carotid bifurcation or dorsal surface of the ECA. Its proximal aspect is usually well visualized on straight or slightly oblique lateral views of common carotid angiograms (Figs. 2-10, 2-12, and 2-13), whereas its more cephalad segment is best delineated on selective APA injections (Fig. 2-14; also see Fig. 17-15). The anterior division of the APA has an

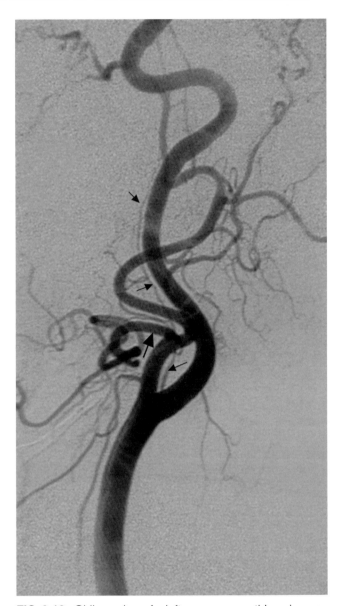

FIG. 2-13. Oblique view of a left common carotid angiogram. Most of the ascending pharyngeal artery (*small arrows*) is evident. In this patient the lingual and facial arteries arise from a common trunk (*large arrow*).

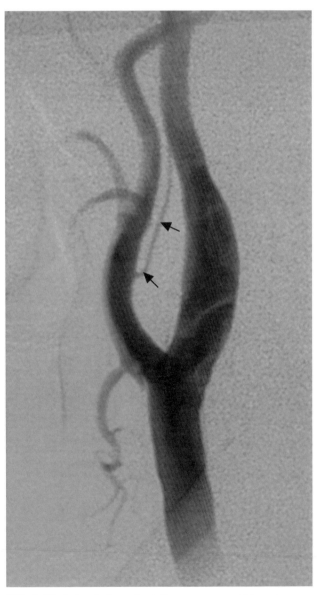

FIG. 2-12. Lateral view of a left common carotid angiogram. The ascending pharyngeal artery is depicted particularly well (*arrows*).

anteriorly directed right-angle bend near the skull base. Selective APA injection may cause a pronounced pharyngeal mucosal vascular blush.

Lingual Artery

The lingual artery, the second branch arising from the anterior aspect of the ECA, has a distinctive U-shaped appearance on both anteroposterior (AP) and lateral angiograms (Fig. 2-10). Its distal branches supply the tongue in a fan-shaped pattern (Figs. 2-7 and 2-15). A dense vascular blush of the tongue and adjacent oral mucosa can sometimes be seen on late arterial phase views of external carotid angiograms (Fig. 2-16D).

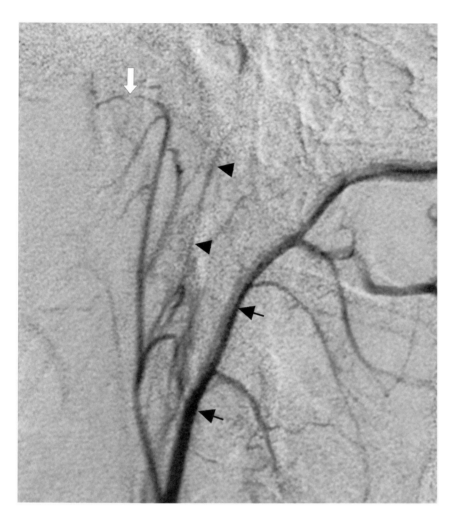

FIG. 2-14. Selective injection of the ascending pharyngeal artery, lateral view, shows some of its anteriorly directed pharyngeal branches (*white arrow*) as well as the posteriorly directed neuromeningeal branch (*arrowheads*). As it does in this case, the occipital artery (*large black arrows*) often arises from a common trunk with the ascending pharyngeal artery.

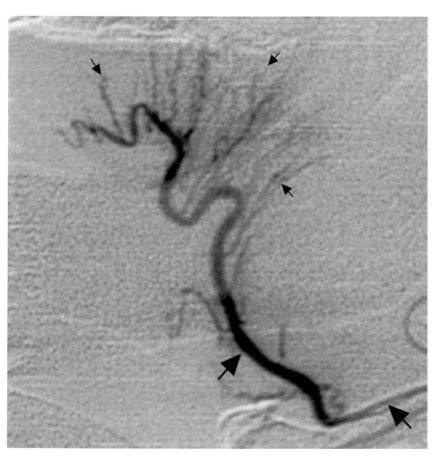

FIG. 2-15. Selective injection of a lingual artery, lateral view, demonstrates the characteristic U-shaped configuration of its proximal trunk (*large arrows*). Note the fanlike array of small branches to the tongue (*small arrows*).

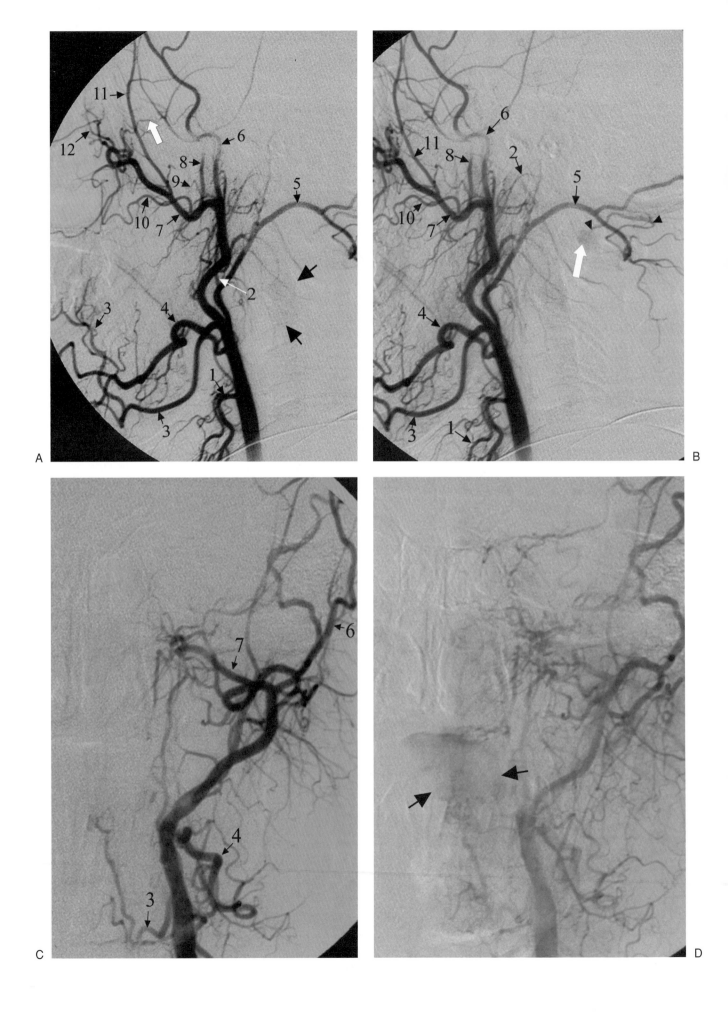

FIG. 2-16. Early phase **(A)** and mid-arterial phase **(B)** (lateral views) and early phase **(C)** and late arterial phase **(D)** (anteroposterior views) of a left common carotid angiogram. The internal carotid artery is occluded at the bifurcation so the ECA branches are especially well seen. Note normal vascular blushes of the cervical musculature (**A**, *large black arrows*) and the tongue (**D**, *arrows*). Of special importance is transient opacification of the vertebral artery (**B**, *open arrow*) by muscular collaterals (*arrowheads*) from the occipital artery. The artery of the foramen rotundum (**A**, *large white arrow*) is also opacified, indicating another potential site for extra- to intracranial blood flow.

1, Superior thyroid artery
2, Ascending pharyngeal artery
3, Lingual artery
4, Facial artery
5, Occipital artery
6, Superficial temporal artery
7, Maxillary artery
8, Middle meningeal artery
9, Accessory meningeal artery
10, Transverse facial artery
11, Middle deep temporal artery
12, Anterior deep temporal artery

Facial Artery

The facial artery, the third anterior ECA branch, initially courses inferiorly but eventually turns superolaterally as it follows a tortuous course across the face toward the nose (Figs. 2-7 and 2-16). It supplies branches to the mandible, palate, and submandibular gland as well as the cheek, nose, and lips. Opacification of submandibular gland lobules with selective facial artery injection may cause a prominent vascular blush below the mandibular angle.

Occipital Artery

The occipital artery (OccA) is the largest branch that arises posteriorly from the ECA. It follows a serpentine, obliquely superior course toward the occiput (Figs. 2-16 and 2-17A). The OccA sometimes has prominent muscular

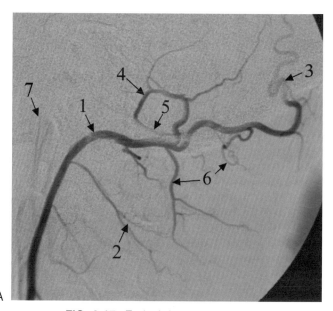

A

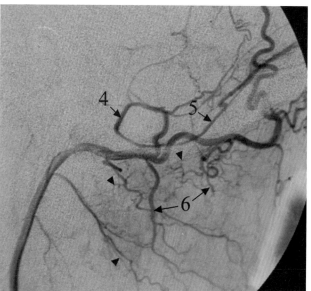

B

FIG. 2-17. Early **(A)** and later **(B)** arterial phase films, lateral view, from a selective occiptial artery angiogram are shown.

1, Occipital artery (main trunk)
2, Muscular branches
3, Scalp branches
4, Transosseous branch
5, Posterior meningeal artery
6, Muscular branches
7, Stylomastoid branches

and meningeal branches that anastomose with the vertebral artery (Figs. 2-16B and 17-14 and Table 2-1). Some small but important OccA branches that are sometimes visualized on selective injection of this vessel include the *stylomastoid artery* (Fig. 2-17A) and the *posterior meningeal artery* (Fig. 2-17B).

Opacification of the OccA during selective or ECA injection often causes a vascular blush in the cervical musculature (Fig. 2-17B). This appearance should not be mistaken for a mass lesion.

Posterior Auricular Artery

The posterior auricular artery (PAA) is usually a small, somewhat tortuous branch that arises near the terminal ECA bifurcation. The PAA courses superiorly and then posteriorly toward the ear (Fig. 2-18A). A curvilinear vascular blush that represents the pinna can appear very prominent on the later arterial phase of ECA angiograms (Fig. 2-18B).

Superficial Temporal Artery

The superficial temporal artery (STA) is the smaller of the two terminal ECA branches (Fig. 2-18A). It often forms a prominent anterior hairpin turn as it loops over the zygomatic arch (Figs. 2-7, 2-9, and 2-19). Distal branches of the STA ramify over the scalp and have a corkscrew appearance on lateral angiograms (Figs. 2-18 and 2-19).

The *transverse facial artery* (TFA), a major horizontal branch of the STA, follows a course that parallels the zygoma (Figs. 2-7 and 2-8). The TFA should not be confused with another horizontally directed ECA branch, the

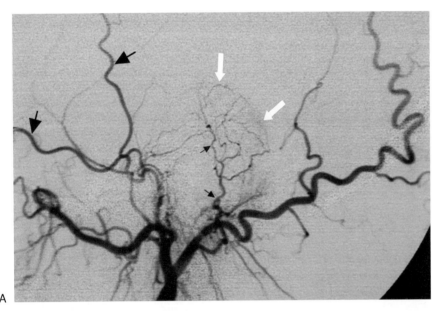

A

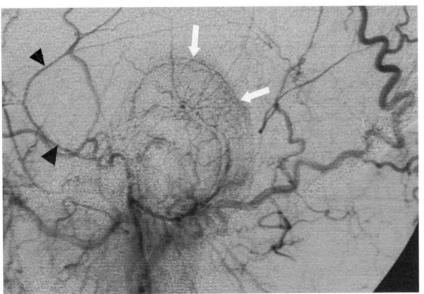

B

FIG. 2-18. Early **(A)** and late **(B)** arterial phase studies of an external carotid angiogram, lateral view. Note the corkscrew appearance of the superficial temporal artery branches (*large black arrows*). The posterior auricular artery (*small black arrows*) is clearly evident. Note prominent but normal vascular blush of the pinna (*white arrows*). The middle meningeal artery branches (**B**, *arrowheads*) typically opacify somewhat later in the angiogram.

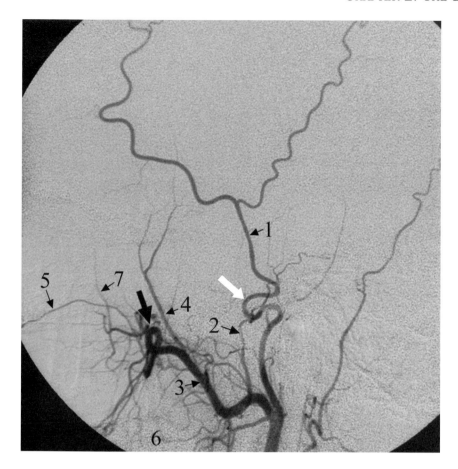

FIG. 2-19. Lateral view of a selective external carotid angiogram shows its terminal branches particularly well.

1, Superficial temporal artery (white arrow indicates the hairpin-shaped turn where the STA crosses the zygoma)
2, Middle meningeal artery
3, Maxillary artery (large black arrow indicates its loop within the pterygopalatine fossa)
4, Middle deep temporal artery
5, Infraorbital artery
6, Buccal arteries
7, Anterior deep temporal artery

internal maxillary artery (IMA). The TFA has a tortuous, corkscrew-shaped appearance and follows a near-horizontal course (Fig. 2-16A,B; see also Fig. 2-24). In contrast, the IMA appears straighter and is directed somewhat anterosuperiorly (Fig. 2-16).

Maxillary Artery

The (internal) maxillary artery is the larger of the terminal ECA branches. The IMA originates behind the neck of the mandible at the distal ECA bifurcation. It then turns anteromedially toward the deep face (Figs. 2-9 and 2-19). The IMA terminates within the pterygopalatine fossa, where it divides into numerous branches that supply the deep face.

Normal Variants

The origins, vascular territories, branches, and hemodynamic balance of the external carotid vessels are quite variable. The numerous arteries that supply the face, orbit, and meninges all exist in a functional hemodynamic balance. Each major pedicle with its corresponding vascular territory can be supplied by one of several possible arterial trunks. The origin, course, and size of each feeding trunk is in turn determined by the pattern of

vascular regression and recruitment that occurred during embryologic development (10).

Anomalies

Variations in the ECA are common, whereas true anomalies are rare. Only the most important patterns are considered here.

Anomalous Origin of the ECA

In rare cases the ECA arises directly from the aortic arch. In other cases a so-called *nonbifurcating carotid artery* is present (see Chapter 3). In this arrangement the common carotid artery has no true bifurcation and the ECA branches arise directly from the common carotid trunk (see Figs. 3-12 and 3-23). This pattern is often seen when other significant anomalies such as an aberrant internal carotid artery are also present.

Anomalous Origins of ECA Branches

Here branches arise from vessels other than the ECA. Variants include *origin of the occipital artery from the cervical internal carotid or vertebral arteries* (Fig. 2-20; see also Fig. 3-13) and *origin of the middle meningeal artery from the ophthalmic artery* (Fig. 2-21).

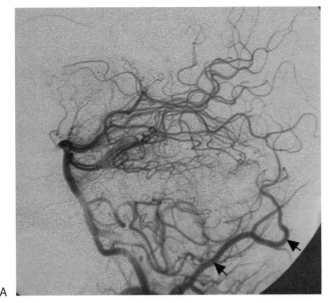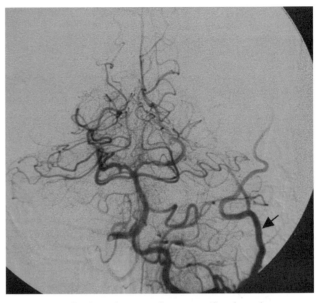

A

B

FIG. 2-20. Lateral **(A)** and anteroposterior **(B)** views of a left vertebral angiogram show opacification of the occipital artery (*arrows*). It has an anomalous origin from the extracranial vertebral artery.

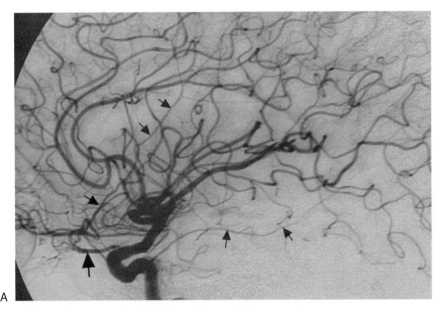

A

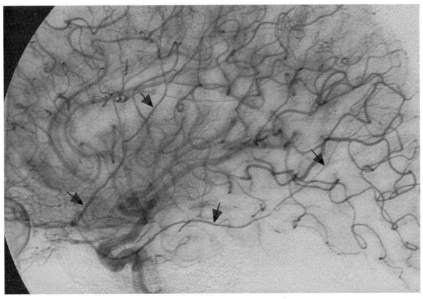

B

FIG. 2-21. Early **(A)** and late **(B)** arterial phase studies, lateral view, from a left internal carotid angiogram show anomalous origin of the middle meningeal artery (*small arrows*) from the ophthalmic artery (*large arrow*).

DEEP (MAXILLARY) BRANCHES OF THE EXTERNAL CAROTID ARTERY

Normal Gross and Angiographic Anatomy

The internal maxillary artery (IMA) is divided into three main segments: (a) a proximal or mandibular segment, (b) a middle or pterygoid segment, and (c) a terminal or pterygopalatine segment (22).

Proximal (Mandibular) Segment

From its origin, the IMA courses anteriorly along the lower border of the lateral pterygoid muscle, where it gives rise to the *middle meningeal artery* (MMA) (Figs. 2-22 and 2-23). The MMA is the largest and most proximal major branch of the IMA. It courses superiorly to the foramen spinosum, where it makes a sharp right-angle bend as it enters the skull. The MMA has frontal, parietal, and petrosal branches. The frontal branch is easily identified by its anteriorly convex curve along the greater sphenoid wing.

The *accessory meningeal artery* (AMA) is a small but important branch that arises from the proximal IMA or the MMA (Figs. 2-22 and 2-23). A small ascending branch of the AMA enters the cranial cavity through the foramen ovale or through the sphenoid emissary foramen (foramen of Vesalius). It may supply part of the trigeminal ganglion, cavernous sinus, and adjacent dura adjacent to the foramen ovale. Distal branches of the AMA often anastomose with the inferolateral trunk of the internal carotid artery (23).

From its origin the AMA follows an oblique anteromedial course to supply the nasopharynx and palate. Despite its name, the major supply of the AMA is extracranial (23).

The *inferior alveolar (dental) artery* descends toward the mandibular foramen to supply the lower teeth and mandible (Figs. 2-9, 2-22, 2-23, and 2-24).

Middle (Pterygoid) Segment

The second IMA segment extends medially across the high deep masticator space (infratemporal fossa) to the pterygopalatine fossa. Important branches that arise from this segment are the *anterior and posterior deep temporal arteries* and the *masseteric and buccal arteries* (Figs. 2-22, 2-23, and 2-24).

Distal (Pterygopalatine) Segment

The distal IMA terminates by looping within the pterygopalatine fossa, a teardrop-shaped opening bordered anteriorly by the posterior wall of the maxillary sinus and posteriorly by the pterygoid plates (Figs. 2-9, 2-25, and 2-26). Branches that arise from this IMA segment ramify around the maxillary sinus to supply the deep face and nose (Figs. 2-26, 2-27, and 2-28).

The *posterior superior alveolar (dental) artery* usually arises just before the IMA enters the pterygopalatine fossa. It courses laterally and inferiorly around the maxillary sinus to supply the maxillary antrum and teeth (Figs. 2-26 and 2-28).

The *infraorbital artery* enters the orbit through the inferior orbital fissure and runs anteriorly along the infraorbital groove, exiting through the infraorbital foramen to supply the cheek, lower eyelid, upper lip, and part of the nose. Its branches anastomose with the buccal, anterior deep temporal, transverse facial, facial, and ophthalmic arteries (Figs. 2-7, 2-9, 2-26, and 2-28) (24).

The *greater (descending) palatine artery* courses inferiorly through the incisive canal to supply the soft palate and tonsils. Its branches outline the posterior wall and floor of the maxillary antrum, which they supply (Fig. 2-28).

The *sphenopalatine artery*, the termination of the maxillary artery, passes medially through the sphenopalatine foramen to supply the nose (Fig. 2-28). Selective injection of the IMA or even the main ECA trunk may cause a very prominent vascular blush in the nasal mucosa.

Other distal IMA branches include three small posteriorly directed branches. From lateral to medial they are the *artery of the foramen rotundum*, the *vidian artery (artery of the pterygoid canal)*, and the *pterygovaginal (pharyngeal) arteries* (Figs. 2-25 and 2-27A) (25,26).

The distal IMA has numerous anastomoses with other ECA branches such as the facial artery (Fig. 2-7). It also has various anastomoses with the ICA and its branches (see Chapters 3, 4, and 17). Some of these anastomoses are the petrous ICA (via the vidian artery), the cavernous ICA (via the artery of the foramen rotundum to the inferolateral trunk), and supraclinoid ICA (ophthalmic artery via ethmoidal branches) (26) (see Table 2-1 and box 17-4).

Functional Angiographic Anatomy

Delineating vascular territories, identifying potential collateral flow patterns, and mapping vascular constraints on regional hemodynamics is called functional angiography. Only the most basic principles of functional neuroangiography can be considered here. For more extensive consideration of this important topic, readers are referred to the excellent review article on functional angiography of the head and neck by Russell (10) and the definitive works of Lasjaunias and Berenstein and co-workers (6,11,17,19,20).

Functional angiography is based on the concept of hemodynamic balance between arterial pedicles, trunks, and anastomotic channels.

Arterial Pedicles

Each anatomic region is nourished by a constant terminal vascular territory called a pedicle. In the face,

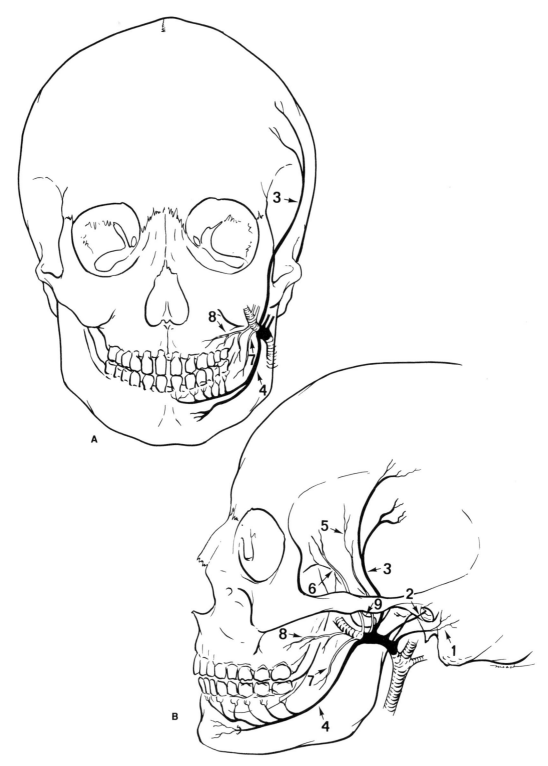

FIG. 2-22. Anteroposterior and lateral anatomic diagrams show the first (mandibular) and second (pterygoid) segments of the internal maxillary artery. The first segment and its branches are indicated by solid black lines; the second segment and its branches are shown by the open lines.

1, Deep auricular artery
2, Anterior tympanic artery
3, Middle meningeal artery
4, Inferior alveolar artery
5, Middle deep temporal artery
6, Anterior deep temporal artery
7, Masseteric branches
8, Buccal branches
9, Accessory meningeal artery

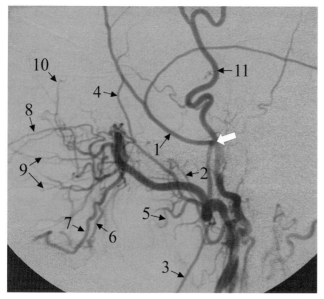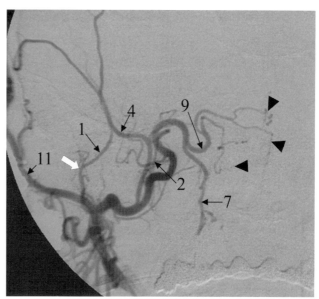

FIG. 2-23. Lateral **(A)** and anteroposterior **(B)** views of a selective external carotid angiogram show the maxillary artery with its three segments and their major branches:

1, Middle meningeal artery (white arrow denotes abrupt angulation as the MMA passes through the foramen spinosum)
2, Accessory meningeal artery
3, Inferior alveolar (dental) artery
4, Middle deep temporal artery
5, Buccal branches
6, Posterior superior alveolar (dental) artery
7, Greater (descending) palatine artery
8, Infraorbital artery
9, Sphenopalatine artery with nasal branches (**B**, *arrowheads*)
10, Anterior deep temporal artery
11, Superficial temporal artery

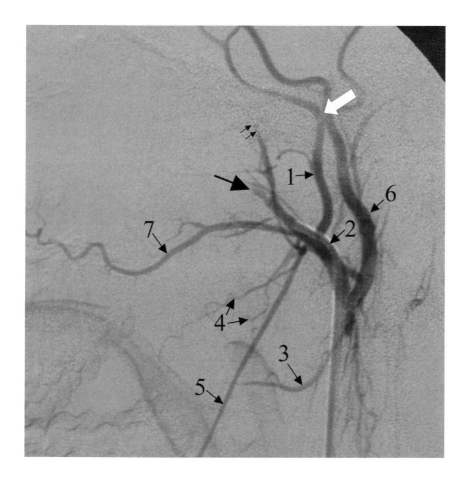

FIG. 2-24. Lateral view of a selective maxillary artery angiogram during therapeutic embolization for epistaxis. The distal maxillary (*large black arrow*) and accessory meningeal (*double arrows*) arteries are occluded. Many of the deep branches from the first and second maxillary segments are well visualized.

1, Middle meningeal artery (white arrow indicates passage through foramen spinosum)
2, Internal maxillary artery (main trunk)
3, Masseteric artery
4, Buccal arteries
5, Inferior alveolar artery
6, Superficial temporal artery
7, Transverse facial artery

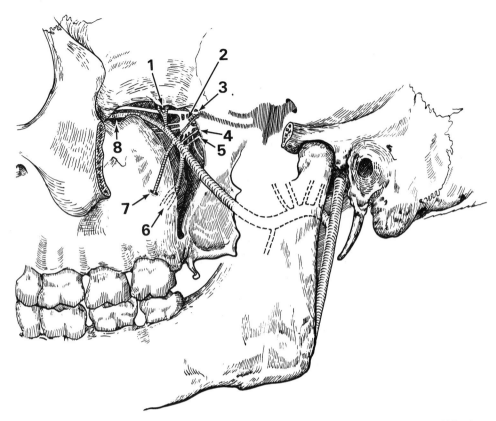

FIG. 2-25. Anatomic diagram depicts the terminal internal maxillary artery branching within the pterygopalatine fossa (PTPF). The zygoma has been cut away to expose the PTPF.

1, Sphenopalatine artery (courses medially to the nose, passing through the sphenopalatine foramen)

2, Sphenopalatine ganglion

3, Maxillary nerve (CN V2) passing from trigeminal ganglion (shown with long dashed lines) through the foramen rotundum, accompanied by the artery of the foramen rotundum (a branch of the cavernous internal carotid artery)

4, Vidian artery

5, Pterygovaginal (pharyngeal) artery

6, Descending palatine artery

7, Posterior superior alveolar artery

8, Infraorbital artery

major pedicles include the mandibular, labial, jugal (cheek), nasal, infraorbital, and ophthalmic territories (6,10,17). A simplified diagram that depicts these major facial pedicles is illustrated in Fig. 2-29.

Arterial Trunks

Each arterial pedicle is supplied by a proximal vessel called a trunk. The source, size, and course of an arterial trunk are highly variable. They are determined by embryonic patterns of vascular regression, recruitment, and assimilation (27,28).

The size as well as the precise structure of each definitive arterial trunk depends on which arterial territories (pedicles) were annexed by that trunk during fetal devel-

opment (6,10). For example, if the facial artery is hypoplastic, much of its territory will be supplied by the masseteric/buccal system (from the IMA), the infraorbital/transverse facial system (from the IMA and STA), or ophthalmic branches of the ICA.

Arterial Anastomoses

Adjacent pedicles may be interconnected to other vascular territories by collateral networks (see Table 2-1 and box on p. 397). Potentially dangerous collateral blood flow toward normal neural tissue may exist (see Fig. 17-15). These regional arterial patterns and possible collateral routes determine the potential risk and efficacy of embolization (10).

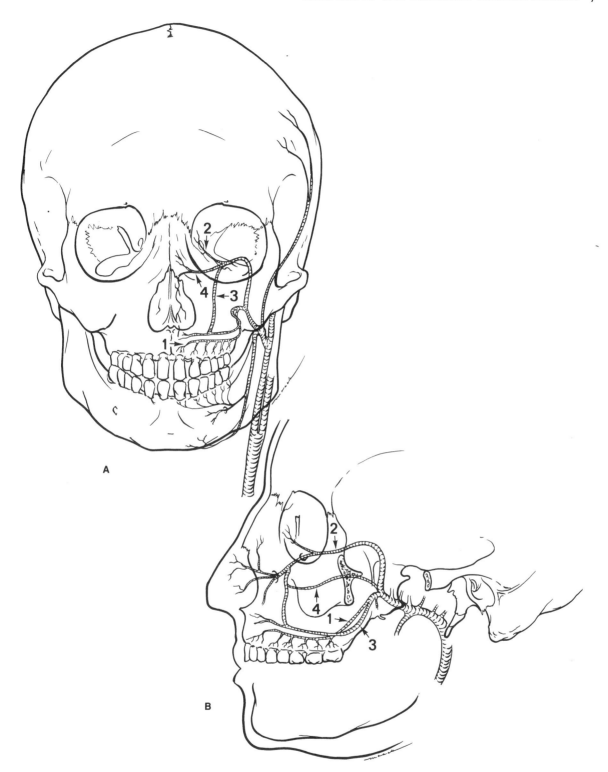

FIG. 2-26. Anteroposterior and lateral anatomic diagrams show the maxillary sinus, orbit, and third (pterygopalatine) segment of the maxillary artery.

1, Posterior superior alveolar artery
2, Infraorbital artery
3, Greater (descending) palatine artery
4, Sphenopalatine artery

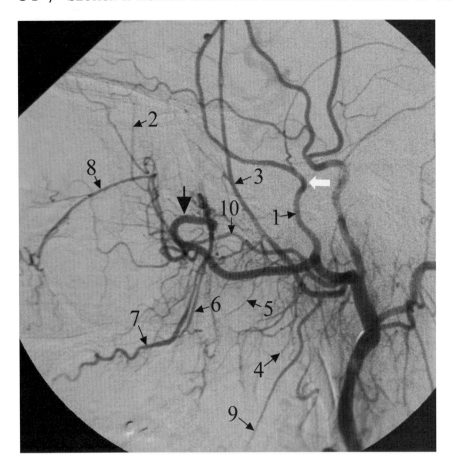

FIG. 2-27. Lateral view of an external carotid angiogram shows the maxillary artery branches. The large black arrow denotes the pterygopalatine fossa.

1, Middle meningeal artery (white arrow demarcates abrupt angulation as the artery passes through the foramen spinosum)
2, Anterior deep temporal artery
3, Middle deep temporal artery
4, Masseteric branches
5, Buccal branches
6, Posterior superior alveolar artery
7, Descending palatine artery
8, Infraorbital artery
9, Inferior alveolar artery
10, Transverse facial artery (a branch of the superficial temporal artery)

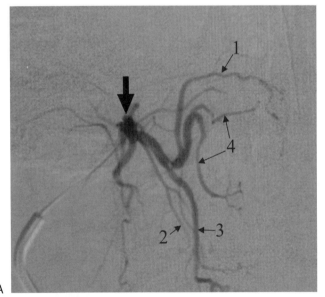

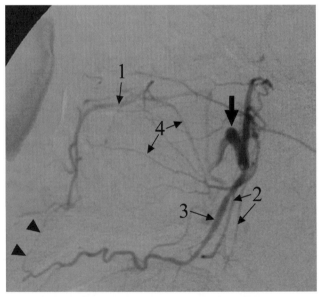

A   B

FIG. 2-28. Lateral **(A)** and anteroposterior **(B)** views of a superselective distal maxillary artery angiogram. The termination of the maxillary artery in the pterygopalatine fossa is indicated by the large arrow. The maxillary sinus and nose are especially well delineated by their surrounding vessels. An anastomosis between the incisive branch of the descending palatine artery (*arrowheads*) and branches of the infraorbital artery shows how different vascular pedicles may communicate with each other via collaterals between their distal branches.

1, Infraorbital artery
2, Posterior superior alveolar arteries
3, Descending (greater) palatine artery
4, Sphenopalatine arteries

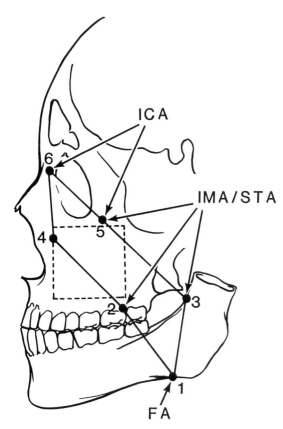

FIG. 2-29. The concept of hemodynamic balance between vascular pedicles is illustrated. Schematic diagram depicts functional anatomy of the facial artery (FA). The facial artery can collect vascular territories (pedicles) at several points (1–6). If a facial artery is hypoplastic, much of its territory is supplied by the masseteric/buccal system (from the internal maxillary artery, IMA), the infraorbital/transverse facial system (from the IMA and superficial temporal artery, STA), or the ophthalmic system (from the internal carotid artery, ICA). For comparison, see the anatomic diagram with anastomoses between branches of different pedicles (Fig. 2-3).

1, Mandibular point
2, Labial point
3, Jugal point
4, Nasal point
5, Infraorbital point
6, Ophthalmic point (Modified and adapted from ref. 17.)

Prior to interventional procedures, a complete functional angiographic map must be drawn by performing and then thoroughly evaluating individual superselective injections of all ECA arterial pedicles that supply the territory in question (10).

REFERENCES

1. Lambiase RE, Haas RA, Carney WI Jr, Roger J. Anomalous branching of the left common carotid artery with associated atherosclerotic changes: a case report. *AJNR* 1991;12:187–189.
2. Dilenge D, Aschaerl GF Jr. Variations of the ophthalmic and middle meningeal arteries: relationship to the embryonic stapedial artery. *AJNR* 1980;1:45–53.
3. Jinkins JR. The vidian artery in childhood tonsillar hypertrophy. *AJNR* 1988;9:141–143.
4. Larsen WJ. Development of the vasculature. In: *Human embryology*, 2nd ed. New York: Churchill Livingstone, 1997.
5. Williams PL, ed. Embryonic circulation. In: *Gray's anatomy*, 38th ed. New York: Churchill Livingstone, 1995:310–315.
6. Lasjaunias PL, Choi IS. The external carotid artery: functional anatomy. *Riv Neuroradiol* 1991;4(suppl 1):39–45.
7. Rodesch G, Choi IS, Lasjaunias P. Complete persistence of the hyoido-stapedial artery in man. *Surg Radiol Anat* 1991;13:63–65.
8. Williams PL, ed. Carotid system of arteries. In: *Gray's anatomy*, 38th ed. New York: Churchill Livingstone, 1995:1513–1523.
9. Salamon G, Faure J, Rayband C, Grisdi F. Normal external carotid artery. In: Newton TH, Potts DG, eds. *Radiology of the skull and brain: angiography*. Vol. 2. St. Louis: Mosby, 1974:1246–1274.
10. Russell EJ. Functional angiography of the head and neck. *AJNR* 1986;7:927–936.
11. Berenstein A, Lasjaunias P, Kricheff II. Functional anatomy of the facial vasculature in pathologic conditions and its therapeutic application. *AJNR* 1983;4:149–153.
12. Gailloud P, Khan KG, Khaw N, et al. The supraisthmic anastomotic arch: a potential pitfall in Doppler sonography of the thyroid gland. *AJR* 1998;170:497–498.
13. Banna M, Lasjaunias P. The arteries of the lingual thyroid: angiographic findings and anatomic variations. *AJNR* 1990;11:730–732.
14. Djindjian R, Merland J-J. *Super-selective arteriography of the external carotid artery*. Berlin: Springer-Verlag, 1978.
15. Lasjaunias P, Moret J. The ascending pharyngeal artery: normal and pathological radioanatomy. *Neuroradiology* 1996;11:77–82.
16. Lasjaunias P, Doyon D. The ascending pharyngeal artery and the blood supply of the lower cranial nerves. *J Neuroradiol* 1978;5:287–301.
17. Lasjaunias P, Berenstein A. *Surgical neuroangiography*. Vol. 1. Functional anatomy of craniofacial arteries. Berlin: Springer-Verlag, 1987.
18. Midy D, Mauruc B, Vergnes P, Caliot P. A contribution to the study of the facial artery, its branches and anastomoses; application to the anatomic vascular bases of facial flaps. *Surg Radiol Anat* 1986;8:99–107.
19. Lasjaunias P, Berenstein A, Doyon D. Normal functional anatomy of the facial artery. *Radiology* 1979;133:631–639.
20. Lasjaunias P, Theron J, Moret J. The occipital artery. *Neuroradiology* 1978;15:31–37.
21. Crabbe JP, Brooks SL, Lillie JH. Gradient-echo MR imaging of the temporomandibular joint: diagnostic pitfall caused by the superficial temporal artery. *AJNR* 1995;164:451–454.
22. Allen WE III, Kier EL, Rothman SLG. The maxillary artery in craniofacial pathology. *AJR* 1974;121:124–138.
23. Vitek JJ. Accessory meningeal artery: an anatomic misnomer. *AJNR* 1989;10:569–573.
24. Lenoble R, Maillot C. L'artère infra-orbitaire. *J Radiol* 1994;75:177–186.
25. Borden NM, Dungan D, Dean BL, Flom RA. Posttraumatic epistaxis from injury to the pterygovaginal artery. *AJNR* 1996;17:1148–1150.
26. Osborn A. The vidian artery: normal and pathologic anatomy. *Radiology* 1980;136:373–378.
27. Pretterkieber ML, Krammer EB, Mayr R. A bilateral maxillofacial trunk in man: an extraordinary anomaly of the carotid system of arteries. *Acta Anat* 1991;141:206–211.
28. Bold EL, Wanamaker HH, Hughes GB, et al. Magnetic resonance angiography of vascular anomalies of the middle ear. *Laryngoscope* 1994;104:1404–1411.

CHAPTER 3

The Internal Carotid Artery

Cervical, Petrous, and Lacerum Segments

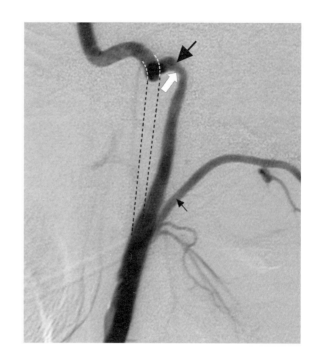

The paired internal carotid arteries (ICAs), two of the four major arteries that supply the brain, provide most of the blood flow to the cerebral hemispheres. Several systems for classifying the ICA segments have been proposed. Although there is no consensus regarding either the nomenclature or numbering of these segments, the classification proposed by Bouthillier and co-workers is practical, takes into account new anatomic information and clinical considerations, and utilizes a logical numerical scale in the direction of normal blood flow (1).

The new classification identifies the ICA segments according to their adjacent structures and the compartments they traverse. Seven anatomically distinct segments are described (Fig. 3-1):

C1 = cervical
C2 = petrous
C3 = lacerum
C4 = cavernous
C5 = clinoid
C6 = ophthalmic
C7 = communicating

In this chapter we will discuss the first three ICA segments. The cavernous, clinoid, ophthalmic, and communicating segments will be considered in Chapter 4.

C1 (CERVICAL) INTERNAL CAROTID ARTERY

Normal Development

The first or C1 (cervical) ICA segment is derived primarily from the fetal third aortic arches (see box on page 58). All other ICA segments, namely the C2 to C7 (petrous to communicating) portions, represent cranial extensions of the embryonic dorsal aortae (see Fig. 2-5) (2).

Gross Anatomy

The ICA normally originates from the common carotid artery (CCA) at the C3–4 or C4–5 level (see Figs. 1-8 and 2-7). It is usually the larger of the two terminal CCA branches. The first ICA segment has two parts: (a) the carotid bulb and (b) the ascending cervical segment (Fig. 3-1).

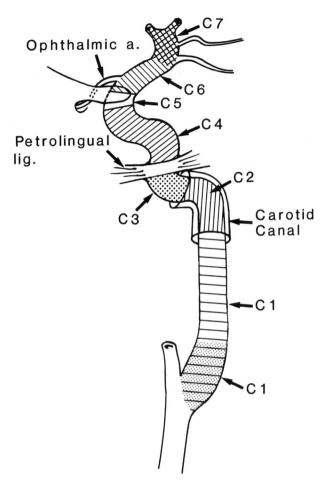

FIG. 3-1. Lateral anatomic diagram depicts the seven internal carotid artery segments.

C1, Cervical segment (the bulb is shown as dotted, and the ascending segment is indicated by the horizontal lines)
C2, Petrous segment
C3, Lacerum segment
C4, Cavernous segment
C5, Clinoid segment
C6, Ophthalmic segment
C7, Communicating (terminal) segment

Cervical Internal Carotid Artery: Normal Anatomy and Variations

---

Normal Development
From embryonic third aortic arch
Gross Anatomy
Also known as C1 or extracranial ICA segment
Two components
Carotid bulb
Ascending cervical ICA
Key relationships
Contained within the carotid space (CS)
Posterolateral, then medial to external carotid artery (ECA) as ICA ascends
Anteromedial to internal jugular vein (IJV)
Separated from IJV by cranial nerves (CNs) IX to XII
Branches
None
Normal variants
Bifurcation (normally at C4 vertebral level) may be high (up to C1) or unusually low (down to T2)
Medial (instead of lateral) origin from common carotid artery (CCA) in 10% to 15%
Anomalies
Absence, hypoplasia, duplication, fenestration (rare)
"Nonbifurcating" carotid artery (no bulb; ECA branches arise separately)
Carotid–basilar anastomoses (see box on page 65)
Persistent hypoglossal artery (PHA)
Proatlantal intersegmental artery (PIA)

CCA, common carotid artery; ICA, internal carotid artery; ECA, external carotid artery; IJV, internal jugular vein; CNs, cranial nerves.

Carotid Bulb

The carotid bulb is the most proximal aspect of the cervical ICA. The bulb forms a significant focal dilatation where the ICA originates from the CCA at a slight angle. The diameter of the normal bulb is approximately 7.5 mm compared with diameters of 7.0 mm for the CCA and 4.7 mm for the ICA distal to the bulb (3).

Blood flow in the ICA compared with the external carotid artery (ECA) occurs in a ratio of approximately 70:30. Recent studies have demonstrated that flow dynamics around the carotid bifurcation and within the bulb itself are complex. Functionally there are two compartments in the bulb: a posterior one that contains slowly swirling retrograde fluid eddies and a more anterior slipstream that accelerates with systole. Blood flow beyond the bulb initially follows a helical pattern before it assumes a more laminar configuration (Fig. 3-2) (3).

Ascending Segment

From the bulb the cervical ICA courses cephalad within the carotid space (CS), a fascially defined tubular-shaped sheath that contains all three layers of the deep cervical fascia (Fig. 3-3). The CS extends from the mediastinum to the skull base (4).

The CS contents include the *internal carotid artery*, the *internal jugular vein*, *lymph nodes* (jugulodigastric nodes of the high deep cervical chain), postganglionic

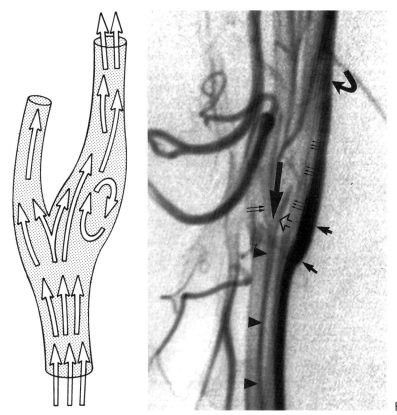

A   B

FIG. 3-2. A: Diagram depicts flow dynamics in the normal human carotid artery. Slipstreams from the common carotid artery are diverted at the bifurcation. Note the recirculation within the carotid bulb (*curved arrows*) and the helical pattern of flow above the bulb (modified and adapted from ref. 3). **B:** Late arterial phase view of a common carotid angiogram, lateral view, shows the intravascular flow patterns described by Kerber. The central slipstream (*arrowheads*) strikes the carina of the CCA bifurcation (*large arrow*), then sends most of its flow (*open arrow*) into the anterior part of the proximal ICA. The remainder (*double arrows*) of the stream passes into the ECA. Relatively stagnant flow in the carotid bulb (*small arrows*) pushes the posterior slipstream (*triple arrows*) anteriorly. Normal laminar flow is reestablished distally in the distal ascending ICA segment (*curved arrow*) (reprinted with permission from Osborn A. *Diagnostic Neuroradiology*. St. Louis: Mosby, 1994).

sympathetic nerves, and several of the lower *cranial nerves*. Above the nasopharynx, CNs IX to XII course within the CS, but only the vagus nerve (CN X) extends throughout its entire length.

The C1 segment terminates as the ICA enters the carotid canal in the petrous temporal bone. At the skull base the CS splits into two layers. The inner layer continues as the periosteum of the carotid canal, whereas the outer layer blends in with the periosteum of the exocranium (1).

Relationships

The cervical ICA is anatomically related to a number of important structures (Fig. 3-3; also see Figs. 1-8 and 2-7) (5).

Anterior

The ICA and CS are covered anterolaterally by the sternomastoid muscle.

Posterior

The longus capitis muscle, superior cervical sympathetic ganglion, and vagus (CN X) nerve lie behind the cervical ICA.

Medial

The ICA initially lies posterolateral to the ECA (see Fig. 2-6). As it ascends, it usually courses medial to the main ECA trunk. The pharyngeal mucosal and parapharyngeal spaces are also anteromedial to the ICA (Fig. 3-3) (4).

Lateral

Except near the skull base, the internal jugular vein and vagus nerve (CN X) are lateral and slightly posterior to the ICA. Below the level of the digastric muscle, the hypoglossal nerve (CN XII), part of the ansa cervicalis, and the lingual and facial veins are also lateral to the ICA. More superiorly, the ICA is crossed by the occipital and posterior auricular branches of the ECA. The styloid process, glossopharyngeal nerve (CN IX),

deep lobe of the parotid gland, and internal jugular vein are all lateral to the ICA as it approaches the skull base (5).

Summary

Thus, the cervical ICA:

1. Initially lies *posterolateral* to the ECA but then courses *medial* to the ECA as it ascends toward the skull base.
2. Lies *in front of* the internal jugular vein and slightly medial to it.

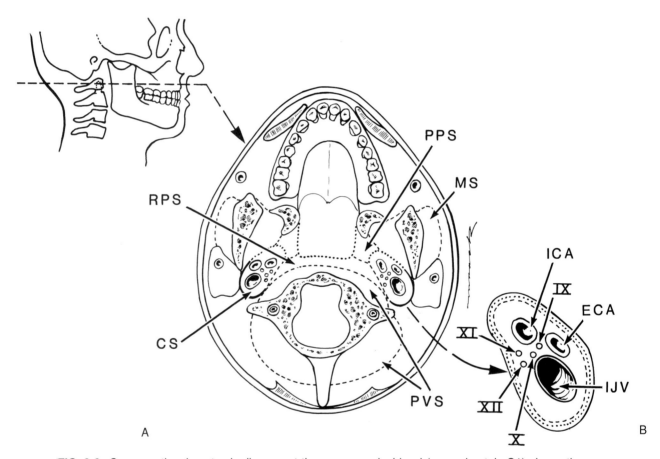

A   B

FIG. 3-3. Cross-sectional anatomic diagram at the upper cervical level (approximately C1) shows the carotid space (CS), its contents, and relationship to adjacent spaces. **A:** Overview diagram illustrates all three layers of deep cervical fascia contributing to the carotid sheath. Note that the parotid space (PS) is lateral to the CS. The parapharyngeal space (PPS), shaded black, is anterior to the CS. The retropharyngeal space (RPS) is anterior and medial to the CS. **B:** Magnified view of the distal CS shows the internal carotid artery (ICA). The external carotid artery (ECA) has already given off many of its branches and appears relatively small. In the upper neck the ICA is medial to the ECA and lies anteromedial to the internal jugular vein (IJV). At this level, the glossopharyngeal (CN IX), vagus (CN X), spinal accessory (CN XI), and hypoglossal (CN XII) nerves are all contained within the CS. Lower in the neck, near the soft palate level, all but the vagus nerve exit the CS. The sympathetic plexus is shown here as a series of small dots anteromedial to the ICA. A few lymph nodes from the high deep cervical chain are present at this level but are not shown.

3. Is separated from the IJV by cranial nerves IX to XII.

Branches

No named branches arise from the carotid bulb or cervical ICA segment. However, a number of anomalous vessels may originate from the extracranial ICA.

Normal Angiographic Anatomy

Except for the carotid bulb, the cervical ICA maintains a smooth, relatively constant diameter throughout its course. The proximal portion of the ICA initially lies posterolateral to the ECA, then the ICA courses medial to the ECA as it passes upward toward the skull base (Fig. 3-4).

The cervical ICA has no angiographically identifiable normal branches.

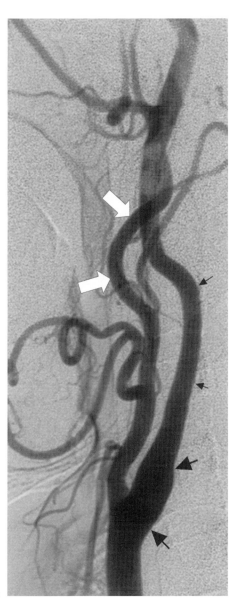 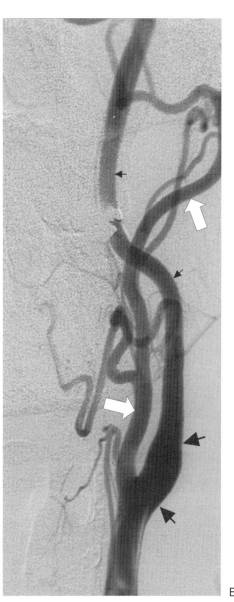

A   B

FIG. 3-4. Lateral **(A)** and anteroposterior **(B)** common carotid angiograms show the normal extracranial internal carotid artery (ICA). The carotid bulb is indicated by the large black arrows. The ICA initially lies behind and lateral to the external carotid artery (ECA). As the cervical ICA (*small black arrows*) ascends, it crosses behind and then courses anteromedially to the main ECA trunk (*white arrows*).

Normal Variants

Variations in the origin, course, and position of the cervical ICA are common, whereas variations in size are rare.

Bifurcation

The normal CCA bifurcation is at or near the level of the thyroid cartilage (approximately C4) (see Fig. 2-7). Bifurcations may occur as high as C1 or as low as T2 (Fig. 3-5). A so-called nonbifurcating carotid artery is a rare but significant anomaly, not a normal variation, and is usually associated with other vascular anomalies.

Position

The proximal ICA is usually lateral to the ECA. The medial origin of the ICA is a common variant and is found in 8% to 15% of normal carotid angiograms. Here the internal and external carotid arteries appear superimposed in the lateral projection (Fig. 3-6A). In such cases the carotid bifurcation can be profiled using oblique (Fig. 3-6B) or anteroposterior (Fig. 3-6C) views. A tortuous,

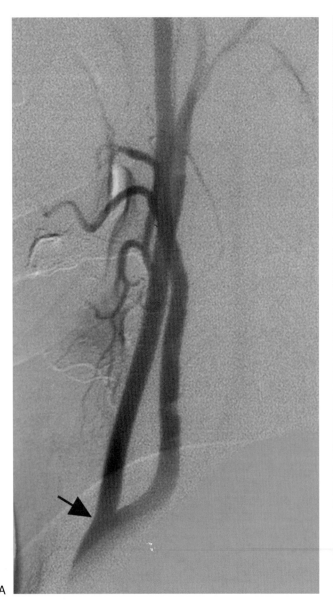
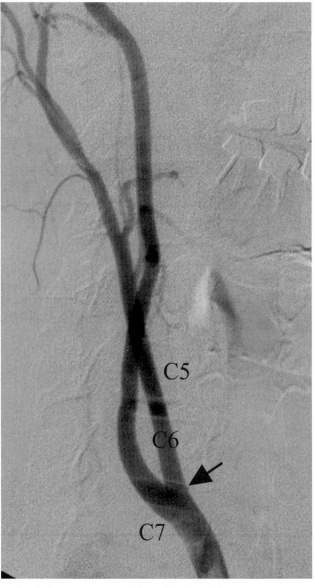

A

B

FIG. 3-5. Lateral **(A)** and slightly oblique anteroposterior **(B)** common carotid angiograms show an unusually low common carotid artery bifurcation (*arrow*). The lower cervical vertebral bodies (C5–7) are indicated. The CCA bifurcation lies at the C6–7 level.

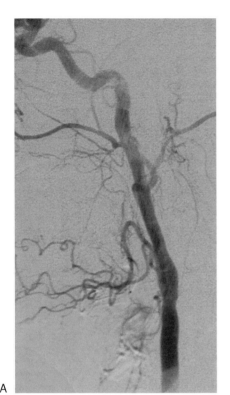
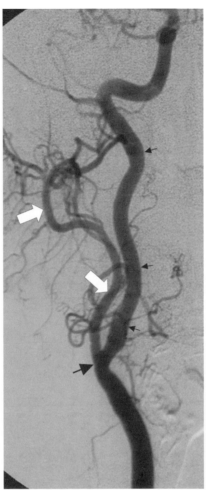
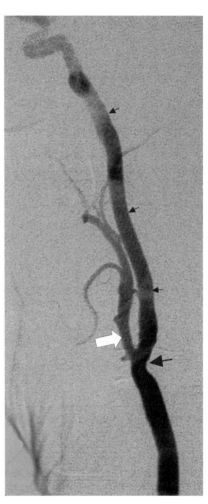

FIG. 3-6. Medial origin of the ICA from the CCA bifurcation is illustrated. **A:** Note that on the standard lateral projection the external (ECAs) and internal carotid arteries (ICAs) are superimposed and cannot be distinguished from each other. **B** and **C:** The carotid bifurcation (*large black arrow*) as well as the origin and course of the ECA (*white arrows*) and ICA (*small black arrows*) are profiled using anteroposterior (**B**) and oblique (**C**) views.

medially projecting ICA can present clinically as a retropharyngeal pulsatile mass (Fig. 3-7).

Course

Tortuosity (Fig. 3-8) or kinking (Fig. 3-9) of the cervical ICA is relatively common in both young children and older adults. Coiling or even complete looping of the ICA occurs in 5% to 15% of patients in unselected angiographic series (Fig. 3-10). This appearance is thought to be at least partially developmental, unrelated to either age or hypertension (6).

Anomalies

Congenital anomalies of the cervical ICA are relatively rare and include anomalous origin, hypoplasia or aplasia, anomalous branches, and persistent primitive carotid–basilar anastomoses.

Anomalous Origin

Rarely, the ECA and ICA each originates directly from the aortic arch instead of the common carotid bifurcation.

Agenesis

Congenital absence of the ICA is rare, with an estimated prevalence of 0.01% (7). Absent ICA is usually unilateral; bilateral ICA agenesis occurs but is extremely uncommon. Agenesis can be distinguished from acquired ICA occlusion by examining the skull base. In cases of true agenesis the bony carotid canal is absent (8).

Congenital absence of an ICA may be asymptomatic due to collateral circulation through the circle of Willis or an intercavernous anastomosis with the contralateral ICA. However, recognition of this anomaly does have clinical significance because there is an increased prevalence of associated abnormalities such as intracranial aneurysm in these cases (9).

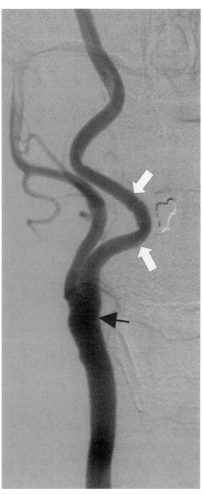

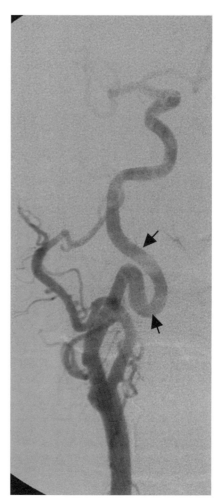

FIG. 3-7. Anteroposterior view of a right common carotid angiogram shows the medial origin of the ICA from the CCA bifurcation (*large black arrow*). The tortuous, medially projecting ICA (*white arrows*) presented cinically as a retropharyngeal pulsatile mass.

FIG. 3-8. Anteroposterior view of a right common carotid angiogram shows an unusually tortuous ICA (*arrows*), a striking but normal variant.

Hypoplasia

Hypoplasia of the ICA has been reported both as an isolated anomaly and in conjunction with other abnormalities such as anencephaly and basal telangectasia (10). Diffuse ICA narrowing is more often acquired and occurs with reduced flow, dissecting aneurysm, fibromuscular dysplasia, or segmental stenosis (see Chapter 16). A developmentally small ICA is associated with a small bony carotid canal (Fig. 3-11) (8).

Duplication and Fenestration

Duplication of the extracranial ICA is a rare anomaly that, if unsuspected, may complicate vascular surgery (11). Duplication and *fenestration* of craniocerebral arteries probably occur when there is incom-

plete fusion of plexiform embryonic vessels (see Chapters 1 and 2).

Anomalous Branches

A so-called *nonbifurcating* carotid artery occurs when the carotid artery extends directly from the aortic arch to the skull base without dividing. In such cases the external carotid branches arise separately from the main carotid trunk and there is no carotid bulb (12). A nonbifurcating cervical carotid artery may be associated with other clinically significant anomalies such as aberrant course of the ICA through the middle ear (Fig. 3-12).

Anomalous branches reported as arising from the extracranial ICA include vessels that normally originate from the ECA (e.g., the ascending pharyngeal and occipital arteries) (Fig. 3-13), other ICA segments (vidian artery), or the vertebrobasilar circulation (e.g., cerebellar and posterior meningeal arteries) (13,14).

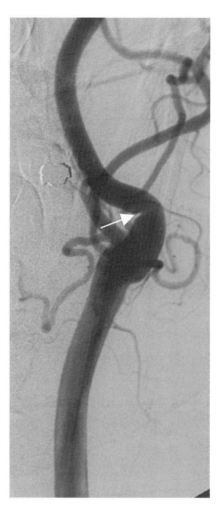

FIG. 3-9. Anteroposterior view of a left common carotid angiogram shows kinking (*arrow*) of the ICA distal to the carotid bulb.

Carotid–Basilar Anastomoses

During development of the fetal craniocerebral circulation, transient segmental connections between the primitive carotid and hindbrain circulations appear (see Fig. 1-2B). With the exception of the extracranial proatlantal intersegmental arteries, these vessels are named according to the cranial nerves they parallel. From top down they are (a) the persistent trigeminal, (b) otic, (c) hypoglossal, and (d) proatlantal intersegmental arteries (Fig. 3-14).

Normally these fetal anastomoses disappear as the posterior communicating arteries develop (see Fig. 1-3). If a segmental anastomosis fails to obliterate and persists into adulthood, it is called a carotid–basilar anastomosis. Two of the four embryonic vessels—the persistent hypoglossal artery and the proatlantal intersegmental artery—connect the cervical ICA to the vertebrobasilar system (see box next column).

Carotid–Basilar Anastomoses: Embryology and Anatomy

Posterior communicating artery (PCoA)
  From caudal division of embryonic internal
    carotid artery (ICA)
  Connects cranial division of primitive ICA
    to developing vertebrobasilar
    circulation
  Partially regresses
  Variants
    "Fetal" origin of posterior cerebral arteries
    "Infundibulum" (junctional dilatation at origin
      from ICA)
Primitive trigeminal artery (PTA)
  Embryonic carotid–basilar anastomosis
  Connects cavernous ICA with embryonic
    dorsal longitudinal neural
    arteries
  Normally regresses completely
  Most common "persistent embryonic
    carotid–basilar anastomosis"
Persistent otic artery (POA)
  Embryonic carotid–basilar anastomosis
  From petrous ICA to embryonic dorsal
    longitudinal neural arteries
  Normally regresses completely
  Extremely rare; almost never identified
    angiographically
Persistent hypoglossal artery (PHA)
  Embryonic carotid basilar anastomosis
  Connects cervical ICA with embryonic dorsal
    longitudinal neural arteries
  Normally regresses completely
  Second most common persistent embryonic
    carotid–basilar anastomosis but <<PTA
  Identified angiographically by
    Origin from C1–2 level of cervical ICA
    Does not pass through foramen magnum
    Hypoglossal (anterior condyloid) canal is
      enlarged
Proatlantal intersegmental artery (PIA)
  Embryonic carotid basilar anastomosis
  Connects cervical ICA with embryonic dorsal
    longitudinal neural arteries (occasionally
    arises from external carotid)
  Normally regresses completely
  Identified angiographically by
    Origin from C2–3 level of cervical ICA
    Lower origin, more vertical course compared
      with PHA
    Horizontal suboccipital course along C1 ring
  Two types (type II arises from ECA, is less
    common)

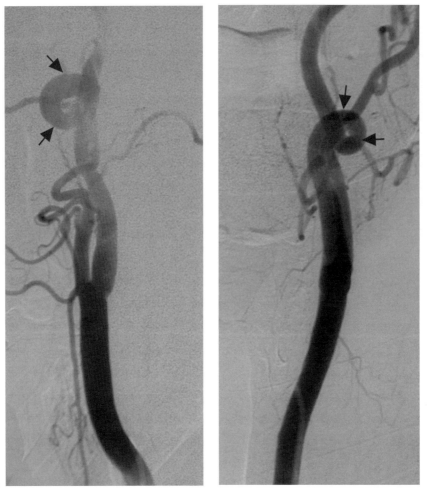

FIG. 3-10. Lateral **(A)** and anteroposterior **(B)** common carotid angiograms show that the cervical ICA forms a complete 360 degree loop (*arrows*).

A *persistent hypoglossal artery (PHA)* is the second most common carotid–basilar anastomosis (trigeminal artery is the most frequent), occurring with an estimated prevalence of 0.027% to 0.26% (15). In this anomaly the persistent embryonic vessel arises from the cervical ICA, usually at the C1–2 level, and curves posteromedially toward an enlarged anterior condyloid (hypoglossal) canal (Fig. 3-15) (16). The PHA penetrates the canal and then joins the basilar artery without passing through the foramen magnum (Fig. 3-16) (17). The posterior communicating arteries are absent (18).

A *proatlantal intersegmental artery (PIA)* originates from the dorsal aspect of the ICA at about the C2–3 level, slightly below the origin of a persistent hypoglossal artery.

The most common type of PIA (a so-called type I PIA) runs upward and dorsolaterally, ascending to the occipitoatlantal (the first cervical or proatlantal) space without passing through the transverse foramen of any cervical vertebra (19). The type I PIA courses horizontally above the atlas to enter the skull through the foramen magnum, giving off the ipsilateral vertebral artery (Figs. 3-17 and 3-18).

A type II PIA is less common. This variant often arises from the ECA and joins the vertebral artery below C1. It then curves dorsally to pass through the transverse process of the atlas.

Most reported examples of PIA are found incidentally at angiography, although one case with a "top of the basilar" syndrome has been reported (19).

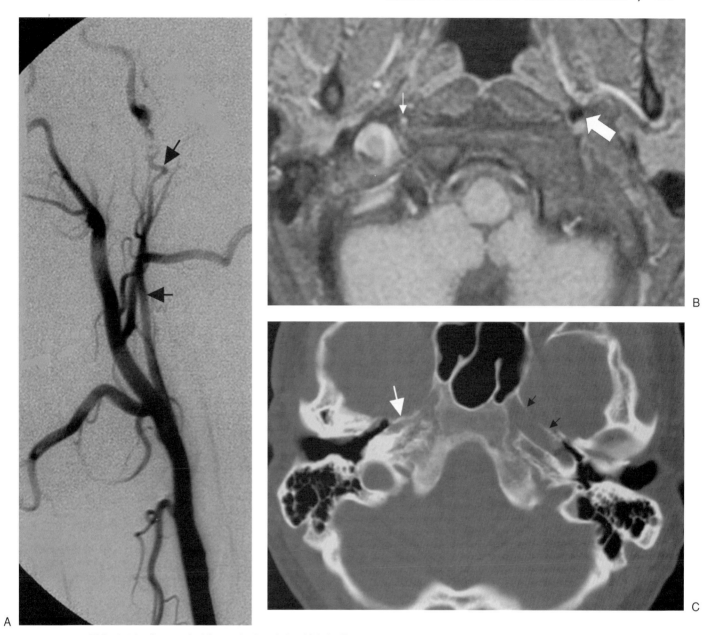

FIG. 3-11. Congenital hypoplasia of the ICA is illustrated. **A:** Lateral view of a right common carotid angiogram shows a very small ICA (*arrows*). **B:** Axial fat-suppressed T1-weighted MR scan shows a normal flow void in the left ICA (*large white arrow*). Compare the absence of flow void in the right ICA (*small white arrow*). **C:** High-resolution CT scan through the skull base shows a very small right carotid canal (*white arrow*). Compare with the normal-sized left carotid canal (*small black arrows*).

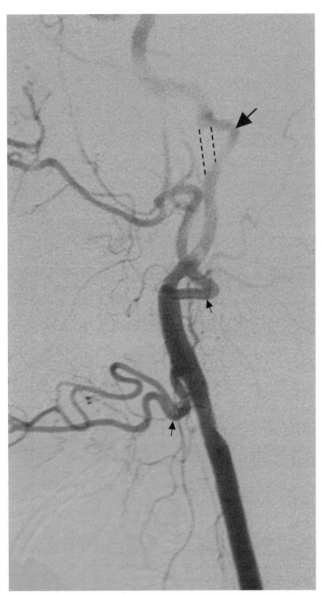

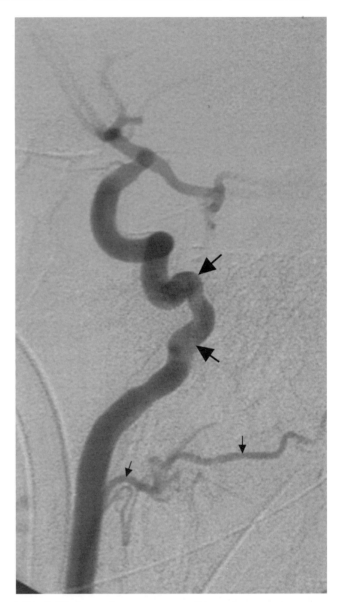

FIG. 3-12. Lateral common carotid angiogram demonstrates a nonbifurcating carotid artery. There is no identifiable carotid bulb or bifurcation. The external carotid branches (*small black arrows*) originate separately and directly from the carotid artery. Note aberrant course of the petrous ICA segment (*large black arrow*). The normal position of the C2 segment is indicated by the dotted lines.

FIG. 3-13. Lateral common carotid angiogram shows an occipital artery (*small arrows*) that arises directly from the cervical ICA. The petrous ICA has an unusual course and is probably aberrant (*large arrows*).

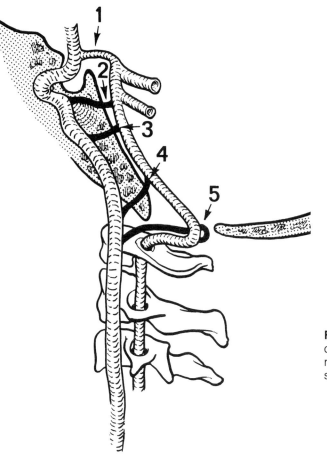

FIG. 3-14. Anatomic diagram depicts the embryologic carotid–basilar and carotid–vertebral anastomoses. The posterior communicating artery is the only vessel that normally persists; the other four, shown in black, usually regress completely.

1, Posterior communicating artery
2, Trigeminal artery
3, Otic artery
4, Hypoglossal artery
5, Proatlantal intersegmental artery

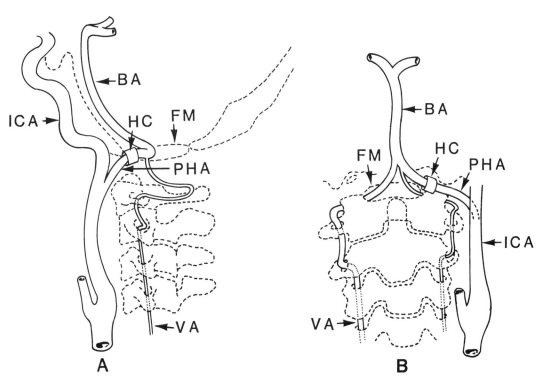

FIG. 3-15. Lateral **(A)** and anteroposterior **(B)** anatomic sketches depict a left persistent primitive hypoglossal artery (PHA). A PHA is a robust vessel that arises from the posterior aspect of the cervical internal carotid artery (ICA), usually at the C1–2 level. The PHA passes through an enlarged anterior condyloid foramen (hypoglossal canal, HC) and does not traverse the foramen magnum (FM). The PHA supplies the basilar artery (BA). The posterior communicating arteries are absent and the ipsilateral vertebral artery (VA) is hypoplastic.

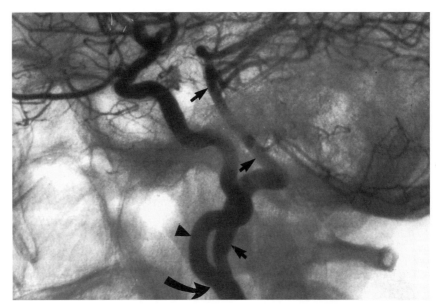

FIG. 3-16. Left common carotid angiogram, lateral view, shows a typical persistent hypoglossal artery (*arrows*) that arises from the cervical ICA (*arrowhead*) and supplies the posterior fossa vasculature. Note point at which the PHA originates from the ICA (*curved arrow*) (from the archives of the Armed Forces Institute of Pathology).

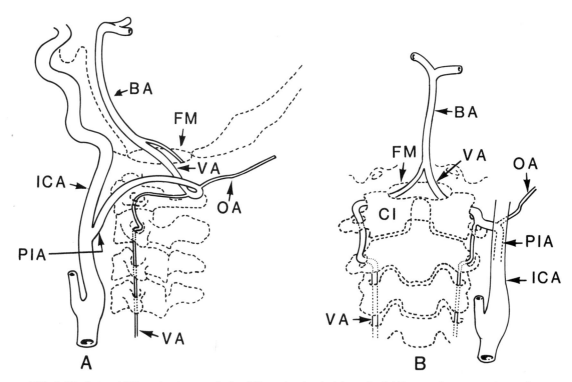

FIG. 3-17. Lateral **(A)** and anteroposterior **(B)** anatomic sketches depict the most common type of persistent proatlantal intersegmental arteries (PIA). In this arrangement, a so-called type I PIA, the PIA arises from the internal carotid artery (ICA) at the C2 or C3 level and courses posterosuperiorly in the first cervical (occipitoatlantal) space. The PIA does not pass through the transverse process of any vertebra. It joins the distal vertebral artery (VA) above the atlas and courses through the foramen magnum (FM) to supply the basilar artery (BA). The PIA often gives origin to the occipital artery (OA).

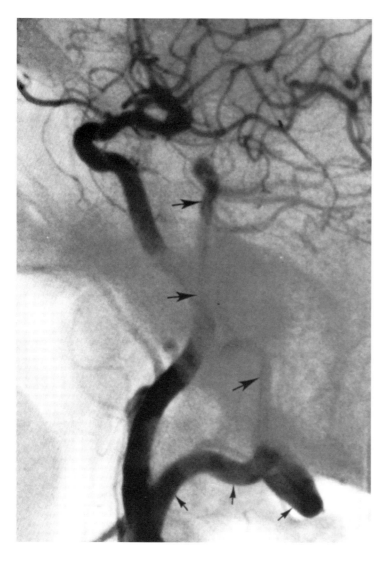

FIG. 3-18. Left common carotid angiogram, lateral view, shows a proatlantal intersegmental artery (*small arrows*) arising from the cervical ICA and filling the basilar artery (*large arrows*).

C2 (PETROUS) INTERNAL CAROTID ARTERY

Development

All ICA segments above the exocranial opening of the carotid canal are derived from the embryonic dorsal aorta (see box below). A remnant of the second aortic arch, the hyoid artery, forms the caroticotympanic artery (see Fig. 2-5) (20).

Petrous Internal Carotid Artery: Normal Anatomy and Variations

Normal development
  Cranial extension of embryonic dorsal aorta
Gross anatomy
  Also known as C2 ICA segment
  Subsegments
    Vertical segment
    Horizontal segment
  One "knee" (genu)

(continues)

Key relationships
  Contained within petrous carotid canal
  Vertical segment is anterior to internal jugular
    vein
  Genu is below, slightly in front of cochlea and
    tympanic cavity
  Horizontal segment exits canal at petrous apex,
    above foramen lacerum (FL)
Branches
  Caroticotympanic artery
  Vidian artery (inconstant)
Normal variants
  None
Anomalies
  Aberrant course through middle ear
    Presents as retrotympanic pulsatile mass
      (may mimic glomus tympanicum
      tumor)
  Persistent stapedial artery (PSA; causes Y-shaped
    enlargement of geniculate fossa, small/absent
    foramen spinosum)

Gross Anatomy

The C2 ICA segment enters the skull base at the periosteal-lined carotid canal and is contained throughout its course by the petrous temporal bone (Fig. 3-19). Within the bony canal the ICA is surrounded by a venous plexus that represents a lateral extension from the cavernous sinus (21). Some rootlets from the carotid autonomic plexus, derived from the internal carotid branch of the superior cervical ganglion, also surround the ICA (5).

The petrous ICA has two distinct subsegments: a vertical or ascending segment and a horizontal segment. The junction between the two segments forms a knee or "genu" that is easily identified at cerebral angiography.

Vertical Segment

The ICA ascends within the vertical segment, then turns anteromedially at the genu. The vertical segment averages approximately 10 mm in length (21).

Horizontal Segment

From the genu, the ICA turns anteromedially toward the apex of the petrous temporal bone. The horizontal

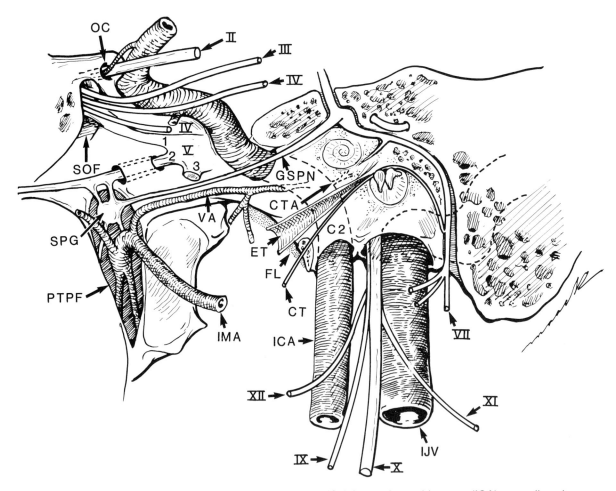

FIG. 3-19. Diagrammatic sketch depicts the petrous (C2) internal carotid artery (ICA) as well as its branches and adjacent structures. As it enters the bony carotid canal, the ICA lies anterior to the internal jugular vein. The eustachian tube (ET) is lateral and anterior. Note that the C2 ICA has an ascending segment, a posterolateral genu, and a longer horizontal segment. The posterior genu of the intrapetrous ICA lies just in front of and below the cochlea. The two significant C2 ICA branches are the caroticotympanic artery (CTA) and the vidian artery (VA). The C3 (lacerum) ICA segment is a short segment that extends from the endocranial opening of the carotid canal to the petrolingual ligament (PL). It typically lies just above the foramen lacerum, (FL), which in life is filled with fibrocartilage. PTPF, pterygopalatine fossa; IMA, internal maxillary artery (ECA branch); SOF, superior orbital fissure; OC, optic canal; SPG, sphenopalatine ganglion; GSPN, greater superficial petrosal nerve; CT, chorda tympani; ET, eustachian tube. FL is indicated by the dotted area. Cranial nerves are indicated by the Roman numerals. Carotid segments are indicated by the Arabic numbers.

segment of the petrous ICA is nearly twice the length of its vertical segment (21).

Relationships

The petrous ICA segment is adjacent to many important structures (Fig. 3-19) (22).

Posterior

The ICA enters the carotid canal anterior to the jugular fossa and internal jugular vein. Within the temporal bone the ICA lies in front of and just below the tympanic cavity and cochlea (Fig. 3-19). The ICA and tympanic cavity are normally separated by a thin bony lamella that may be cribriform in childhood and is often resorbed in old age (23).

Superior

The geniculate ganglion and cochlea lie above the roof of the horizontal canal segment. The greater superficial petrosal nerve parallels the course of the petrous ICA and lies lateral to it (Fig. 3-19).

Inferior

As the ICA exits the petrous temporal bone it lies above the foramen lacerum.

Lateral

The ICA enters the temporal bone medial to the styloid process. The eustachian tube lies lateral and somewhat anterior to the horizontal C2 segment.

Medial

As it courses upward toward the cavernous sinus, the inferior petrosal sinus lies medial and slightly posterior to the petrous ICA.

Summary

Thus, the petrous ICA:

1. Enters the temporal bone *in front of* the internal jugular vein, *medial* to the styloid process.
2. Angles anteromedially *below* and slightly *anterior* to the cochlea and tympanic cavity.
3. Lies *above* the cartilage-filled foramen lacerum as it exits the carotid canal at the petrous apex.

Branches

The intrapetrous ICA branches, the vidian and caroticotympanic arteries, are small and inconstant but nevertheless important. They may provide some collateral blood flow from the ECA if ICA occlusion occurs. More importantly, they are sometimes encountered in translabyrinthine and transmastoid surgical approaches to middle ear tumors or infections.

Vidian Artery

The vidian artery, also termed the *artery of the pterygoid canal*, usually arises from the ECA. However, it also may originate from the horizontal petrous ICA segment just as it emerges from the temporal bone. The vidian artery passes anteroinferiorly through the foramen lacerum and anastomoses with branches from the ECA (see Figs. 4-2A and 4-3) (22). A vidian artery can be identified on 30% of temporal bone dissections (21).

Caroticotympanic Artery

The caroticotympanic artery, a vestige of the embryonic hyoid artery, is a small branch that arises from the ICA near its genu. It passes superiorly through the stapes to supply the middle ear cavity. The caroticotympanic artery also anastomoses with the *inferior tympanic artery*, a small branch from the ascending pharyngeal artery (Fig. 3-19; see also Fig. 2-5) (24,25).

Normal Angiographic Anatomy

As it enters the carotid canal, the ICA ascends for approximately 1 cm, then angles sharply forward as it courses anteromedially toward the petrous apex (Fig. 3-20). The vidian artery is occasionally visualized on some high-resolution digital subtraction angiograms (Fig. 3-21). In contrast, the caroticotympanic artery is rarely identified unless it is abnormally enlarged (25).

Anomalies

Two rare but important anomalies of the petrous ICA have been described: (a) aberrant ICA (aICA) and (b) persistent stapedial artery. A third potential anomaly, persistent otic artery, is extremely uncommon and has been documented convincingly only once (26).

Aberrant Petrous Internal Carotid Artery

An aICA traverses the middle ear cavity and presents clinically as a retrotympanic pulsatile mass. In this anomaly

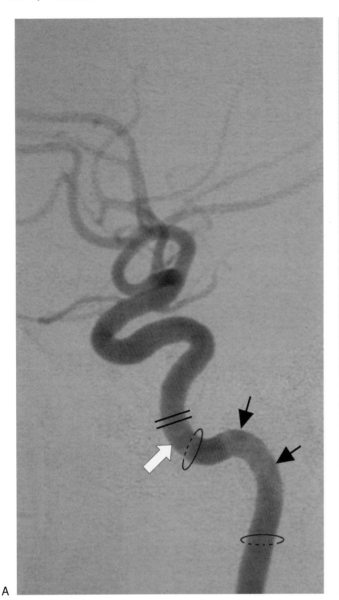
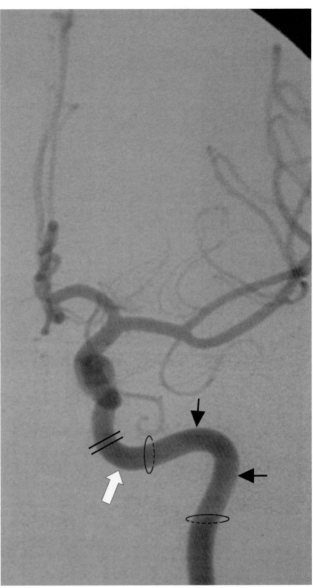

A   B

FIG. 3-20. Lateral **(A)** and anteroposterior **(B)** selective internal carotid angiograms show the upside-down L-shaped configuration of the intrapetrous ICA (*black arrows*). The exo- and endocranial openings of the carotid canal are indicated by the circles. The approximate location of the petrolingual ligament is shown by the parallel black lines. The C3 (lacerum) ICA segment is indicated by the white arrow.

the aICA enters the temporal bone posterior to the external auditory meatus, ascending between the facial canal and the jugular bulb. As it enters the middle ear cavity, the aICA angles sharply laterally and anteriorly (Fig. 3-22).

Some investigators postulate that an aICA represents underdevelopment or abnormal regression of the intrapetrous ICA during embryogenesis (26). In such cases collateral circulation develops between the caroticotympanic artery and an enlarged inferior tympanic artery, a branch of the ascending pharyngeal artery. This

creates an aberrant course of the internal carotid artery ICA in the middle ear (27,28). The aberrant vessel often appears narrowed as it passes through the inferior tympanic canaliculus (Figs. 3-22 and 3-23) (27).

Noninvasive diagnosis of an aICA can be established with magnetic resonance (MR) angiography (Fig. 3-24) or high-resolution computed tomography (CT). CT scans disclose absence of the normal vertical carotid canal and presence of a soft-tissue mass in the tympanic cavity that abuts the cochlea (Fig. 3-25).

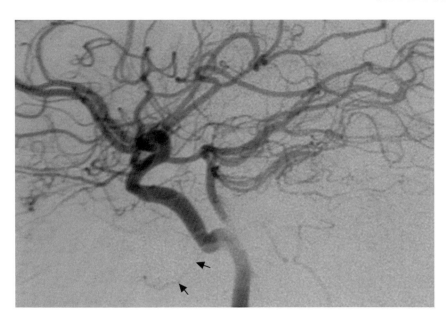

FIG. 3-21. Lateral view of a selective internal carotid angiogram demonstrates a small vidian artery (*arrows*) arising from the horizontal ICA segment. The vidian artery passes anteroinferiorly through the foramen lacerum.

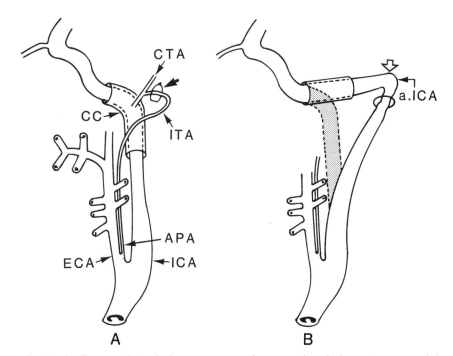

FIG. 3-22. Anatomic diagram, lateral view, compares the normal and aberrant course of the internal carotid artery (ICA) through the petrous temporal bone. **A:** The normal carotid canal (CC) is L-shaped, with an ascending (vertical) and a horizontal segment. The caroticotympanic artery (CTA) arises from the genu and sends branches superomedially to the middle ear cavity. The CTA also sends a branch inferolaterally to anastomose with the inferior tympanic artery (ITA), a small branch from the ascending pharyngeal artery (APA) that passes upward through the inferior tympanic canaliculus (*curved arrow*). **B:** When the petrous ICA follows an aberrant course through the middle ear (aICA), the vertical segment of the carotid canal is absent. The ICA courses more posteriorly and laterally than usual, then at its genu (*open arrow*) the aICA angles sharply downward to pass through an enlarged inferior tympanic canaliculus (*curved arrow*). The aICA is often narrowed at this point (compare with the angiogram shown in Fig. 3-23). The normal carotid canal and usual ICA course are indicated by the dotted and shaded area. Also illustrated here is a nonbifurcating cervical carotid artery with origin of the individual external carotid branches directly from the carotid trunk (compare with Fig. 3-23).

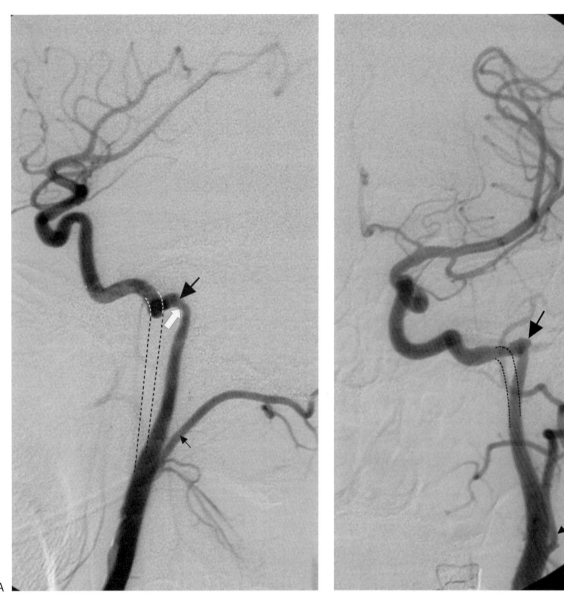

A

B

FIG. 3-23. Selective injection of a nonbifurcating carotid artery demonstrates the aberrant course of the intrapetrous ICA (same case as Fig. 3-12). Lateral **(A)** and anteroposterior **(B)** views show the abnormal posterolateral position of the genu (*large arrow*). Note narrowing of the intrapetrous ICA at this point (*outlined arrow*). The usual, i.e., normal, course of the ICA is indicated by the dotted lines. In this anomaly the external carotid artery branches (*curved arrow*) arise directly and separately from the ICA.

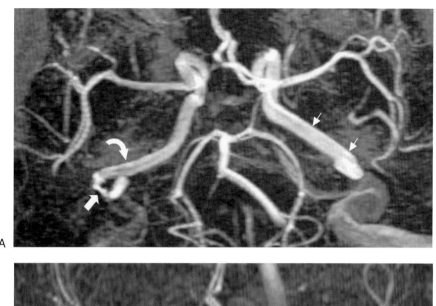

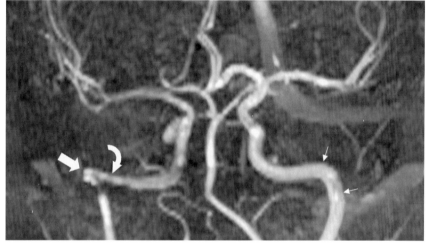

FIG. 3-24. Submentovertex **(A)** and anteroposterior **(B)** views of a multiple overlapping thin slab MR angiogram (MOTSA) show an aberrant right ICA (*curved white arrow*). Compare the abnormal size and position of the aICA with the normal ICA on the left (*small white arrows*). Note narrowing of the aICA genu (*straight white arrow*) where the aICA passes through the inferior tympanic canaliculus (compare with Fig. 3-22B).

Failure to recognize an aICA may cause serious complications if this anomaly is mistaken for a vascular middle ear neoplasm (glomus tympanicum tumor) and submitted for biopsy (29).

Persistent Stapedial Artery

A persistent stapedial artery (PSA) is a rare anomaly. If the embryonic stapedial artery fails to involute, the PSA courses from the vertical ICA segment through the obturator foramen of the stapes (30). The PSA exits from a bony canal on the cochlear promontory and crosses the footplate of the stapes (31). It enlarges the tympanic facial nerve canal en route to the middle cranial fossa, where it terminates as the middle meningeal artery (32).

Persistent stapedial arteries are usually not visualized at angiography. On CT scans they can be identified as a Y-shaped enlargement of the geniculate fossa with accompanying deformity of the anterior epitympanic recess (Fig. 3-26).When a PSA is present, the foramen spinosum is small or absent.

Persistent Otic Artery

The primitive otic artery is the first of the four transient carotid–basilar anastomoses to disappear, perhaps accounting for its exceptional rarity. Only a few cases of persistent otic artery (POA) have been reported in the literature, with only one demonstrated at angiography (33).

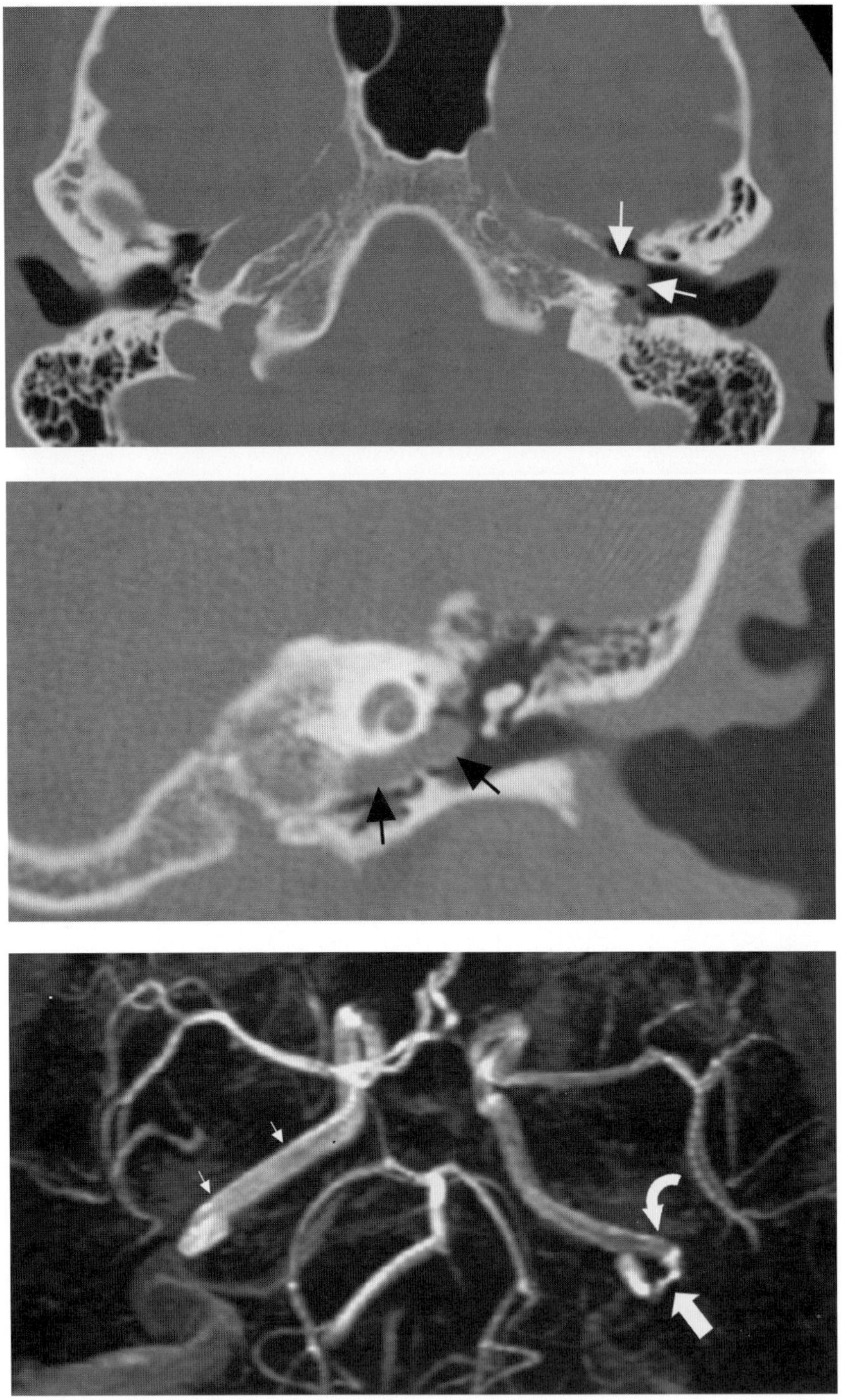

FIG. 3-25. Another aICA is illustrated. Axial **(A)** and coronal **(B)** temporal bone tomograms show a soft-tissue mass in the middle ear (*arrows*) caused by the aICA. **C:** MR angiogram shows the aberrant left ICA (*curved white arrow*). Note the stenosis where the aICA passes through the inferior tympanic canaliculus (*large white arrow*). Compare with the normal right ICA (*small white arrows*).

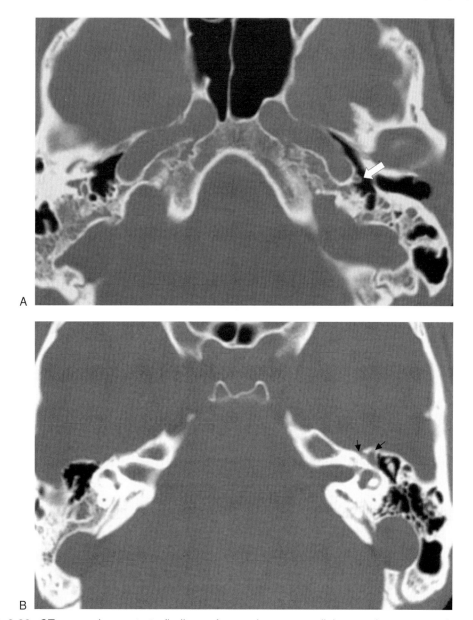

FIG. 3-26. CT scans demonstrate findings of a persistent stapedial artery. Lower scans (not shown) demonstrated absence of the left foramen spinosum. Axial scans through the carotid canal show a vessel (**A**, *arrow*) that coursed from the intrapetrous ICA genu along the carotid promontory, passing superiorly into an enlarged, Y-shaped facial nerve canal (**B**, *small arrows*). The vessel, a PSA, becomes the middle meningeal artery.

C3 (LACERUM) INTERNAL CAROTID ARTERY SEGMENT

Development

The C3 ICA segment is derived from the dorsal aorta between the first aortic arch and primitive maxillary artery (see box below and Chapter One).

Gross Anatomy

The C3 (lacerum) segment begins where the petrous carotid canal ends (Fig. 3-19). Here the ICA courses above (not through) the cartilage-filled FL. The ICA is surrounded by a layer of periosteum and fibrocartilaginous tissue that covers the FL, forming a closed floor and open roof through which the ICA exits. The ICA then ascends in a posterior extension of the carotid sulcus, part of the basisphenoid. The lacerum segment ends at the petrolingual ligament, a small reflection of periosteum that runs between the lingula of the sphenoid bone anteriorly and the petrous apex posteriorly (see Fig. 3-1; also see Fig. 4-1) (1).

Relationships

Like the cervical and petrous ICA segments, the C3 segment is surrounded by areolar tissue, a venous plexus, and small branches of the carotid autonomic plexus (derived from the internal carotid branch of the superior cervical ganglion) (5,21). The greater superficial petrosal nerve courses anteriorly, crossing lateral to the ICA (34).

Lacerum Internal Carotid Artery: Normal Anatomy and Variations

---

Normal development
  Cranial extension of embryonic dorsal aorta
Gross anatomy
  Also known as C3 ICA segment
  Extends from petrous endocranial carotid canal to petrolingual ligament
Key relationships
  Covered by trigeminal ganglion
  Courses above (not through) the foramen lacerum
  Crossed laterally by greater superficial petrosal nerve
Branches
  Usually none (may give origin to vidian artery)
Normal variants
  None
Anomalies
  None

Branches

The C3 segment usually has no branches, although the vidian artery sometimes arises near the junction between the C2 and C3 segments.

Angiographic Anatomy

The C3 segment begins where the carotid canal ends, near the posterolateral margin of the FL. It turns upward, ascending toward the cavernous sinus. The C3 segment ends at the petrolingual ligament, approximately a centimeter below the posterior genu of the C4 (cavernous) ICA (Fig. 3-20).

REFERENCES

1. Bouthillier A, van Loveren HR, Keller JT. Segments of the internal carotid artery: a new classification. *Neurosurgery* 1996;38:425–433.
2. Larsen WJ. *Human embryology*, 2nd ed. New York: Churchill Livingstone, 1997.
3. Kerber CW, Knox K, Hecht ST, Buxton RB. Flow dynamics in the human carotid bulb. *International Journal of Neuroradiology* 1996;2:422–429.
4. Harnsberger HR. The carotid space. In: *Handbook of head and neck imaging*, 2nd ed. St. Louis: Mosby–Year Book, 1995:75–88.
5. Williams P, ed. Internal carotid artery. In: *Gray's anatomy,* 38th ed. New York: Churchill Livingstone, 1995:1523-1529.
6. Vannix RS, Joergenson EJ, Carter R. Kinking of the internal carotid artery. Clinical significance and surgical management. *Am J Surg* 1977; 134:82–89.
7. Chen CJ, Chen ST, Hsieh FY, et al. Hypoplasia of the internal carotid artery with intercavernous anastomosis. *Neuroradiology* 1998;40: 252–254.
8. Quint DJ, Boulos RS, Spera TD. Congenital absence of the cervial and petrous internal carotid artery with intercavernous anastomosis. *AJNR* 1989;10:435–439.
9. Czarnicki EJ, Silbergleit R, Mehta BA, Sanders WP. Absence of the supraclinoid internal carotid artery in association with intracranial aneurysms. *Neuroradiology* 1998;140:11–14.
10. Pascual-Castroviejo I, Viaño J, Pascual-Pascual SI, Martinez V. Facial haemangioma, agenesis of the internal carotid artery and dysplasia of the cerebral cortex: case report. *Neuroradiology* 1995;37:692–695.
11. Chess MA, Barsotti JB, Chang J-K, et al. Duplication of the extracranial internal carotid artery. *AJNR* 1995;16:1545–1547.
12. Morimoto T, Nitta K, Kazekawa K, Hashizume K. The anomaly of a non-bifurcating cervical carotid artery. *J Neurosurg* 1990;72:130–132.
13. Teal JS, Rumbaugh CL, Bergeron RT, et al. Persistent carotid-superior cerebellar artery anastomosis: a variant of persistent trigeminal artery. *Radiology* 1972;103:335–341.
14. Littooy NN, Baker WH, Field TC, et al. Anamalous branches of the cervical internal carotid artery: two cases of clinical importance. *J Vasc Surg* 1988;8:634–637.
15. Kanai H, Nagai H, Wakabayashi S, Hashimoto N. A large aneurysm of the persistent primitive hypoglossal artery. *Neurosurgery* 1992;30: 794–797.
16. Wardell GA, Goree JA, Jimenez JP. The hypoglossal artery and hypoglossal canal. *AJR* 1973;118:528–533.
17. Fujita N, Shimada N, Takimoto H, Satou T. MR appearance of the persistent hypoglossal artery. *AJNR* 1995;16:990–992.
18. Brismar J. Persistent hypoglossal artery, diagnostic criteria. *Acta Radiol Diagn* 1976;17:160–166.
19. Bahsi YZ, Uysal H, Peker S, Yurdakul M. Persistent primitive proatlantal intersegmental artery (proatlantal artery I) results in "top of the basilar" syndrome. *Stroke* 1993;24:2114–2117.
20. Lasjaunias PL, Choi IS. The external carotid artery: functional anatomy. *Riv Neuroradiol* 1991;4(suppl 1):39–45.
21. Paullus WS, Pait TG, Rhoton AL Jr. Microsurgical exposure of the petrous portion of the carotid artery. *J Neurosurg* 1977;47:713–726.

22. Osborn AG. The vidian artery: normal and patholological anatomy. *Radiology* 1980;131:133–136.
23. Sekhar LN, Schramm VL Jr, Jones NF, et al. Operative exposure and management of the petrous and upper cervical internal carotid artery. *Neurosurgery* 1986;19:967–982.
24. Quisling RG, Rhoton AL. Intrapetrous carotid artery branches: radioanatomic analysis. *Radiology* 1979;131:133–136.
25. Quisling RG. Intrapetrous carotid artery branches: pathological application. *Radiology* 1980;134:109–113.
26. Kemp LG, Smith DR. Trigeminal neuralgia, facial spasms, intermedius and glossopharyngeal neuralgia with persistent carotid basilar anastomosis. *Neurosurgery* 1969;31:445–451.
27. Lo WWM, Solti-Bohman LG, McElveen JT Jr. Aberrant carotid artery: radiological diagnosis with emphasis on high-resolution computed tomography. *Radiographics* 1985;5:985–993.
28. Koenigsberg RA, Zito JL, Patel M, et al. Fenestration of the internal carotid artery: a rare mass of the hypotympanum associated with persistence of the stapedial artery. *AJNR* 1995;16:908–910.
29. Glasscock ME III, Seshul M, Seshul MB Sr. Bilateral aberrant internal carotid artery case presentation. *Arch Otolaryngol* 1993;119: 335–339.
30. Lasjaunias P, Moret J. Normal and non-pathological variations in the angiographic aspects of the arteries of the middle ear. *Neuroradiology* 1978;15:213–219.
31. Pahor AL, Hussain SSM. Persistent stapedial artery. *J Laryngol Otol* 1992;106:254–257.
32. Petrus LV, Lo WWM. The anterior epitympanic recess: CT anatomy and pathology. *AJNR* 1997;18:1109–1114.
33. Reynolds AFJr, Stovring J, Turner PT. Persistent otic artery. *Surg Neurol* 1980;13:115–117.
34. Sen C, Chen CS, Post KD. The internal carotid artery. In: *Microsurgical anatomy of the skull base*. New York: Thieme, 1997:15-41.

CHAPTER 4

The Internal Carotid Artery

Cavernous, Clinoid, Ophthalmic, and Communicating Segments

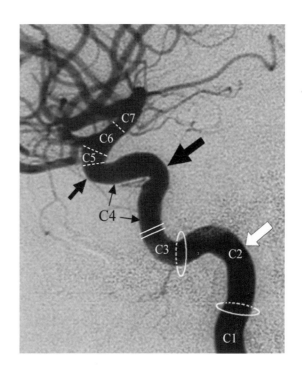

In this chapter the C4–7 internal carotid artery (ICA) segments are discussed. The cervical (C1), petrous (C2), and lacerum (C3) segments were considered previously in Chapter 3.

C4 (CAVERNOUS) INTERNAL CAROTID ARTERY SEGMENT

Gross Anatomy

The C4 (cavernous) ICA segment begins at the superior margin of the petrolingual ligament (1). The C4 ICA has three subsegments: (a) a posterior ascending or vertical portion, (b) a longer horizontal segment, and (c) a short anterior vertical portion (Fig. 4-1). At their junctions with the horizontal segment the two vertical portions form gently rounded curves. These bends are

called the posterior genu and the anterior genu. The C4 segment exits the cavernous sinus through a dural ring in the superior wall (2,2a) (see box on page 84).

Relationships

The C4 ICA segment is surrounded by areolar tissue, variable amounts of fat, the interconnecting venous plexi of the cavernous sinus, and postganglionic sympathetic nerves (1). The cavernous ICA lies adjacent to a number of important structures.

Lateral

The *gasserian (trigeminal) ganglion* covers the C3 (lacerum) and posterior (vertical) C4 segments (Fig. 4-2A). The trigeminal ganglion is separated from the cav-

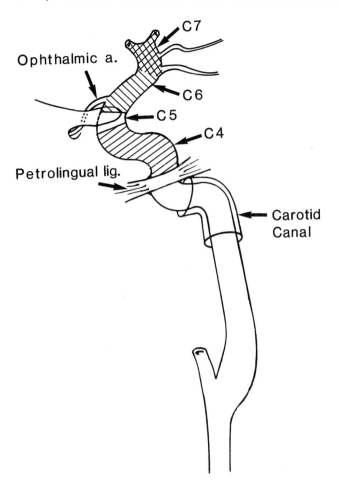

FIG. 4-1. Anatomic diagram depicts the cavernous and supraclinoid internal carotid artery (ICA) segments. C4, cavernous segment (note vertical and horizontal segments, anterior and posterior bends); C5, clinoid segment (open area); C6, ophthalmic segment; C7, communicating segment (cross-hatched area).

Cavernous Internal Carotid Artery: Normal Anatomy and Variations
Normal development
Cranial extension of embryonic dorsal aorta
Gross anatomy
Also known as C4 ICA
Subsegments
Posterior ascending segment
Horizontal segment
Anterior vertical segment
Two "knees"
Posterior (more medial) genu
Anterior (more lateral) genu
Key relationships
Covered by trigeminal ganglion
Abducens nerve (CN VI) is inferolateral
Medial to CNs III, IV, V_1, V_2 (in lateral dural wall)
Branches
Posterior trunk (meningohypophyseal artery)
Inferolateral trunk
Capsular arteries (small, inconstant)
Normal variants
Paramedian course (into sella turcica)
Exaggerated tortuosity
Anomalies
Primitive trigeminal artery (a persistent embryonic carotid–basilar anastomosis)

ernous carotid artery by a well-defined dural layer that forms the floor of Meckel's cave (1). More anteriorly, the third (oculomotor), fourth (trochlear), and sixth (abducens) nerves (cranial nerves *[CNs] III, IV, and VI)* all course lateral to the cavernous ICA. CNs III and IV are contained within the lateral dural wall; only the abducens nerve (CN VI) courses within the cavernous sinus proper.

The C4 segment exits the cavernous sinus medial to the *anterior clinoid process.* The anterior clinoid process, a short bony projection from the lesser sphenoid wing, anchors the anterior continuation of the tentorium and the dura of the cavernous sinus wall.

Medial

The carotid artery itself is the most medial structure within the cavernous sinus proper (Fig. 4-2B). Sur-

rounded by *endothelial-lined sinusoids* and *thin-walled venules,* the ICA runs anteriorly in a shallow groove along the basisphenoid bone called the *carotid sulcus.* The *sphenoid sinus* is medial to the cavernous ICA. Nearly two thirds of anatomic dissections have less than a 1-mm thickness of bone that separates the ICA and sphenoid sinus; 4% of specimens are covered only by periosteum (i.e., the outer layer of dura mater) (3,4).

Superior

The tentorial edge courses above the cavernous ICA. Anteriorly the dural reflection from the cavernous sinus and tentorium splits into *proximal* and *distal dural rings* that surround the anterior clinoid process and partially enclose the ICA as it exits from the cavernous sinus (Fig. 4-2A). These dural rings demarcate the transition between the extradural C4 (cavernous) and the C5 (clinoid) ICA segments (see Fig. 4-13) (1).

The *sella turcica* and the *pituitary gland* lie superomedially to the C4 segment, separated from it by a bony lamina and the thin medial dural wall of the cavernous sinus (Fig. 4-2B).

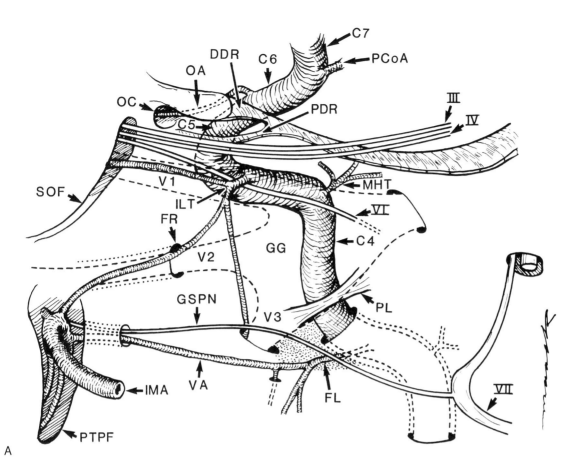

A

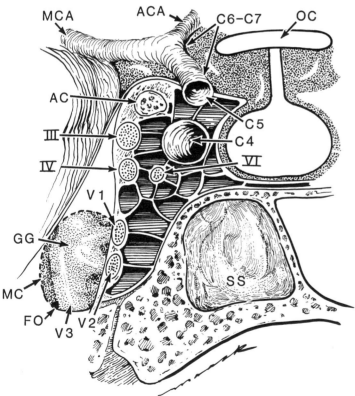

B

FIG. 4-2. A: Lateral anatomic diagram depicts the distal internal carotid artery (ICA) and its relationship to adjacent structures. The lateral dural wall of the cavernous sinus has been removed. The C4 (cavernous) ICA segment begins as the ICA passes under the petrolingual ligament (PL) and enters the cavernous sinus. The C5 (clinoid) segment lies between the proximal dural ring (PDR) and the distal dural ring (DDR). The C6 (ophthalmic) and C7 (communicating) segments are also shown. The gasserian ganglion (GG), indicated by the dotted lines, normally covers much of the posterior intracavernous ICA. Cranial nerves are indicated by the Roman numerals. GSPN, greater superficial petrosal nerve; FL, foramen lacerum; FO, foramen ovale; FR, foramen rotundum; PTPF, pterygopalatine fossa; SOF, superior orbital fissure; PC, pterygoid (vidian) canal; OC, optic canal; IMA, internal maxillary artery; VA, vidian artery; MHT, meningohypophyseal trunk; PCoA, posterior communicating artery. **B:** Anteroposterior anatomic drawing shows the internal carotid artery (ICA) and cavernous sinus (CS) in coronal section. The C4 ICA segment is surrounded by the endothelial-lined venous sinusoids that comprise the cavernous sinus. C4–C7 indicates the different carotid segments that are shown in these diagrams. The abducens nerve (VI) is the only cranial nerve that lies within the cavernous sinus proper; the other cranial nerves (III, IV, V_1, V_2) are contained within the lateral dural wall. The mandibular division of the trigeminal nerve (V_3) does not enter the cavernous sinus but exits Meckel's cave (MC) through the foramen ovale (FO). GG, gasserian (trigeminal) ganglion; AC, anterior clinoid process; SS, sphenoid sinus (**B** modified with permission from Osborn AG. *Diagnostic neuroradiology.* St. Louis: Mosby, 1994).

Inferior

The bony floor of the carotid sulcus, part of the *basisphenoid*, lies under the ICA. The *first and second divisions of the trigeminal nerve*, the ophthalmic (CN V$_1$) and maxillary (CN V$_2$) nerves, run within the lateral cavernous sinus wall and are inferolateral to the ICA (Fig. 4-2B).

Anterior

The *optic strut* and *anterior clinoid process* lie in front of, and slightly superolateral to, the anterior genu (see Figs. 3-19 and 4-2A).

Summary

Thus, the C4 ICA:

1. Courses *within* the cavernous sinus, surrounded by venous channels.
2. Is *medial* to the abducens nerve (CN VI).
3. Is covered *laterally* by the trigeminal ganglion (CN V).

Branches

Several small but very important branches arise from the C4 ICA segment (Fig. 4-2A). These branches are named according to their topographic origins from the

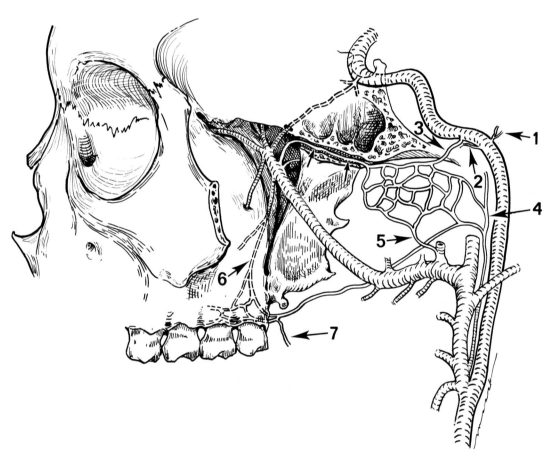

FIG. 4-3. Anatomic diagram depicts anastomoses between branches of the petrous and cavernous ICA segments and the external carotid artery. The usual origin of each vessel is also indicated below (in parentheses). Note that the vidian artery may terminate in the oropharynx or continue anteriorly as the artery of the pterygoid canal (*small arrows*).

    1, Caroticotympanic artery (petrous ICA)
    2, Periosteal branches (petrous ICA)
    3, Vidian artery (petrous or lacerum ICA segment)
    4, Ascending pharyngeal artery (ECA)
    5, Accessory meningeal artery (internal maxillary artery)
    6, Descending palatine artery (internal maxillary artery)
    7, Ascending palatine artery (facial artery)

artery; their divisions are named according to the territories that they supply (5).

Posterior Trunk

The posterior trunk, also sometimes called the *meningohypophyseal artery*, is found in almost all anatomic specimens. It arises from the superior aspect of the first bend (i.e., the posterior genu) of the C4 segment (Fig. 4-2A). It supplies branches to the pituitary gland *(inferior hypophyseal artery)*, tentorium *(marginal tentorial artery)*, and clivus *(clival branches)* (5,6).

Lateral Trunk

The lateral trunk, also sometimes called the *inferolateral trunk* (ILT) or the artery of the inferior cavernous sinus, is found in 66% to 84% of anatomic dissections (5–9). The ILT originates from the lateral aspect of the horizontal segment and usually crosses the abducens (CN VI) nerve within the cavernous sinus (Fig. 4-2A) (2).

The ILT gives rise to two or three small but important branches. These branches provide blood supply to the third, fourth, and sixth cranial nerves as well as the gasserian ganglion and cavernous sinus dura (6,7).

The ILT has important anteroinferiorly directed anastomoses with the maxillary artery through the *artery of the foramen rotundum* (Figs. 4-2A and 4-3). A posterior branch supplies part of cavernous sinus wall and the tentorium *(tentorial branch)* as well as the gasserian ganglion. It anastomoses with branches of the middle meningeal artery (through the foramen spinosum) and the maxillary artery (through the *artery of the foramen ovale*) (Fig. 4-2) (9,10).

Medial Branches

These small, inconstant branches, the so-called *capsular arteries of McConnell*, are found in only 28% of anatomic specimens (8). They supply the pituitary gland.

Normal Angiographic Anatomy

Cavernous (C4) ICA

On lateral views the C4 ICA has a horizontal segment and two distinct bends: a posterior genu (formed by the junction between the comparatively short vertical and the longer horizontal aspects of the cavernous ICA) and an anterior genu (Fig. 4-4A).

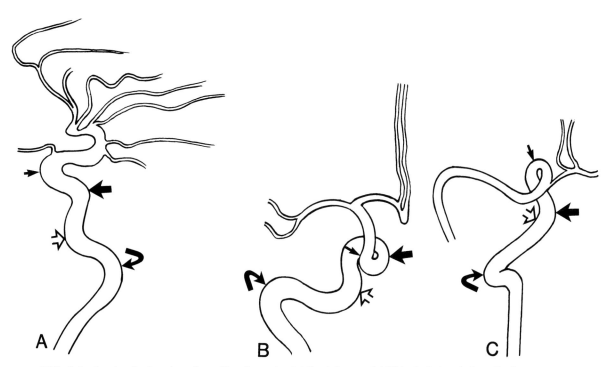

FIG. 4-4. Anatomic drawings in outline form depict the intracranial ICA. **A:** Lateral view. **B:** Anteroposterior (AP) view. **C:** Submentovertex (SMV) projection. The posterior genu of the cavernous ICA (C4 segment) is indicated by the large black arrows; the small black arrows point to the anterior genu. Note that on AP and SMV views the posterior part of the cavernous ICA is actually medial to the anterior genu. The genu between the vertical and horizontal petrous ICA (C2) segments is indicated by the curved arrows. The open arrows indicate the point at which the C3 (lacerum) ICA segment turns superiorly and ends near the petrolingual ligament (compare with Fig. 4-2A).

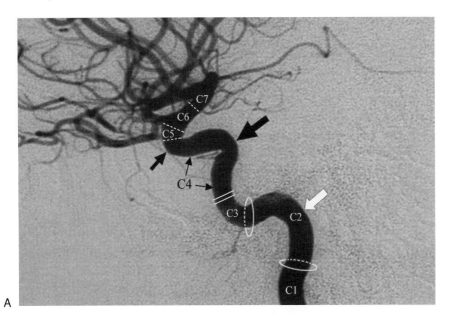

A

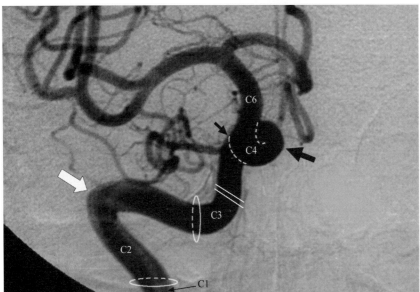

B

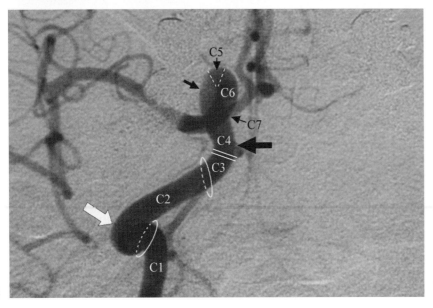

C

FIG. 4-5. Normal selective internal carotid angiograms in different patients demonstrate the ICA segments. Lateral (A), anteroposterior (B), and submentovertex (C) views are shown. The circles indicate the exo- and endocranial openings of the petrous carotid canal; the white lines denote approximate position of the petrolingual ligament. The white arrow indicates the genu of the petrous ICA. The large black arrow indicates the posterior genu of the cavernous ICA; the small black arrow points to its anterior genu.

As the horizontal ICA courses anteriorly, it also courses slightly laterally. Thus, on anteroposterior (AP) and submentovertex views of internal carotid angiograms, the bend formed by the posterior genu is usually compared with the more laterally located anterior genu (Figs. 4-4B and C and 4-5). Submentovertex views nicely demonstrate the C4 segment (Fig. 4-5C).

Branches

The posterior and inferolateral trunks are normally small. The posterior trunk (meningohypophyseal artery) is often seen as a small vessel that arises from the superior aspect of the posterior genu (Fig. 4-6A). A prominent vascular blush of the posterior pituitary gland is frequently present on the late arterial phase of selective internal carotid angiograms (Fig. 4-7) and should not be mistaken for a neoplasm (compare Fig. 4-6B).

The ILT is inconstantly visualized, even on high-resolution digital subtraction angiograms.

Normal Variants

Exaggerated Tortuosity

The cavernous ICA may become quite tortuous, with exaggerated loops at its posterior and anterior bends and a sharply sloping horizontal segment (Fig. 4-8).

Paramedian ("Kissing") Internal Carotid Arteries

In this normal anatomic variant the cavernous ICAs run medially within the sella turcica instead of coursing

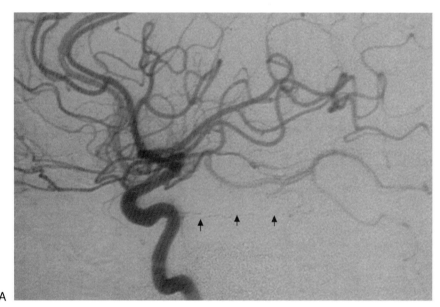

A

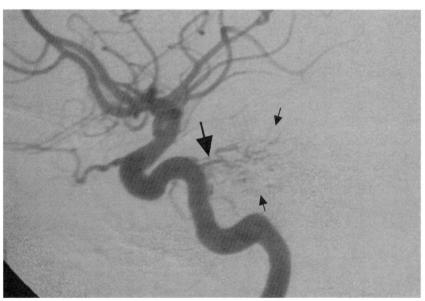

B

FIG. 4-6. A: Lateral internal carotid angiogram shows a prominent but normal meningohypophyseal trunk (*small black arrows*). **B:** Another case shows an enlarged meningohypophyseal trunk (*large black arrow*) that supplies a clivus meningioma (*small black arrows*).

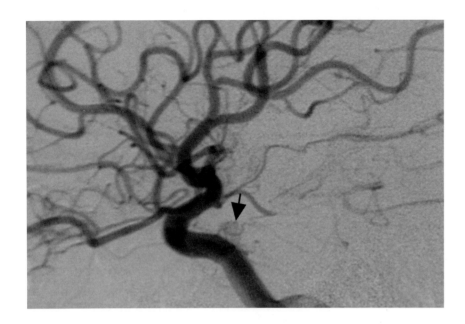

FIG. 4-7. Lateral view of a selective internal carotid angiogram shows a prominent but normal posterior pituitary vascular blush (*arrow*).

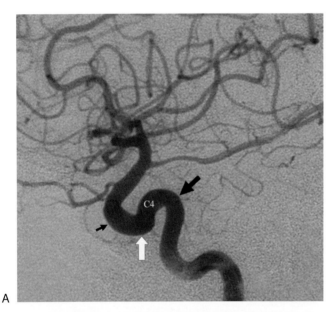

A

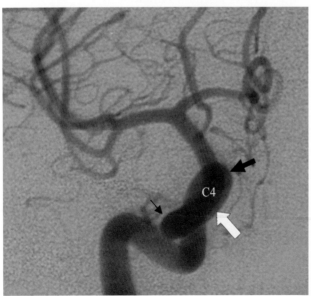

B

FIG. 4-8. Lateral **(A)** and anteroposterior **(B)** selective internal carotid angiograms show a tortuous but normal intracavernous ICA (C4 segment). Note that in this case most of the "horizontal" portion of the C4 segment (*white arrow*) is actually nearly vertical. Here the posterior genu (*large arrow*) is so ectatic it lies above the level of the anterior genu (*small arrow*).

laterally along the carotid sulcus. These so-called kissing internal carotid arteries pose a potential hazard during transsphenoidal hypophysectomy.

Anomalies

Persistent Trigeminal Artery

The trigeminal arteries are the most cephalad of the transient embryonic anastomoses that connect the fetal carotid arteries to the paired dorsal longitudinal neural arteries, precursors of the vertebrobasilar system (see Fig. 1-2B) (11,12). A persistent trigeminal artery (PTA) is the most common of these four primitive carotid–basilar anastomoses and is found in approximately 0.02% to 0.6% of cerebral angiograms (see Fig. 3-14).

A PTA arises from the cavernous ICA near the posterior genu and may follow either a para- or an intrasellar course. A parasellar PTA curves laterally and posteriorly around the dorsum sellae, following the trigeminal nerve. An intrasellar PTA passes directly posteriorly, piercing the dorsum sellae and anastomosing with the basilar artery in the midline (Fig. 4-9) (13).

Several anatomic variants of PTA have been described. In the so-called Saltzman type I variant, the PTA supplies the entire vertebrobasilar system distal to the anastomosis. The basilar artery proximal to the anastomosis is usually hypoplastic and the posterior communicating arteries (PCoAs) are often absent (Fig. 4-10). In the Saltzman type II variant, the PTA fills the superior cerebellar arteries but the posterior cerebral arteries are supplied via patent PCoAs. The relative prevalence of the two types is approximately equal (14). Numerous variations on these common patterns also have been described (15).

Conventional MR scans, MR angiography, and CT angiography with multiplanar reconstructions from thin section axial data sets can all provide excellent visualization of these anomalous vessels (Fig. 4-11).

PTAs are associated with an increased prevalence of other vascular abnormalities such as aneurysm (see Chapter 12). The incidence of vascular anomalies associated with PTA approaches 25%; aneurysms are found in nearly 14% of all cases (Fig. 4-12) (16).

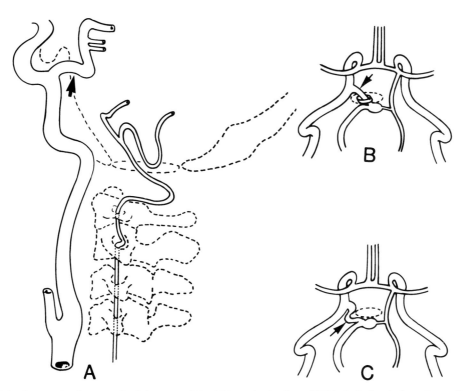

FIG. 4-9. Anatomic diagram depicts a persistent trigeminal artery (PTA). **A:** Lateral view shows the typical "trident" configuration formed by the PTA (*arrow*) as it arises from the cavernous internal carotid artery. **B** and **C:** Axial (submentovertex) drawings depict the two possible courses of a PTA. The PTA may parallel the course of the trigeminal nerve (CN V) and pass posterolaterally around the dorsum sellae (**C**, *arrow*). In another variant, the PTA passes posteriorly and medially (**B**, *arrow*), piercing the dorsum sellae and anastomosing with the basilar artery.

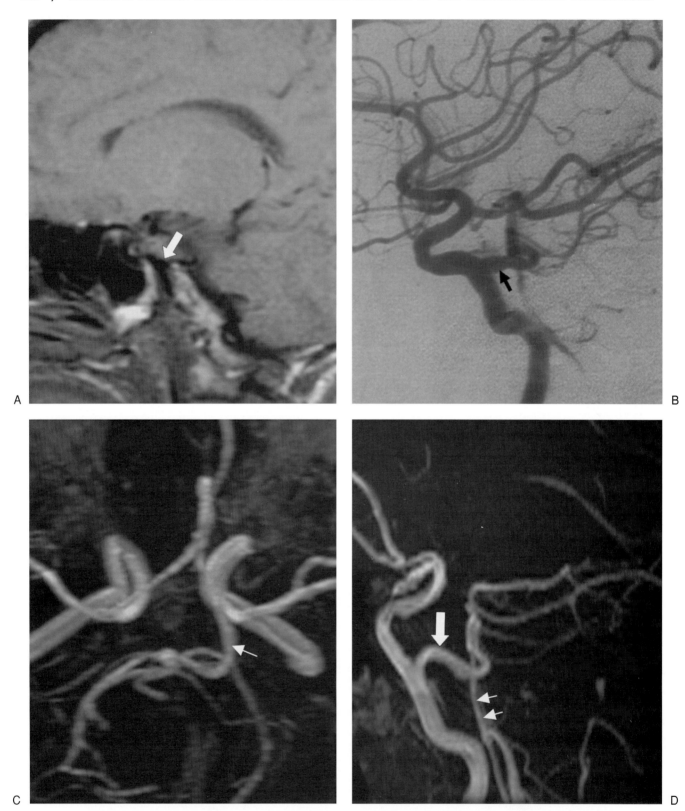

FIG. 4-10. A: 47-year old woman with severe headaches underwent standard imaging via magnetic resonance (MR) angiography. A: Sagittal T1-weighted scan shows the trident shape of a typical persistent trigeminal artery arising from the cavernous ICA (*white arrow*). **B:** Lateral view of a conventional angiogram depicts the PTA (*black arrow*). Submentovertex **(C)** and lateral **(D)** MR angiograms in another patient show a PTA (*large white arrow*) that courses laterally and posteriorly around the dorsum sellae to supply the basilar artery (BA). The BA proximal to the persistent embryonic anastomosis is hypoplastic (*small white arrows*) and the posterior communicating arteries are absent. This is a Saltzman type I PTA.

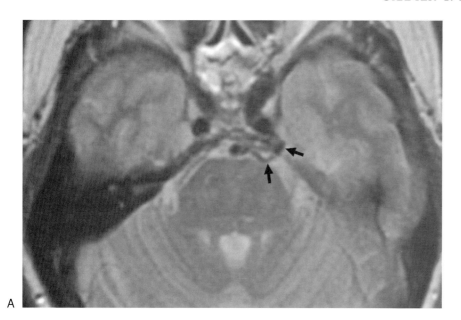

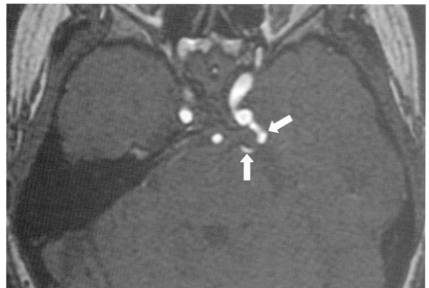

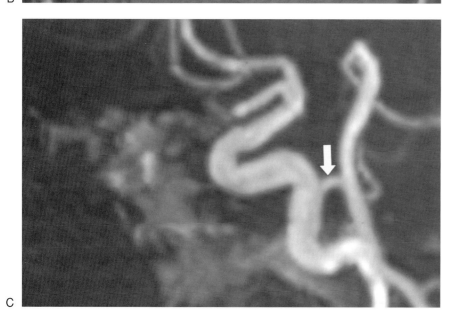

FIG. 4-11. A persistent trigeminal artery (PTA) was discovered incidentally in this 69-year-old woman. **A:** Axial T2-weighted MR scan shows an unusual vessel (*arrows*) that passes posterolaterally around the dorsum sellae to the basilar artery. Source images **(B)** and a sagittal reformatted view **(C)** of her MR angiogram show a PTA (*arrows*). The posterior communicating artery is absent, making this a Saltzman type I PTA.

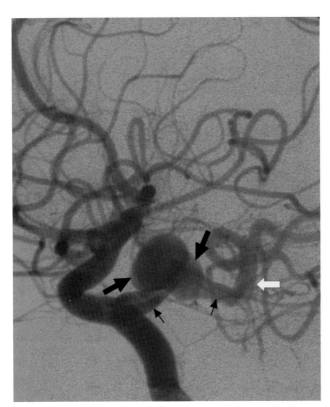

FIG. 4-12. Lateral view of a selective internal carotid angiogram shows a large persistent trigeminal artery (*small arrows*) that supplies the distal basilar artery (*white arrow*). A bilobed aneurysm (*large arrows*) is associated with the anomalous vessel. A small posterior communicating artery (*arrowheads*) is present.

Clinoid Internal Carotid Artery: Normal Anatomy and Variations

Normal development
  Cranial extension of embryonic dorsal aorta
Gross anatomy
  Also known as C5 ICA
  Small wedge-shaped segment (forms part of anterior genu)
  Interdural structure (between proximal and distal dural rings)
Key relationships
  Anterior clinoid is superior, lateral
  Venous tributaries of cavernous sinus course in dural rings
Branches
  Usually none (may have some capsular branches)
  Occasionally ophthalmic artery has interdural origin
Normal variants
  None
Anomalies
  Hypoplasia or absence is rare
  May have intercavernous anastomotic vessel connecting the ICAs

---

Intercavernous Anastomoses

ICA aplasia is an uncommon anomaly (see Chapter 3). If an ICA fails to develop, collateral flow is usually provided through the circle of Willis. Less commonly, the affected hemisphere is supplied by an intracavernous anastomosis that connects the ICAs (17).

C5 (CLINOID) ICA SEGMENT

Gross Anatomy

The clinoid (C5) segment is the shortest of all the ICA segments. It comprises only a small, wedge-shaped area along the superior aspect of the anterior genu (18) (see box next column). The C5 segment begins at the proximal dural ring, just above the curve of the anterior ICA genu. It ends at the distal dural ring where the ICA enters the subarachnoid space (Fig. 4-13) (19). The C5 segment is thus an interdural structure, located in a collar of dura through which course venous tributaries of the cavernous sinus (20). The dural collar is most prominent along its lateral and anterior border. It is less distinct medially and disappears posteriorly (20).

Relationships

Lateral

The *anterior clinoid process* lies above and lateral to the C5 ICA segment.

Medial

The carotid sulcus of the *basisphenoid bone* is medial.

Superior

Posterosuperiorly, the C5 segment is covered by *dura* that reflects over the posterior clinoid process and is continuous with the cavernous sinus roof and diaphragma sellae. If the anterior and middle clinoid processes fuse, the C5 ICA segment may be entirely surrounded by bone (1).

Branches

This part of the ICA usually has no discernible branches, although a few tiny capsular arteries may arise from the C5 segment. In rare instances the ophthalmic artery (OA) can originate from this segment.

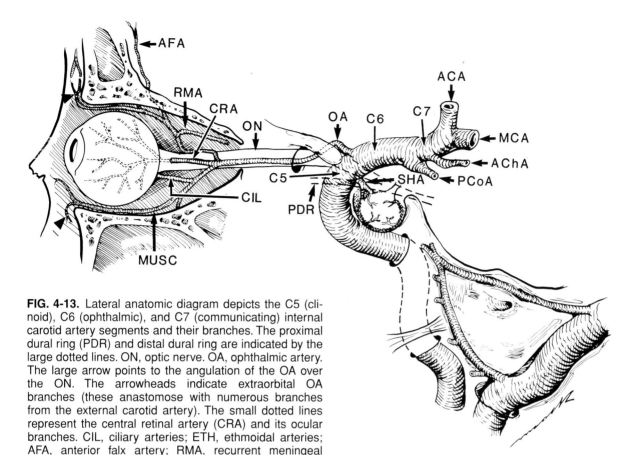

FIG. 4-13. Lateral anatomic diagram depicts the C5 (clinoid), C6 (ophthalmic), and C7 (communicating) internal carotid artery segments and their branches. The proximal dural ring (PDR) and distal dural ring are indicated by the large dotted lines. ON, optic nerve. OA, ophthalmic artery. The large arrow points to the angulation of the OA over the ON. The arrowheads indicate extraorbital OA branches (these anastomose with numerous branches from the external carotid artery). The small dotted lines represent the central retinal artery (CRA) and its ocular branches. CIL, ciliary arteries; ETH, ethmoidal arteries; AFA, anterior falx artery; RMA, recurrent meningeal artery; MUSC, muscular branches; SHA, superior hypophyseal arteries; PCoA, posterior communicating artery (small arrow points to an infundibulum, junctional widening at the PCoA origin from the ICA); ACA, anterior cerebral artery; MCA, middle cerebral artery.

Normal Angiographic Anatomy

The C5 segment forms the superior aspect of the anterior cavernous carotid genu (Fig. 4-14A).

C6 (OPHTHALMIC) ICA SEGMENT

Gross Anatomy

The ophthalmic ICA segment begins at the distal dural ring and terminates just proximal to the posterior communicating artery origin (Fig. 4-13). This segment arches posteriorly and slightly superiorly, completing the anterior ICA genu (see box next column). The C6 segment represents the most proximal intradural portion of the supraclinoid ICA. A loosely adherent dural evagination called the carotid cave is often seen adjacent to the ophthalmic ICA segment (1,19,21).

Relationships

Lateral

The *distal dural ring* lies lateral to the C6 segment.

Medial

Cerebrospinal fluid within the *suprasellar subarachnoid space* surrounds the intradural ICA.

Ophthalmic Internal Carotid Artery: Normal Anatomy and Variations

Normal development
 Cranial extension of embryonic dorsal aorta
 Ophthalmic artery branches may arise from, or anastomose with, ECA orbital branches derived from the embryonic hyoidostapedial trunk
Gross anatomy
 Also known as C6 ICA
 Forms superior aspect of anterior genu
 Most proximal intradural part of supraclinoid ICA
Key relationships
 Optic nerve courses above, medial to ICA
 Surrounded by CSF
Branches
 Ophthalmic artery (origin is intradural in >90% of cases)
 Superior hypophyseal arteries
Normal variants/anomalies
 Middle meningeal artery originates from ophthalmic artery
 Ophthalmic artery originates from middle meningeal artery

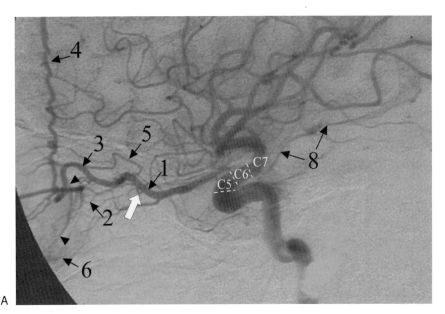

A

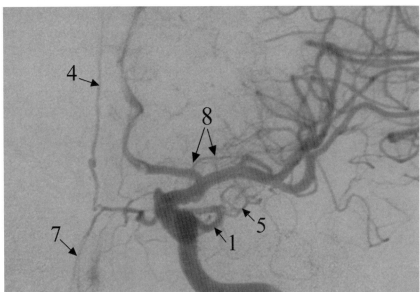

B

FIG. 4-14. Lateral **(A)** and slightly oblique anteroposterior **(B)**. late arterial phase views of a selective internal carotid angiogram are shown. The C5 (clinoid), C6 (ophthalmic), and C7 (communicating) ICA segments and their branches are indicated.

1, Ophthalmic artery (OA) (arrow indicates the abrupt angulation where the OA passes up and over the optic nerve)
2, Ocular OA branches (arrowheads indicate the vascular choroid blush)
3, Orbital OA branches
4, Anterior falx artery (an extraorbital OA branch)
5, Lacrimal artery
6, Muscular branches
7, Anterior ethmoid arteries
8, Anterior choroidal artery

Superior

The *optic nerve* (CN II) courses superomedial to the ophthalmic ICA segment.

Inferior

The *sphenoid sinus* is anteroinferior to the C6 segment. In nearly 80% of cases, the bone that separates the optic nerve and sheath from the sphenoid sinus is less than 0.5 mm thick (4).

Anterior

The ophthalmic artery (OA) originates from the anterosuperior aspect of the C6 segment and, accompa-

nied by the optic nerve, courses inferolaterally through the optic canal into the orbit (Figs. 4-1 and 4-13).

Branches

Two important branches arise from the C6 ICA segment. They are the ophthalmic artery and the superior hypophyseal arteries.

Ophthalmic Artery

The ophthalmic artery arises medial to the anterior clinoid process as the ICA exits the cavernous sinus. Therefore, the OA is typically the first major intracranial ICA branch (Fig. 4-13). The OA originates from the antero- or superomedial surface of the ICA near the junction between the C5 and C6 segments. The OA origin is intradural in approximately 90% of anatomic dissections (22).

From its origin the OA enters the orbit and courses anteriorly through the optic canal. Initially the OA lies inferolateral to the optic nerve and medial to the oculomotor (CN III) and abducens (CN VI) nerves. It then crosses between the optic nerve and superior rectus muscle, running to the medial orbital wall between the superior oblique and medial rectus muscles (23,24).

The OA has three types of branches: (a) ocular, (b) orbital, and (c) extraorbital branches. The ocular branches include the *central retinal artery* and the *ciliary arteries*. Ocular branches supply the retina and choroid of the eye. They also may supply some collateral branches to the optic nerve.

The major orbital branches of the OA are the *lacrimal artery* and a group of unnamed *muscular branches* that supply the extraocular muscles and orbital periosteum. The lacrimal artery is a prominent branch that leaves the OA near its exit from the optic canal. It courses along the upper border of the lateral rectus muscle and supplies the lacrimal gland and conjunctiva. An important branch of the lacrimal artery, the *recurrent meningeal artery*, passes backward through the superior orbital fissure and anastomoses with branches of the middle meningeal artery (23).

A number of extraorbital branches arise from the OA. These include the *supraorbital, anterior and posterior ethmoidal, dorsal nasal, palpebral, medial frontal, and supratrochlear arteries* (22,24). Extraorbital OA branches have extensive anastomoses with ethmoidal and facial branches of the external carotid artery. These anastomoses may become an important source of collateral blood flow to the intracranial ICA in the event of more proximal occlusion (see Chapter 17).

A prominent OA branch, the *anterior falx artery*, arises from the anterior ethmoidal arteries and supplies part of the falx cerebri.

Superior Hypophyseal Arteries

One or more superior hypophyseal arteries (SHAs) arise from the posteromedial aspect of the C6 ICA. In nearly half of all cases, a single large dominant SHA branches like a candelabra to supply the anterior pituitary lobe, pituitary stalk, optic nerve, and chiasm (Fig. 4-13). In the absence of a large dominant branch, two or three separate smaller vessels supply these areas (6,25,26).

Normal Angiographic Anatomy

Intradural ICA

The C6 ICA segment is best visualized on lateral cerebral angiograms. From its junction with the C5 (clinoid) segment the distal ICA curves upward and backward to complete the so-called angiographic *carotid siphon*, an S-shaped curve that is formed by the cavernous and supraclinoid ICA segments (Figs. 4-14 and 4-15). On AP views the distal intracavernous and proximal intradural ICA segments often overlap one another (Fig. 4-14B).

The absence of a reliable angiographic landmark for entry of the ICA into the subarachnoid space makes it difficult to distinguish between the end of the C5 (interdural) and the beginning of the C6 (intradural) segments (27). Practically speaking, lesions such as aneurysms that are at or above the OA level are usually at least partially intradural. Kobayashi and co-workers have referred to aneurysms at this location as *carotid cave* aneurysms. These lesions may rupture into the subarachnoid space (21).

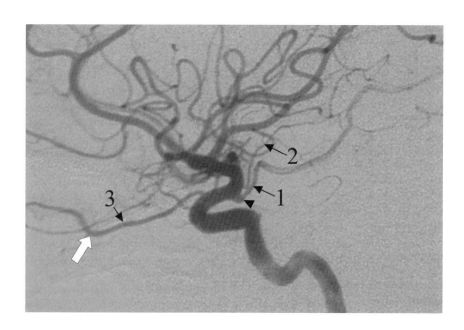

FIG. 4-15. Lateral view of a selective internal carotid angiogram shows the C6 (ophthalmic) and C7 (communicating) ICA segments and their major branches.

1, Posterior communicating artery (from C7 segment). Note the funnel-shaped infundibulum at its origin, indicated by the arrowhead (compare with Fig. 4-13A)

2, Anterior choroidal artery

3, Ophthalmic artery (from C6 segment). White arrow indicates normal angulation over the optic nerve

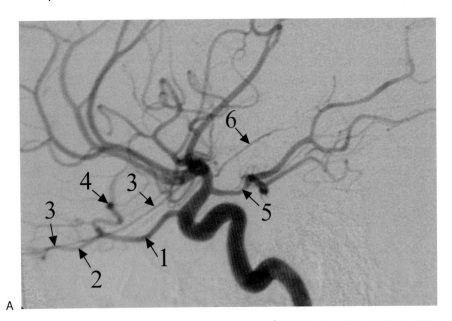

A

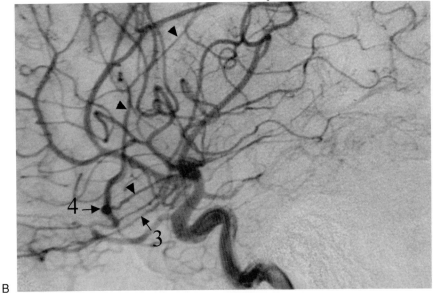

B

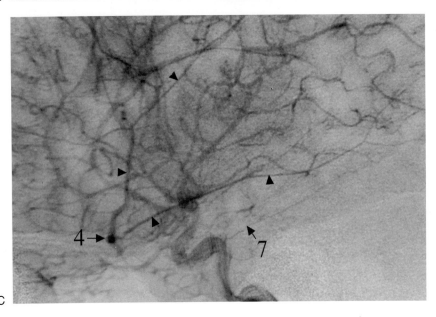

C

FIG. 4-16. Early **(A)**, middle **(B)**, and late **(C)** arterial phase films of an internal carotid angiogram, lateral view, show aberrant origin of the middle meningeal artery from the ophthalmic artery. Other meningeal and supraclinoid ICA branches are also demonstrated.

1, Ophthalmic artery
2, Lacrimal artery
3, Recurrent meningeal artery (courses backward through the superior orbital fissure)
4, Middle meningeal artery (arrowheads, **C**, indicate distal branches)
5, Posterior communicating artery
6, Anterior choroidal artery
7, Tentorial branch of the meningohypyseal trunk

Ophthalmic Artery

The OA is seen in nearly all cases and is best delineated on lateral views (Figs. 4-15 and 4-16). From its origin, the OA courses superiorly for 1 or 2 mm, then turns and runs directly anteriorly. Near the mid-point between its origin and the globe, the OA often angles abruptly where it passes over the optic nerve (Fig. 4-15).

Although the *central retinal artery* is rarely visualized even on high-resolution studies, the vascular plexus of the *ocular choroid* can almost always be identified as a distinct crescent-shaped vascular blush on mid-arterial phase views of internal carotid angiograms (Fig. 4-14A).

The *anterior falx artery* arises from the anterior ethmoidal arteries and follows a relatively straight course, curving superiorly along the falx cerebri (Fig. 4-14). *Nasal* and *anterior ethmoidal branches* from the OA also may cause a distinct vascular blush on the late arterial phase of internal carotid angiograms (Fig. 4-14B).

Although the *superior hypophyseal arteries* are rarely visualized, even on high-resolution digital subtraction studies, they may be a site for aneurysm formation (18).

Normal Variants

The definitive OA develops from primitive arteries that may be annexed by either the internal or external carotid systems (see Chapter 2). The orbital and extraorbital branches of these two vessels exist in hemodynamic balance. Thus, either vessel may provide the dominant blood supply to the orbit (28,29). In cases where the ophthalmic artery is embryologically dominant and annexes part of the fetal hyoidostapedial artery, the OA supplies part of the usual ECA territory. An example of this arrangement is *ophthalmic origin of the middle meningeal artery*, seen in 0.5% of cases. Here the middle meningeal artery arises from the recurrent meningeal branch of the OA (Fig. 4-16).

Anomalies

A number of anomalous OA origins have been described. *Ophthalmic artery origin from the middle meningeal artery* is the most common anomaly reported in the literature. Here the OA passes into the orbit through the superior orbital fissure or a foramen in the greater sphenoid wing instead of through the optic canal (22). *Cavernous origin of the ophthalmic artery* is a less common anomaly, found in 8% of anatomic dissections (22).

C7 (COMMUNICATING) SEGMENT

Gross Anatomy

The C7 (communicating) segment begins just proximal to the origin of the posterior communicating artery (PCoA) and ends as the ICA bifurcates into its two terminal branches, the anterior and middle cerebral arteries (Figs. 4-1 and 4-13A) (see box next column).

Communicating Internal Carotid Artery: Normal Anatomy and Variations

Normal development
Cranial extension of embryonic dorsal aorta
Gross anatomy
Also known as C7 internal carotid artery
Key relationships
Passes between optic, oculomotor nerves
Terminates below anterior perforated substance
Bifurcates into anterior, middle cerebral arteries
Branches
Posterior communicating artery (PCoA)
Anterior choroidal artery (AChA)
Normal variants
"Fetal" origin of posterior cerebral artery from ICA
Junctional dilatation (infundibulum) at origin of PCoA from ICA
Anomalies
AChA origin proximal to PCoA

Relationships

Medial

The ICA passes between the optic (CN II) and oculomotor (CN III) nerves. The optic nerve is superomedial to the ICA.

Superior

The ICA terminates below the anterior perforated substance at the medial end of the Sylvian fissure (lateral cerebral sulcus) (23).

Branches

Two major branches, the posterior communicating artery and the anterior choroidal artery, arise from the C7 segment (Fig. 4-13).

Posterior Communicating Artery

For a detailed description of the PCoA, see the discussion on the circle of Willis (Chapter 5). The PCoA arises from the posterior aspect of the intradural ICA and anastomoses with the posterior cerebral artery (PCA), a branch of the basilar artery. The PCoA therefore connects the anterior (carotid) and posterior (vertebrobasilar) circulations.

From its origin the PCoA courses posteriorly, running above the oculomotor (CN III) nerve. The PCoA gives rise to several small branches, the *anterior thalamoperforating arteries*, that pass through the posterior perforated substance to supply the medial thalamus and walls of the third ventricle (23).

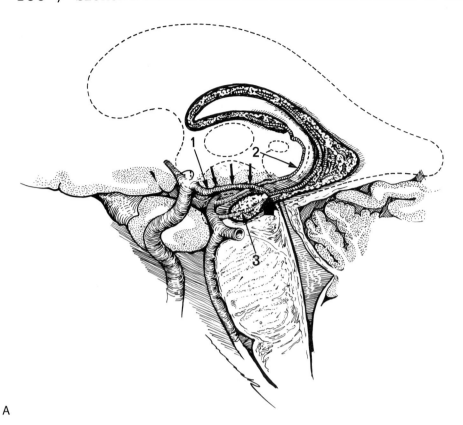

A

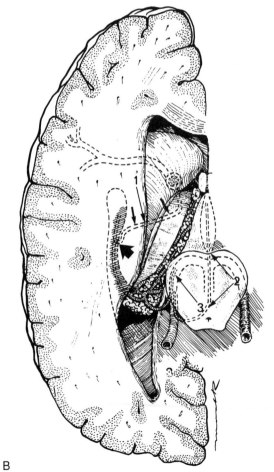

B

FIG. 4-17. Lateral **(A)** and superior **(B)** anatomic diagrams depict the anterior choroidal artery (AChA) and its relationship with the posterior choroidal arteries (branches of the PCA). Small arrows indicate the cisternal AChA segment. The large black arrow indicates the plexal point where the AChA enters the choroidal fissure of the temporal horn. (Modified from Osborn A, *Diagnostic Neuroradiology* CV Mosby, 1994)

1, Anterior choroidal artery
2, Medial posterior choroidal artery
3, Lateral posterior choroidal artery

Anterior Choroidal Artery

The anterior choroidal artery (AChA) is a small but relatively constant vessel that arises from the posteromedial aspect of the supraclinoid ICA a short distance above the PCoA origin (Fig. 4-17A). The AChA may exist either as a single trunk or a plexus of small vessels.

The AChA has two main segments. These are (a) a proximal (cisternal) segment and (b) a distal (intraventricular) segment (Fig. 4-17). From its origin, the cisternal AChA first courses posteromedially below the optic tract and superomedial to the temporal lobe uncus. Turning laterally, the AChA continues its course through the crural cistern and curves around the cerebral peduncle toward the lateral geniculate body. Near the lateral geniculate body, the AChA angles sharply as it enters the temporal horn through the choroidal fissure (30–33).

The distal AChA segment begins at the choroidal fissure and continues posteriorly within the supracornual cleft of the temporal horn. The ACHA follows the choroid plexus, typically curving around the pulvinar of the thalamus and then running anteriorly for a variable distance. In some cases it extends to the foramen of Monro, where it anastomoses with branches of the medial posterior choroidal artery.

The AChA supplies many important structures in an arc-shaped zone that lies between the corpus striatum anterolaterally and the thalamus posteromedially (33). The AChA territory is quite variable but may include part or any of the following structures: the optic tract, posterior limb of the internal capsule, cerebral peduncle, choroid plexus, and medial temporal lobe.

Anterior and Middle Cerebral Arteries

The anterior (ACA) and middle (MCA) cerebral arteries are the two terminal ICA branches (Fig. 4-13). These vessels are discussed in Chapters 6 and 7.

Normal Angiographic Anatomy

C7 (Communicating) ICA Segment

As it courses upward and backward from the anterior clinoid process, the supraclinoid ICA also courses slightly laterally (Fig. 4-15).

Posterior Communicating Artery

The PCoA arises from the dorsal aspect of the distal ICA and courses posteriorly toward the PCA.

Anterior Choroidal Artery

The AChA can be identified on approximately 95% of all internal carotid angiograms and may be observed on both standard lateral and AP views.

On lateral views the cisternal AChA segment ends in a definite lateral angulation or kink where the AChA enters the choroidal fissure (Fig. 4-18A). This angulation is termed the angiographic plexal point. From its entry into the temporal horn, the AChA follows a gently undulating course as it accompanies the choroid plexus within the lateral ventricle. The intraventricular AChA first curves laterally, then gradually turns superomedially to reach the atrium and lateral geniculate body. The AChA then follows a broad, anteriorly concave course as it extends around the pulvinar of the thalamus (Fig. 4-18B).

The choroid plexus of the lateral ventricle may appear as a dense homogeneous stain or blush that persists well into the capillary or early venous phase of carotid angiograms (Fig. 4-18C and D).

In the AP projection the AChA is seen arising from the medial aspect of the supraclinoid ICA. The proximal AChA segment first curves medially and then posteriorly within the suprasellar cistern. It courses around the uncus, then turns laterally to enter the temporal horn (Fig. 4-14B; also see Fig. 5-13).

Normal Variants

Posterior Communicating Artery

The PCoA varies greatly in size. It may be absent or very large. If the horizontal (P1) PCA segment is hypoplastic or absent, the PCoA may supply the entire PCA territory. This is termed "fetal origin" of the PCA (see Chapter 8). The PCoA itself is often hypoplastic or absent (see Chapter 5). A funnel-shaped dilatation called an infundibulum may be present at the PCoA origin (Fig. 4-13A).

Anterior Choroidal Artery

The AChA exists in hemodynamic balance with the posterolateral and medial posterior choroidal arteries (branches of the vertebrobasilar system). Branches of the AChA anastomose freely and frequently with these vessels. Because of this reciprocal relationship, the AChA varies considerably in size and vascular territory. The usual AchA territory is shown in Fig. 4-19.

An ectopic origin of the AChA is found in 4% of anatomic dissections (32).

Anomalies

Normal variations in the PCoA and AChA are common, but true anomalies are rare. Hypoplasia of the AChA is seen in only 3% of cerebral angiograms (33). A hyperplastic anomalous AChA supplies part of the PCA territory in 2.3% of cases (32). In rare cases, the AChA

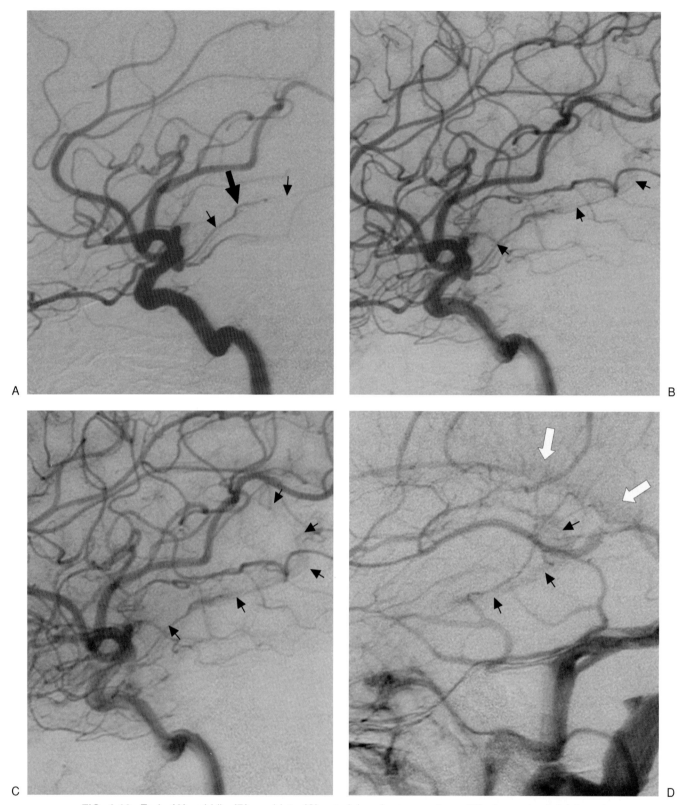

FIG. 4-18. Early **(A)**, middle **(B)**, and late **(C)** arterial and venous phase **(D)** views of a left internal carotid angiogram. **A–C:** The anterior choroidal artery (AChA) is indicated by the small black arrows. The plexal point where the AChA enters the temporal horn of the lateral ventricle is shown (**A,** *large black arrow*). **D:** There is a distinct vascular blush of the choroid plexus (*small black arrows*) during the venous phase of the study. Prominent but normal medullary (white matter) veins are indicated by the white arrows.

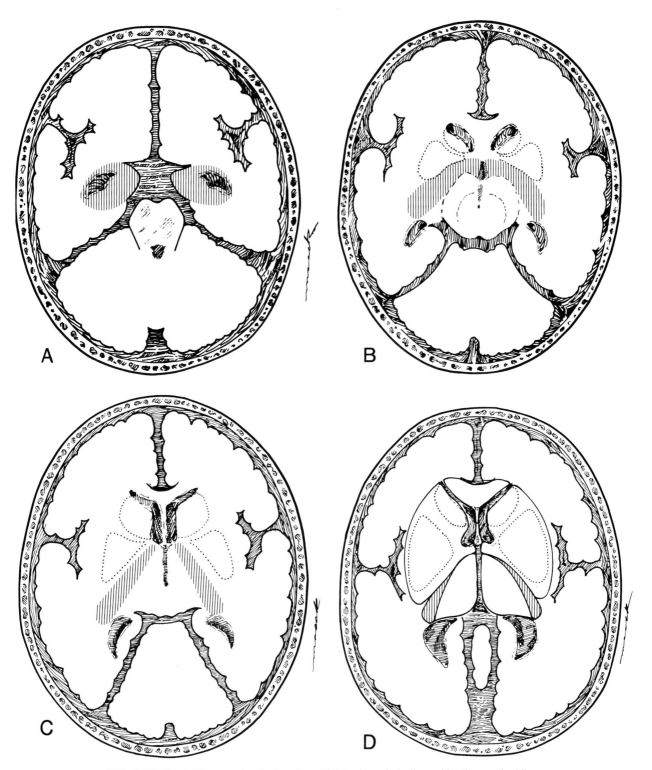

FIG. 4-19. A–D: The usual anterior choroidal territory is indicated by the vertical lines.

originates from the ICA proximal to the PCoA (instead of distal). Failure to appreciate this uncommon anomaly preoperatively may result in a clinically devastating infarct if the AChA is mistaken for the PCoA and occluded during aneurysm clipping.

REFERENCES

1. Bouthillier A, van Loveren HR, Keller JT. Segments of the internal carotid artery: a new classification. *Neurosurgery* 1996;38:425–433.
2. Sen C, Chen CS, Post KD. The internal carotid artery. In: *Microsurgical anatomy of the skull base.* New York: Thieme, 1997:15–41.
2a. Oikawa S, Kyoshima K, Kobayashi S. Surgical anatomy of the juxta-dural ring area. *J Neurosurg* 1998;89:250–254.
3. Renn WH, Rhoton AL Jr. Microsurgical anatomy of the sellar region. *J Neurosurg* 1975;43:288–298.
4. Fujii K, Chambers SM, Rhoton AL Jr. Neurovascular relationships of the sphenoid sinus. *J Neurosurg* 1979;50:31–39.
5. Tran-Dinh H. Cavernous branches of the internal carotid artery: anatomy and nomenclature. *Neurosurgery* 1987;20:205–210.
6. Krisht A, Barnett DW, Barrow DL, Bonner G. The blood supply of the intracavernous cranial nerves: an anatomic study. *Neurosurgery* 1994;34:275–279.
7. Capo H, Kupersmith MJ, Berenstein A, et al. The clinical importance of the inferolateral trunk of the intimal carotid artery. *Neurosurgery* 1991;28:733–738.
8. Harris FS, Rhoton AL. Anatomy of the cavernous sinus: a microsurgical study. *J Neurosurg* 1975;45:169–180.
9. Yamaki T, Tanabe S, Hashi K. Prominent development of the inferolateral trunk of the internal carotid artery as a collateral pathway to the external carotid system. *AJNR* 1989;10:206.
10. Willinsky R, Lasjaunias P, Berenstein A. Intracavernous branches of the internal carotid artery (ICA): comprehensive review of the variations. *Surg Radiol Anat* 1987;9:201–215.
11. Caldemeyer KS, Carrico JB, Mathews VB. The radiology and embryology of anomalous arteries of the head and neck. *AJR* 1998;270:297–304.
12. Boyko OB, Curnes JT, Blatter DD, Parker DL. MRI of basilar artery hypoplasia associated with persistent primitive trigeminal artery. *Neuroradiology* 1996;38:11–14.
13. Schuierer G, Laub G, Huk WJ. MR angiography of the primitive trigeminal artery: report on two cases. *AJNR* 1990;11:1131–1132.
14. McKenzie JD, Dean BL, Flom RA. Trigeminal-cavernous fistula: Saltzman anatomy revisited. *AJNR* 1996;17:280–282.
15. Oushiro S, Inoue T, Hamada Y, Matsuno H. Branches of the persistent primitive trigeminal artery—An autopsy case. *Neurosurgery* 1993;32:144–148.
16. Ahmad I, Tominaga T, Suzuki M, et al. Primitive trigeminal artery associated with cavernous aneurysm: case report. *Surg Neurol* 1994;41:75–79.
17. Midkiff RB, Boykin MW, McFarland DR, Bauman JA. Agenesis of the internal carotid artery with intercavernous anastomosis. *AJNR* 1995;16:1356–1399.
18. Roy D, Raymond J, Bouthillier A, et al. Endovascular treatment of ophthalmic segment aneurysms with Guglielmi detachable coils. *AJNR* 1997;18:1207–1215.
19. Knosp E, Müller G, Perneczky A. The paraclinoid carotid artery: anatomical aspects of a microneurosurgical approach. *Neurosurgery* 1988;22:896–901.
20. Seoane E, Rhoton AL Jr, de Oliveira E. Microsurgical anatomy of the dural collar (carotid collar) and rings around the clinoid segment of the internal carotid artery. *Neurosurgery* 1998;42:869–886.
21. Kobayashi S, Koike G, Orz Y, Okudera H. Juxta-dural ring aneurysms of the internal carotid artery. *J Clin Neurosci* 1995;2:345–349.
22. Hayreh SS. The ophthalmic artery. In: Newton TH, Potts DG, eds. *Radiology of the skull and brain: angiography.* St. Louis: Mosby, 1974:1333–1390.
23. Williams P, ed. Internal carotid artery. In: *Gray's anatomy,* 38th ed. New York: Churchill Livingstone, 1995:1523–1529.
24. Long J, Kageyama I. The ophthalmic artery and its branches, measurements and clinical importance. *Surg Radiol Anat* 1990;12:83–90.
25. Gibo H, Hobayashi S, Kyoshima K, Hokama M. Microsurgical anatomy of the arteries of the pituitary gland as viewed from above. *Acta Neurochir (Wien)* 1988;90:60–66.
26. Krisht AF, Barrow DL, Barnet DW, et al. The microsurgical anatomy of the superior hypophyseal artery. *Neurosurgery* 1994;35:899–903.
27. Kraemer JL, Schneider FL, Raupp SF, Ferreira NP. Anatomoradiological correlation of the intersection of the carotid siphon with the dura mater. *Neuroradiology* 1989;31:408–412.
28. Schumacher M, Wakhloo AK. An orbital arteriovenous malformation in a patient with origins of the ophthalmic artery from the basilar artery. *AJNR* 1994;15:550–553.
29. Dilenge D, Ascherl DGF Jr. Variations of the ophthalmic and middle meningeal arteries: relation to the embryonic stapedial artery. *AJNR* 1980;1:45–53.
30. Fujii K, Lenkey C, Rhoton AL Jr. Microsurgical anatomy of the choroidal arteries: lateral and third ventricles. *J Neurosurg* 1980;52:165–188.
31. Rhoton AL Jr, Fujii K, Fradd B. Microsurgical anatomy of the anterior choroidal artery. *Surg Neurol* 1979;12:171–187.
32. Morandi X, Brassier G, Darnault P, et al. Microsurgical anatomy of the anterior choroidal artery. *Surg Radiol Anat* 1996;18:275–280.
33. Takahashi S, Suga T, Kawata Y, Sakamoto K. Anterior choroidal artery: angiographic analysis of variations and anomalies. *AJNR* 1990;11:719–729.

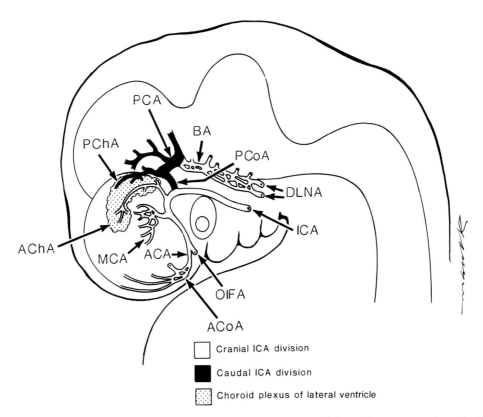

FIG. 5-1. Lateral anatomic sketch depicts the embryonic intracranial arteries at approximately 5 to 6 weeks of gestation. The primitive internal carotid arteries (ICAs) each have a cranial and a caudal division. The cranial divisions give rise to the primitive olfactory arteries (OlfA) as well as the anterior cerebral arteries (ACAs), anterior choroidal arteries (AChA), and middle cerebral arteries (MCAs). The anterior communicating artery (ACoA) forms from coalescence of a midline plexiform network. The caudal divisions will become the posterior communicating arteries (PCoAs) and also supply the stems of the posterior cerebral arteries (PCAs). The basilar artery (BA) will be formed from fusion of the paired dorsal longitudinal neural arteries (DLNAs).

Basilar Artery

The basilar artery (BA) normally terminates near the pontomesencephalic junction by dividing into its two terminal branches, the right and left posterior cerebral arteries. The PCAs are laterally directed branches of the distal BA. Their proximal segments are also called the precommunicating or *P1 segments* (see Chapter 8). These segments course laterally in front of the upper pons and lower mid-brain. At a variable distance from their origin, each PCA is joined by its ipsilateral PCoA to close the circle of Willis.

A complete circle of Willis thus consists of *two ICAs, two ACAs, the ACoA, two PCoAs, the BA,* and *two PCAs.*

Relationships

The circle of Willis lies above the sella turcica within the interpeduncular and suprasellar cisterns. The circle of Willis surrounds the ventral surface of the diencephalon and lies adjacent to the optic nerves and tracts as well as a number of other important structures (Fig. 5-2) (3,4).

Superior

The circle of Willis lies below and lateral to the hypothalamus and the anterior recesses of the third ventricle. The optic tracts course above the posterior communicating arteries (PCoAs). From its origin, each horizontal ACA (A1 segment) courses medially below the anterior perforated substance and gyrus rectus.

Inferior

The pituitary gland, diaphragma sellae, and basisphenoid bone lie below the circle of Willis. The oculomotor nerves (CN III) course obliquely anteriorly under the PCoAs.

From their origin, the two A1 segments pass medially above the optic nerves to the interhemispheric (longitudinal) fissure. The ACoA junction with the two A1 segments lies above either the optic chiasm (70% of cases) or optic nerves (30%) (5).

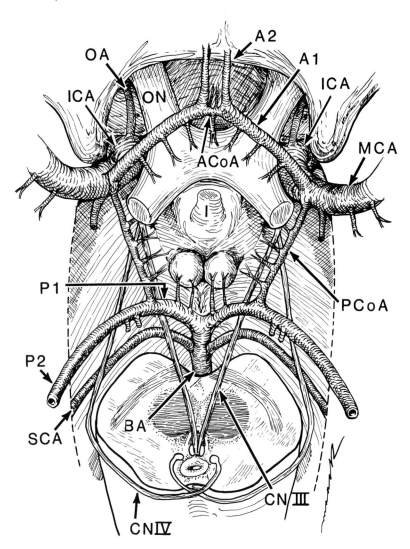

FIG. 5-2. Anatomic diagram depicts the circle of Willis and its relationship to adjacent structures as seen from above. Note that innumerable perforating branches arise from every part of the circle of Willis to supply vital structures at the base of the brain. A1, horizontal (precommunicating) anterior cerebral artery (ACA) segment; A2, vertical (postcommunicating) ACA segment; P1, horizontal (precommunicating) posterior cerebral artery (PCA); P2, ambient PCA segment; SCA, superior cerebellar artery; OA, ophthalmic artery; ON, optic nerve; I, infundibulum; CN III, oculomotor nerve; CN IV, trochlear nerve.

Posterior

The basilar bifurcation lies within the interpeduncular fossa in front of the mid-brain.

Lateral

The tentorial incisura and the temporal lobes lie lateral to the circle of Willis.

Medial

The circle of Willis surrounds the infundibular stalk and mammillary bodies.

Summary

Thus, the circle of Willis:

1. Lies *in* the suprasellar cistern, *below* the hypothalamus and third ventricle.
2. *Surrounds* the infundibular stalk.

3. Passes *above* the optic and oculomotor nerves (CN III) but *under* the optic tracts.
4. Is *medial* to the tentorium and temporal lobes.

Normal Angiographic Anatomy

Noninvasive imaging studies such as spiral computed tomographic angiography (CTA), high-resolution magnetic resonance angiography (MRA), and transcranial color Doppler flow imaging can provide an overview of the carotid siphon and major arteries at the base of the brain (Fig. 5-3) (6–8). However, detailed examination of the circle of Willis and especially its small but important perforating branches is still largely the domain of high-resolution conventional angiography (9).

Circle of Willis

The entire circle of Willis is rarely seen on a single cerebral angiogram, and its components are usually visualized sequentially. However, on occasion a patient with a

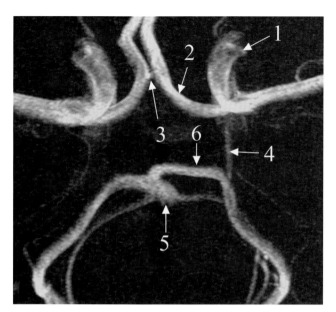

FIG. 5-3. High-resolution MR angiogram, submentovertex view, depicts the circle of Willis. The small left posterior communciating artery (PCoA) is visualized; the right PCoA is absent.

1, Interior carotid artery
2, A1 anterior cerebral artery segment
3, Anterior communicating artery
4, Posterior communicating artery
5, Basilar artery
6, P1 posterior cerebral artery segment

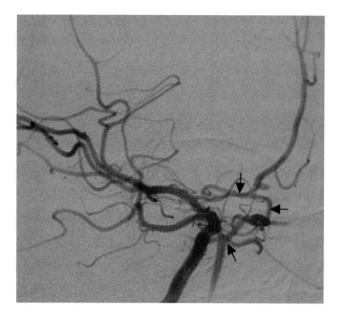

FIG. 5-4. Right internal carotid angiogram, oblique view, demonstrates transient opacification of the circle of Willis (*arrows*).

ACoA clearly without the presence of overlapping vessels (Figs. 5-6 and 5-7) (10). Temporary cross-compression of the contralateral common carotid artery during contrast injection is sometimes necessary to demonstrate the ACoA (Fig. 5-6).

favorable anatomic configuration may have transient, partial filling of the circle of Willis (Fig. 5-4). The circle of Willis is also sometimes seen when three of the four major arteries that supply the brain are occluded and the sole remaining patent vessel fills the arterial circle (see Chapter 17).

Anterior Cerebral Arteries

The contour of the A1 ACA segment varies. From its origin, an ACA normally follows a relatively straight or sinusoidal course toward the interhemispheric fissure (Fig. 5-5). In very young patients, it may ascend slightly; in older patients, it usually courses inferiorly. Because the horizontal ACA segment is overlapped by the MCA on lateral views, the A1 segment is best visualized on anteroposterior (AP) or submentovertex projections (see Chapter 6) (10).

Anterior Communicating Artery

Because the ACoA is typically oriented in a somewhat oblique (rather than strictly anteroposterior) plane, it often cannot be visualized optimally on either standard AP and lateral views (Fig. 5-5). Oblique, Water's, or submentovertex views may be required to demonstrate the

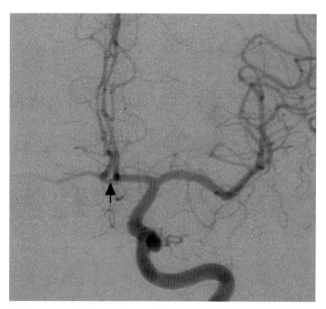

FIG. 5-5. Left internal carotid angiogram, AP view, shows the anterior communicating artery (ACoA) complex (*arrow*). The small lucency is present because the ACoA is fenestrated. The ACoA is visualized in this projection because it lies in the straight coronal plane. More often, the ACoA is oriented obliquely within the interhemispheric fissure, and oblique or submentovertex views are needed to profile this vessel (see Figs. 5-6 and 5-7).

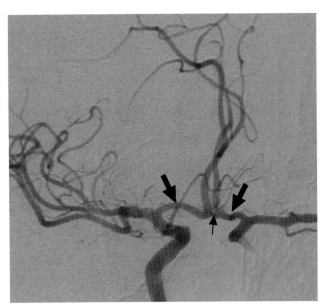

FIG. 5-6. A right internal carotid angiogram, oblique view, performed with temporary cross-compression of the left common carotid artery is shown. Both horizontal (A1) anterior cerebral artery segments are opacified (*large arrows*). The short anterior communicating artery (*small arrow*) is also easily observed.

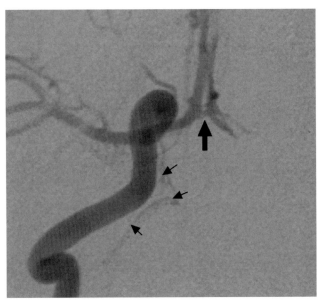

FIG. 5-7. Right internal carotid angiogram, submentovertex view, depicts the anterior communicating artery (*large arrow*). Note transient filling of the right posterior communicating and posterior cerebral arteries (*small arrows*).

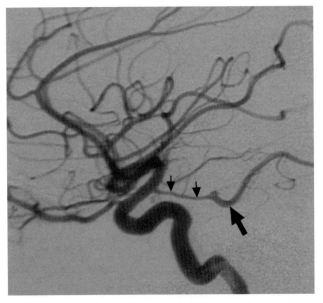

FIG. 5-8. Left internal carotid angiogram, lateral view, shows transient filling of the posterior communicating artery (*small arrows*). The ipsilateral posterior cerebral artery (*large arrow*) is also seen.

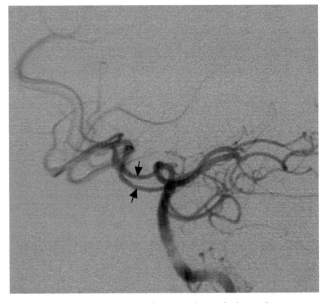

FIG. 5-9. Left vertebral angiogram, lateral view, shows transient filling of both posterior communicating arteries (*arrows*).

Posterior Communicating Arteries

Transient reflux of contrast into the PCoA during injection of either the ICA (Fig. 5-8) or a vertebral artery (Fig. 5-9) often occurs. Temporary compression of the ipsilateral common carotid artery during contrast injection into the vertebral artery may improve reflux into

the PCoA. The lateral or submentovertex views usually best depict PCoA anatomy (Fig. 5-10).

Basilar Artery and Posterior Cerebral Arteries

Angiographic anatomy of the BA and PCAs is considered in detail in Chapters 8 and 9. The BA bifurcation and

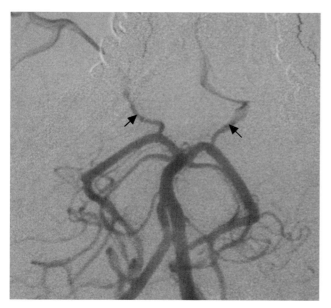

FIG. 5-10. Left vertebral angiogram, shallow submentovertex view, demonstrates transient contrast reflux into both posterior communicating arteries (*small arrows*). Partial filling of the left anterior cerebral and right middle cerebral arteries also has occurred.

horizontal (P1) PCA segments are optimally seen on steep Towne or shallow submentovertex projections of vertebral angiograms (Fig. 5-10). Failure to visualize a PCA when the vertebrobasilar system is opacified is most often because a "fetal" PCA is present. Injection of the ipsilateral ICA confirms this common variation (Fig. 5-11D; see also Fig. 5-15).

Normal Variants

Anatomic variations in the circle of Willis are the rule, not the exception. A so-called complete circle of Willis, with well-developed symmetric components, is present in less than half of all cases (Fig. 5-11) (8). In 90% of cases a complete circular channel is present, but in at least 60% of anatomic specimens one or more vessels is sufficiently narrowed to reduce its role as a potential collateral route (1,2).

Common circle of Willis variations are described below.

Hypoplastic or Absent A1 Segment

The anterior portion of the circle of Willis, composed of the paired A1 (horizontal) segments and the ACoA, is a common site for congenital circle of Willis variations. *A1 hypoplasia* is identified in approximately 10% of anatomic dissections (Figs. 5-11C and 5-12) (5). True *absence of an A1 segment* is much less common, found in only 1% to 2% of cases (Figs. 5-11E and 5-13) (see Chapter 6).

ACoA Variations

A single ACoA is present in approximately 60% of cases. *Multiple vascular channels ("plexiform" ACoAs)* are present in 10% to 33% of anatomic dissections (Fig. 5-11G) (5,11). A *duplicated ACoA* (Fig. 5-11F) occurs in 18% of cases, whereas a *fenestrated ACoA* is seen in 12% to 21% of cases (Figs. 5-5 and 5-11G) (5,11,12). An *absent ACoA* occurs in only 5% of cases (Fig. 5-11H) (13).

Hypoplastic or Absent PCoA

Anomalies of the posterior circle of Willis are even more frequent, occurring in nearly half of all anatomic specimens. The posterior communicating arteries are the most common site of these variations (8,14).

The PCoAs are typically smaller than the internal carotid arteries and posterior cerebral arteries (Figs. 5-7 to 5-9). In many patients one or both PCoAs are small or absent (Fig. 5-11B). *Hypoplasia of one or both PCoAs* is seen in one fourth of MR angiograms and one third of all anatomic dissections (Fig. 5-11B) (8,14,15).

PCoA Infundibulum

Funnel-shaped dilations at the origin of the PCoA at its junction with the ICA have been detected on angiography or at autopsy in approximately 6% to 17% of cases (16). This type of "junctional" dilatation is referred to as a *PCoA infundibulum* (see Fig. 4-13A). Such widening is typically round or conical, is 2 mm or less in diameter, is symmetric, and has a wide base at its origin from the ICA. The PCoA arises from its apex (Fig. 5-14). A PCoA infundibulum is considered a normal variant but must be distinguished from an ICA–PCoA aneurysm (see Fig. 12-32).

Fetal Origin of the PCA

In some cases a PCoA has the same diameter as the PCA. It is then referred to as a *fetal PCA* (Fig. 5-11D). If the embryonic PCoA fails to regress, the dominant blood supply to the occipital lobes comes from the ICA via the fetal PCA instead of from the vertebrobasilar system (Fig. 5-15) (1). This primitive or fetal configuration is found in approximately 20% to 30% of cases (14,17).

Hypoplastic or Absent P1

The P1 segments vary considerably in both length and diameter and are more often asymmetric than are the A1 segments. If a fetal PCA configuration is present, an ipsilateral *hypoplastic P1 segment* occurs (Figs. 5-11D and 5-15B). This configuration is seen in 15% to 22% of cerebral angiograms (see Chapter 8) (18). An *absent P1 segment* is very uncommon (14).

Summary

Circle of Willis variations are common, especially in the posterior part of the circle. Many of these variations

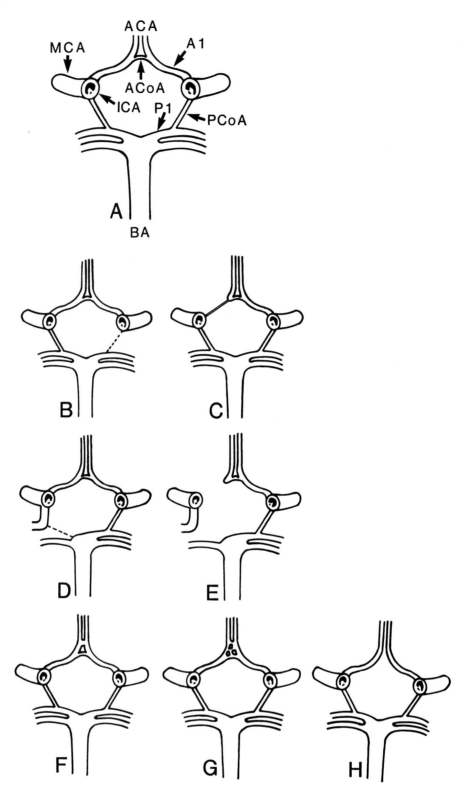

have little significance. One exception is a small (less than 1 mm in diameter) or absent PCoA, which is an independent risk factor for ischemic cerebral infarction in patients with ICA occlusion (19).

Other variations also may restrict or eliminate collateral blood flow in vascular occlusive disease. One exam- ple is an anatomically *isolated* internal carotid artery. This occurs when a fetal PCA and absent A1 ACA seg- ment are both present on the same side (Figs. 5-11E and 5-16). Here the ICA supplies the ipsilateral MCA and PCA but cannot receive collateral blood flow from either the contralateral ICA or the vertebrobasilar circulation.

FIG. 5-11. Anatomic diagrams depict the circle of Willis **(A)** and its common variations **(B–H)**. **A:** A "complete" circle of Willis is present. Here all components are present and none are hypoplastic. This configuration is seen in less than half of all cases. **B:** Hypoplasia (right) or absence (left) of one or both posterior communicating arteries (PCoAs) is the most common circle of Willis variant, seen in 25% to 33% of cases. **C:** Hypoplasia or absence of the horizontal (A1) anterior cerebral artery segment is seen in approximately 10% to 20% of cases. Here the right A1 segment is absent. **D:** Fetal origin of the posterior cerebral artery (PCA) with hypoplasia of the precommunicating (P1) PCA segment, seen in 15% to 25% of cases. **E:** If both a fetal PCA and an absent A1 occur together, the internal carotid artery (ICA) is anatomically isolated with severely restricted potential collateral blood flow. Here the right ICA terminates in an MCA and fetal-type PCA. **F:** Multichanneled (two or more) anterior communicating artery segments, seen in 10% to 15% of cases. Here the duplicated ACoAs are complete and both extend across the entire ACoA. **G:** In a fenestrated ACoA, the ACoA has a more plexiform appearance. **H:** Absence of an ACoA is shown. ACA, distal anterior communicating artery segments; A1, horizontal ACA segment; P1, horizontal (precommunicating) PCA segment.

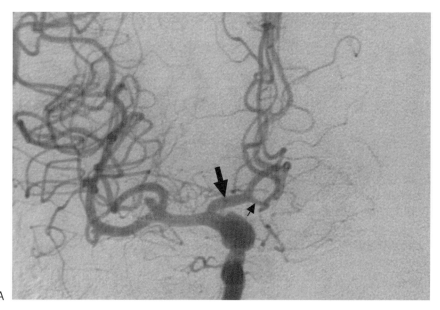

A

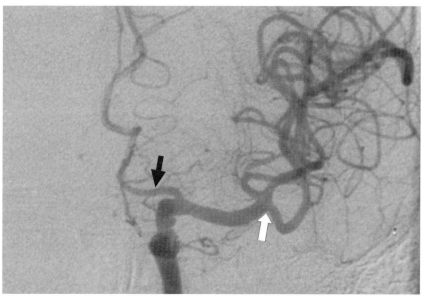

B

FIG. 5-12. Anteroposterior views of selective right **(A)** and left **(B)** internal carotid angiograms in a patient with subarachnoid hemorrhage. **A:** The right carotid study demonstrates two aneurysms, a larger right supraclinoid internal carotid aneurysm and a smaller middle cerebral artery (MCA) trifurcation aneurysm. Note that the right A1 anterior cerebral artery (ACA) segment is unusually large (*large arrow*), almost equal in size to the MCA. The anterior communicating artery (ACoA) is also prominent (*small arrow*). Both distal ACAs are supplied primarily via the right carotid circulation. **B:** The left carotid angiogram shows a hypoplastic A1 segment (*large black arrow*) that continues as the callosomarginal artery. Note the prominent but normal MCA trifurcation on this side (*large white arrow*).

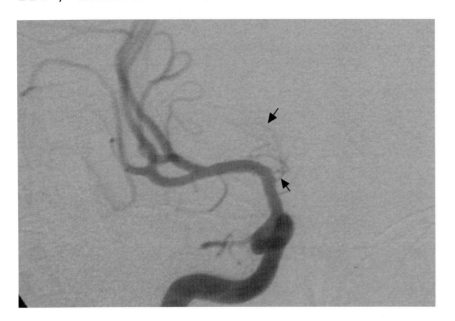

FIG. 5-13. Right internal carotid angiogram, anteroposterior view, shows an absent horizontal (A1) anterior cerebral artery (ACA) segment. In this case the internal carotid artery essentially terminates by becoming the middle cerebral artery. Because the ACA is absent, the anterior choroidal artery (*arrows*) is unusually well seen.

Anomalies

Variations in the circle of Willis are common, but true anomalies are rare. Anomalous circles of Willis are associated with an increased prevalence of intracranial aneurysm (see Chapter 12), but normal developmental variations in the circle of Willis do not have this association (20).

Anomalies of the ACA–ACoA Complex

Rare anomalies of the ACA include *infraoptic origin of the ACA* from the ICA. In this condition the ACA arises from the ICA near the ophthalmic artery origin. It follows a characteristic course, passing anterior to the optic chiasm and between the two optic nerves before ascending in the interhemispheric fissure. This anomaly is associated with a high prevalence of intracranial aneurysms (7,21).

Fenestration of the ACA has been associated with increased risk of aneurysm formation by some investigators (22,23).

An *azygous ACA* is a solitary, unpaired vessel that arises as a single trunk from confluence of the right and left horizontal (A1) segments. In this situation the ACoA is absent. Associated anomalies may include an increased prevalence of intracranial aneurysm (24). A true azygous ACA is also found in various forms of holoprosencephaly (see Chapter 6).

Anomalies of the PCoA–BA–PCA Complex

True posterior circulation anomalies are rare. *Persistent carotid–basilar anastomoses* are considered in Chapters 2 and 3.

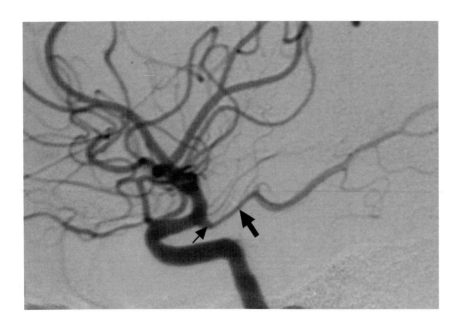

FIG. 5-14. Left internal carotid angiogram, lateral view, demonstrates a posterior communicating artery (PCoA) infundibulum, a funnel-shaped dilatation at its origin from the internal carotid artery (*small arrow*). Note that the PCoA (*large arrow*) arises directly from the apex of the infundibulum. This configuration and its small size distinguish an infundibulum from a PCoA aneurysm.

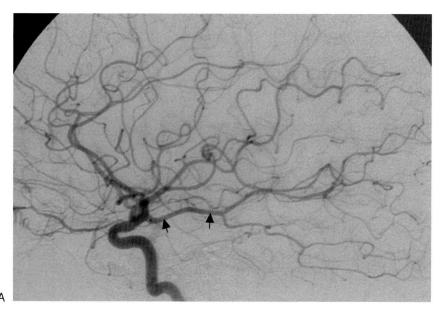

A

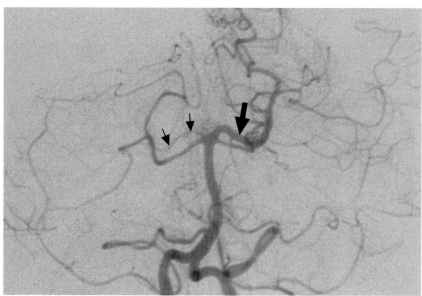

B

FIG. 5-15. A: Lateral view of a right internal carotid angiogram shows a fetal posterior cerebral artery (PCA) (*arrows*). In this case the embryonic posterior communicating artery (PCoA) did not regress. The PCoA has the same diameter as the PCA, and the PCA thus appears to arise directly from the ICA. B: Anteroposterior view of the right vertebral angiogram in the same patient shows a hypoplastic P1 PCA segment (*small arrows*). The right PCA distal to the PCoA is not opacified (compare with the normal left PCA, indicated by the large arrow). The most common reason that a PCA is not visualized on vertebrobasilar angiograms is the presence of a fetal PCA. In these cases injection of the ipsilateral ICA demonstrates the "missing" vessel (see A).

PERFORATING BRANCHES OF THE CIRCLE OF WILLIS

Without exception, important perforating branches arise from every part of the circle of Willis (Fig. 5-2). These are briefly summarized here and are considered in detail with their respective parent arteries (see Chapters 6,8, and 9).

Anterior Cerebral Arteries

Small ACA perforating branches, the *medial lenticulostriate arteries*, and the *recurrent artery of Heubner* supply the caudate nucleus head, anterior limb of the internal capsule, and part of the basal ganglia (25).

Anterior Communicating Artery

Several small but important perforating branches arise from the ACoA to supply the superior surface of the optic chiasm and anterior hypothalamus (5,26). These branches may have a significant vascular territory that includes part of the corpus callosum, columns of the fornix, parolfactory areas, lamina terminalis, and hypothalamus (27,28).

Posterior Communicating Arteries

A number of small but important perforating branches, the *anterior thalamoperforating arteries*, arise from the PCoA to supply part of the thalamus, the infralenticular limb of the internal capsule, and optic tracts (14).

Basilar Artery and Posterior Cerebral Arteries

The distal BA and proximal PCAs give rise to numerous small perforating arteries. These branches, the *posterior thalamoperforating arteries* and the *thalamogeniculate arteries*, supply the mid-brain and thalamus (30).

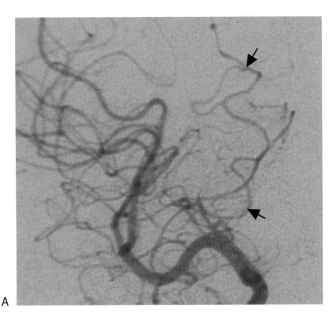 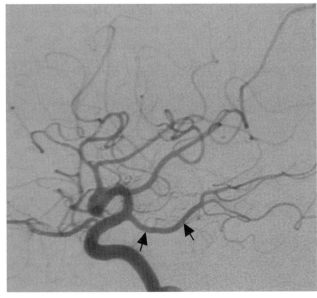

A   B

FIG. 5-16. Anteroposterior **(A)** and lateral **(B)** views of a right internal carotid angiogram demonstrate an anatomically isolated internal carotid artery (ICA). The anterior cerebral artery (ACA) is not visualized because the A1 segment on this side is absent and both ACAs filled from the left ICA. There is a fetal posterior cerebral artery (PCA) (*arrows*), i.e., the proximal PCA did not involute during fetal development. In this arrangement the PCA originates directly from the ICA and the precommunicating (P1) segment is hypoplastic or absent. When both P1 and A1 segments are absent, the ICA is functionally and anatomically isolated. With severely limited potential collateral flow from other parts of the circle of Willis, occlusion of such an isolated ICA usually results in a major neurologic deficit.

REFERENCES

1. Williams P, ed. Embryonic circulation. In: *Gray's anatomy*, 58th ed. New York: Churchill Livingstone, 1995:315.
2. Wolpert SM. The circle of Willis. *AJNR* 1997;18:1033–1034.
3. Williams P, ed. Circle of Willis. In: *Gray's anatomy*, 58th ed. New York: Churchill Livingstone, 1995:1528.
4. Destrieux C, Kakou MK, Velut S, et al. Microanatomy of the hypophyseal fossa boundaries. *J Neurosurg* 1998;88:743–752.
5. Perlmutter D, Rhoton AL Jr. Microsurgical anatomy of the anterior cerebral-anterior communicating-recurrent artery complex. *J Neurosurg* 1976;45:259–272.
6. Brown JH, Lustrin ES, Lev MH, Taveras JM. CT angiography of the circle of Willis: is spiral technology always necessary? *AJNR* 1997;18:1974–1976.
7. Barboriak DP, Provenzale JM. Pictorial review: magnetic resonance angiography of arterial variants at the circle of Willis. *Clin Radiol* 1997;52:429–439.
8. Krabbé-Hartkamp MJ, van der Grond J, de Leeuw F-E, et al. Circle of Willis: morphologic variation on three-dimensional time-of-flight MR angiograms. *Radiology* 1998;207:103–111.
9. Katz DA, Marks MP, Napel SA, et al. Circle of Willis: evaluation with spiral CT angiography, MR angiography, and conventional angiography. *Radiology* 1995;195:445–449.
10. Lin JP, Kricheff II. The anterior cerebral artery complex. In: Newton TH, Potts DG, eds. *Radiology of the skull and brain,* vol. 2, book 2. St. Louis: Mosby, 1974:1391–1420.
11. Serizawa T, Saeki N, Yamaura A. Microsurgical anatomy and clinical significance of the anterior communicating artery and its perforating branches. *Neurosurgery* 1997;40:1211–1218.
12. Finlay HM, Canham PB. The layered fabric of cerebral artery fenestrations. *Stroke* 1994;25:1799–1806.
13. Rhoton AL Jr, Saeki N, Perlmutter D, Zeal A. Microsurgical anatomy of common aneurysm sites. *Clin Neurosurg* 1979;26:248–306.
14. Saeki N, Rhoton AL Jr. Microsurgical anatomy of the upper basilar artery and the posterior circle of Willis. *J Neurosurg* 1977;46:563–578.
15. Pedroza A, Dujovny M, Artero JC, et al. Microanatomy of the posterior communicating artery. *Neurosurgery* 1987;20:228–235.
16. Endo S, Furuichi S, Takaba M, et al. Clinical study of enlarged infundibular dilation of the origin of the posterior communicating artery. *J Neurosurg* 1995;83:421–425.
17. Bisaria KK. Anomalies of the posterior communicating artery and their potential significance. *J Neurosurg* 1984;60:572–576.
18. Wollschlaeger G, Wollschlaeger PB. The circle of Willis. In: Newton TH, Potts DG, eds. *Radiology of the skull and brain,* vol. 2, book 2. St. Louis: Mosby, 1974:1171–1201.
19. Schomer DF, Marks MP, Steinberg GK, et al. The anatomy of the posterior communicating artery as a risk factor for ischemic cerebral infarction. *N Engl J Med* 1994;330:1565–1570.
20. Mackenzie JM: The anatomy of aneurysm-bearing circles of Willis. *Clin Neuropathol* 1991;10:187–189.
21. Bollar A, Martinez R, Gelabert M, Garcia A. Anomalous origin of the anterior cerebral artery associated with aneurysm: embryological considerations. *Neuroradiology* 1988;30:86.
22. San-Galli F, Leman C, Kien P, et al. Cerebral arterial fenestrations associated with intracranial saccular aneurysms. *Neurosurgery* 1992;30:279–283.
23. Sanders WP, Sorek PA, Mehta BA. Fenestration of intracranial arteries with special attention to associated aneurysms and other anomalies. *AJNR* 1993;14:657–680.
24. Schick RM, Rumbaugh CL. Saccular aneurysm of the azygous anterior cerebral artery. *AJNR* 1989;10:273.
25. Ghika JA, Bogousslavsky J, Regli F. Deep perforations from the carotid system. *Arch Neurol* 1990;47:1097–1100.
26. Mercier P, Fournier D, Brassier G, et al. The perforating arteries of the anterior part of the circle of Willis. *Riv Neuroradiol* 1994;7(Suppl 4):79–83.
27. Vincentelli F, Lehman G, Caruso G, et al. Extracerebral course of the perforating branches of the anterior communicating artery. Microsurgical anatomical study. *Surg Neurol* 1991;35:98–104.
28. Marinkovic S, Gibo H, Milisavljevic M. The surgical anatomy of the relationships between the perforating and the leptomeningeal arteries. *Neurosurgery* 1996;39:72–83.
29. Grand W, Hopkins LN. The microsurgical anatomy of the basilar artery bifurcation. *Neurosurgery* 1977;1:128–131.
30. Brassier G, Morandi X, Fournier D, et al. Origin of the perforating arteries of the interpeduncular fossa in relation to the termination of the basilar artery. *Interv Neuroradiol* 1998;4:109–120.

CHAPTER 6

The Anterior Cerebral Artery

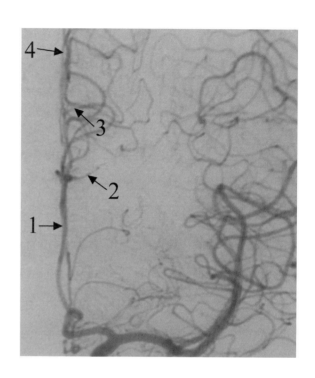

The vascular complex formed by the anterior cerebral artery (ACA), anterior communicating artery (ACoA), and recurrent artery (of Huebner) is a common site for aneurysm formation. Penetrating branches from these vessels also supply important basal brain structures such as the lentiform nucleus and the internal capsule. Familiarity with the normal anatomy, variants, anomalies, and vascular territories of this vascular complex is very important for planning microsurgical approaches to the anterior basal brain.

The ACA has been subdivided in different ways by different investigators. Between three and five anatomic segments are described (1–3). The first two segments (A1 and A2) represent the proximal ACA, whereas the others (variably numbered A3 to A5) represent the distal ACA.

The most common, simplest classification describes three ACA segments:

A1 = horizontal or precommunicating segment
A2 = vertical or postcommunicating segment
A3 = distal ACA and cortical branches

The first section in this chapter delineates the anatomy and normal imaging appearance of the proximal ACA (A1 and A2 segments) and the basal perforating branches. The second section covers the distal ACA and its terminal branches.

ANTERIOR CEREBRAL ARTERY: PROXIMAL (A1 AND A2) SEGMENTS

Normal Development

At 5 weeks' gestation, the anterior cerebral artery (ACA) appears as a secondary branch of the *primitive olfactory artery*, which is in turn derived from the *primitive internal carotid artery*. By 6 weeks, each ACA is advancing toward the midline, where it is joined with its counterpart from the opposite side by a plexiform anastomosis that in turn forms the future anterior communicating artery (ACoA) (see Fig. 5-1) (4,5).

A small embryonic branch known as the *median artery of the corpus callosum* arises from the ACoA and extends toward the lamina terminalis. This vessel normally involutes as the ACA segments distal to the ACoA develop (6). By 7 weeks' gestation, the *definitive ACA* extends superiorly between the cerebral hemispheres.

Basal perforating arteries that arise from the ACA, i.e., the medial striate arteries and the recurrent artery of Huebner, are formed either from the primitive olfactory artery or components of an anastomosis between this artery and its collateral anterior cerebral branch (5).

Normal Gross Anatomy

The internal carotid artery (ICA) terminates below the anterior perforated substance by bifurcating into the ante-

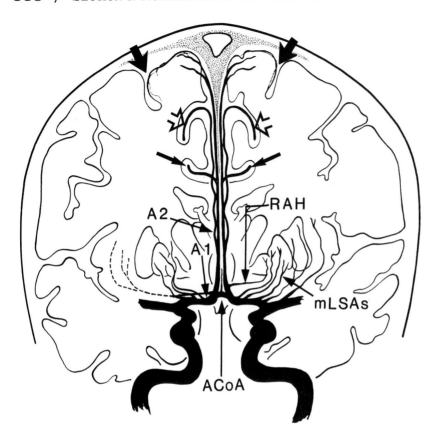

FIG. 6-1. Anteroposterior (AP) diagrammatic sketch shows the anterior cerebral arteries (ACAs) and their branches. A1, horizontal or precommunicating segment. ACoA, anterior communicating artery (note perforating branch; also shows position of an anatomic variant, the median artery of the corpus callosum); A2, vertical segment; mLSAs, medial lenticulostriate arteries (perforating branches); RAH, recurrent artery of Heubner (the usual course is shown on the left; on the right, the RAH—indicated by the dotted lines—is shown extending laterally almost to the sylvian fissure). The large black arrows indicate the vascular "watershed" zone. The small black arrows indicate the pericallosal arteries within the callosal sulci. On AP angiograms these vessels have the appearance of a smile. The open arrows indicate the callosomarginal branches as they course within the cingulate sulci. On AP angiograms these vessels have the appearance of a moustache (compare with Fig. 6-17B).

Proximal Segments of the Anterior Cerebral Artery: Normal Anatomy and Variations

Normal development
  ACAs from primitive olfactory, internal carotid
    arteries
  ACoA from fusion of midline plexus of
    vessels
Gross anatomy
  Horizontal or precommunicating ACA segment
    (A1)
  Vertical or postcommunicating ACA segment
    (A2)
Key relationships
  A1 segments course medially over optic nerves or
    chiasm
  A2 segments course superiorly within
    interhemispheric fissure, anterior to corpus
    callosum rostrum
Branches
  Perforating branches
    Medial lenticulostriate arteries
    Recurrent artery of Heubner (RAH)
    Callosal perforating arteries (ACoA may have a
      large "median artery of the corpus
      callosum")

  Cortical branches
    Orbital branches (e.g., orbitofrontal artery)
    Frontal branches (e.g., frontopolar artery)
Vascular territory
  Perforating branches
    Head of caudate nucleus
    Anteromedial, inferior basal ganglia
    Inferomedial internal capsule
    Anterior commissure
    Rostrum of corpus callosum
  Cortical branches
    Olfactory bulb and tract
    Gyrus rectus
    Ventromedial frontal lobe
Variants
  A1 hypoplasia or aplasia
Anomalies
  Infraoptic origin of ACA (high prevalence of
    aneurysms)
  Accessory ACA
  Bihemispheric ACA
  Azygous ACA (associated with holoprosencephaly,
    migration anomalies, aneurysms)
  Persistent primitive olfactory artery

rior and middle cerebral arteries. The ACA is the smaller of these two terminal branches (Fig. 6-1; see box on facing page).

A1 Segment

The A1 segment is also called the precommunicating segment. This segment extends horizontally from the ACA origin to its junction with the ACoA.

A2 Segment

The A2 segment is also called the postcommunicating segment. This segment extends vertically from the ACoA to the corpus callosum genu.

Relationships

Summary

1. As the A1 segment courses medially toward the interhemispheric fissure, it passes *over* the optic chiasm (70%) or optic nerves (30%) and *below* the anterior perforated substance (see Fig. 5-2).

2. The ACA–ACoA junction lies *within* or just *below* the longitudinal (interhemispheric) fissure (Fig. 6-2).
3. The A2 segment curves upward within the interhemispheric fissure, *anterior* to the lamina terminalis and corpus callosum rostrum (Fig. 6-2).

Branches

The proximal ACA has both perforating and cortical branches.

Perforating Branches

From one to 12 *medial lenticulostriate arteries* arise from the A1 ACA segment and course posterosuperiorly through the anterior perforated substance to supply important parts of the anterobasal brain (Fig. 6-1) (7–10). Smaller perforating branches course inferiorly to supply the optic chiasm and optic nerves (see Fig. 5-2). *Perforating branches* also may arise from the ACoA and A2 segments to supply the corpus callosum genu, septum pellucidum, and columns of the fornix (11).

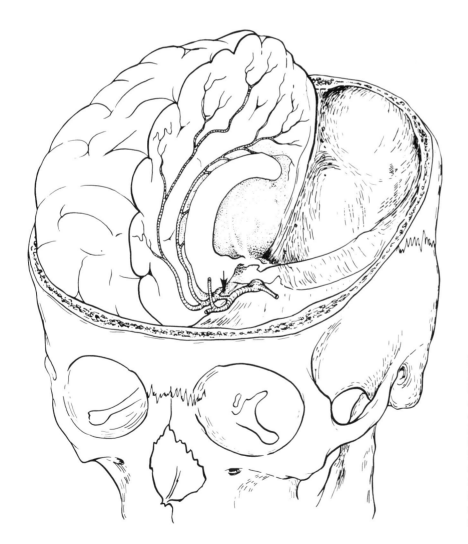

FIG. 6-2. Anatomic sketch of the anterior cerebral arteries (ACAs) and their relationship to the corpus callosum. The A1 (horizontal or precommunicating) ACA segments initially course anteromedially toward the interhemispheric fissure, where they are joined together by the anterior communicating artery (*arrow*). The A2 (vertical or postcommunicating) segments course anteriorly and superiorly within the interhemispheric fissure, curving around the genu of the corpus callosum.

The *recurrent artery of Huebner* (RAH) is the largest and longest ACA penetrating branch (12). The RAH arises either from the proximal A2 segment (seen in 34% to 50% of cases) or the A1 segment (seen in 17% to 45% of cases). It also may arise from the ACoA (5% to 20% of cases) (8). From its origin the RAH doubles back on its parent artery at an acute angle (Fig. 6-1). The RAH usually terminates dorsal and slightly lateral to the carotid bifurcation (8). In some cases it runs laterally almost to the sylvian fissure before turning superiorly to enter the anterior perforated substance (12).

Cortical Branches

Anterior cerebral artery (ACA) branching patterns are quite variable. The ACA cortical branches are now named by the territory they supply (13).

Cortical branches normally do not arise from the precommunicating ACA. The first cortical branches arise from the proximal A2 segment. These are two or three *orbital branches* (such as the *orbitofrontal artery*) that ramify on the orbital surface of the frontal lobe (Fig. 6-3).

The second group of branches that arises from the A2 segment is represented by the *frontal branches* (14). The most prominent of these branches is the *frontopolar artery*. This vessel arises below the corpus callosum rostrum or genu and extends anteriorly to the frontal pole (Fig. 6-3).

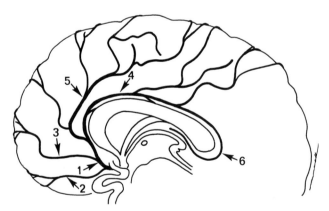

FIG. 6-3. Lateral anatomic drawing of the medial surface of the right cerebral hemisphere shows the anterior cerebral artery (ACA) and its major cortical branches.

1, A2 (vertical or postcommunicating) ACA segment
2, Orbitofrontal artery
3, Frontopolar artery
4, Pericallosal artery
5, Callosomarginal artery
6, Splenial branch (Reprinted with permission from Osborn AG, Tong KA. *Handbook of neuroradiology,* 2nd ed. St. Louis: Mosby–Year Book, 1996.)

Vascular Territory and Anastomoses

Perforating Branches

Distribution of the ACA basal perforating arteries (ACoA and callosal perforators, medial lenticulostriate arteries, and RAH) is illustrated in Fig 6-4. Small but important structures supplied by these vessels include the caudate nucleus head, anteromedial part of the putamen and globus pallidus, inferior and medial aspects of the anterior limb of the internal capsule, corpus callosum rostrum, and part of the anterior commissure (15).

Cortical Branches

Typical, minimal, and maximal vascular distributions of all the ACA cortical branches is shown in Fig. 6-5. The orbital branches supply the olfactory bulb and tract, gyrus rectus, and medial orbital gyrus. The frontal branches supply the ventromedial surface of the frontal pole and a band of brain parenchyma that extends for several centimeters onto the frontal convexity (14,16–18).

Anastomoses

The normal ACA–ACoA complex is one in which a communicating artery (the ACoA) connects two horizontal ACA segments that are equal in size (see Fig. 5-11A). In this arrangement both A1 segments and the ACoA facilitate potential cross-circulation between the two carotid arteries via the circle of Willis.

The basal perforating ACA branches are usually single unpaired end vessels with few anastomoses and little potential for collateral flow from other small deep arteries.

Normal Angiographic Anatomy

Anteroposterior View

The ICA bifurcation into the anterior and middle cerebral arteries forms a T on the anteroposterior (AP) view of carotid angiograms. The horizontal ACA is the smaller, more medial arm of the T (Fig. 6-1). The A1 segment varies in angiographic appearance. It may follow a nearly horizontal course as it runs medially toward the interhemispheric fissure (Fig. 6-6A). It also may ascend, descend, or describe a sinusoidal course (Figs. 6-6B–D). The two A1 segments may be asymmetric in size, position, or both (Fig. 6-7).

In the AP projection, the ACA should be located in the interhemispheric fissure at the midpoint along a line drawn between the orbital rims (Fig. 6-8). Shallow side-to-side undulations of the A2 segments are common. Normal undulations are gentle and short, and return to or

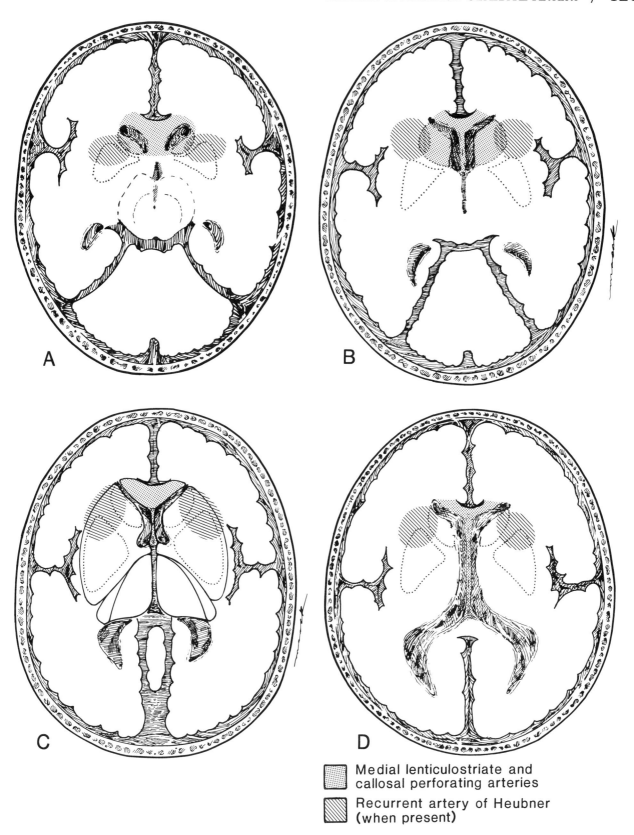

Medial lenticulostriate and
callosal perforating arteries

Recurrent artery of Heubner
(when present)

FIG. 6-4. Axial anatomic drawings depict the vascular territories of the perforating branches that arise from the anterior cerebral artery. These include the medial lenticulostriate arteries, callosal perforating branches, and the recurrent artery of Huebner (when present).

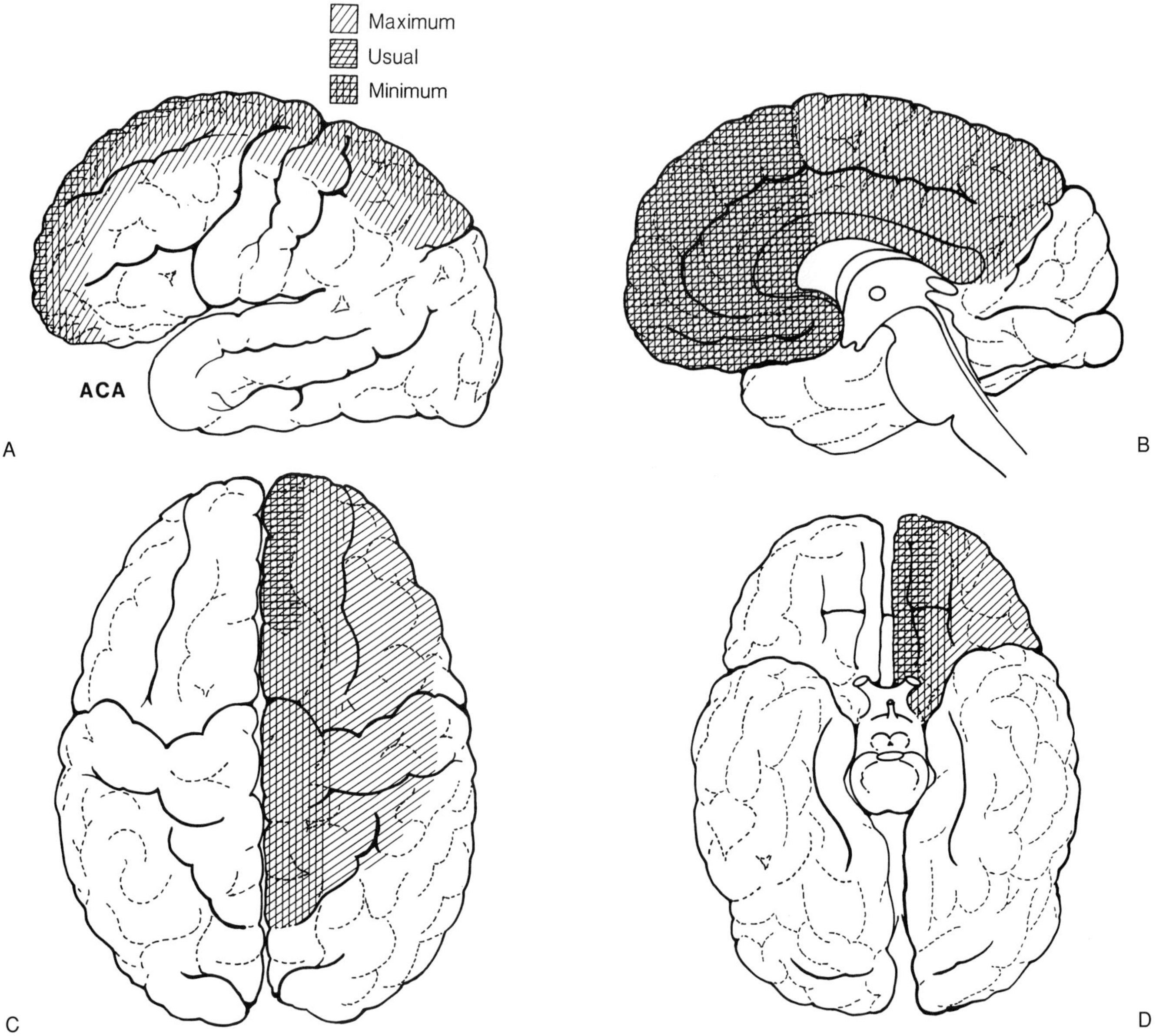

FIG. 6-5. Vascular territories of the cortical (hemispheric) ACA branches with maximum, usual, and minimum distributions as delineated by van der Zwan (16). **A:** Lateral view. **B:** Medial view. **C:** Superior view. **D:** Base view. (Reprinted with permission from Osborn AG. *Diagnostic neuroradiology.* St. Louis: Mosby, 1994.)

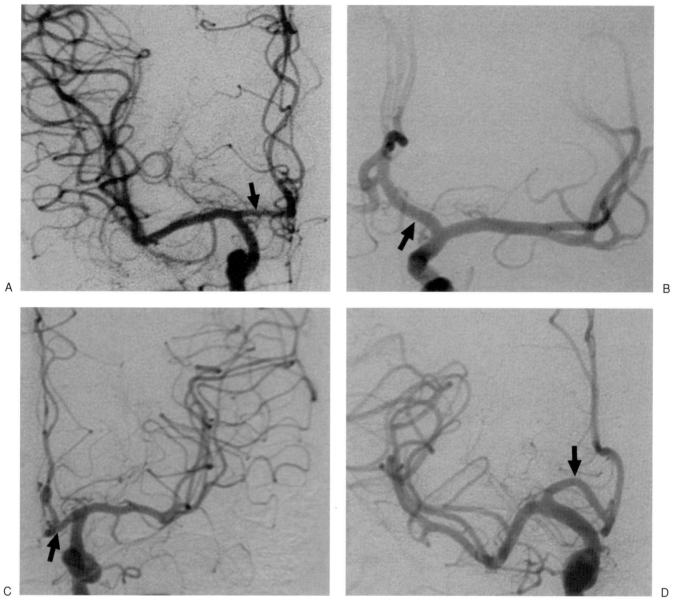

FIG. 6-6. Anteroposterior views of the internal carotid angiograms in four different patients illustrate normal variations in the course of the A1 (horizontal or precommunicating) ACA segments (*arrows*).

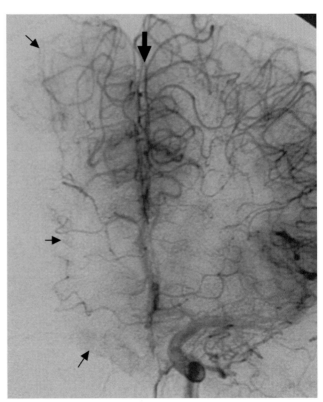

FIG. 6-7. A: Left internal carotid angiogram, anteroposterior view, illustrates asymmetry in size and position of the two A1 (horizontal or precommunicating) ACA segments (*small arrows*). **B:** Late arterial phase clearly illustrates the vascular watershed zone (*small arrows*) between the ACA and the other cerebral arteries. The interhemispheric fissure is indicated by the large arrows. Note midline position of the distal ACAs in both views (compare with Fig. 6-8).

even cross the midline (Fig. 6-9A). In many cases where the ACA appears tortuous, the "brain blush" on the late arterial phase of digital subtraction angiograms will demonstrate that the medial hemisphere is in the midline (Fig. 6-9B). Persistent displacement of the ACA across the midline is abnormal (see Chapter 14).

Oblique View

Thirty degree to 45 degree oblique transorbital views are often the optimal projection for visualizing the A1 segment and its junction with the ACoA (Fig. 6-10) (19).

Lateral View

The A1 segment is not well visualized on lateral views. However, the A2 segment is clearly seen in this projection as the ACA passes anterior to the lamina terminalis and courses superiorly toward the corpus callosum genu.

On lateral carotid angiograms the course of the postcommunicating (A2) segment is quite variable. It often follows a gentle, anteriorly convex curve (Fig. 6-11A). It also may assume a "humped" or inferiorly concave course, or even an acutely angled one (Fig. 6-11B and C). Occasionally it may even appear somewhat blunt or squared off at its most anterior extent. If the ACA essentially terminates by becoming the callosomarginal artery, the A2 segment may assume a "bull nose" appearance (Fig. 6-11D).

Normal Variants

A1 Hypoplasia

The A1 segment is hypoplastic (Fig. 6-12A) or absent (Fig. 6-12B) in 10% to 25% of all anatomic dissections (1). The contralateral ACA then supplies part or all of the normal ACA vascular territory in the opposite hemisphere via a large ACoA and two normal distal (A2) segments (see Fig. 5-11C and E).

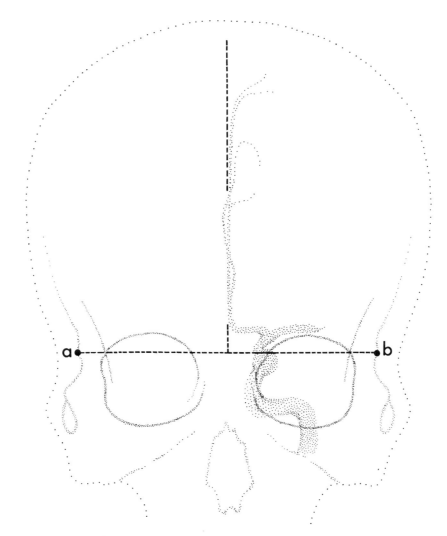

FIG. 6-8. Diagrammatic sketch of a left internal carotid angiogram (arterial phase, anteroposterior view). Two dots, a and b, are placed on the lateral margins of the orbital rims. A line is drawn between these two points, bisected, and a perpendicular constructed at its midpoint. The A2 ACA segments should lie along this line.

Anomalies and Associated Conditions

Anomalous Anterior Cerebral Artery Origin

Anomalous origin of the ACA is rare (see Chapter 5). A carotid–ACA anastomosis, also called *infraoptic origin of the ACA*, has been reported. In this anomaly the ACA arises a few millimeters above the intradural ICA, usually at the level of the ophthalmic artery. It courses medially below (not above) the optic nerve and then curves superiorly, where it anastomoses with the ACoA. This anomaly has frequent association with other anomalies such as

aneurysm, carotid agenesis, and agenesis or hypoplasia of the A1 segment (20–23).

A so-called *accessory* ACA is a branch that arises from the ICA and courses under the optic nerve to supply the medial–basal part of the frontal lobe (24).

Bihemispheric Anterior Cerebral Artery

If one A2 segment is hypoplastic and the other A2 divides into branches that provide the major blood supply to both hemispheres, a so-called bihemispheric ACA is present (Fig. 6-13A). This anomaly is found in 2% to 7% of anatomic specimens (2). A bihemispheric ACA may be

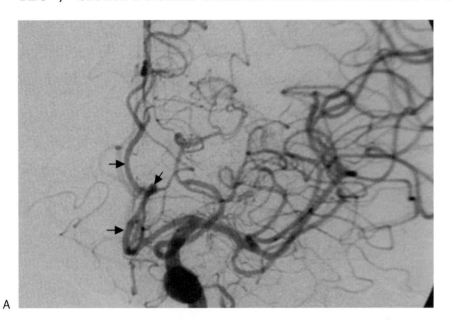

A

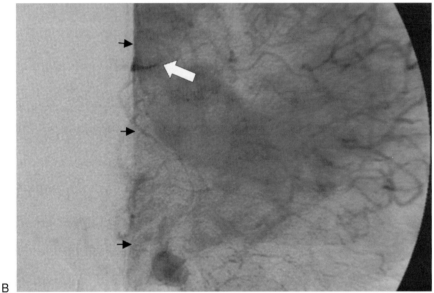

B

FIG. 6-9. A: Left internal carotid angiogram, anteroposterior view, illustrates a tortuous A2 ACA segment (*arrows*). Note that the vertical portion of the ACA may normally course back and forth across the midline. These undulations are shallow, relatively short, and approximately equidistant on both sides of the midline. **B:** Late arterial phase view shows that the brain blush (*small arrows*) is midline. Note the vascular blush of the pericallosal artery (*white arrow*), a normal finding.

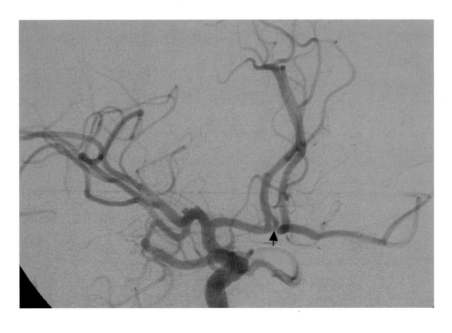

FIG. 6-10. Right internal carotid angiogram, transorbital oblique view, performed with temporary manual cross-compression of the left common carotid artery. The horizontal ACA segments are well delineated. The anterior communicating artery has a large branch (*arrow*) that arises from it and courses superiorly, paralleling the two A2 (vertical) ACA segments. This represents either ACA duplication or a large median branch of the corpus callosum.

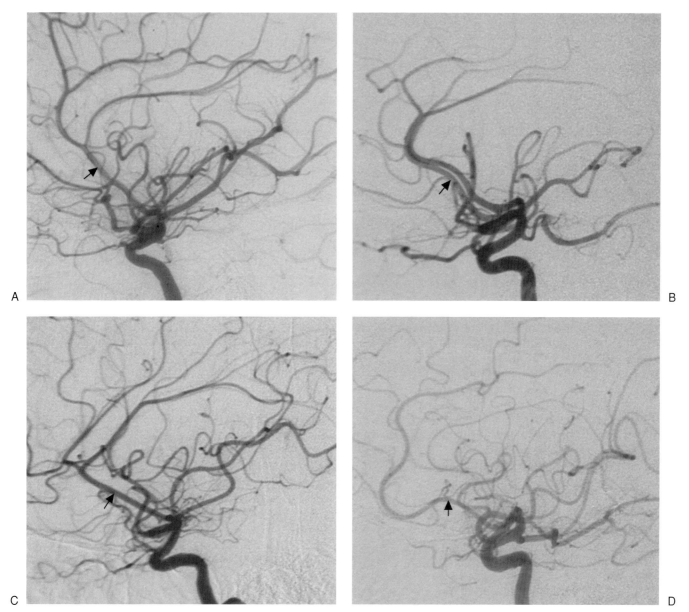

FIG. 6-11. A-D: Lateral views of the internal carotid angiograms in four different patients illustrate the wide variability in the A2 (vertical or postcommunicating) ACA segments (*arrows*). In **D,** the ACA essentially continues as the callosomarginal artery.

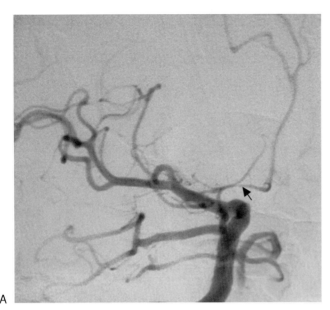
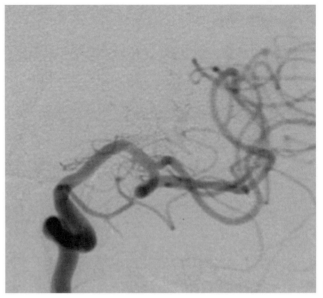

A
B

FIG. 6-12. A: Right internal carotid angiogram, arterial phase, oblique view, shows a very hypoplastic A1 (horizontal or precommunicating)(*arrow*) ACA segment. **B:** AP left common carotid angiogram in another patient is shown for comparison. The A1 segment is absent. The supraclinoid internal carotid artery essentially continues as the middle cerebral artery. In this case the right internal carotid artery supplied both ACAs via a large A1 and anterior communicating artery (ACoA).

difficult to distinguish angiographically from a true azygous ACA unless the hypoplastic contralateral A2 segment can be identified (Fig. 6-13B).

Azygous Anterior Cerebral Artery

If the embryonic median artery of the corpus callosum persists, an azygous ACA is formed. Here a single unpaired ACA arises as a solitary midline trunk that supplies both ACA territories. The reported prevalence of an azygous ACA is between 0.2% and 4% (25).

Azygous ACAs may be observed as an incidental finding with little clinical significance. They also have been reported in association with holoprosencephaly, neuronal migration anomalies, and an increased risk of aneurysm formation (Fig. 6-14) (6).

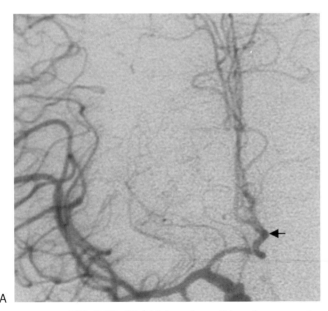
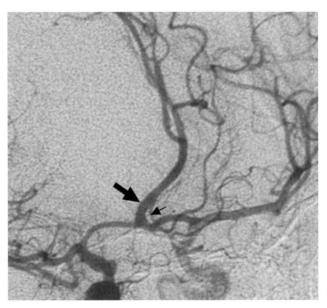

A
B

FIG. 6-13. Right internal carotid angiogram, anteroposterior **(A)** and oblique **(B)** views, shows a single midline ACA (*large arrows*) that supplies most of the cortical branches to both hemispheres. This is a bihemispheric ACA. Note that on the oblique study **(B)**, performed with temporary manual cross-compression of the left common carotid artery, a very small left A2 segment (*small arrow*) is present.

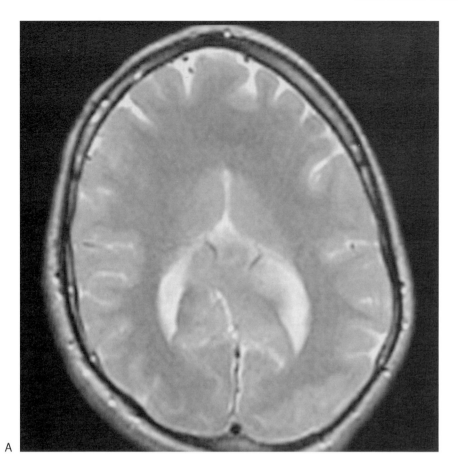

A

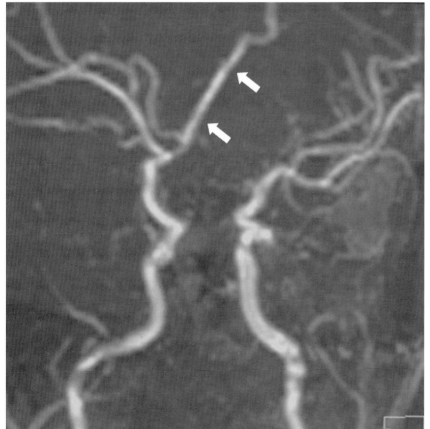

B

FIG. 6-14. A: Axial T2-weighted MR scan in a patient with lobar holoprosencephaly shows absence of the anterior interhemispheric fissure. The frontal lobes are fused across the midline. **B:** MR angiogram, frontal view, in the same patient shows that a single (azygous) ACA (*arrows*) arises from the right internal carotid artery and supplies both frontal lobes.

Multichanneled Anterior Cerebral Artery

More than two A2 segments may be found in some cases. A triple ACA probably represents two normal A2 segments plus persistence of the embryonic median artery of the corpus callosum (Fig. 6-10). The reported incidence of a so-called duplicated ACA varies from 2% to 13% (26).

Persistent Primitive Olfactory Artery

Persistence of a primitive olfactory artery results in an anomalous vessel that is associated with a longer than usual ACoA. The recurrent artery of Heubner is absent. There is a high prevalence of aneurysm formation associated with this and other ACA anomalies (5).

Aberrant Branches

Occasionally vessels with an aberrant origin from the ACA occur. Reported cases include an *ophthalmic artery* and *accessory middle cerebral artery* originating from the A1 segment.

ANTERIOR CEREBRAL ARTERY: DISTAL (A3 TO A5) SEGMENTS

Normal Gross Anatomy

A3 Segment

This segment extends around the corpus callosum genu. Many investigators include both the distal ACA and its cortical branches as the A3 segment (see box below) (26).

A4 and A5 Segments

Other investigators have described two addition segments (A4 and A5) that course above the corpus callosum and are separated by the plane of the coronal fissure (3).

Relationships

Summary

1. The A3 segment curves *around* the corpus callosum genu (Fig. 6-3).
2. As it courses above the corpus callosum, the distal ACA runs *under* the inferior free margin of the falx cerebri (Fig. 6-15).
3. The cortical branches that arise from the distal ACA run along the surface of the medial hemisphere *adjacent* to the falx (Fig. 6-1).

Branches

The A2 segments terminate near the junction of the corpus callosum rostrum and genu. At this point the distal ACA often appears to bifurcate into two main vessels. The larger of these two vessels, the *pericallosal artery*, represents the continuation of the main ACA trunk. It courses posteriorly at a variable distance above the corpus callosum (Fig. 6-3).

The *callosomarginal artery* passes over the cingulate gyrus and runs posteriorly within the cingulate sulcus. A discrete callosomarginal artery is present in approximately 50% of cerebral angiograms.

The last, most distal group of ACA branches supplies much of the medial cortex. Collectively this group of vessels is called the *parietal branches*. These vessels supply the

---

Distal Segments of the Anterior Cerebral Artery: Normal Anatomy and Variations

Normal development
  Outgrowths from primitive internal carotid arteries
Gross anatomy
  Distal ACA and cortical branches (A3 segments)
  ACA curves around and above corpus callosum genu
  Runs posterosuperiorly within interhemispheric fissure
Key relationships
  Distal ACA runs under falx cerebri
Branches
  Pericallosal artery
    Distal continuation of main ACA trunk
    Courses above corpus callosum body
    Splenial branches anastomose with corresponding branches from PCA

Callosomarginal artery
  Present in 50% of cases
  Runs posteriorly within cingulate sulcus
Parietal branches
  Terminal cortical branches
Vascular territory
  Anterior two thirds of medial hemisphere
  Variably sized (usually small) strip of cortex over convexity
  Corpus callosum body
Variants
  Distal ACA may supply part of contralateral hemisphere
Anomalies
  Rare

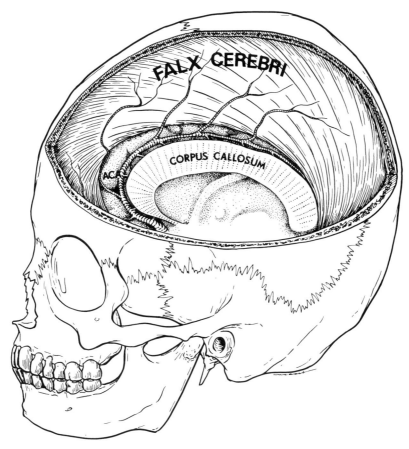

FIG. 6-15. Diagrammatic sketch depicts the distal anterior cerebral artery (ACA) and its relationship with the falx cerebri and corpus callosum. Note that the distance between the pericallosal artery and the inferior (free) edge of the falx decreases as the ACA courses posteriorly. When a mass lesion is present, the relatively rigid falx will prevent significant midline displacement of brain and blood vessels posteriorly. But anteriorly, the height of the falx is comparatively attenuated. This permits considerable displacement of brain and vessels under its free edge near the corpus callosum genu.

precuneus and the adjacent convexity as well as the medial surface of the hemisphere above the corpus callosum (14).

Vascular Territory and Anastomoses

The ACA typically supplies the anterior two thirds of the medial brain surface and a small strip of cortex that extends a variable distance over the convexity (see Fig. 6-5). Via small pial branches, the ACA cortical branches anastomose with other cerebral arteries across the so-called vascular *watershed* zone. The watershed zone represents the confluence of the anterior, middle, and posterior cerebral artery territories (14,16–18,27–30) (Fig. 6-10B; also see Fig. 7-12).

Normal Angiographic Anatomy

Lateral Views

The two main distal ACA branches, the callosomarginal and pericallosal arteries, can usually be identified in

this projection. The callosomarginal artery courses above the cingulate gyrus, whereas the pericallosal artery runs in the callosal sulcus, just above the body of the corpus callosum (Figs. 6-2, 6-3, and 6-16) (27).

The distal ACA branches are usually overlapped by the middle cerebral artery branches on the lateral view, making it difficult to identify and name the smaller cortical branches. In addition, distal branching of the pericallosal and callosomarginal arteries is quite variable. ACA branches are now named by their terminal area of distribution instead of by their proximal origin (e.g., orbitofrontal, frontal, and parietal branches).

Anteroposterior View

The pericallosal and callosomarginal arteries may be difficult to distinguish from each other in this projection. The callosomarginal artery is often more serpentine in appearance, whereas the pericallosal artery usually has a somewhat straighter course (Figs. 6-1, 6-6, and 6-17A).

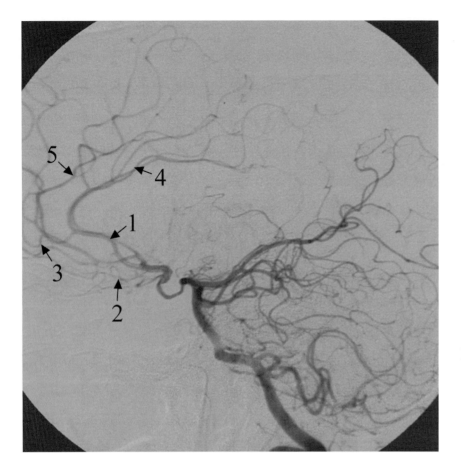

FIG. 6-16. Left vertebral angiogram, arterial phase, lateral view. Contrast reflux through a large posterior communicating artery opacifies the anterior cerebral arteries (ACAs) and their branches. The middle cerebral artery does not fill, permitting an unobstructed view of the ACAs. Compare with Fig. 6-3.

1, A2 (vertical or postcommunicating) ACA segment
2, Orbitofrontal branches
3, Frontopolar arteries
4, Pericallosal arteries
5, Callosomarginal arteries

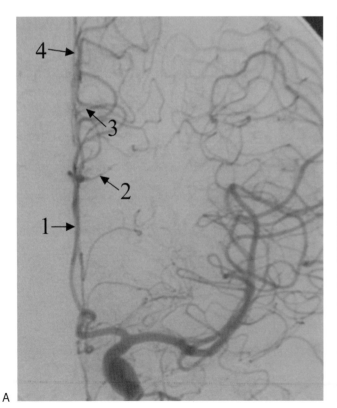

A

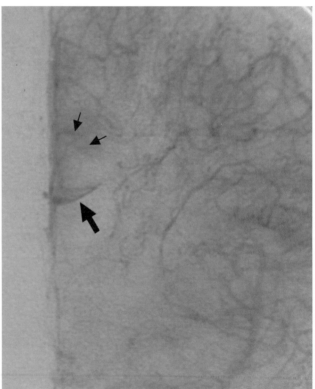

B

FIG. 6-17. Left internal carotid angiogram, early (A) and late (B) arterial phase, anteroposterior view. The distal ACA segment and branches are shown.

1, A2 ACA
2, Pericallosal artery (note the "smile" on the late arterial phase (B, *large arrow*)
3, Callosomarginal artery. Note the "moustache" on the late arterial phase (B, *small arrows*)
4, Cortical branches

A vascular pial plexus that covers the dorsal aspect of the corpus callosum arises from the pericallosal artery. On the late arterial phase of cerebral angiograms, this pial plexus may have a striking vascular blush that resembles a smile; the callosomarginal branches may form a "moustache" (Fig. 6-17B).

Variations and Anomalies

Normal Variants

Variations of the distal ACA are common, reported in one fourth to two thirds of anatomic specimens (2). In the most common variation, a distal ACA on one side sends some branches to a small area on the medial surface of the contralateral hemisphere. This can be seen in 64% of brain dissections (2).

Anomalies

True anomalies of the distal ACA are uncommon. An unusual communication between the two distal ACAs near the corpus callosum has been described. This anomaly, a *superior anterior communicating artery*, has been associated with an increased risk of aneurysm (31).

REFERENCES

1. Perlmutter D, Rhoton AL Jr. Microsurgical anatomy of the anterior-cnerebral-anterior communicating-recurrent artery complex. *J Neurosurg* 1976;45:259–272.
2. Perlmutter D, Rhoton AL Jr. Microsurgical anatomy of the distal anterior cerebral artery. *J Neurosurg* 1978;49:204–228.
3. Morris P. The anterior cerebral artery. In: *Practical neuroangiography.* Baltimore: Williams & Wilkins, 1997:165–181.
4. Padget DH. Development of cranial arteries in human embryo. *Contrib Embryol* 1948;32:205–262.
5. Tsuji T, Abe M, Tabuchi K. Aneurysm of a persistent primitive olfactory artery. *J Neurosurg* 1995;83:138–140.
6. Truwit CL. Embryology of the cerebral vasculature. *Neuroimag Clin North Am* 1994;4:663–689.
7. Dunker RO, Harris AB. Surgical anatomy of the proximal anterior cerebral artery. *J Neurosurg* 1976;44:359–367.
8. Marinkovic S, Milisavljevic M, Kovacevic M. Anatomical bases for surgical approach to the initial segment of the anterior cerebral artery. *Surg Radiol Anat* 1986;8:7–18.
9. Marinkovic S, Gibo H, Milisavljevic M. The surgical anatomy of the relationships between the perforating and leptomeningeal arteries. *Neurosurgery* 1996;39:72–83.
10. Serizawa T, Saeki N, Yamaura A. Microsurgical anatomy and clinical significance of the anterior communicating artery and its perforating branches. *Neurosurgery* 1997;40:1211–1218.
11. Ture U, Yasargil G, Krisht AF. The arteries of the corpus callosum: a microsurgical anatomic study. *Neurosurgery* 1996;39:1075–1085.
12. Mercier Ph, Fournier D, Brassier G, et al. The perforating arteries of the anterior part of the circle of Willis. *Riv Neuroradiol* 1944;7(Suppl): 79–83.
13. Williams PL, ed. Internal carotid artery. In: *Gray's anatomy*, 38th ed. New York: Churchill Livingstone, 1995:1523–1529.
14. Gloger S, Gloger A, Vogt H, Kretschmann H-J. Computer-assisted 3D reconstruction of the terminal branches of the cerebral arteries. I. Anterior cerebral artery. *Neuroradiology* 1995;36:173–180.
15. Ghika JA, Bogousslavsky J, Regli F. Deep perforators from the carotid system: template of the vascular territories. *Arch Neurol* 1990;47: 1097–1100.
16. van der Zwan A, Hillen B, Tulleken CAF, et al. Variability of the major cerebral arteries. *J Neurosurg* 1992;77:927–940.
17. Hayman LA, Taber KH, Hurley RA, Naidich TP. An imaging guide to the lobar and arterial vascular divisions of the brain. Part I: Sectional anatomy. *IJNR* 1997;3:175–179.
18. Hayman LA, Taber KH, Hurley RA, Naidich TP. An imaging guide to the lobar and arterial vascular divisions of the brain. Part II: Surface brain anatomy. *IJNR* 1997;3:256–261.
19. Graves VB. Advancing loop technique for endovascular access to the anterior cerebral artery. *AJNR* 1998;19:778–780.
20. Bollar A, Martinez R, Gelabert M, Garcia A. Anomalous origin of the anterior cerebral artery associated with aneurysm—embryological considerations. *Neuroradiology* 1988;30:86.
21. Mancuso P, Chiaramonte I, Alessandrello R, et al. Infraoptic course of the anterior cerebral artery. *Riv Neuroradiol* 1996;9:329–332.
22. Mercier PH, Velut S, Fournier D, et al. A rare embryologic variation: carotid-anterior cerebral artery anastomosis or infraoptic course of the anterior cerebral artery. *Surg Radiol Anat* 1989;11:73–77.
23. Odake G. Carotid-anterior cerebral artery anastomosis with aneurysm: case report and review of the literature. *Neurosurgery* 1988;23:654–658.
24. Ladzinski P, Maliszewski M, Majchrzak H. The accessory anterior cerebral artery: case report and anatomic analysis of vascular anomaly. *Surg Neurol* 1997;48:171–174.
25. Cinnamon J, Zito J, Chalif DJ, et al. Aneurysm of the azygos pericallosal artery: diagnosis by MR imaging and MR angiography. *AJNR* 1992;13:280–282.
26. Osborn AG. The anterior cerebral artery. In: *Diagnostic neuroradiology*. St. Louis: Mosby, 1994:132–136.
27. Ring BA, Waddington MM. Roentgenographic anatomy of the pericallosal arteries. *AJR* 1968;104:109–118.
28. Berman SA, Hayman LA, Hinck VC. Correlation of CT cerebral vascular territories with function: I. Anterior cerebral artery. *AJNR* 1980;1:259–263.
29. Savoiardo M. The vascular territories of the carotid and vertebrobasilar systems. Diagrams based on CT studies of infarcts. *Ital J Neurol Sci* 1986;7:405–409.
30. Kazui S, Sawada T, Naritomi H. Angiographic evaluation of brain infarction limited to the anterior cerebral artery territory. *Stroke* 1993; 24:549–553.
31. Yasargil MG, Carter LP. Saccular aneurysms of the distal anterior cerebral artery. *J Neurosurg* 1974;40:218–223.

CHAPTER 7

The Middle Cerebral Artery

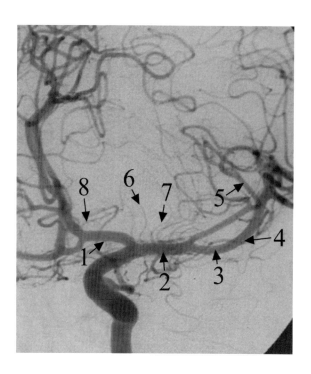

The middle cerebral artery (MCA) is the larger of the two terminal internal carotid artery branches. Because it supplies an extensive area that includes most of the lateral surface of the cerebral hemispheres, ischemic disease and infarcts most commonly involve this vascular territory. The MCA is also a common site for aneurysms and vascular malformations. Therefore, thorough knowledge of the normal gross and angiographic anatomy of the MCA is requisite for complete, correct interpretation of cerebral angiograms.

The MCA is divided anatomically into four segments (Fig. 7-1) (1):

M1 = horizontal segment
M2 = insular segments
M3 = opercular segments
M4 = cortical branches, also termed the M4 segments

In this chapter, the proximal (M1) segment and its penetrating branches are first considered. Also included are the MCA trunks (M2 segments) that lie deep within the lateral (sylvian) fissure. The second section delineates the opercular (M3) segments. This chapter closes with a brief discussion of the cortical (M4) MCA branches and their vascular territories.

THE MIDDLE CEREBRAL ARTERY: PROXIMAL (M1 AND M2) SEGMENTS

Normal Development

Middle cerebral artery development is intimately related to development of the sylvian (lateral cerebral) fissure and insula (2).

Sylvian (Lateral Cerebral) Fissure and Insula

Between 8 and 12 weeks' gestation a slight triangular-shaped depression appears on the lateral aspect of each developing cerebral hemisphere (Fig. 7-2A). Further deepening and infolding of this shallow fossa forms the future insula (island of Reil). As the infolding progresses, the frontal and parietal lobes begin to overlap the insula from above while the temporal lobe overlaps it from below (Fig. 7-2B). Eventually, apposition of the superiorly located frontoparietal and the inferiorly located temporal lobe operculae completely covers the insula and forms the lateral cerebral fissure (Fig. 7-2C and D). The fully developed sylvian fissure has both a superficial and a deep component. The superficial part is visible on the brain surface. The deep part, sometimes referred to as the sylvian cistern, is buried by the over-

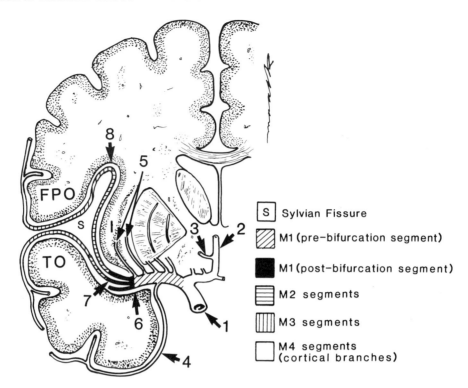

FIG. 7-1. Anteroposterior anatomic diagram depicts the middle cerebral artery (MCA) and its four main segments. For purposes of simplification, only one or two branches are depicted and the sylvian fissure is exaggerated. The main MCA trunk (also called the horizontal or M1 segment) extends from the internal carotid artery bifurcation to the sylvian fissure and includes both pre- and postbifurcation segments. The MCA genu or knee is the point at which the MCA begins to curve posterosuperiorly over the insula. The M2 segments extend from the genu to the top of the sylvian fissure and circular sulcus. The M3 segments begin here and extend laterally through the sylvian fissure. The M4 segments represent the cortical MCA branches as they exit the sylvian fissure and curve over the frontal, temporal, and parietal operculae. FPO, frontoparietal operculae; TO, temporal operculum; I, insula.

1, Internal carotid artery
2, Anterior cerebral artery
3, Recurrent artery of Heubner (ACA branch)
4, Anterior temporal artery (MCA branch)
5, Lateral lenticulostriate arteries (MCA branches)
6, MCA bifurcation/trifurcation
7, MCA knee (genu)
8, Top of the sylvian fissure (and upper limit of the circular sulcus)

lapping operculae and is thus hidden below the surface (1).

Middle Cerebral Artery

Before the insula and sylvian fissure form, cortical branches of the MCA ramify directly over the lateral surfaces of the cerebral hemispheres. At this stage of development these branches appear to course almost vertically from their origin at the terminal internal cerebral artery (ICA) bifurcation (Fig. 7-2A). As the frontal, parietal, and temporal lobes are formed and the lateral fissure begins to develop, the MCA branches follow the deepening depression that will form the insula (Fig. 7-2B).

Progressive infolding of the insular cortex and the overlying MCA branches causes these vessels first to curve into the sylvian fissure and course over the insula, then to turn laterally through the lips of the apposed frontal, parietal, and temporal operculae to ramify over the lateral surface of the cerebral hemispheres. At birth, the MCA has essentially attained an adult configuration (Fig. 7-2C and D).

Gross Anatomy

The MCA arises as the larger of the two terminal branches of the internal carotid artery (Fig. 7-3). At its

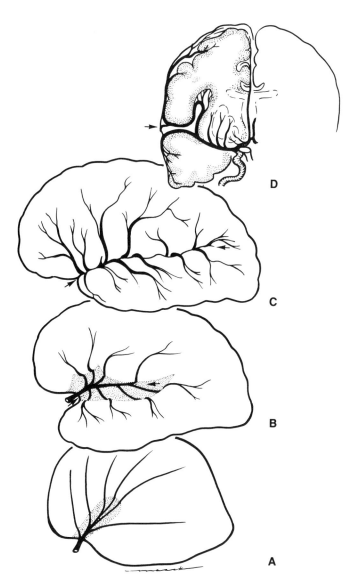

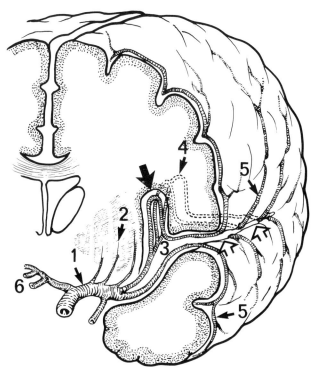

FIG. 7-3. Cutaway anatomic drawing shows the middle cerebral artery (MCA) and its relationship to adjacent structures. The sylvian fissure has been exaggerated so that the MCA loops over the insula, and operculae can be depicted clearly. The top of the sylvian fissure is indicated by the large black arrow. Exit of the MCA branches from the lateral aspect of the sylvian fissure is indicated by the open arrows.

1, M1 (horizontal) MCA segment
2, Lateral lenticulostriate arteries
3, Sylvian fissure (large black arrow indicates the top of the circular sulcus, where the M3 segments begin by turning inferolaterally to course toward the surface of the brain)
4, MCA loops within the sylvian fissure (*solid and dotted lines*). These loops form the top of the angiographic sylvian triangle
5, Opercular (M4 or cortical) MCA branches
6, Anterior cerebral arteries (cut off; shown for perspective)

FIG. 7-2. Anatomic drawing depicts formation of the insula and sylvian fissure (*arrows*) in the fetal brain. Note the effect that alteration in these underlying structures has on the developing middle cerebral artery (MCA). **A:** Fetal brain at 13 to 14 gestational weeks, seen from the lateral perspective. The MCA branches follow nearly a straight course over the surface of the brain. The insula (*dotted area*) is beginning to appear as a small fossa or shallow depression on the cortical surface. **B:** At 24 weeks the sylvian fissure deepens and begins to cover the insula (*dotted area*). The MCA branches, following the surface of the brain, also begin to invaginate inward. **C:** Brain at term. The insula is completely buried within the sylvian fissure. Branches of the MCA course upward over the insula to the top of the sylvian fissure (circular sulcus) but then must turn laterally to escape the sylvian fissure. **D:** Cutaway view of the brain in frontal section. Note how the horizontal part of the MCA (M1 segment) courses laterally. When it reaches the limen insulae, it forms a knee or genu as it curves around this structure. The M2 segment curves upward and over the insula. The M3 segments start at the top (and, in the case of the temporal branches, the bottom) of the insula and course laterally through the sylvian fissure. They become the M4 segments (cortical branches) when they exit the fissure and ramify over the hemispheres.

origin, the MCA is approximately twice the size of the anterior cerebral artery (ACA).

M1 Segment

The horizontal (M1) segment extends from its origin at the ICA bifurcation to the sylvian fissure (Figs. 7-1 and 7-3) (See box on page 138). It consists of two parts, pre- and postbifurcation segments. The prebifurcation segment comprises a single main trunk that extends laterally from the MCA origin to its bifurcation. This segment runs just below the APS.

MCA trunks turn upward in a gentle curve, forming its so-called *genu* or "knee" (Fig. 7-1).

Proximal Segments of the Middle Cerebral Artery: Normal Anatomy and Variations

Normal development
MCAs are derived from primitive internal carotid arteries
MCAs begin as vessels on surface of embryonic telencephalon
Formation of insula causes progressive infolding of MCAs
Gross anatomy
Horizontal or proximal MCA (M1 segment)
Prebifurcation segment
Postbifurcation segment
MCA bi- or trifurcates before reaching genu
Insular part of MCA (M2 segment)
Turns posterosuperiorly at genu
Divides into six to eight major stem arteries
Key relationships
M1 segments course laterally under anterior perforated substance (APS)
M2 segments course within sylvian fissure, over insula
Branches
Perforating branches
Lenticulostriate arteries (mostly lateral)
Cortical branches
Anterior temporal artery
Vascular territory
Perforating branches
Most of caudate nucleus, internal capsule
Most of basal ganglia
Cortical branches
Anterior pole of temporal lobe
Normal variants
Early bifurcating MCA
Anomalies
Accessory MCA (may have increased prevalence of aneurysm)
Duplicated or fenestrated MCA
Hypoplasia, aplasia very rare

M2 Segment

The M2 (insular) segments begin as the main MCA trunks turn posterosuperiorly at the genu (Fig. 7-1). The greatest branching of the MCA occurs near the anterior part of the insula just distal to the genu (1). The M2 part of the MCA thus consists of six to eight major *stem arteries* that lie over the insula and terminate at the top of the circular sulcus (Figs. 7-3 and 7-4).

Relationships

Summary

The proximal MCA:

1. Originates from the ICA bifurcation near the medial end of the lateral cerebral (sylvian) fissure.
2. The M1 segment is *lateral* to the optic chiasm and *behind* the olfactory trigone.
3. The M1 segment courses horizontally *below* the anterior perforated substance (APS).
3. At the limen insulae, the M1 segment ends by turning *posterosuperiorly* to form the knee or genu.
4. The six to eight stem arteries that comprise the M2 segments course *within* the lateral cerebral fissure, *over* the insula.
5. The M2 segments end at the top of the sylvian fissure when they reach the limits of the circular sulcus.

Branches

The proximal MCA has both central (penetrating) and cortical branches.

Penetrating Branches

A number of small but important central perforating arteries called the *lenticulostriate arteries* arise from the M1 segment. These vessels course superiorly through the APS to supply the basal ganglia and other deep structures of the brain (Fig. 7-1) (3).

The lenticulostriate arteries are divided into a smaller medial group that arises from the proximal MCA near the ICA bifurcation and a larger lateral group that originates from the distal half of the M1 segment. The *medial (lenticulo)striate arteries* enter the APS and ascend directly through the lentiform nucleus to supply it, the caudate nucleus, and the internal capsule. The *lateral (lenticulo)striate arteries* curve over the lentiform nucleus as they ascend within the external capsule. They then turn medially to traverse the basal ganglia and supply the caudate nucleus.

The MCA divides approximately 10 to 12 mm from its origin. The postbifurcation trunks of the M1 segment follow a nearly parallel course, diverging only minimally prior to reaching the MCA genu. In the majority of cases, the MCA divides proximal to the genu. The main MCA trunk *bifurcates* in 78% of anatomic specimens and *trifurcates* in 12%. In 10% of cases, it divides by giving rise to multiple trunks (1).

Near the limen insulae (a small gyrus located near the anteroinferior corner of the insula), the postbifurcation

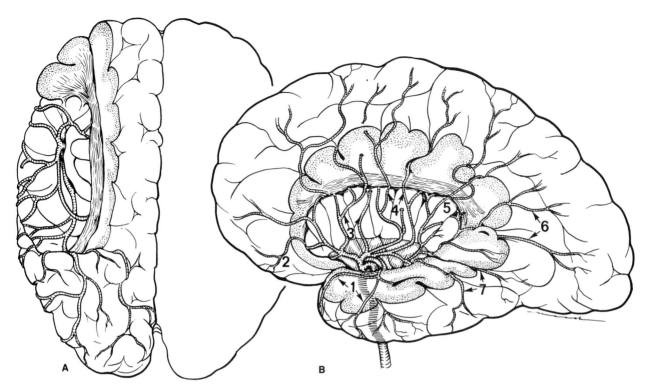

FIG. 7-4. Anatomic drawings depict the relationship of the MCA branches to the insula, sylvian fissure, and cortical surfaces of the hemisphere. The operculae have been partially dissected to display the MCA. **A:** Superior view. **B:** Lateral view.

1, Anterior temporal artery
2, Orbitofrontal artery
3, Operculofrontal arteries (sometimes called the "candelabra" because their angiographic appearance resembles a branched candlestick)
4, Central sulcus arteries (rolandic group)
5, Posterior parietal artery
6, Angular artery and branches
7, Posterior temporal artery

One or more large perforating arteries arise from the MCA after its bifurcation in nearly half of all anatomic dissections (4).

Cortical Branches

Cortical branches arise both from the main (M1) MCA segment and the two or more trunks that are formed by its bifurcation, trifurcation, or division into multiple trunks (Fig. 7-1).

The *anterior temporal artery* is a variably sized branch that usually arises from the M1 segment before its bifurcation (see Figs. 7-1 and 7-12). The anterior temporal artery arises from the main MCA trunk at approximately the same level as the lenticulostriate arteries. It passes directly anteriorly and inferiorly over the temporal tip and usually does not enter the sylvian fissure itself.

Vascular Territory

The vascular territory of all the MCA segments and their branches is described in the last section of this chapter (see Figs. 7-13 and 7-14).

Normal Angiographic Anatomy

Anteroposterior Projection

The proximal (M1) MCA segment and its bifurcation or trifurcation is best visualized on either anteroposterior (AP) or submentovertex views. The M1 segment usually follows a relatively straight horizontal course from its origin at the ICA to its entrance into the lateral cerebral (sylvian) fissure (Fig. 7-5A). However, in neonates or very young patients the M1 segment may course quite superiorly (Fig. 7-5B), whereas in older patients it often describes a pronounced sinusoidal or inferior oblique curvature (Fig. 7-5C).

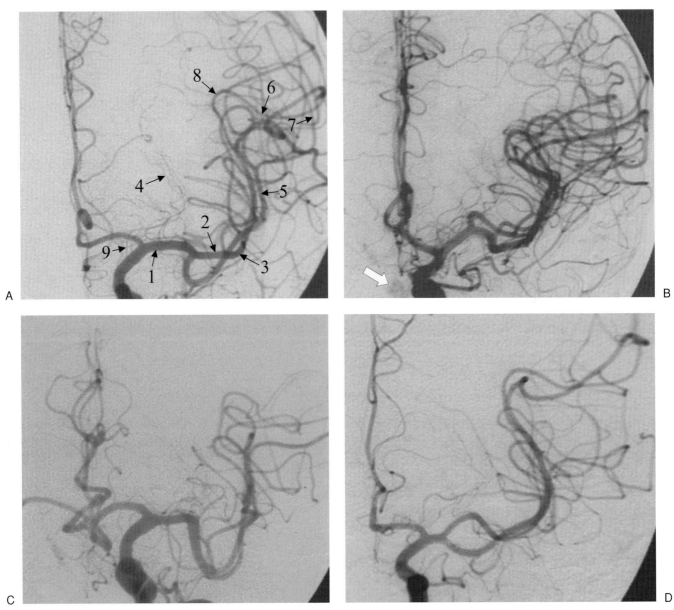

FIG. 7-5. A series of carotid angiograms obtained in the anteroposterior (AP) projection demonstrates the wide but normal variability in the proximal middle cerebral artery (MCA). **A:** In the usual configuration, the first (horizontal or M1) MCA segment follows a relatively straight course toward the sylvian fissure. **B:** In a 19-year-old patient the proximal M1 segment angles superiorly (the pituitary gland, indicated by the open arrow, has a prominent but normal vascular blush). **C:** In this elderly patient the horizontal segments of both the anterior and middle cerebral arteries are very tortuous. D: If an MCA bifurcates within 10 mm of its origin from the internal carotid artery, it is called an early bifurcating MCA. This is a normal variant.

1, M1 segment (prebifurcation segment)
2, M1 segment (postbifurcation segment)
3, MCA genu
4, Penetrating MCA branches (lateral lenticulostriate arteries)
5, M2 segment
6, M3 segment
7, M4 segment (cortical branches as they ramify over the hemisphere)
8, Apex of sylvian fissure (angiographic sylvian point)
9, Anterior choroidal artery (a branch of the distal internal carotid artery)

The lenticulostriate arteries are well seen on both AP and shallow oblique projections. They course superomedially for a short distance as they pierce the APS, then turn superolaterally through the basal ganglia and external capsule following a gentle, laterally convex curve (Fig. 7-6).

The M2 segments begin as the MCA makes a pronounced superior turn at the limen insulae, forming the genu or knee (Figs. 7-1 and 7-3). These segments assume a medially convex configuration as they course upward and over the insula (Figs. 7-5 and 7-6). The M2 branches turn inferolaterally as they reach the apex of the circular sulcus (the cerebrospinal cistern that courses around the insula). They then become the M3 segments.

Lateral Projection

The M1 segment is not easily observed in the lateral projection. However, the M2 (insular) branches are seen as they course posterosuperiorly across the insula to reach the top of the sylvian fissure (Fig. 7-7A).

Sylvian Point and Sylvian Triangle

The highest and most medial point where the last cortical MCA branch (usually the angular artery) turns infer-olaterally to exit the sylvian fissure is termed the *angiographic sylvian point*. This point approximates the apex of the insula and represents the posterior limit of the lateral cerebral sulcus (Fig. 7-7B).

On anteroposterior views the sylvian points of both MCAs should appear similar in position (Fig. 7-8). Significant asymmetry indicates either volume loss or a mass (see Chapter 14). On lateral cerebral angiograms the *angiographic sylvian triangle* is demarcated by the superior insular line (a line tangent to the tops of the insular loops), the main MCA trunk (which forms the posterior-inferior margin of the triangle), and the most anterior branch of the ascending frontal complex (which forms the anterior border of the triangle) (Fig. 7-7B). Displacements of the angiographic sylvian point and triangle commonly occur with intracranial masses (see Chapter 14).

Brain Stain

A prominent vascular blush in the basal ganglia and cortex can sometimes be seen during the late arterial phase of carotid angiograms (see Fig. 7-12). This is a normal finding and should not be mistaken for a neoplasm.

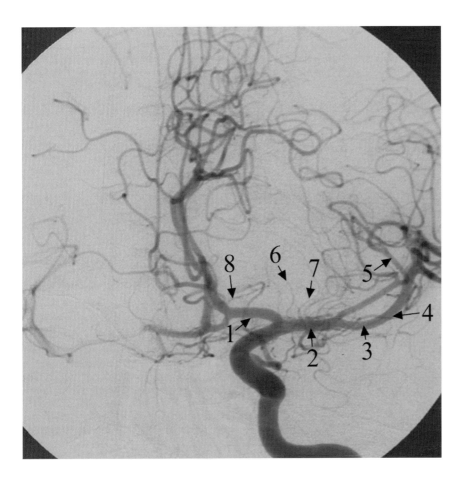

FIG. 7-6. Left internal carotid angiogram, oblique view, shows the striate arteries unusually well. The medial lenticulostriate arteries arise from the horizontal (A1) segment of the anterior cerebral artery (ACA); the lateral lenticulostriate arteries arise from the M1 segment of the middle cerebral artery (MCA). The lateral striate arteries course through the external capsule and putamen, describing a gentle laterally convex curve.

1, A1 segment, ACA
2, Prebifurcation M1 segment, MCA
3, Postbifurcation M1 segment, MCA
4, MCA genu
5, M2 MCA segments
6, Medial lenticulostriate arteries
7, Lateral lenticulostriate arteries
8, Recurrent artery of Heubner (this vessel usually arises from the A2 ACA segment, as it does here)

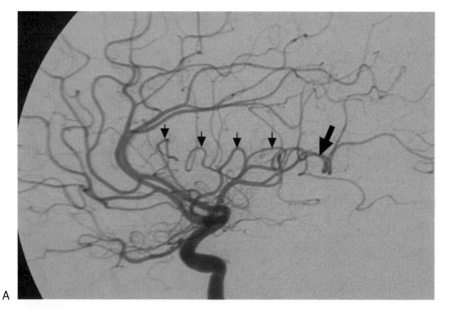

A

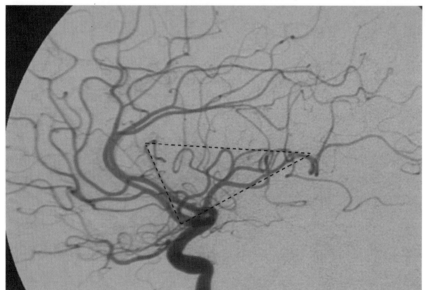

B

FIG. 7-7. Left internal carotid angiogram, lateral view, shows the MCA within the sylvian fissure. **A:** The M2 segments (*solid arrows*) course superiorly toward the top of the circular sulcus. The M2 segments loop within the roof of the sylvian fissure and demarcate the insula. These loops, indicated by open arrows, should form a relatively straight line. This line forms the top of the so-called angiographic sylvian triangle. The sylvian point (*large arrow*) is the highest and most medial point where the last cortical branch (usually the angular artery) turns to exit the sylvian fissure. **B:** The same view is now shown with the sylvian triangle indicated by dotted lines. The top of the triangle is formed by a line drawn tangential to the insular loops. This superior insular line should lie about half way between the petrous internal carotid artery and the inner table of the skull. Displacement or deformation of the angiographic sylvian triangle usually indicates an intracranial mass (see Chapter 16).

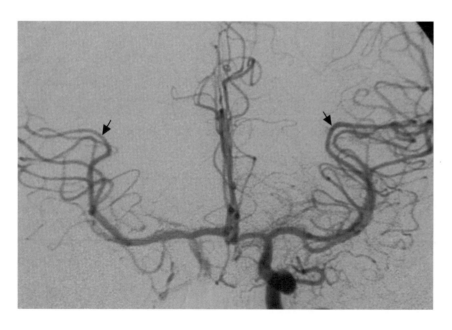

FIG. 7-8. Left internal carotid angiogram, anteroposterior view, performed with temporary cross-compression of the right common carotid artery. Contrast has refluxed across the anterior communicating artery and opacified the right middle cerebral artery. Note that the angiographic sylvian points (*arrows*) appear symmetrically positioned.

Normal Variants and Anomalies

Middle cerebral artery branching patterns are normally quite variable, whereas true anomalies of this vessel are uncommon, seen in only 1% to 3% of anatomic dissections (1,5) and less than 1% of cerebral angiograms (6).

Normal Variants

In most patients the MCA bifurcates (50% of cases) or trifurcates (25% of cases) near the insula (see Fig. 5-12B). So-called early division of the M1 segment is not unusual (Fig. 7-5D). A large anterior temporal artery may arise from the proximal M1 segment (Fig. 7-9). This normal variant should not be mistaken for an accessory MCA (an anomaly that is associated with an increased risk of aneurysm formation).

Anomalies

Hypoplasia and *aplasia* of the MCA are rare anomalies (7). *MCA duplication* occurs when a large MCA branch arises from the ICA prior to its terminal bifurcation. The duplicated vessel parallels the course of the main M1 segment, running below it (Fig. 7-10A) (8). This anomaly occurs in 1% to 3% of anatomic dissections. A duplicated MCA typically supplies the anterior temporal lobe (6). A duplicated MCA should not be confused with early branching of the MCA. In the latter configuration, considered a normal variant, the MCA bifurcates close to its origin from the ICA (Fig. 7-10B). An *accessory middle cerebral artery* (AccMCA) is an MCA branch that arises from the ACA and parallels the M1 segment. An AccMCA supplies the anterior-inferior frontal lobe. This anomaly is identified in 2.7% of cases (9). An AccMCA should be distinguished from a large recurrent artery of Heubner (10). MCA anomalies such as AccMCA have been associated with aneurysm formation (7,10,11).

Other uncommon MCA anomalies include partial duplication or *fenestrated MCA* (Fig. 7-11A), *anomalous origin of MCA branches* (Fig. 7-11B), and a *single nonbifurcating MCA trunk* (5).

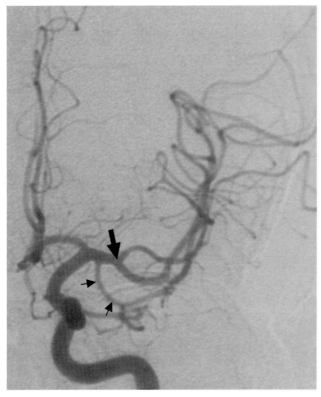

FIG. 7-9. Left internal carotid angiogram, anteroposterior view, shows an early bifurcating middle cerebral artery (*large arrow*). Note the prominent anterior temporal artery (*small arrows*) that arises from the M1 segment just after its origin from the internal carotid artery. This should not be mistaken for an accessory or duplicated MCA (see Fig. 7-10).

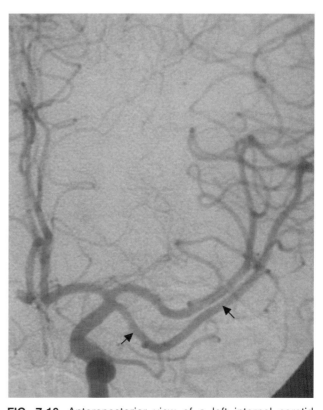

FIG. 7-10. Anteroposterior view of a left internal carotid angiogram shows a duplicated middle cerebral artery (MCA) (*arrows*). In this anomaly a large branch arises from the distal ICA just before its terminal bifurcation. The duplicated MCA branch parallels the main MCA trunk.

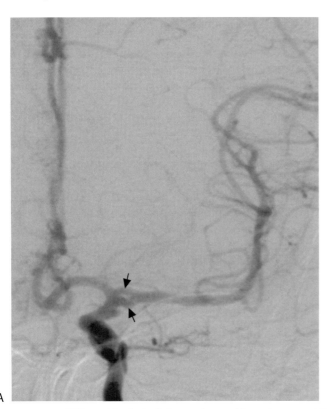
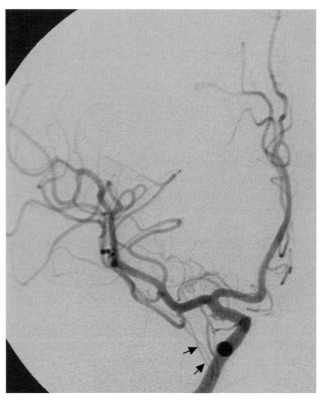

A

B

FIG. 7-11. A: Left internal carotid angiogram, AP view, shows a fenestrated middle cerebral artery (*arrows*) (case courtesy of J. Rees). **B:** Right internal carotid angiogram (oblique view) in another patient shows a number of small vessels (*arrows*) that arise from the cavernous internal carotid artery. These vessels are anomalous middle cerebral branches that supply the temporal pole.

MIDDLE CEREBRAL ARTERY: OPERCULAR (M3) SEGMENTS

Normal Gross Anatomy

The M3 (opercular) segments begin at the top of the circular sulcus as the M2 stems turn laterally within the sylvian fissure. The M3 segments end at the surface of the lateral cerebral fissure (see Fig. 7-1 and Box below).

**Distal Segments of the Middle Cerebral Artery:
Normal Anatomy and Variations**

Normal development
  Cortical MCA branches sprout from primitive
    ICAs
  Deepening of sylvian fissure folds MCA over
    insula
Gross anatomy
  Opercular MCA (M3 segment; from top of insula
    to lateral end of sylvian fissure)
  Cortical MCA branches (M4 segments)
Key relationships
  Overhanging frontal, temporal, and parietal
    operculae cause M3 segments to loop at top

of sylvian fissure, then turn laterally to exit
    fissure and course over hemispheres
  Tops of M3 loops form angiographic sylvian
    triangle
Branches
  Anterior cortical branches
    Orbitofrontal artery
    Prefrontal arteries
  Intermediate (central) cortical branches
    Precentral sulcus artery
    Central sulcus (rolandic) artery
    Postcentral sulcus (anterior parietal) artery
  Posterior cortical branches
    Posterior parietal artery
    Angular artery
    Temporooccipital artery
    Temporal arteries (posterior, medial, anterior
      temporal, temporopolar)
Vascular territory
  Most of lateral surface of brain
  Anterior temporal lobe (variable)
Variants, anomalies
  Variations in cortical branching, territories
    common
  True anomalies are rare

Normal Angiographic Appearance

Anteroposterior View

On AP views the M3 segments overlap each other. As a group they can be identified by their lateral course from the insula through the sylvian fissure to the hemisphere surface (Fig. 7-5).

Lateral View

As depicted on lateral cerebral angiograms, the M3 branches often have a characteristic double curve (compare Figs. 7-12 and 7-16). The first curve occurs where the M2 vessels that course upward over the insular surface turn 180 degrees to pass downward under the frontoparietal operculae (Figs. 7-1 and 7-12). These loops

form the top of the angiographic sylvian triangle (Fig. 7-7). The second curve occurs as the MCA branches turn again to exit the sylvian fissure and become the M4 (cortical) branches (see Fig. 7-1).

MIDDLE CEREBRAL ARTERY: CORTICAL BRANCHES (M4 SEGMENTS)

Normal Gross Anatomy

The cortical or *M4 segments* begin at the surface of the sylvian fissure as the distal MCA branches extend over the cortical surface of the hemisphere (Fig. 7-12). The more anterior branches turn sharply upward or downward after exiting the lateral fissure. The intermediate branches follow a gradual posterior incline away from the fissure, and the posterior branches pass backward in nearly the same direction as the long axis of the sylvian fissure (1).

Branches

The proximal MCA (M1 segment) usually bifurcates into six or eight major stem arteries per hemisphere. In turn, each individual stem artery (M2 or M3 segment) typically gives rise to one to five cortical (M4) branches (Fig. 7-12) (1). These branches are conveniently divided into anterior, intermediate, and posterior groups.

Anterior Branches

The *orbitofrontal (lateral frontobasal) artery* supplies the inferior surface of the frontal lobe (Fig. 7-12, arrow 2). The *prefrontal arteries* branch off in a "candelabra" form around the frontal operculum before coursing to the frontal lobe convexity (Fig. 7-12, arrow 3). The prefrontal arteries supply much of the lateral aspect of the frontal lobe anterior to the sylvian triangle. The prefrontal and orbitofrontal territories often overlap (Fig. 7-13) (12).

Intermediate (Central) Branches

The *precentral sulcus (precentral, prerolandic) artery* appears on the posterior part of the frontal lobe or the anterior edge of the parietal operculum. It courses superiorly, giving off one or two main branches between the precentral and central sulci (Fig. 7-12, arrow 4) (13).

The *central sulcus (central, rolandic) artery* consists of one or two branches that extend onto the convexity and course posterosuperiorly between the pre- and postcentral sulci toward the superior margin of the hemisphere (Fig. 7-12, arrow 5). The *anterior parietal (postcentral sulcus) artery* initially follows the postcentral sulcus, then courses in the intraparietal sulcus (Fg. 7-12, arrow 6) (13).

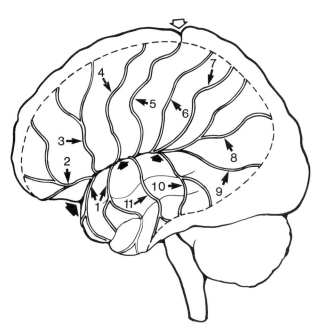

FIG. 7-12. Anatomic drawing depicts the left cerebral hemisphere as seen from the lateral perspective. The central sulcus and sylvian fissure are indicated by the large open and solid arrows, respectively. The M4 MCA segments emerge from the sylvian fissure and ramify over the lateral surface of the hemisphere. Eight to 12 named cortical MCA branches are usually present. The watershed zone, the border between the MCA vascular territory and that of the anterior and posterior cerebral arteries, is shown by the dotted line.

1, Anterior temporal and temporopolar arteries
2, Orbitofrontal artery
3, Prefrontal arteries
4, Precentral sulcus artery
5, Central sulcus artery
6, Anterior parietal (postcentral sulcus) artery
7, Posterior parietal artery
8, Angular artery
9, Temporooccipital artery
10, Posterior temporal arteries
11, Intermedial temporal artery

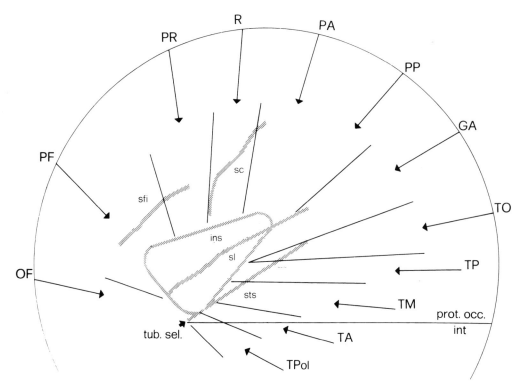

FIG. 7-13. Diagrammatic template depicts cortical (M4) branches of the middle cerebral artery and their vascular territories. tub sel, tuberculum sellae; prot occ int, internal occipital protuberance; OF, orbitofrontal artery; PF, prefrontal artery; PR, precentral or prerolandic artery; R, central or rolandic artery; PA, anterior parietal artery; PP, posterior parietal artery; GA, angular artery; TO, temporooccipital artery; TP, posterior temporal artery; TM, middle temporal artery; TA, anterior temporal artery; TPol, temporal polar artery; Sfi, inferior frontal sulcus; SC, central sulcus; INS, insula; LS, lateral sulcus; Sts, superior temporal sulcus. (Reprinted with permision from Michoty P, Mosco NP, Salamon G. Anatomy of the cortical branches of the MCA. In: Newton TH, Potts DG, eds. *Radiology of the skull and brain.* Vol. 2. St. Louis: Mosby, 1974:1476.)

Posterior Branches

The posterior MCA branches supply much of the parietal lobe as well as part of the temporal and occipital lobes (Fig. 7-13).

The *posterior parietal artery* crosses onto the convexity at the posterior end of the lateral sulcus (sylvian fissure). It courses in a posterosuperior direction and marks the anterior border of the supramarginal gyrus (Fig. 7-12, arrow 7). The *angular artery* is the major terminal MCA branch. It leaves the lateral sulcus in its most posterosuperior portion and crosses Heschl's (transverse temporal) gyrus (Fig. 7-12, arrow 8) (13).

The *temporooccipital artery* courses posteriorly in the superior temporal sulcus to supply the superior temporal gyrus, then branches in the occipital region to supply the lateral surface of the occipital lobe (Fig. 7-12, arrow 9). The *posterior temporal artery* traverses the superior temporal gyrus in a hairpinlike ascent and descent before coursing in the superior temporal sulcus. This branch crosses the middle temporal gyrus into the inferior temporal sulcus to supply the posterior part of the temporal lobe (Fig. 7-12, arrow 10) (13).

The *intermedial temporal (medial temporal) artery* courses across the superior temporal gyrus to the corresponding sulcus, then crosses the middle temporal gyrus to terminate in the inferior temporal sulcus (Fig. 7-12, arrow 11). The *anterior temporal artery*, usually a branch of the M1 segment, crosses the temporal lobe to supply the anterolateral parts of the superior, middle, and inferior temporal gyri (Figs. 7-1 and 7-12, arrow 1) (13). The *temporopolar artery* supplies the temporal pole and may arise separately or as a branch from the anterior temporal artery (Fig. 7-13).

Vascular Territory and Anastomoses

Central (Perforating) Branches

The lenticulostriate branches of the MCA supply the substantia innominata, lateral aspect of the anterior commissure, most of the putamen and lateral globus pallidus, the superior half of the internal capsule and adjacent corona radiata, and the body and head (except the anterior inferior portion) of the caudate nucleus. Portions of the optic radiations and arcuate fasciculus are also supplied by these branches (Fig. 7-14).

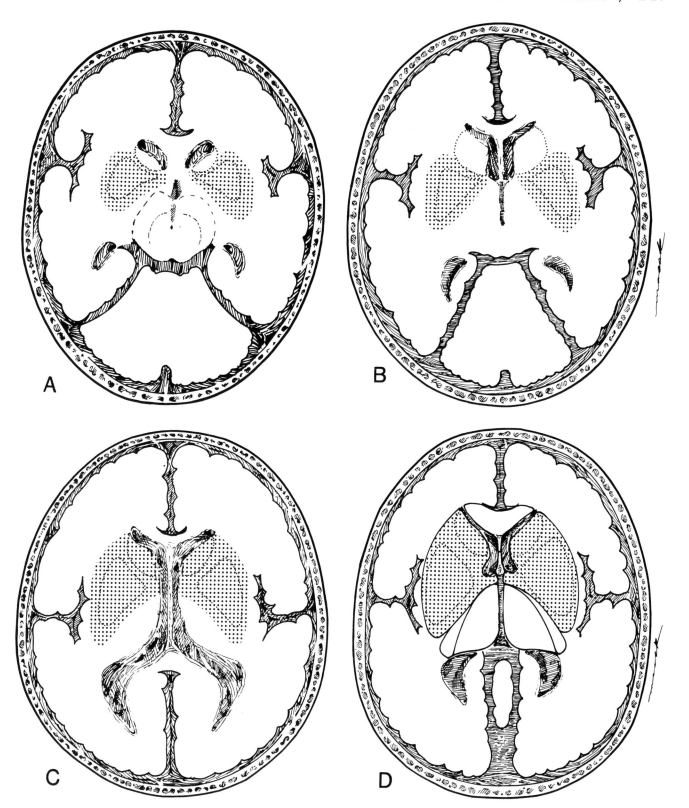

FIG. 7-14. Axial anatomic drawings depict the vascular territory of the MCA perforating branches (mostly the lateral lenticulostriate arteries).

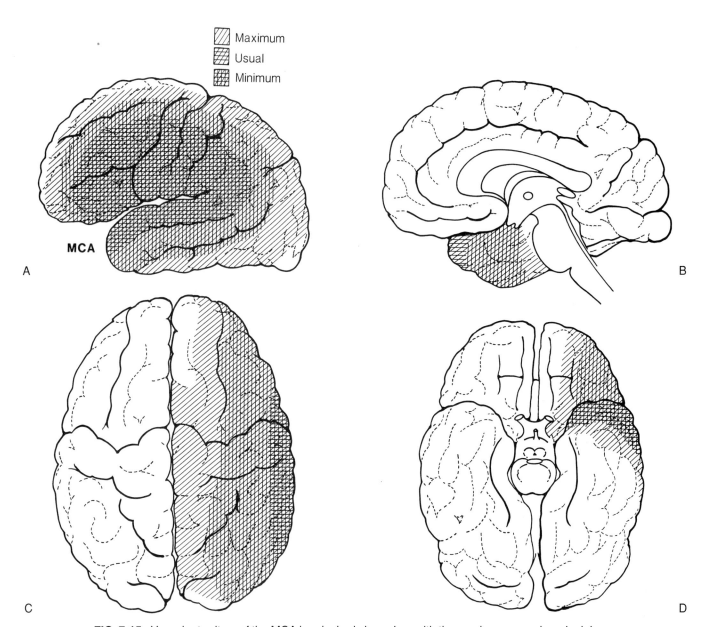

FIG. 7-15. Vascular territory of the MCA hemispheric branches with the maximum, usual, and minimum distributions as delineated by van der Zwan (15). **A:** Lateral view. **B:** Medial view. **C:** Superior view. **D:** Base view. (Reprinted with permission from Osborn AG. *Diagnostic neuroradiology.* St. Louis: Mosby, 1994:138.)

If a large recurrent artery of Heubner or anterior choroidal artery is present, the territory normally supplied by the striate arteries is proportionately smaller (14).

Cortical (Hemispheric) Branches

There is considerable variation in the number, size, and vascular territory of individual MCA cortical branches (15). In general, one (or less commonly, two) cortical arteries supplies each of the 12 major cortical areas (16,17). These cortical regions are shown schematically in Fig. 7-13. The typical, maximum, and minimal MCA cortical territories are shown in Fig. 7-15.

Anastomoses

Cortical MCA branches terminate at the so-called vascular "watershed" or border zone, where they have small pial anastomoses with their counterparts from the anterior and posterior cerebral arteries (Fig. 7-12; also see Figs. 17-1 and 17-3).

Normal Angiographic Appearance

Anteroposterior View

The M4 segments overlap and generally cannot be distinguished from one another on this projection (Fig. 7-16A and B).

Lateral View

The M4 branches are often overlapped by the ACA on this projection. A vascular template (Fig. 7-13) may be helpful in naming the individual branches and delineating their vascular territories. If the ipsilateral ACA is not opacified, the M4 segments are easier to identify (Figs. 7-16C–E).

Normal Variants and Anomalies

Cortical MCA branching patterns vary widely, but true anomalies of the M4 segments are rare.

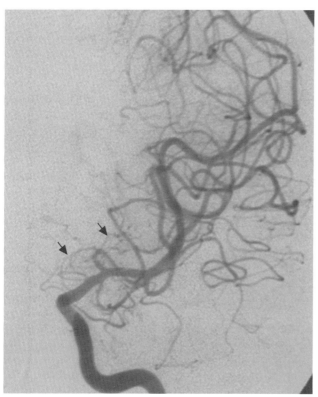
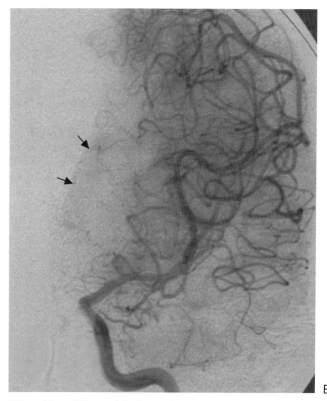

A   B

FIG. 7-16. Left internal carotid angiogram with early **(A)** and late **(B)** arterial phase views performed in the anteroposterior projection show absence of the A1 anterior cerebral artery segment. Therefore, the internal carotid artery essentially ends by becoming the middle cerebral artery (MCA). The lenticulostriate arteries (**A**, *arrows*) are particularly well depicted. Note the prominent vascular "stain" in the basal banglia (**B**, *arrows*), a normal finding that should not be mistaken for ischemia or neoplasm.

(Continued)

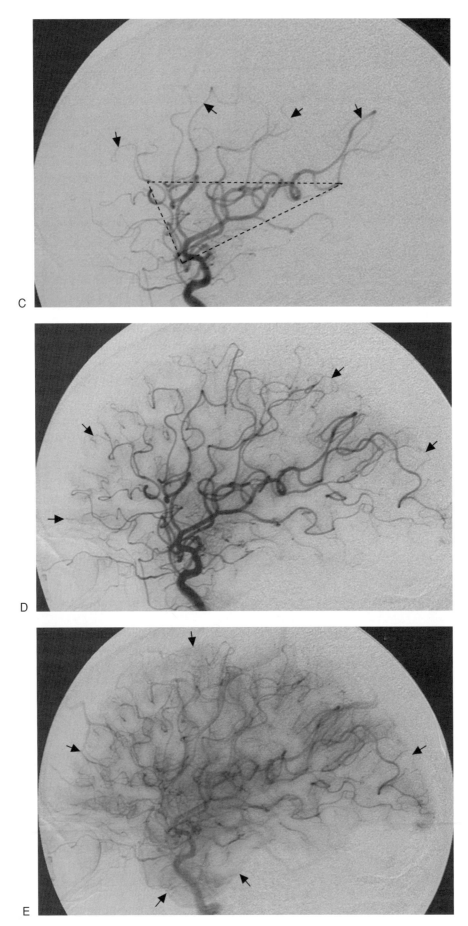

FIG. 7-16. *Continued.* On early **(C)**, mid- **(D)**, and late **(E)** arterial phase views, the vascular distribution of the entire MCA can be appreciated. **C:** The M2 and M3 MCA segments form the angiographic sylvian triangle, indicated here by the dotted lines. Because there is no filling of overlying ACA branches, the M4 segment (MCA cortical branches) is especially well depicted (*arrows*). **D:** On a later phase, the cortical branches are shown as they ramify over the hemisphere and terminate about 1 cm from the cerebral convexity (*arrows*). **E:** The late arterial phase has a distinctive but normal "brain stain" that corresponds to the MCA vascular territory (compare with Figs. 7-12 and 7-14). The edge of the brain stain demarcates the vascular watershed zone, the boundary between the MCA and cortical branches from the anterior and posterior cerebral arteries.

REFERENCES

1. Gibo H, Carver CC, Rhoton AL Jr, et al. Microsurgical anatomy of the middle cerebral artery. *J Neurosurg* 1981;54:151–169.
2. Ring BA. The middle cerebral artery. I. Normal middle cerebral artery. In: Newton TH, Potts DG, eds. *Radiology of the skull and brain: angiography.* St. Louis: Mosby, 1974:1442–1470.
3. Marinkovic S, Gibo H, Milisavljevic M. The surgical anatomy of the relationship between the perforating and the leptomeningeal arteries. *Neurosurgery* 1996;39:72–82.
4. Grand W. Microsurgical anatomy of the proximal middle cerebral artery and the internal carotid artery bifurcation. *Neurosurgery* 1980;7:215–218.
5. Umansky F, Dujovny M, Ausman JI, et al. Anomalies and variations of the middle cerebral artery: a microanatomical study. *Neurosurgery* 1988;22:1023–1027.
6. Komiyama M, Nakajima H, Nishikawa M, Yasui T. Middle cerebral artery variations: duplicated and accessory arteries. *AJNR* 1998;19:45–49.
7. Han DH, Gwak HS, Chung CK. Aneurysm at the origin of accessory middle cerebral artery associated with middle cerebral artery aplasia: case report. *Surg Neurol* 1994;42:388–391.
8. Teal JS, Rumbaugh CL, Bergeron RT, Segall HD. Anomalies of the middle cerebral artery: accessory artery, duplication, and early bifurcation. *AJR* 1973;118:567–575.
9. Tacconi L, Johnston FG, Symon L. Accessory middle cerebral artery. *J Neurosurg* 1995;83:916–918.
10. Takahashi S, Hoshino F, Vemura K, et al. Accessory middle cerebral artery: is it a variant form of the recurrent artery of Heubner? *AJNR* 1989;10:563–568.
11. Takahashi T, Suzuki S, Okkuma H, Iwabuchi T. Aneurysm at a duplication of the middle cerebral artery. *AJNR* 1994;15:1166–1168.
12. Michotey P, Moscow NP, Salamon G. The middle cerebral artery. II. Anatomy of the cortical branches of the middle cerebral artery. In: Newton TH, Potts DG, eds. *Radiology of the skull and brain: angiography.* St. Louis: Mosby, 1974:1471–1478.
13. Gloger SA, Hayman LA, Hinck VC, Kretschmann H-J. Computer-assisted 3D reconstruction of the terminal branches of the cerebral arteries. II. Middle cerebral artery. *Neuroradiology* 1994;36:181–187.
14. Berman SA, Hayman LA, Hinck VC. Correlation of CT cerebral vascular territories with function. 3. Middle cerebral artery. *AJNR* 1984;5:161–166.
15. van der Zwan A, Hillen B, Tulleken CAF, et al. Variability of the territories of the major cerebral arteries. *J Neurosurg* 1992;77:927–940.
16. Hayman LA, Taber KH, Hurley RA, Naidich TP. An imaging guide to the lobar and arterial vascular divisions of the brain. Part I: Sectional brain anatomy. *IJNR* 1997;3:175–179.
17. Hayman LA, Taber KH, Hurley RA, Naidich TP. An imaging guide to the lobar and arterial vascular divisions of the brain. Part II: Surface brain anatomy. *IJNR* 1997;3:256–261.

CHAPTER 8

The Posterior Cerebral Artery

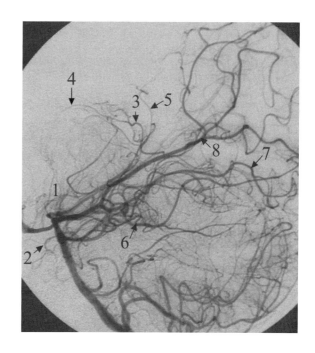

The two posterior cerebral arteries (PCAs) are the main terminal branches of the basilar artery. More than any other cranial vessel, the PCA subserves the comprehensive functions of "seeing and looking" (1). In addition to supplying the visual cortex itself, the PCA also subserves other visual functions, including ocular reflexes, eye movements, and the transmission and integration of visual information and memory (2). The PCA also supplies most of the limbic system and many of the vital structures at the base of the brain (3).

The PCA is divided anatomically into four segments (Fig. 8-1) (4):

    P1 = precommunicating (mesencephalic) segment
    P2 = ambient segment
    P3 = quadrigeminal segment
    P4 = calcarine segment

The proximal (i.e., P1 and P2) PCA segments and their branches are discussed in the first section of this chapter. The second section of this chapter covers the distal PCA (P3 and P4 segments).

THE POSTERIOR CEREBRAL ARTERY: PROXIMAL (P1,P2) SEGMENTS

Normal Development

The PCA does not appear until the later stages of fetal development. Several prominent embryonic vessels that supply the mesencephalon, diencephalon, and choroid plexus arise from a common stem at the caudal end of the posterior communicating artery (PCoA; see Fig. 6-1). Fusion of these primitive vessels forms the proximal segment of the future PCA (Fig. 8-2) (1).

By the 40-mm stage, the PCA can be identified as a posterior continuation of the PCoA (caudal division of the internal carotid artery [ICA]). The PCoA normally regresses in caliber as the vertebrobasilar system develops (see Chapters 1 and 5).

Gross Anatomy

The PCAs originate from the terminal basilar bifurcation ventral to the mid-brain (Fig. 8-3) (5). In over 90% of normal cases the basilar bifurcation lies either in the interpeduncular cistern (adjacent to the dorsum sellae) or the suprasellar cistern (below the third ventricular floor) (4).

P1 Segment

The P1 (mesencephalic or precommunicating) PCA segment lies within the interpeduncular cistern. This segment represents the most proximal aspect of the PCA. It extends from the basilar bifurcation to the junction with the PCoA (see Fig. 8-1 and box below). As it curves posterolaterally around the mid-brain, the P1 segment gives rise to a number of important perforating branches that supply the brainstem and thalamus (see box on next page).

Proximal Segment of the Posterior Cerebral Artery: Normal Anatomy and Variations

Normal development
Develops somewhat later than anterior, middle cerebral arteries
Proximal PCAs, branches initially sprout from caudal division of embryonic ICA
PCoA regresses as vertebral, basilar arteries form as dorsal longitudinal neural arteries fuse and establish anastomoses with the PCA stems

Gross anatomy
Horizontal (mesencephalic or "precommunicating") PCA = P1 segment (from basilar bifurcation to junction with PCoAs)
Ambient PCA = P2 segment (from PCoA junction to posterior mid-brain)

Key relationships
PCAs sweep around, behind mid-brain
Lie above oculomotor and trochlear nerves (cranial nerves [CNs] III and IV)
Course medial to incisura and above tentorium

Branches
Central (perforating) branches
Thalamoperforating, thalamogeniculate arteries (TGAs)
Peduncular perforating arteries (PPAs)
Ventricular and choroid plexus branches
Medial posterior choroidal artery (MPChA)
Lateral posterior choroidal arteries (LPChAs)
Cerebral (cortical) branches
Anterior temporal artery (ATA)
Posterior temporal artery (PTA)
Splenial branches (to corpus callosum)

Vascular territory
Perforating branches
Posterior thalamus, hypothalamus
Posterior limb of internal capsule
Mid-brain
Oculomotor, trochlear nuclei
Choroidal branches (reciprocal relationship with AChA)
Cortical branches
Inferolateral surface of temporal lobe

Normal variants
P1 segments often differ in size and position
Hypoplastic P1 with "fetal" origin of PCA

Anomalies
Carotid–basilar anastomoses (persistent primitive trigeminal, hypoglossal, or proatlantal intersegmental artery)

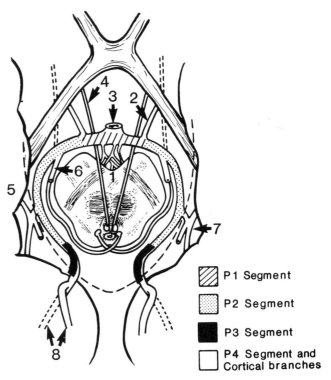

P1 Segment
P2 Segment
P3 Segment
P4 Segment and Cortical branches

FIG. 8-1. Anatomic diagram, superior view, depicts segmental anatomy of the posterior cerebral artery (PCA) and its relationship to adjacent structures. Approximate position of the tentorial incisura is indicated by the large dotted lines.

1, Peduncular perforating branches
2, Posterior communicating artery
3, Basilar artery
4, Oculomotor nerve (CN III)
5, Trochlear nerve (CN IV)
6, Posterior choroidal arteries (cut off)
7, Temporal branches
8, Calcarine artery (*solid line*) and parietooccipital artery (*dotted line*)

P2 Segment

The P2 (ambient) segment extends from the junction between the PCoA and PCA to the posterior aspect of the mid-brain (see box above). The P2 segment sweeps around the cerebral peduncle just above the tentorium (Fig. 8-1). This segment of the PCA courses posteriorly within the ambient cistern, paralleling the optic tract and basal vein of Rosenthal. The P2 segment has perforating, ventricular, and cortical branches.

Relationships

Summary

The PCA:

1. Begins in the interpeduncular cistern *anterior* to the mid-brain, then sweeps *around* and *behind* the mid-brain.

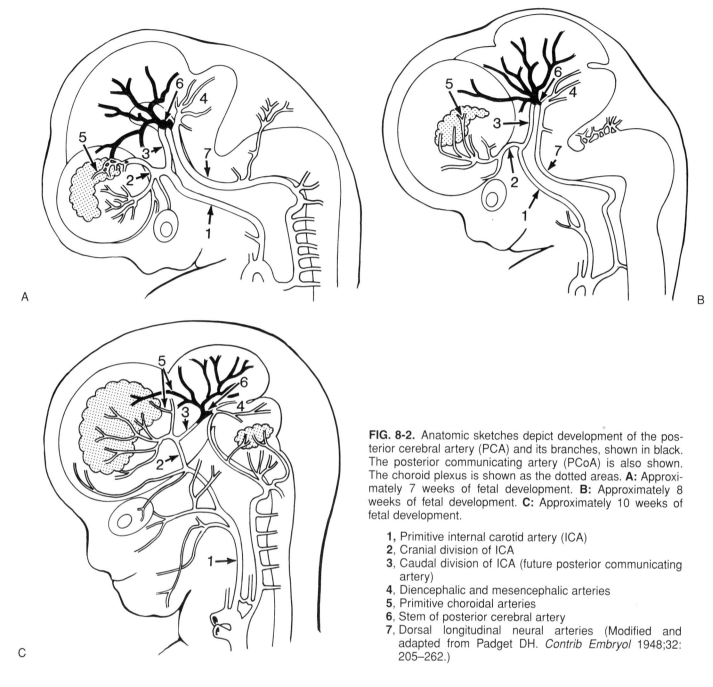

FIG. 8-2. Anatomic sketches depict development of the posterior cerebral artery (PCA) and its branches, shown in black. The posterior communicating artery (PCoA) is also shown. The choroid plexus is shown as the dotted areas. **A:** Approximately 7 weeks of fetal development. **B:** Approximately 8 weeks of fetal development. **C:** Approximately 10 weeks of fetal development.

1, Primitive internal carotid artery (ICA)
2, Cranial division of ICA
3, Caudal division of ICA (future posterior communicating artery)
4, Diencephalic and mesencephalic arteries
5, Primitive choroidal arteries
6, Stem of posterior cerebral artery
7, Dorsal longitudinal neural arteries (Modified and adapted from Padget DH. *Contrib Embryol* 1948;32: 205–262.)

2. Lies *above* the oculomotor nerve (CN III) and, more laterally, the trochlear nerve (CN IV).
3. Courses *medial* to the tentorial incisura and optic tracts, then runs posteriorly *above* the tentorium.
4. Terminates by running *below* the occipital and posterior temporal lobes.

Branches

The PCA gives rise to three main types of branches: (a) central (perforating) branches; (b) ventricular and choroid plexus branches; and (c) cerebral branches (6). The PCA also may supply branches to the corpus callosum splenium.

Central (Perforating) Branches

The PCA gives rise to three main groups of central perforating branches: (a) thalamoperforating arteries; (b) thalamogeniculate arteries, and (c) peduncular perforating arteries.

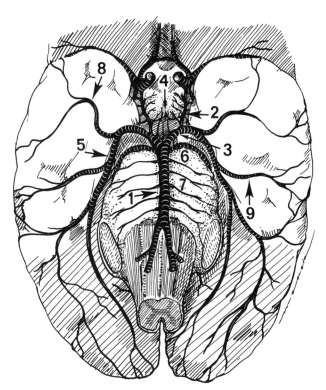

FIG. 8-3. Anatomic drawing of the proximal posterior cerebral artery (PCA) and adjacent structures, anteroinferior view. The distal PCA bifurcation and its terminal branches overlie the shaded area.

1, Basilar artery
2, Posterior communicating artery
3, P1 (horizontal or precommunicating) PCA segment
4, Perforating branches
5, P2 (ambient) segment
6, Superior cerebellar artery
7, Pontine branches of basilar artery
8, Anterior temporal artery
9, Posterior temporal artery

The first group of perforating arteries arises from the posterior or superior aspect of the P1 segment. These vessels are known as the *posterior thalamoperforating arteries* (PTPAs) (6). The PTPAs initially course posterosuperiorly within the interpeduncular fossa (Fig. 8-4). Passing through the posterior perforated substance, they enter the brain just behind the mammillary bodies.

In 42% of anatomic dissections, a PTPA is the largest branch that arises from the P1 segment (7). In 80% of cases, one to six anastomotic channels are present between the PTPAs; these channels are absent in 20% of anatomic dissections (8).

The second group of PCA perforating branches is the *thalamogeniculate arteries* (TGAs). In 80% of cases these vessels originate from the ambient (P2) segment (Fig. 8-4); in the remaining 20% they arise from the P3 segment. The number of TGAs present varies from two to 12. The TGAs may arise as individual vessels (two thirds of cases) or may originate from a common stem (one third of cases) (9).

Anastomotic channels between the TGAs and the medial posterior choroidal artery or other mesencephalothalamic branches are found in 33% of anatomic dissections (9).

The third group of PCA perforating branches is the *peduncular perforating arteries* (PPAs). These are small branches that arise from the P2 segment and pass directly from the PCA into the cerebral peduncles (Fig. 8-1) (9a). The PPAs vary in number from none to six per anatomic specimen (6).

Ventricular and Choroid Plexus Branches

Two major ventricular and choroid plexus arteries arise from the PCA: the medial posterior choroidal artery and the lateral posterior choroidal artery.

The *medial posterior choroidal artery* (MPChA) typically arises as a single vessel (Fig. 8-4; also see Fig. 4-17); multiple MPChAs are present in 10% to 45% of dissections. In 70% of cases the MPChA arises from the P2 segment. It also may arise from the precommunicating (P1) segment (12% of cases) or the parietooccipital artery (POA) (10% of cases) (6).

After its origin, the MPChA courses around the brainstem, then turns superomedially and runs forward to enter the roof of the third ventricle between the thalami. The MPChA terminates by passing through the foramen of Monro to enter the choroid plexus of the lateral ventricle (6).

A group of *lateral posterior choroidal arteries* (LPChAs) arises either from the P2 segment or from various cortical PCA branches. In contrast to the MPChAs (which are usually single), multiple LPChAs are the rule.

After their origin, the LPChAs pass laterally through the choroidal fissure to enter the choroid plexus of the temporal horn and atrium. Together with the choroid plexus, the LPChAs curve around the pulvinar of the thalamus within the lateral ventricle (Fig. 8-5). The LPChAs anastomose with branches of the anterior choroidal artery (an internal artery branch) as well as the MPChA (see Fig. 4-17).

Cerebral Branches

The proximal PCA has two main cortical branches: the anterior and posterior temporal arteries (Fig. 8-4; see also Fig. 8-13).

The *anterior temporal artery* (ATA) is the first cortical PCA branch. It arises either as multiple separate branches or a single trunk from the ambient (P2) segment. The ATA courses anterolaterally under the hippocampal gyrus and anastomoses with anterior temporal branches of the middle cerebral artery (10).

The *posterior temporal artery* (PTA) is the second major cortical PCA branch (see Fig. 8-12). It arises from the middle of the P2 segment. As it courses posteriorly and laterally along the hippocampal gyrus, the PTA gives off numerous small branches to the inferior aspect of the

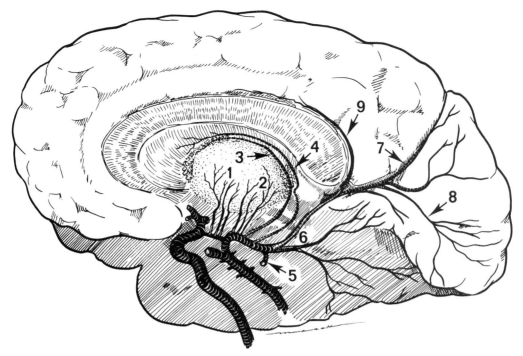

FIG. 8-4. Anatomic drawing of the proximal cerebral artery and some of its branches, medial view. The brainstem has been removed to demonstrate the cortical branching pattern.

1, Anterior thalamoperforating arteries (from the posterior communicating artery)
2, Posterior thalamoperforating and thalamogeniculate arteries
3, Medial posterior choroidal artery
4, Lateral posterior choroidal artery
5, Anterior temporal artery (cut off)
6, Posterior temporal artery
7, Parietooccipital artery
8, Calcarine artery
9, Splenial artery

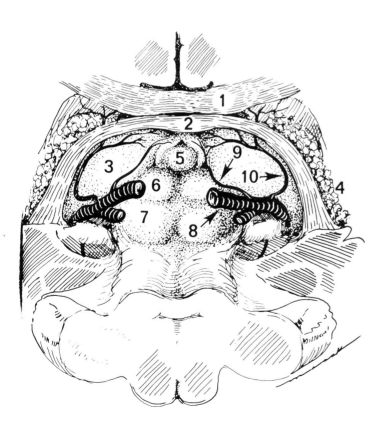

FIG. 8-5. Anatomic drawing of the brainstem, quadrigeminal plate, and corpus callosum as seen from behind. The relationship between the choroidal branches of the posterior cerebral artery (PCA) and their adjacent structures is depicted.

1, Corpus callosum
2, Fornix
3, Pulvinar of thalamus
4, Choroid plexus of the lateral ventricle
5, Pineal gland
6, Superior colliculi
7, Inferior colliculi
8, Posterior cerebral artery (beginning of P3 segment)
9, Medial posterior choroidal artery
10, Lateral posterior choroidal artery

posterior temporal lobe and adjacent occipital lobe. In 20% of cases the PTA extends to the occipital pole and supplies the macular area of the visual cortex (10).

Vascular Territory and Anastomoses

The vascular territory of all the PCA segments and their branches is described in the second section of this chapter.

Normal Angiographic Appearance

Lateral View

Because they course laterally in front of the mid-brain, the P1 segments are not easily observed on this projection (Fig. 8-6). In contrast, the P2 segments are visualized clearly as they curve posterolaterally around the mid-brain within the ambient cistern. The P2 segments often have a slight inferiorly convex configuration. The PCAs curve upward as they approach each other behind the mid-brain. This point demarcates the beginning of the P3 segments (Fig. 8-6).

Penetrating and peduncular PCA branches are also best seen in the lateral view. The thalamoperforating and thal-amogeniculate arteries initially follow a tortuous course within the interpeduncular cistern. They often assume a straighter configuration as they penetrate the mid-brain and thalamus (Fig. 8-7; see also Fig. 8-13B).

The choroidal arteries also are easily observed on the lateral projection of vertebral angiograms. The MPChA appears to curve posteriorly around the pineal gland, resembling the number "3" (Fig. 8-8A). The MPChA courses anteriorly to supply the choroid plexus in the roof of the third ventricle. It terminates by running through the foramen of Monro to anastomose with branches from the LPChAs and supply the choroid plexus in the body of the lateral ventricle (Fig. 8-8B).

The LPChAs follow a gentle, anteriorly concave course around the thalami. On lateral views the LPChAs appear to course several millimeters above the MPChA (Figs. 8-7 and 8-9A). Occasionally a distinct choroid plexus blush can be seen on the late arterial phase of vertebral angiograms (Figs. 8-8B and 8-9B). This normal finding should not be mistaken for a vascular malformation or neoplasm.

Most cortical PCA branches are easily observed on lateral vertebral angiograms. The anterior temporal arteries appear to course in front of the basilar artery, then curve

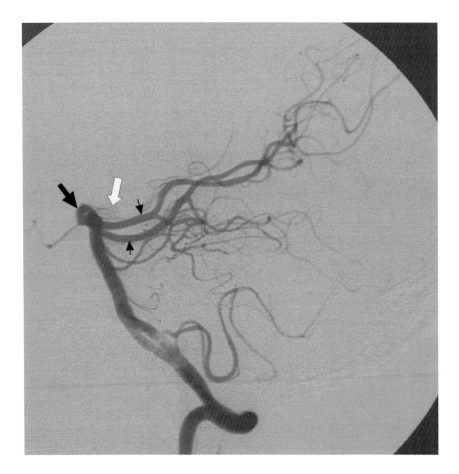

FIG. 8-6. Left vertebral angiogram, early arterial phase, lateral view. The P1 segments (*large black arrow*) are not easily seen as they course laterally. The P2 segments (*small black arrows*) are visualized as they course posterolaterally around the mid-brain. Penetrating branches (*white arrow*) arise from the top of the basilar artery and proximal P1 segments and course superiorly to supply the mid-brain and thalami.

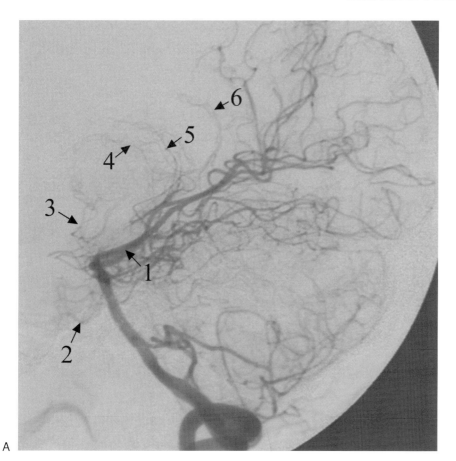

A

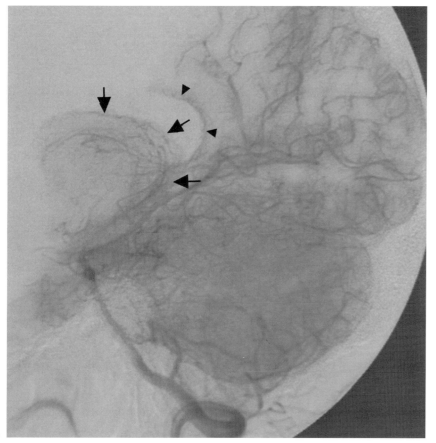

B

FIG. 8-7. A: Early arterial phase of a vertebral angiogram, lateral view, demonstrates many of the posterior cerebral artery (PCA) branches. The perforating arteries are especially evident. Note their more tortuous proximal course within the interpeduncular cistern (*curved arrow*). As they traverse the midbrain and thalami, they assume a straighter configuration (*open arrows*).

1, P2 (ambient) PCA segments
2, Anterior temporal branches
3, Thalamoperforating and thalamo-geniculate arteries
4, Medial posterior choroidal artery
5, Lateral posterior choroidal arteries
6, Splenial branches (posterior pericallosal artery)

B: Late arterial phase shows prominent but normal vascular blushes in the choroid plexus (*large black arrows*) and along the dorsal surface of the posterior corpus callosum (*arrowheads*).

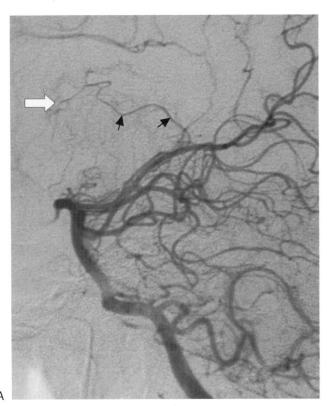

A

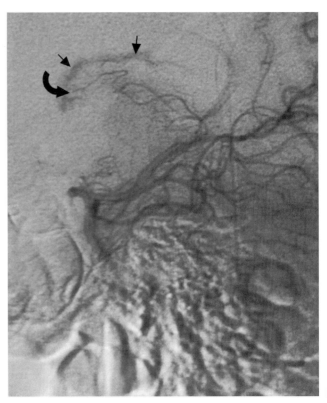

B

FIG. 8-8. Early **(A)** and late **(B)** arterial phase films of a lateral vertebral angiogram show a prominent but normal medial posterior choroidal artery (MPChA). The MPChA somewhat resembles the number "3" (**A**, *small arrows*). Note the sharp "hairpin" turn as the MPChA turns upward and backward through the foramen of Monro (**B**, *curved arrow*). A prominent vascular blush is seen in the choroid plexus of the lateral ventricles (**B**, *small black arrows*).

inferiorly in the middle cranial fossa (Fig. 8-7A). The posterior temporal artery courses posteriorly and inferiorly below the calcarine and parietooccipital arteries (Fig. 8-8A).

Anteroposterior View

The P1 segments are best delineated on anteroposterior (AP) Towne (Fig. 8-10A) or submentovertex views (Fig. 8-11) of vertebral angiograms. Considerable side-to-side asymmetry between the two P1 segments is common. The two P2 segments first curve laterally around the mid-brain, then turn medially. The P3 segments begin at the dorsal mid-brain as the PCAs approach each other within the quadrigeminal cistern (Fig. 8-9; compare with Fig. 8-1).

Of all the penetrating PCA branches, only the lateral posterior choroidal arteries (LPChAs) are seen clearly in the AP projection. The LPChAs first course laterally to enter the choroidal fissure of the temporal horn. They then turn superiorly and medially around the pulvinar of the thalamus. A prominent curvilinear blush often can be identified on the late arterial phase of vertebral

angiograms (Fig. 8-10B). This represents the choroid plexus as it courses within the posterior temporal horn, atrium, and body of the lateral ventricle.

Occasionally a small midline vascular blush is seen just above the basilar bifurcation on AP views. This normal appearance is caused by the peduncular perforating branches (Fig. 8-10A).

Some cortical branches are best seen in the frontal projection. The posterior temporal artery is especially well visualized as it extends laterally from its origin in the ambient cistern. The PTA then courses posteriorly as the most lateral of all the PCA cortical branches (Fig. 8-10A) (10).

Normal Variants, Anomalies, and Associated Conditions

Normal Variants

Considerable side-to-side asymmetry as well as variation in course between the P1 and P2 segments of the PCAs is not uncommon (Fig. 8-12).

In the typical configuration, the P1 (precommunicating) PCA segment has a diameter that is larger than the ipsilat-

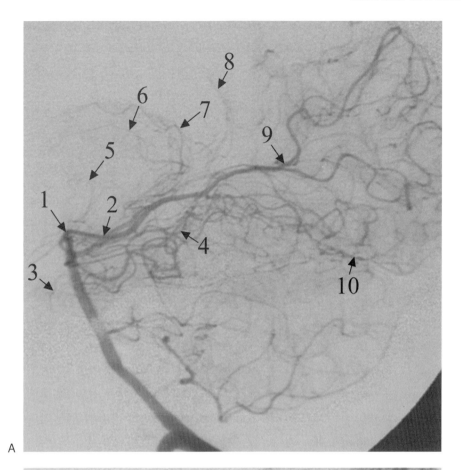

A

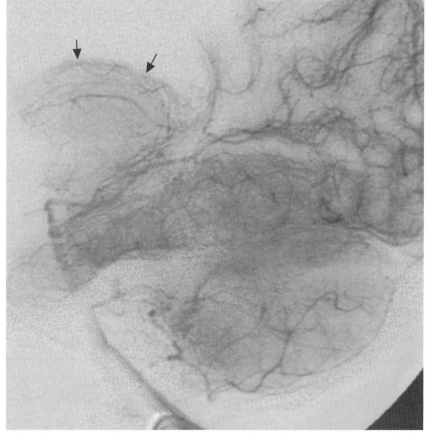

B

FIG. 8-9. Early (A) and late (B) arterial phase films of a vertebral angiogram, lateral view, show the choroidal arteries and some of the cortical PCA branches. Note the prominent choroidal blush on the late phase of the angiogram (B, *small arrows*).

1, P1 PCA segments
2, P2 segments
3, Anterior temporal artery
4, Posterior temoral artery
5, Perforating branches
6, Medial posterior choroidal artery
7, Lateral posterior choroidal arteries
8, Splenial branches (posterior pericallosal artery)
9, Parietooccipital artery
10, Calcarine artery

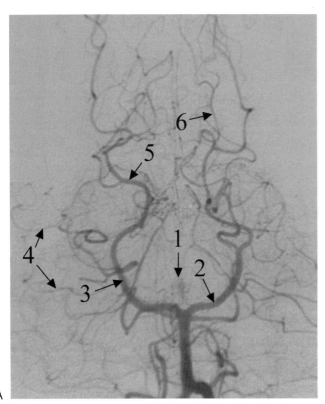
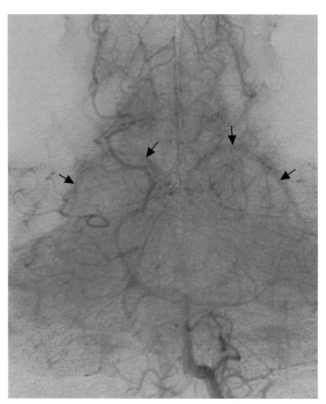

A   B

FIG. 8-10. Early **(A)** and late **(B)** arterial phase films of a vertebral angiogram, anteroposterior view, show the choroidal arteries and some of the cortical PCA branches. Note the very prominent choroidal blush on the late phase of the angiogram (**B**, *small arrows*). The small midline blush (**A**, *arrow 1*) is caused by the thalamoperforating arteries and is normal.

1, Thalamoperforating arteries
2, P1 PCA segment
3, P2 PCA segment
4, Inferior temporal arteries
5, Parietooccipital artery
6, Calcarine artery.

eral PCoA. In 20% of cases the P1 segment is smaller than the PCoA (7). In this arrangement, blood supply to the occipital lobe is mainly from the internal carotid artery via the PCoA instead of from the vertebrobasilar system (see Fig. 5-11). This variant has been called "embryonic" or *"fetal origin of the PCA"* (as opposed to "adult" origin from the basilar artery). Recent studies have shown that the so-called embryonic configuration is no more common in fetuses than it is in adults (11).

Fetal origin of the PCA must be distinguished from PCA occlusion (Fig. 8-13). Failure to opacify a PCA on a vertebral angiogram usually means that a fetal-type PCA is present (Fig. 8-13A–D), embolic PCA occlusion (Fig. 8-13A and E) is far less common. Injection of the ipsilateral carotid artery confirms the presence of a fetal PCA (Fig. 8-13C and D).

Anomalies

In some *persistent carotid–basilar anastomoses* the PCAs are supplied via a proatlantal intersegmental artery, persistent trigeminal artery, or other anomalous vessel (see Chapters 3 and 4) (1).

Anomalous Origin of PCA Cortical Branches

These anomalies are extremely rare. The parietooccipital, posterior temporal, and calcarine arteries have all been described as originating directly from the ICA (12). In some cases, the temporooccipital territory is supplied by branches from the AChA. This represents a partial embryonic transfer of one vascular territory (the PCA) to another (the AChA) (13).

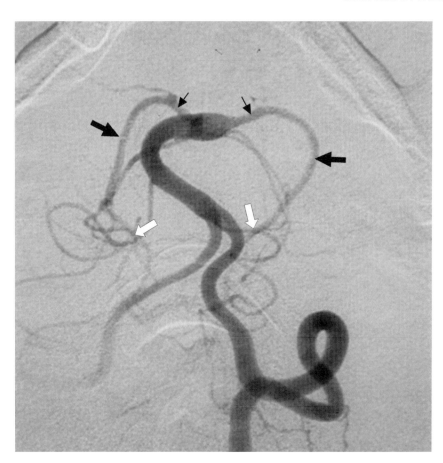

FIG. 8-11. Left vertebral angiogram, arterial phase, submentovertex view, shows the P1 PCA segments (*small black arrows*) as they course laterally from the basilar bifurcation. The P2 segments (*large black arrows*) run postero-laterally in the ambient cistern as they curve around the mid-brain. The P3 segments (*white arrows*) begin at about the dorsal mid-brain level.

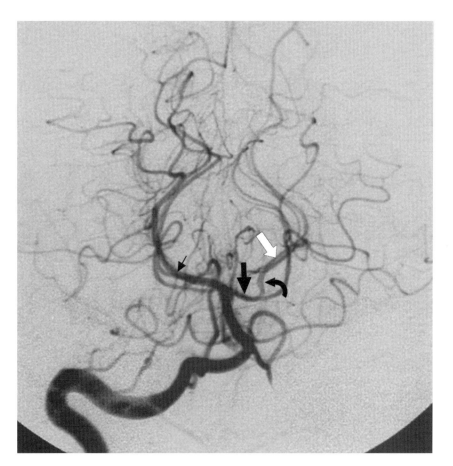

FIG. 8-12. Right vertebral angiogram, arterial phase, anteroposterior view. There is considerable asymmetry in the P1 segments. The right P1 segment (*small arrow*) is higher and larger than the left P1 segment (*open arrow*). The posterior communicating artery (*curved arrow*) and P2 segment (*white arrow*) are both larger than the ipsilateral P1 segment.

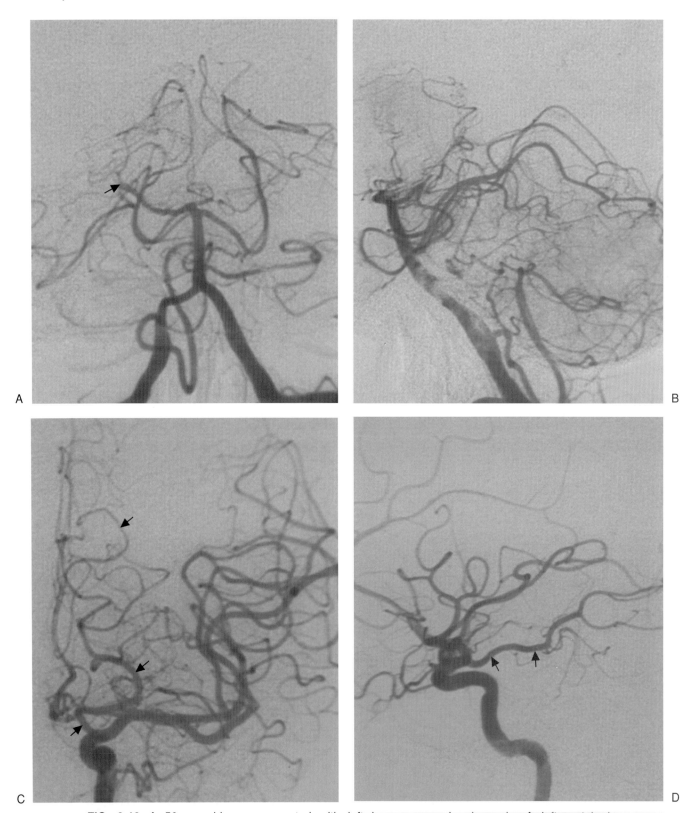

FIG. 8-13. A 56-year-old man presented with left homonymous hemianopsia. A left vertebral angiogram, AP **(A)** and lateral **(B)** views, shows that neither distal posterior cerebral artery (PCA) is opacified. The right P1 segment (*large black arrow*) can be identified, but the P2 segment appears occluded (*small arrow*). The left P1 segment (*white arrow*) is very small, and its distal branches cannot be seen. AP **(C)** and lateral **(D)** views of the left carotid angiogram in this patient indicate the presence of a fetal PCA (*arrows*), a common normal variant.

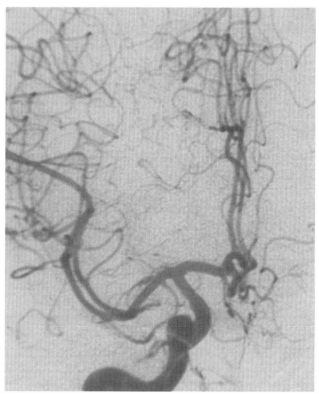

FIG. 8-13. *Continued.* E: The right carotid angiogram, AP view, does not opacify the distal PCA. The "missing" vessel, the right PCA, is therefore occluded.

Posterior Cerebral Artery: Normal Anatomy and Variations

Normal development
Distal PCAs sprout from proximal stems as brain develops
Gross anatomy
Quadrigeminal PCA = P3 segment (from posterior mid-brain to calcarine fissure)
Calcarine (cortical) PCA = P4 segment
Key relationships
Distal PCA division is usually above incisura, below lateral geniculate body
Terminal PCA division is often within calcarine fissure
Branches
Medial branch (medial occipital artery)
Parietooccipital artery
Calcarine artery (CA)
Lateral branch (lateral occipital artery)
Anterior, middle, and posterior inferior temporal arteries
Vascular territory
Medial division supplies posterior third of brain along interhemispheric fissure, part of parietal lobe, most of occipital lobe
Lateral division supplies most of temporal lobe
Variants and anomalies
Branching patterns vary, but true anomalies are rare.

POSTERIOR CEREBRAL ARTERY: DISTAL (P3,P4) SEGMENTS

Normal Development

As the embryo matures and the occipital lobes expand, each PCA stem elongates and increases its caliber. These posterior outgrowths give rise to the definitive distal cortical PCA branches (Fig. 8-2C) (1).

Gross Anatomy

P3 Segment

This relatively short segment represents the PCA continuation within the perimesencephalic cistern (see box below). It extends from the level of the quadrigeminal plate to the calcarine fissure (Figs. 8-1 and 8-14). Both P3 segments curve medially within the perimesencephalic cistern, approaching each other at a variable distance behind the colliculi (6). The PCA often divides into its major terminal branches before reaching the anterior limit of the calcarine fissure.

P4 Segment

This segment represents termination of the PCA within the calcarine fissure (Fig. 8-14). It also includes cortical branches that arise from the distal PCA (see Box above).

Relationships

Summary

The distal PCA usually divides *above* the tentorial incisura and *below* the lateral geniculate body.

Branches

The distal PCA divides into its two terminal trunks at or just before reaching the calcarine fissure. These vessels supply a medial and a lateral set of end branches (Fig. 8-14).

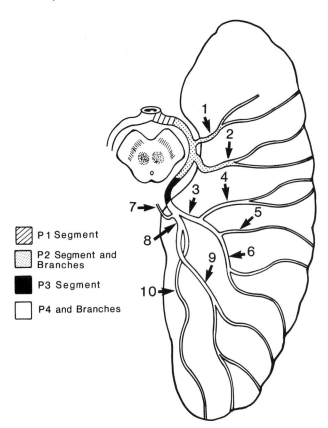

FIG. 8-14. An anatomic diagram depicts segmental anatomy and cortical branches of the posterior cerebral artery.

1, Anterior temporal artery
2, Posterior temporal artery
3, Lateral occipital artery
4, Anterior inferior temporal artery
5, Middle inferior temporal artery
6, Posterior inferior temporal artery
7, Splenial branches (posterior pericallosal artery, cut off)
8, Medial occipital artery
9, Parietooccipital artery
10, Calcarine artery

P1 Segment
P2 Segment and Branches
P3 Segment
P4 and Branches

Medial Branches

The medial distal PCA branch, called the *medial occipital artery* (Fig. 8-14, arrow 8) divides into two main branches. These are the parietooccipital and calcarine arteries (14).

A *parietooccipital artery* (POA) (Fig. 8-14, arrow 9) is present in almost all anatomic dissections. In 95% of cases it arises as a single branch, originating either with the calcarine artery or arising independently from the PCA within the ambient cistern (10). The POA courses posteriorly in the parietooccipital sulcus along the medial surface of the occipital lobe, then curves laterally to supply the brain adjacent to the parietooccipital sulcus. It provides accessory blood supply to the visual cortex in 35% of anatomic specimens (10).

The *calcarine artery* (CA) (Fig. 8-14, arrow 10) is the other major medial PCA branch. The CA arises at the distal PCA bifurcation and follows a posteriorly winding course deep within the calcarine sulcus to reach the visual cortex (10).

The medial PCA trunk also gives rise to a group of *splenial arteries* (Fig. 8-14, arrow 7). These small rami arise either directly from the PCA itself or from the POA. Together they are sometimes termed the posterior pericallosal artery. The splenial arteries ramify over the splenium and dorsal surface of the corpus callosum to anastomose with pericallosal branches from the distal ACA (10).

Lateral Branches

The lateral distal PCA branch, called the *lateral occipital artery* (Fig. 8-14, arrow 3), gives rise to several arteries that supply the inferior surface of the temporal lobe. These branches are the *anterior inferior, middle inferior,* and *posterior inferior temporal arteries* (Fig. 8-14, arrows 4-6) (14).

Vascular Territory and Anastomoses

The vascular territory of the entire PCA and its branches is described in this section.

Central (Penetrating) Branches

The *posterior thalamoperforating arteries* (PTPAs) supply a significant part of the central basal brain. Their area of supply includes most of the thalamus, hypothalamus, posterior aspect of the internal capsule, and part of the mid-brain. The PTAs also supply the oculomotor and trochlear nerve nuclei (Fig. 8-15) (3,15).

The *thalamogeniculate arteries* supply the pulvinar, geniculate bodies, and part of the subthalamus. The *peduncular perforating arteries* also supply the mid-brain (6).

Choroidal and Ventricular Branches

The *medial posterior choroidal arteries* supply the choroid plexus of the third ventricle as well as part of the ventromedial thalamus. In addition to supplying the choroid plexus, the *lateral posterior choroidal arteries* may send a number of small branches to the cerebral peduncle, posterior commissure, parts of the fornix and thalamus, and caudate nucleus body (6).

Splenial Branches

These vessels supply the posterior body and splenium of the corpus callosum. They anastomose with their counterparts from the anterior cerebral artery.

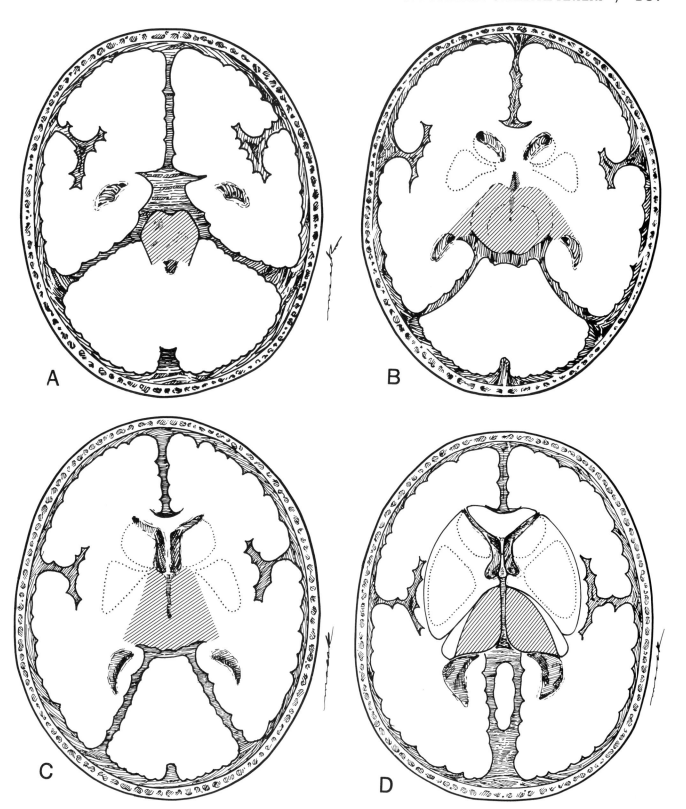

FIG. 8-15. A-D: Axial anatomic drawings depict the vascular territory supplied by perforating branches of the posterior cerebral artery. Part of these territories also may be supplied by penetrating branches that arise from the posterior communicating arteries or the choroidal arteries.

Cortical Branches

In general, the *parietooccipital* and *calcarine arteries* supply the posterior one third of the brain along the interhemispheric fissure, part of the parietal lobe, and most of the occipital lobe (16). Except for its anterior tip, most of the inferior surface of the temporal lobe is supplied by temporal branches from the PCA (17,18). The typical, maximum, and minimal PCA cortical territories are shown in Fig. 8-16 (16).

Anastomoses

Cortical PCA branches terminate at the so-called vascular "*watershed*" or "*border zone,*" where they have small pial anastomoses with their counterparts from the anterior and middle cerebral arteries. The area where all three cortical distributions meet is one of the most vulnerable regions in cerebral hypoperfusion syndromes (see Fig. 7-12).

Normal Angiographic Appearance

Anteroposterior View

The P3 segment extends only a few millimeters from the level of the dorsum of the mid-brain to the anterior aspect of the calcarine fissure. The P3 segment is best visualized on steep AP Towne (Fig. 8-17) or submentovertex views (Fig. 8-11).

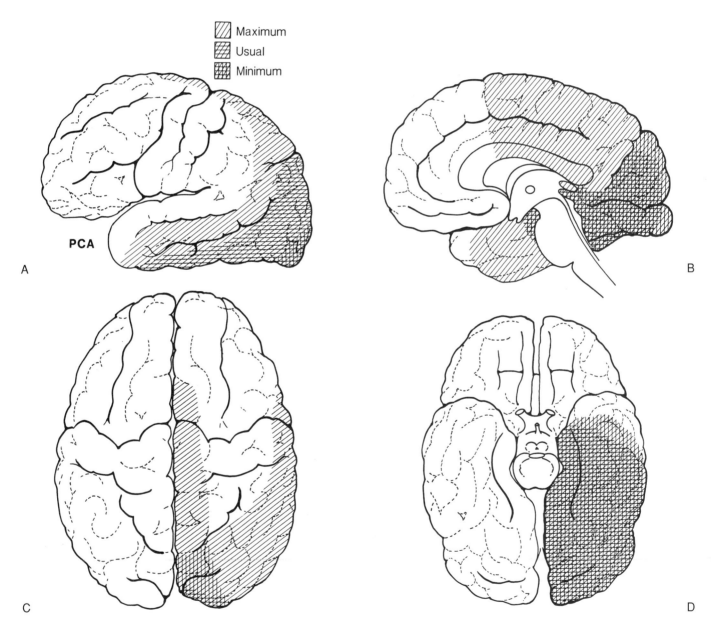

FIG. 8-16. Vascular distribution of the PCA cortical branches with maximum, usual, and minimum territories as delineated by van der Zwan. A: Lateral view. B: Medial view. C: Superior view. D: Base view. (Reprinted with permission from Osborn AG. *Diagnostic neuroradiology.* St. Louis: Mosby, 1994.)

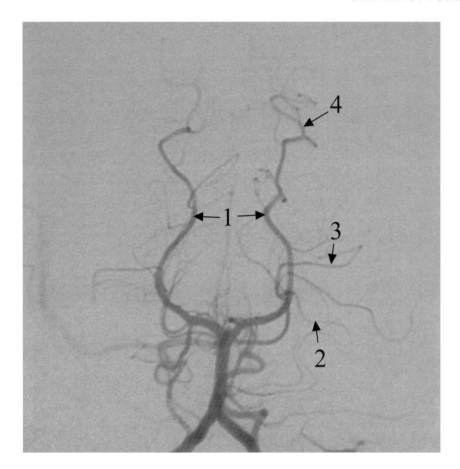

FIG. 8-17. Left vertebral angiogram, steep anteroposterior (Towne) view, shows the P3 segments of the posterior cerebral arteries (PCAs) as well as some of the temporal branches.

1, P3 PCA segments
2, Anterior temporal artery
3, Posterior temporal artery
4, Parietooccipital artery (P4 segment)

The P4 segment represents the distal PCA termination within the calcarine fissure. The P4 segment and its bifurcation into medial and lateral trunks is well seen in the frontal projection (Fig. 8-18). The proximal POA is typically the most medial of the terminal PCA branches; more posteriorly, the distal POA extends superiorly and laterally as it courses deep into the parietooccipital fissure (Fig. 8-19) (10).

In the AP projection the calcarine artery (CA) origin is lateral to the POA and medial to the PTA. The distal CA is usually crossed by the POA branches as they extend laterally into the parietooccipital fissure (Fig. 8-18) (10).

Lateral View

All the terminal PCA cortical branches as well as the posterior pericallosal artery are usually easily observed on this view (Fig. 8-20). The parietooccipital artery courses posteriorly and superiorly as the uppermost of the three posterior cortical branches of the PCA. The calcarine artery is easily identified on lateral views by its relatively straight course between the POA above and the PTA below.

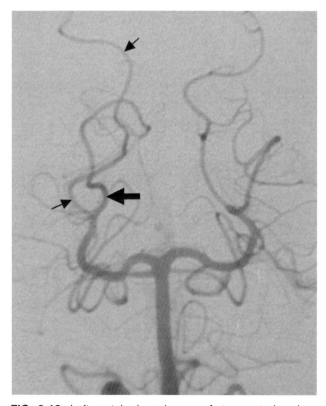

FIG. 8-18. Left vertebral angiogram, Anteroposterior view, shows the distal PCA bifurcation into medial (*large arrow*) and lateral (*small arrow*) trunks.

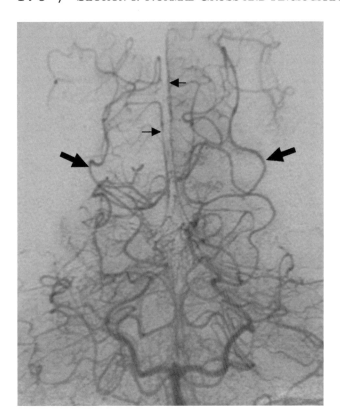

FIG. 8-19. Left vertebral angiogram, anteroposterior view, late arterial phase, shows the parietooccipital (*large arrows*) and calcarine arteries (*small arrows*).

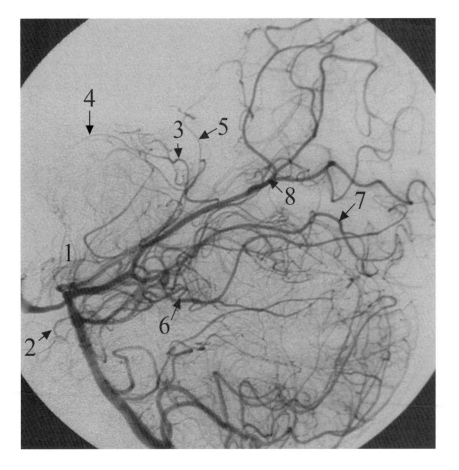

FIG. 8-20. Left vertebral angiogram, mid-arterial phase, lateral view, shows many of the PCA branches.

1, Perforating branches
2, Anterior temporal arteries
3, Medial posterior choroidal artery
4, Lateral posterior choroidal artery
5, Splenial branches (posterior peri-callosal artery)
6, Posterior inferior temporal artery
7, Calcarine artery
8, Parietooccipital artery

REFERENCES

1. Hoyt WF, Newton TH, Margolis MT. The posterior cerebral artery. Section I. Embryology and developmental anomalies. In: Newton TH, Potts DG, eds. *Radiology of the skull and brain*. Vol. 2, book 2. St. Louis: Mosby, 1974:1540–1550.
2. Ardaman MF, Hayman LA, Taber KH, Charletta DA. An imaging guide to neuropsychology. Part I: Visual object and face recognition, spatial perception, voluntary actions and auditory word comprehension. *IJNR* 1996;2:296–308.
3. George AE, Raybaud CH, Salamon G, Kricheff II. Anatomy of the thalamoperforating arteries with special emphasis on arteriography of the third ventricle: Part I. *AJR* 1975;124:220–240.
4. Gerber CJ, Neil-Dwyer G, Evans BT. An alternative surgical approach to aneurysms of the posterior cerebral artery. *Neurosurg* 1993;32:928–931.
5. Smoker WRK, Price MJ, Keyes WD, et al. High-resolution computed tomography of the basilar artery. 1. Normal size and position. *AJNR* 1986;7:55–60.
6. Zeal AA, Rhoton AL Jr. Microsurgical anatomy of the posterior cerebral artery. *J Neurosurg* 1978;48:534–559.
7. Saeki N, Rhoton AL Jr. Microsurgical anatomy of the upper basilar artery and the posterior circle of Willis. *J Neurosurg* 1977;46:563–578.
8. Marinkovic SV, Milisavljevic MM, Kovacevic MS. Anastomoses among the thalamoperforating branches of the posterior cerebral artery. *Arch Neurol* 1986;43:811–814.
9. Milisavljevic MM, Marinkovic SV, Gibo H, Puskas LF. The thalamogeniculate perforators of the posterior cerebral artery: the microsurgical anatomy. *Neurosurgery* 1991;28:523–530.
9a. Brassier G, Morandi X, Fournier D, et al. Origin of the perforating arteries of the interpeduncular fossa in relation to the termination of the basilar artery. *Interv Neuroradiol* 1998;4:109–120.
10. Margolis MT, Newton TH, Hoyt WF. Cortical branches of the posterior cerebral artery. Anatomic-radiologic correlation. *Neuroradiology* 1971; 2:127–135.
11. Van Overbeeke JJ, Hillen B, Tulleken CA. A comparative study of the circle of Willis in fetal and adult life. The configuration of the posterior bifurcation of the posterior communicating artery. *J Anat* 1991;176: 45–54.
12. Furuno M, Yamakawa N, Okada M, Waga S. Anomalous origin of the calcarine artery. *Neuroradiology* 1995;37:658.
13. Lasjaunias P. Correspondence. *Neuroradiology* 1994;36:160.
14. Gloger S, Gloger A, Vogt H, Kretschmann H-J. Computer-assisted 3D reconstruction of the terminal branches of the cerebral arteries. III. Posterior cerebral artery and circle of Willis. *Neuroradiology* 1994;36: 251–257.
15. Barkhof F, Valk J. "Top of the basilar" syndrome: a comparison of clinical and MR findings. *Neuroradiology* 1988;30:293–298.
16. van der Zwan A, Hillen B, Tulleken CAF, et al. Variability of the territories of the major cerebral arteries. *J Neurosurg* 1992;77:927–940.
17. Hayman LA, Taber KH, Hurley RA, Naidich TP. An imaging guide to the lobar and arterial vascular divisions of the brain. Part I: Sectional brain anatomy. *International Journal of Neuroradiology* 1997;3: 175–179.
18. Hayman LA, Tabaer KH, Hurley RA, Naidich TP. An imaging guide to the lobar and arterial vascular divisions of the brain. Part II: Surface brain anatomy. *International Journal of Neuroradiology* 1997;3:256–261.

CHAPTER 9

The Vertebrobasilar System

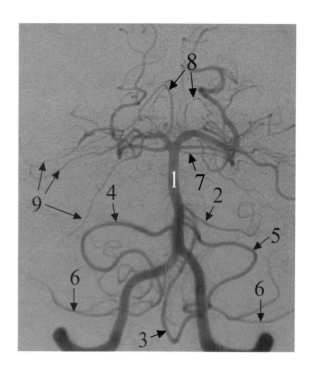

With minor exceptions, the entire blood supply of the medulla, pons, mid-brain, and cerebellum is derived from the vertebrobasilar system (1). Familiarity with its development, gross anatomy, normal imaging appearance, and vascular territory is a prerequisite for understanding pathologic processes that affect the posterior circulation.

The normal development, anatomy, and angiographic appearance of the vertebral arteries (VAs) and their branches are briefly recapped. The basilar artery (BA) and its penetrating and cerebellar branches are delineated in the second section. The two terminal BA branches, the posterior cerebral arteries (PCAs), were discussed in detail in Chapter 8.

VERTEBRAL ARTERIES

Normal Development

Four Weeks of Fetal Development

By the 4-mm (28-day) stage, the *cranial and caudal divisions of the primitive ICAs* are present. Two parallel plexiform arterial arcades, the paired dorsal *longitudinal neural arteries*, appear by day 29 (see Fig. 1-2).

Five Weeks of Fetal Development

The vertebral arteries develop from plexiform anastomoses between the seven embryonic *cervical intersegmental arteries* (see Fig. 1-2) (2).

At this stage the longitudinal neural arteries begin to unite along the sides of the developing rhombencephalon. Temporary anastomoses between these channels and the primitive carotid arteries also develop. The most cephalad of these transient vessels, called *carotid–basilar anastomoses*, is the trigeminal artery. The longitudinal neural arteries are initially supplied from above via the primitive trigeminal arteries and below via the cervical segmental arteries (see Fig. 1-2) (3).

Six Weeks of Fetal Development

The caudal divisions of the internal carotid arteries (ICAs), the future *posterior communicating arteries* (PCoAs), now link the ICAs with the cranial ends of the plexiform longitudinal neural arteries (see Fig. 1-3).

The seventh cervical segments (C7) enlarge and become the definitive *subclavian arteries*. The *vertebral arteries* arise from the enlarging seventh cervical intersegmental arteries (C7) and supply the caudal end of the longitudinal neural arteries. Connections between the first six intersegmental arteries and the dorsal aortae normally regress completely. The primitive carotid–basilar anastomoses also regress (see Figs. 1-4 and 1-5).

Gross Anatomy

The vertebral artery can be conveniently divided into four segments (see box on page 174) (4):

1. The V1 (extraosseous) segment
2. The V2 (foraminal) segment
3. The V3 (extraspinal) segment
4. The V4 (intradural) segment

Vertebral Arteries: Normal Anatomy and Variations

Normal development
  From fusion of the dorsal longitudinal neural arteries
  Anastomose inferiorly with seventh cervical intersegmental artery
Gross anatomy
  Extraosseous segment (subclavian artery to C6) = V1
  Foraminal segment (C6 to axis) = V2
  Extraspinal segment (exit from C1 to foramen magnum) = V3
  Intradural segment (foramen magnum to basilar junction) = V4
Key relationships
  Transverse foramina of C1–6 vertebral segments (vulnerable to injury from fractures)
  Extraspinal segment vulnerable to rotational forces
Branches
  Cervical branches (spinal, muscular)
  Meningeal branches (anterior, posterior meningeal arteries)
  Intracranial branches
    Anterior posterior spinal arteries (PSAs)
    Posterior inferior cerebellar artery (PICA)
Vascular territory
  Lateral medulla, upper spinal cord
  Tonsils, inferior cerebellar hemisphere and vermis
Variants
  Variation in size is normal
  PICA may share or replace trunk with anterior inferior cerebellar artery (AICA)
Anomalies
  Direct origin from aortic arch (5% of cases)
  PICA may originate below the foramen magnum
  Fenestration, duplication (associated with aneurysm)

V1 Segment

The VAs arise from either the superior (47%) or the ventral, caudal, or dorsal (53%) aspect of the subclavian arteries (5,6). The V1 (extraosseous) segments course posterosuperiorly to enter the transverse foramen of the sixth cervical vertebrae (Fig. 9-1A).

V2 Segment

The V2 (foraminal) segments ascend almost vertically, passing through the foramina of the C3–6 transverse processes. They follow an inverted L-shaped course through C2, first briefly ascending before turning laterally to exit from the axis (Fig. 9-1B). The VAs then turn again, running superiorly through the C1 transverse foramina.

V3 Segment

The V3 segments begin as the VAs exit from C1 and end where they penetrate the dura. After they pass through the C1 transverse foramen, each VA follows a sharp posteromedial curve around the atlantooccipital articulation (Fig. 9-1C). This produces a prominent grooving along the posterior ring of the atlas (C1). The V3 segments then turn sharply forward and upward to pierce the dura as they enter the skull via the foramen magnum (Fig. 9-1A and C).

V4 Segment

The intradural V4 segments first course anteromedially through the foramen magnum. They then run superomedially behind the lower clivus. At or near the pontomedullary junction, the two VAs unite to form the BA (7).

Relationships

Summary

From its origin each VA:

1. Initially passes *behind* the anterior scalene muscles and the common carotid arteries.
2. *Ascends* through the foramina of all cervical transverse processes (except C7), lying *anterior* to the ventral rami of the cervical spinal nerves.
3. Exits from C1 to curve *backward* and course *above* the posterior arch of the atlas.
4. Enters the posterior fossa at the foramen magnum, coursing *anterior* to the hypoglossal (cranial nerve [CN] XII) roots.
5. *Terminates* near the pontomedullary junction by uniting with the contralateral VA to form the midline BA (4).

Branches

Each VA has cervical, meningeal, and intracranial branches (7).

Cervical Branches

Vascular supply to the neck is organized segmentally and numbered according to intervertebral level (8). The major spaces are:

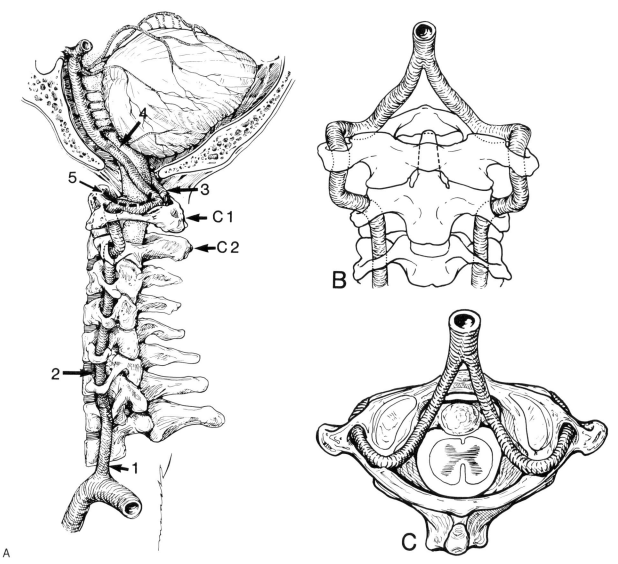

FIG. 9-1. Anatomic drawings depict the proximal vertebral artery segments. **A:** Lateral view. **B:** Antero-posterior view. **C:** Submentovertex view. The VA ascends through the transverse foramina of the C6–3 vertebral bodies. At C2 the VA turns laterally in an inverted L-shaped curve. As it exits from C2, it again ascends toward the transverse foramen of C1. After the VA exits from C1, it turns posteromedially around the atlantooccipital joint, initially running along the ring of C1. It then turns sharply anterosuperiorly to enter the skull through the foramen magnum. This complex bending and turning of the VA explains its appearance on conventional AP and lateral angiograms as well as the submentovertex view of magnetic resonance angiograms.

1, Extraosseous (V1) segment
2, Foraminal (V2) segment
3, Extraspinal (V3) segment
4, Intradural (V4) segment
5, Approximate position of occipital condyle (*dotted lines*)

1. The first space (atlantooccipital).
2. The second space (atlantoaxial).
3. The third space (between C2 and C3).
4. The fourth space (between C3 and C4).

Each upper cervical space is supplied by branches from both the vertebral and external carotid arteries. The VAs give rise to two types of cervical branches: muscular and spinal branches.

During its ascent through the transverse foramina, each V2 segment gives off multiple small unnamed *muscular branches* that supply the deep cervical musculature.

Segmental *spinal branches* supply the spinal cord and its coverings, anastomosing with spinal arteries from other vessels such as the ascending pharyngeal artery and thyrocervical trunk. Branches of the spinal segmental arteries supply the periosteum and vertebral bodies (4). Small rami from each VA also communicate with their counterparts from the opposite VA.

Meningeal Branches

Anterior and posterior meningeal branches arise from the distal extracranial VA to supply part of the posterior fossa dura. The *anterior meningeal artery* arises from the distal portion of the V2 segment. This vessel is usually quite small and only supplies the dura around the foramen magnum. The larger *posterior meningeal artery* originates from the VA at or just below the foramen mag-

num. It follows a relatively straight superomedial course to supply the falx cerebelli and the dura along the medial aspect of the occipital bone (Fig. 9-2).

Intracranial Branches

Intracranial VA branches include a number of small meningeal arteries, the posterior and anterior spinal arteries, perforating arteries, and the posterior inferior cerebellar artery.

The *posterior spinal artery* (PSA) arises from the distal VA or posterior inferior cerebellar artery. It descends along the dorsal surface of the medulla and spinal cord. Together with numerous spinal radicular branches, the PSA forms a vascular network that continues inferiorly along the cord all the way to the cauda equina.

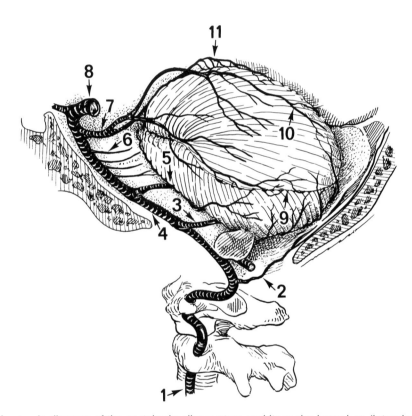

FIG. 9-2. Anatomic diagram of the vertebrobasilar system and its major branches (lateral view).

1, Left vertebral artery
2, Posterior meningeal artery
3, Posterior inferior cerebellar artery
4, Basillar artery
5, Anterior inferior cerebellar artery
6, Lateral pontine branches
7, Superior cerebellar artery (main trunk) (SCA)
8, Posterior cerebral artery (cut off)
9, Cerebellar hemispheric branches in the great horizontal fissure
10, SCA hemispheric branches
11, Superior vermian arteries (SCA branches)

The *anterior spinal artery* (ASA) also arises from the distal VA. The ASA gives off a number of small perforating branches that supply the anterior surface of the medulla, i.e., the pyramid. In approximately 50% of cases, the ASA courses inferomedially to unite with its counterpart from the opposite VA, then runs caudad in the anteromedian sulcus of the spinal cord (Fig. 9-3).

A number of small *perforating arteries* arise directly from the VA to supply the olive and inferior cerebellar peduncle. These branches anastomose extensively with perforators from the BA as well as the anterior inferior and posterior inferior cerebellar arteries (9).

The posterior inferior cerebellar artery (PICA) is the most important, largest, and most variable of all the cerebellar arteries. The PICA arises from the VA at the

anterolateral aspect of the brainstem, near the inferior olive, and passes rostral to or between roots of the glossopharyngeal, vagus, and accessory nerves. The main PICA trunk is divided anatomically into four segments and two distinct loops (Fig. 9-4). The first or anterior medullary segment courses posterolaterally within the medullary cistern, winding around the lower end of the olive. The second or lateral medullary segment continues posteriorly in the cerebellomedullary fissure. This segment loops caudally for a variable distance along the lateral surface of the medulla.

The third or posterior medullary segment is formed when the PICA reaches the posterior border of the medulla and ascends behind the posterior medullary velum. The fourth or supratonsillar segment represents the second or cranial loop of the PICA as it courses above

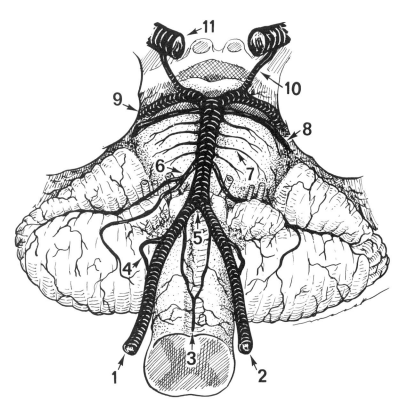

FIG. 9-3. Anatomic diagram of the vertebrobasilar system and its major branches (anteroposterior view).

1, Right vertebral artery (VA)
2, Left VA
3, Anterior spinal artery
4, Posterior inferior cerebellar artery
5, Junction of right and left VAs form the basilar artery
6, Anterior or inferior cerebellar artery
7, Lateral pontine arteries
8, Superior cerebellar artery
9, Posterior cerebellar artery
10, Posterior communicating artery
11, Internal carotid artery

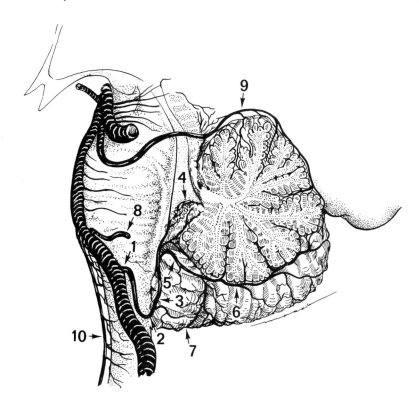

FIG. 9-4. Anatomic diagram of the vertebrobasilar system (lateral view). The left cerebellar hemisphere has been removed to show the relationship of the posterior inferior cerebellar artery (PICA) to the tonsil and vermis.

1, Anterior medullar segment of PICA
2, Lateral medullary segment (caudal loop) of PICA
3, Posterior medullar segment of PICA
4, Choroidal branches of PICA
5, Supratonsillar segment of PICA
6, Hemispheric and vermian branches of PICA
7, Tonsillar branches of PICA
8, Anterior inferior cerebellar artery (cut off)
9, Superior vermian branches of the superior cerebellar artery
10, Anterior spinal artery

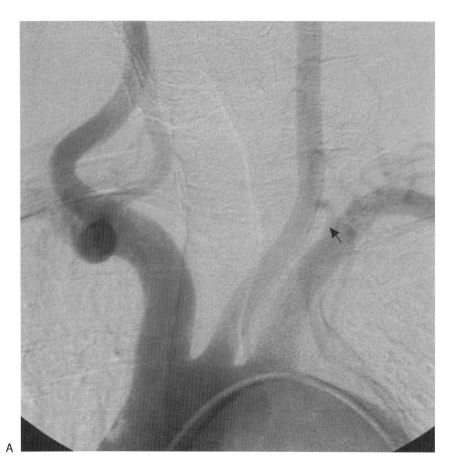

A

FIG. 9-5. Aortic arch angiogram shows the use of multiple oblique projections to profile the vertebral artery (VA) origins. **A:** On the standard left anterior oblique projection, the left VA origin (*small arrow*) is clearly evident, but the dominant right VA origin (*large arrow*) is obscured by overlapping vessels.

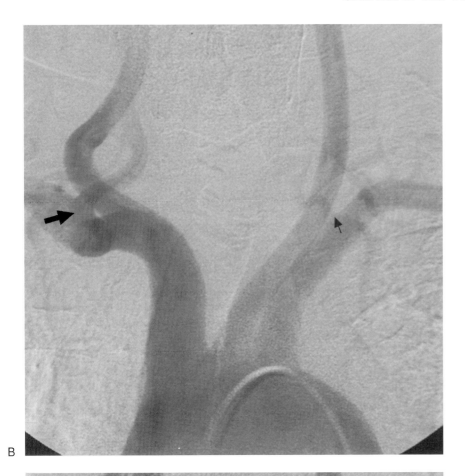

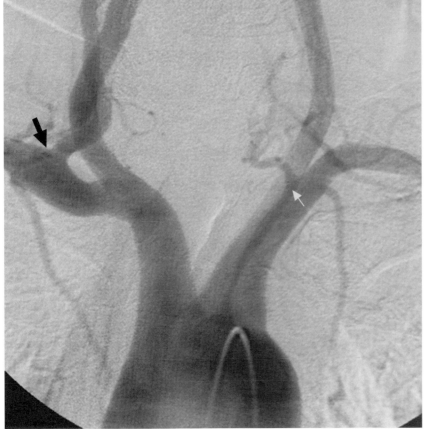

FIG. 9-5. *Continued.* **B** and **C:** Slightly different oblique projections now show the right VA origin (*large arrow*) and proximal segment, but the left VA origin (*small arrow*) is partially obscured.

or across the cerebellar tonsil. The PICA then turns downward in the retrotonsillar fissure and terminates a short distance distal to the apex of the cranial loop by dividing into tonsillohemispheric (lateral) and vermian (medial) branches (10).

The PICA gives off perforating, choroidal, and cortical arteries as well as numerous small perforating branches that supply the lateral medulla. At the apex of its cranial loop, the PICA also sends small branches to the choroid plexus of the fourth ventricle and the tonsil itself. The PICA terminates by dividing into inferior medullary and cerebellar hemispheric arteries.

Vascular Territory

The vascular territory of the VA and its branches is discussed together with the basilar artery (see below).

Normal Angiographic Anatomy

Evaluating the proximal VA and its origin can be difficult. In slightly more than half of all cases, the VA originates from the ventral, caudal or dorsal aspect of the subclavian artery instead of from its superior border. The proximal part of V1 is thus often overlapped by the subclavian artery on aortic arch angiograms (see Fig. 1-12).

Tortuousity of the V1 segment also may result in superimposition of the VA origin and SCA on standard oblique angiographic projections. Multiple projections or selective injection of the subclavian artery may be required to separate overlapping vessels (Fig. 9-5). Ostial lesions as well as stenosis and kinking of the proximal VA can be missed unless the VA origin is profiled completely (5).

Anteroposterior View

The V2 segment typically follows a relatively straight cephalad course through the C3–6 transverse foramina. Segmental branches to the cervical musculature and spinal cord arise along its course (Fig. 9-6A).

The VA course through C2 and C1 has the appearance of a half square. When the VA reaches the transverse process of C2, it turns laterally, forming the first corner and inferior border of the square. It then turns superiorly through the transverse foramen of the atlas, forming the second corner and lateral border of the square. As it turns medially at a 90-degree angle, it forms the third corner and upper border of the square. The V3 segment then bends sharply upward as it courses through the foramen magnum (Fig. 9-6A).

Lateral View

On lateral views of vertebral angiograms, the V2 segment ascends until it reaches C2. Its lateral bend through C2 is often overlapped on this projection by the distal V2 segment. A slight posterior angulation usually demarcates its course through the C2 transverse foramen (Fig. 9-6B).

From C2 the VA turns sharply caphalad to pass upward through the C1 transverse foramen. As it exits from C1, the V3 segment then curves backward, passing posterolaterally around the atlantooccipital joint. The VA then runs posteriorly in a horizontal groove along the arch of C1. Near the posterior limit of the C1 ring, the VA abruptly bends upward and then runs anteriorly, forming a sharp "hairpin" turn. The VA then approaches the midline and enters the skull through the foramen magnum (Fig. 9-6B).

The PICA follows a characteristic course that is generally best depicted on the lateral projection of vertebral angiograms. The caudal and cephalic loops are particularly well delineated on this view (Fig. 9-7), as are the anterior spinal and posterior meningeal arteries (Fig. 9-8).

Normal Variants, Anomalies, and Associated Conditions

Normal Variants

There is significant variability in relative size of the two VAs. The left VA is dominant in the majority of cases (see Chapter 1). In 25% of cases the right VA is larger than the left.

A *shared AICA–PICA trunk* is a common normal variant. Occasionally a *single trunk supplies both PICAs*. In 0.2% of cases a *VA terminates in a PICA* (Fig. 9-9). In such an arrangement the ipsilateral VA is small and the opposite VA provides most of the posterior fossa blood supply (7).

An *extradural origin of the PICA* occurs in 5% to 18% of cases (7,7a). Here the PICA originates from the extracranial vertebral artery instead of its intracranial segment (Fig. 9-10). The PICA then courses superiorly through the foramen magnum to supply the tonsil and inferior segments of the cerebellar hemispheres. In unusual cases the PICA may originate as low as the C1–2 level (Fig. 9-10B). In about a third of all cases the PICA originates normally from the intradural VA, but its caudal loop extends below the foramen magnum for a variable distance (Fig. 9-11).

A *duplicated PICA* has been identified in 2% of anatomic dissections. Here the PICA arises as two or more vessels instead of a single dominant trunk (7).

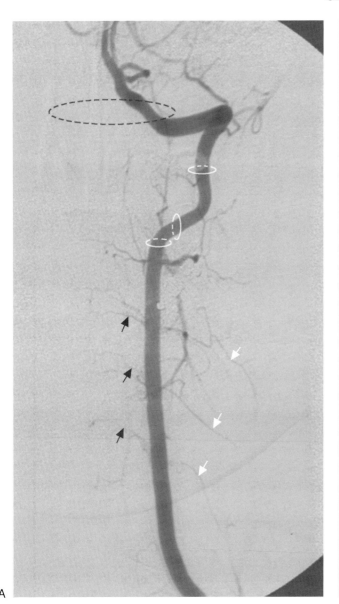
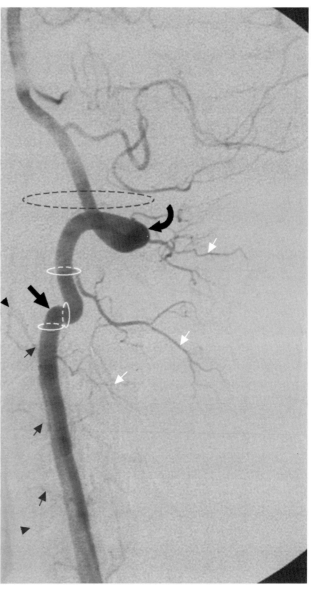

A

B

FIG. 9-6. Left vertebral angiograms in two patients show the V2 (foraminal) and V3 (extraspinal) segments. **A:** Anteroposterior view shows the nearly vertical course of the vertebral artery (VA) as it passes upward through the transverse foramina of the C6 to C3 vertebrae. The vertebral canal of C2 is indicated by the lower two white circles. The VA runs superiorly then turns laterally within C2, forming an inverted L (compare with Fig. 9-1B). After exiting from C2, the VA turns cephalad to pass through the transverse foramen of the atlas (*upper white circle*). It exits from the transverse foramen of C1 and then passes sharply backward along its posterior ring, completing the appearance of a half square. The VA then turns anterosuperiorly through the foramen magnum (*black dotted circle*). Note the numerous segmental spinal (*small arrows*) and muscular branches (*white arrows*) that arise from the V2 segment. **B:** Lateral view also shows the segmental spinal rami (*small black arrows*) supplying the spinal cord (*arrowheads*). The VA angles sharply within the C2 vertebral canal (*large arrow*), then turns upward again to pass through the transverse foramen of C1 (*upper white circle*). It curves backward and medially around the atlantooccipital articulation as it runs along the upper border of the C1 ring (compare with Fig. 9-1C). The VA then bends forward in a tight hairpin turn (*curved arrow*) to pierce the dura as it passes through the foramen magnum (*black dotted circle*) (compare with Fig. 9-1A).

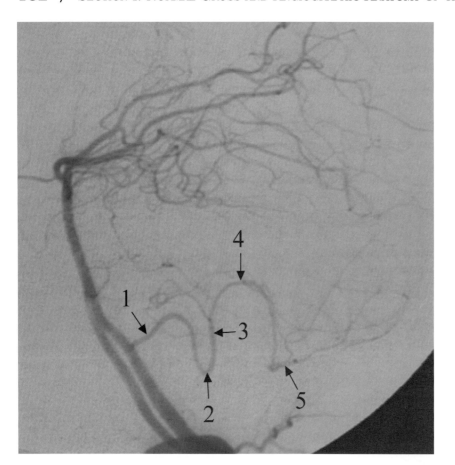

FIG. 9-7. Left vertebral angiogram, lateral view, shows the posterior inferior cerebellar artery (PICA) and some of its branches.

1, Anterior and lateral medullary segments
2, Caudal loop of PICA
3, Posterior medullary segment
4, Supratonsillar segment
5, Hemispheric branches

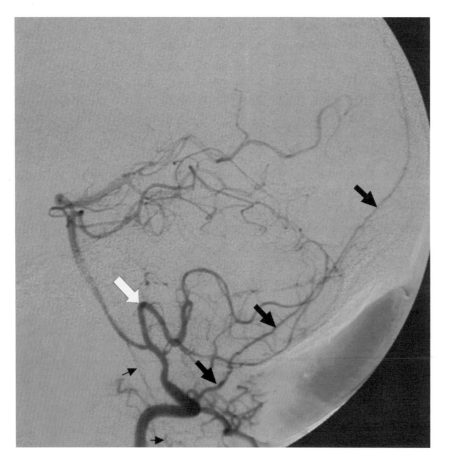

FIG. 9-8. Left vertebral angiogram, lateral view, shows the anterior spinal (*small arrows*) and posterior meningeal (*large arrows*) VA branches. The posterior inferior cerebellar artery (PICA) is indicated by the white arrow.

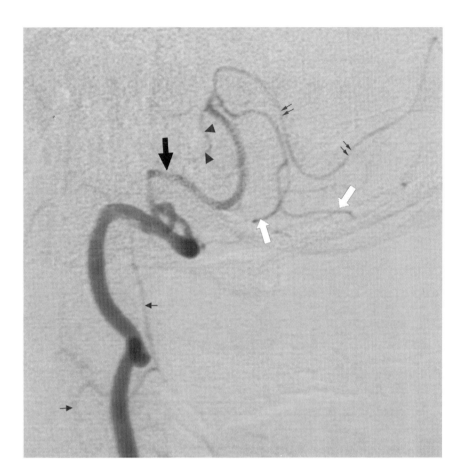

FIG. 9-9. Left vertebral angiogram, lateral view, shows the vertebral artery terminates by becoming the posterior inferior cerebellar artery (PICA) (*large black arrow*). Note opacification of the anterior and posterior spinal arteries (*small arrows*), as well as the tonsillar (*arrowheads*), inferior vermian (*double arrows*), and hemispheric (*white arrows*) PICA branches.

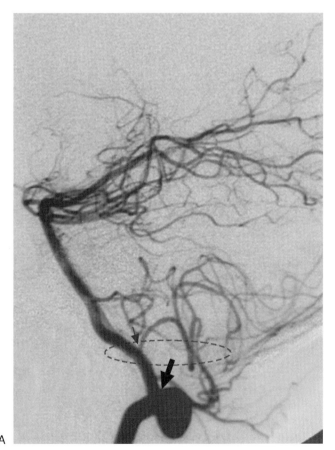

A

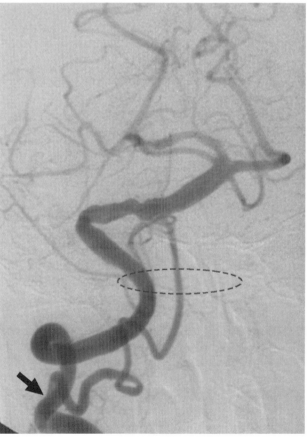

B

FIG. 9-10. Vertebral angiograms in two different patients show extracranial origin of the posterior inferior cerebellar artery (*large arrows*). **A:** Lateral view. **B:** Anteroposterior view. The usual origin of PICA is indicated in **A** by the small arrow.

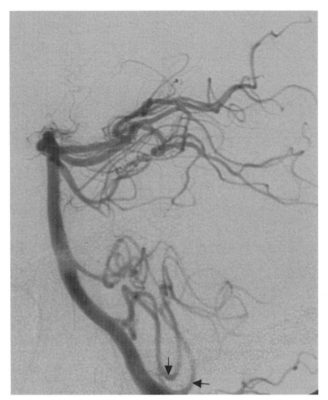

FIG. 9-11. Right vertebral angiogram, lateral view. Both posterior inferior cerebellar arteries (PICAs) are opacified and have normal origins. Their caudal loops (*arrows*) extend below the foramen magnum. This is a normal variant and does not indicate tonsillar herniation.

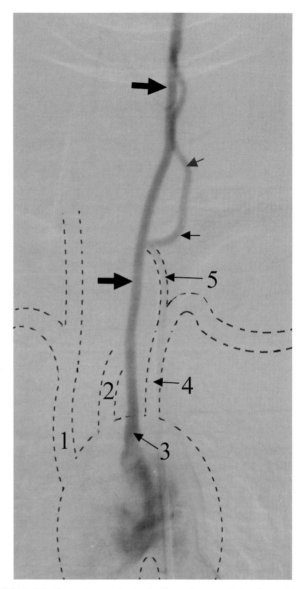

FIG. 9-12. Selective catheterization of a small duplicated left VA was performed. In this anteroposterior view, contrast fills the smaller VA (*small arrows*) and refluxes into a larger ipsilateral VA (*large arrows*) (case courtesy of J. Rees).

1, Innominatge artery
2, Left common carotid artery
3, Left vertebral artery (arch origin)
4, Left subclavian artery
5, Left vertebral artery duplication

Anomalies

The VA has an anomalous origin in 5% to 6% of cases (6). *Aortic arch origin of the VA* is the most common anomaly, present in approximately 5% of angiograms (see Chapter 1). *Anomalous origin of the PICA* is uncommon. The PICA may arise from the posterior meningeal artery or the internal carotid artery (11). Origin of the posterior meningeal artery from the PICA (instead of the VA) also has been reported (12).

Bifid or duplicate origin and *fenestration* of the VA also have been reported (2). Duplication implies that a vessel has two origins that follow a more or less parallel course for a variable distance (Fig. 9-12). Fenestration (sometimes erroneously referred to as segmental duplication) occurs when a vessel has a normal origin and position but has a double lumen for part of its course (Fig. 9-13) (13).

Both duplicated and fenestrated VAs are rare anomalies, found in less than 1% of anatomic dissections (14). They probably represent partial persistence of the plexiform embryonic channels from which these vessels developed.

Associated Conditions

A fenestrated VA is often associated with other anomalies of the brain, spinal cord, and spine. These include *fused vertebrae, other vascular anomalies,* and an *increased prevalence of aneurysms and vascular malformations* (14). An increased prevalence of intracranial aneurysm with aberrant PICA origin from the ICA also has been reported (15,16).

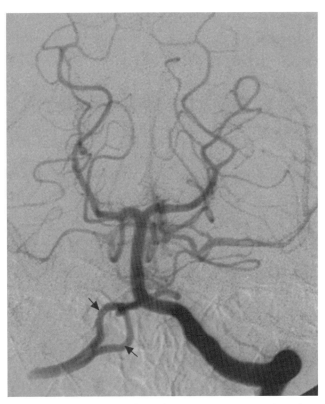

FIG. 9-13. Left vertebral angiogram, anteroposterior view, shows a fenestrated right vertebral artery (*arrows*).

THE BASILAR ARTERY

Normal Development

Five Weeks of Development

The primitive paired longitudinal neural arteries that lie on either side of the developing rhombencephalon slowly appose each other and then fuse in the midline (see Figs. 1-3, 1-4, and 1-5) (3). The definitive BA results from a craniocaudal fusion of the paired dorsal *longitudinal neural arteries*. This typically occurs between the level of the primitive trigeminal and hypoglossal arteries (17). The caudal end of the *definitive basal artery* remains plexiform for a considerable period of time, probably accounting for the presence of fenestrations at this site.

Six Weeks of Development

During earlier stages of brain development the ICA supplies both the anterior and posterior circulations. The embryonic channels that interconnect these two circulations gradually regress as the BA forms. They may persist as the *posterior communicating arteries*. The developing vertebrobasilar system becomes the dominant supply to the posterior fossa.

Four to Five Fetal Months

The cerebellum develops relatively late in embryonic life compared with the cerebral hemispheres. The *superior cerebellar arteries* (SCAs) are the first to appear, followed by the *anterior inferior cerebellar arteries*. The *posterior inferior cerebellar arteries* are the last to evolve. The great variability in these vessels relates to the relatively late persistence of the primordial vascular plexus in the hindbrain region (18).

Normal Gross Anatomy

The BA is a large midline or paramedian vessel that is formed by the confluence of the two VAs (see box below and Fig. 9-3). The BA extends superiorly from its origin near the pontomedullary junction to its terminal bifurcation into the two posterior cerebral arteries (PCAs). In 92% of cases, the terminal BA bifurcation is located in the interpeduncular cistern adjacent to the dorsum sellae

---

Basilar Artery: Normal Anatomy and Variations

Normal development
  From craniocaudal fusion of dorsal longitudinal neural arteries
Gross anatomy
  From vertebral artery confluence to terminal division into posterior cerebral arteries
Key relationships
  Anterior to pons, posterior to clivus
  Courses between abducens nerve (CN VI) at lower pons and oculomotor nerve (CN III) at upper pons
Branches
  Pontine perforating branches
  Anterior inferior cerebellar artery (AICA)
  Superior cerebellar arteries (SCAs)
  Posterior cerebral arteries (PCAs)
Vascular territory
  Most of the brainstem
  Most of mid- and upper cerebellum and vermis
  Occipital and temporal lobes (with PCAs)
  Mid-brain, part of thalamus, posterior internal capsule (PCA perforators)
Variants
  Considerable variation in branches
  May be very tortuous and ectatic
  May have hypoplastic segment(s)
Anomalies
  Duplication and fenestration (associated with aneurysm)
  Embryonic carotid–basilar anastomosis (persistent trigeminal or hypoglossal artery)

or in the suprasellar cistern below the level of the third ventricular floor (19). The normal BA is 3 to 4 mm in diameter and averages 32 mm in length (19–21).

Relationships

Summary

The BA:

1. Occupies a shallow median groove on the pons.
2. Lies *anterior* to the pons and *posterior* to the clivus.
3. Courses *superiorly* within the prepontine cistern.
4. Runs *between* the abducens nerves (CN VI) at the lower pontine border and the oculomotor nerves (CN III) at the upper pons.
5. Divides into the two PCAs in the interpeduncular fossa or posterior half of the suprasellar cistern.

Branches

The BA has labyrinthine (internal auditory), perforating, cerebellar, and cerebral hemispheric branches.

Labyrinthine (Internal Auditory) Arteries

The *labyrinthine arteries* (LAs) are long, slender arteries that arise either directly from the BA (16%) or from the superior (25%) or anterior inferior (45%) cerebellar

arteries. The LAs accompany the facial nerve (CN VII) and vestibulocochlear nerve (CN VIII) into the internal acoustic meati and are distributed to the inner ears (22).

Perforating Branches

The BA is a rich source of perforating arteries. Along its course in the prepontine cistern the BA gives off numerous pontine perforating arteries (see Fig. 9-2). There are two sets of these important pontine branches: (a) median and paramedian branches and (b) lateral or circumferential branches (Fig. 9-14).

The *median and paramedian pontine perforating arteries* arise at right angles from the posterior aspect of the BA. They course directly posteriorly, penetrating the pons and extending to the floor of the fourth ventricle (20). The *lateral pontine arteries* arise from the posterolateral surfaces of the BA and encircle the anterior and lateral borders of the brainstem. Along their course these vessels give rise to many small perforating branches that penetrate the pons at right angles to their parent vessels (23,24).

Cerebellar Arteries

The BA gives rise to two important cerebellar arteries: the anterior inferior and superior cerebellar arteries.

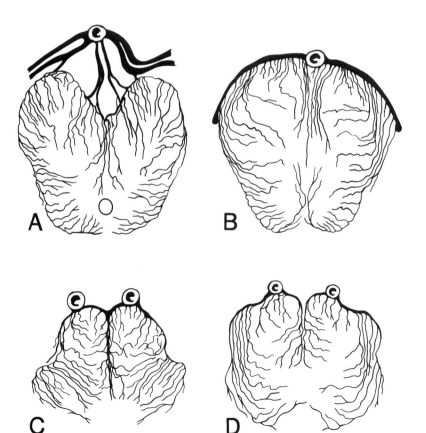

FIG. 9-14. Axial anatomic diagrams depict the numerous perforating branches that arise from the vertebral and basilar arteries.

The *anterior inferior cerebellar arteries* (AICAs) are the smallest of the three cerebellar arteries. Each AICA arises as a single (72%), duplicate (26%), or triplicate (2%) vessel from the proximal BA (25). The AICAs course posteriorly, inferiorly, and laterally across the pons (Figs. 9-2 and 9-3). Within the cerebellopontine angle cistern, each AICA lies ventral and medial to the ipsilateral facial nerve (CN VII) and vestibulocochlear nerve (CN VIII) (22,26).

In two thirds of cases, the AICA loops into the internal acoustic meatus or projects into the canal itself. Thus, vascular loops and elongated arteries of the AICA are normal (22). The AICA almost always gives off labyrinthine (internal auditory) branches (25). The AICA terminates by running over the cerebellum to supply the petrosal (anterolateral) surface of the cerebellum (27). The AICA also may supply a few penetrating branches to the inferolateral parts of the pons and upper medulla (4).

The AICA is variable in size, has a reciprocal relationship with the PICA, and may share a common origin with this vessel. The cerebellar hemispheric branches of the AICA and PICA have numerous anastomoses.

The *superior cerebellar arteries* (SCAs) are the most constant and most rostral infratentorial BA branches. The SCAs arise just prior to the BA bifurcation (Figs. 9-2 and 9-4). Most arise as a single trunk from each side of the BA, although duplicate or even triplicate vessels have been identified (28).

The SCAs course posterolaterally below the oculomotor nerve (CN III), then curve around the cerebral peduncles below the trochlear nerve (CN IV) and above the trigeminal nerve (CN V). An SCA directly contacts the trigeminal nerve in half of all anatomic dissections (29). In their proximal segments the SCAs are separated from the PCAs by the oculomotor nerves. Distally, these vessels are separated by the tentorium cerebelli.

The SCA bifurcation usually occurs about one third of the distance around the upper pons in the ventrolateral region (21). Each SCA has two main terminal branches. A lateral branch supplies the superolateral surface of the cerebellar hemispheres, superior cerebellar peduncle, dentate nucleus, and part of the brachium pontis. The medial SCA branch supplies the superomedial surface of the cerebellar hemisphere and the upper vermis.

Cerebral Arteries

Within the interpeduncular cistern the BA bifurcates into its two terminal branches, the *posterior cerebral arteries* (PCAs). The PCAs are discussed in detail in Chapter 8.

Vascular Territory, Anastomoses, and Flow Patterns

The posterior fossa is supplied entirely by branches from the vertebral and basilar arteries. Discussion of their vascular territories is conveniently divided by anatomic region.

Brainstem

There is significant variation in the extent of perforating arterial supply to the medulla, pons, and tegmentum. The V4 VA segments and their branches supply the lateral medulla; perforating branches from the BA supply the central medulla (Fig. 9-14A). The pons receives its vascular supply from the BA paramedian and circumferential perforating arteries (Figs. 9-14B and C). The upper pons is also perfused by small SCA branches (1).

In the typical pattern, the tegmentum is supplied mainly by branches of the PCAs and SCAs, but it also receives contributions from median and lateral perforating arteries that arise directly from the BA (Fig. 9-14D).

Cerebellar Hemispheres and Vermis

The three cerebellar surfaces are the tentorial or superior surface (which faces the tentorium cerebelli), the petrosal surface (which faces forward toward the petrous bone), and the posterior or occipital portion (which faces the occipital squama) (26).

In general, the SCA supplies the superior surface of the cerebellum and upper vermis (Fig. 9-15C and D). The PICA supplies the posterior and inferior surfaces of the cerebellum and inferior vermis (Fig. 9-14A–C). The AICA has the smallest area of supply, the petrosal surface (Fig. 9-14A–C).

Anastomoses

Numerous anastomoses exist between muscular branches that arise from the extracranial VA and corresponding branches from the occipital and ascending pharyngeal arteries (see box above). These intersegmental anastomoses may provide an important source of collateral blood flow in occlusive vascular disease (see Chapter 17).

The PICA anastomoses with the anterior inferior and superior cerebellar arteries over the cerebellar hemisphere and vermis (see Fig. 9-19B). The central part of the vermis and hemispheres represents a watershed area with variable contributions from all three vessels (30).

Flow Patterns

Recent studies have demonstrated that there is significant nonadmixture of VA flows within the BA. In 80% of cases the contributing vertebral components remain ipsilateral, resulting in a parallel flow pattern. In the remaining 20%, spiral rotation of inflow from each VA results in variable admixture of the two sources (31).

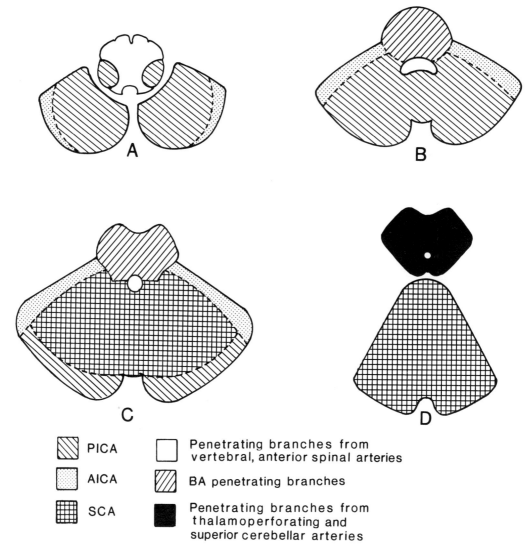

PICA

AICA

SCA

Penetrating branches from
vertebral, anterior spinal arteries

BA penetrating branches

Penetrating branches from
thalamoperforating and
superior cerebellar arteries

FIG. 9-15. Axial anatomic drawings through the lower **(A)** and upper medulla **(B)**, pons and cerebellar hemispheres **(C)**, and upper vermis **(D)** depict vascular territories of the vertebrobasilar circulation.

Normal Angiographic Anatomy

Anteroposterior Views

On anteroposterior (AP) projections the normal BA courses in the midline or in a paramedian position, medial to the lateral margins of the clivus and dorsum sellae (Fig. 9-16A) (19).

The AICAs are usually easily observed on standard AP and Towne projections of vertebral angiograms. The AICAs arise from the proximal BA and course directly laterally toward the cerebellopontine angle cisterns (Fig. 9-16). As they reach the internal auditory meatus, the AICAs often have an outward loop that curves into the canal (Fig. 9-17).

The proximal SCAs are well demonstrated on AP views of vertebral angiograms, although their distal branches are better delineated on lateral views. The initial segments of the SCAs tend to parallel the course of the

PCAs and are separated from them by only a few millimeters (Fig. 9-16A).

As the SCAs sweep around and then behind the brainstem, on steep AP Towne views they appear to approximate each other in the quadrigeminal cistern (Fig. 9-16A). The superior vermian branches of the SCAs then course posteriorly over the culmen, following a relatively straight course (Fig. 9-16B).

The small pontine perforating branches and the labyrinthine branches (internal auditory arteries) are not usually identified, even on high-resolution digital subtraction angiograms.

Lateral Views

On this view the BA typically exhibits a slight anterior convexity, lying several millimeters behind the clivus (Fig. 9-18).

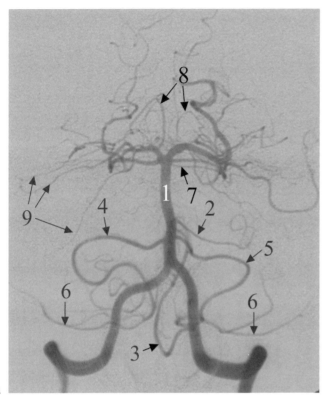 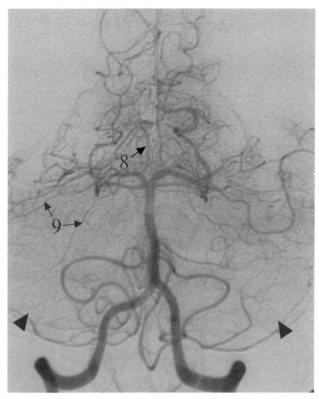

A

B

FIG. 9-16. Early **(A)** and slightly later **(B)** arterial phases, anteroposterior views, of a left vertebral angiogram show the basilar artery and its branches. The arrowheads on **B** indicate the brain blush of the cerebellar hemispheres.

1, Basilar artery
2, Left anterior inferior cerebellar artery (AICA)
3, Caudal loop of the left posterior inferior cerebellar artery (PICA) extends below the foramen magnum
4, Right AICA–PICA trunk
5, Left PICA

6, Hemispheric branches of PICA
7, Superior cerebellar arteries (SCAs)
8, Superior vermian SCA branches
9, Hemispheric branches of the superior cerebellar artery (note "stepladder" configuration)
9, Superior vermian branches of the SCAs

On lateral views the AICAs have a characteristic single or double curve as they loop into the porus acusticus. This double curve often resembles an "N" or "M" on this view (Fig. 9-18) (26). The angiographic appearance of the distal AICA branches is quite variable. They may terminate near the pons or continue laterally to supply the petrosal surface of the cerebellar hemispheres. If the ipsilateral PICA is small or absent, the AICA may give rise to an accessory branch that supplements the usual PICA distribution (Fig. 9-17).

On lateral views of vertebral angiograms the superior vermian arteries appear to lie at or sometimes even a few millimeters above the distal PCAs (Fig. 9-19A). This occurs because the culmen and declive, the most superior lobules of the vermis, lie just under the tentorial apex. The superior vermian arteries then course posteroinferiorly around the vermis to anastomose with inferior vermian branches (usually from the PICA) (Fig. 9-19B).

Hemispheric branches of the SCA ramify over the superior (tentorial) surface of the cerebellum. Occasionally prominent marginal branches of the SCA course into the great horizontal fissure of the cerebellum, providing an angiographic demarcation of this important anatomic landmark (Fig. 9-19A).

Normal Variants, Anomalies, and Associated Conditions

Normal Variants

The AICA may share a common origin with or originate from a single trunk with the PICA, forming an *AICA–PICA trunk* (Figs. 9-17A and 9-19). The PICA also may supply the entire AICA distribution. Occasionally the reverse also occurs.

An *accessory AICA* may supplement or replace part of the normal AICA distribution and has been identi-

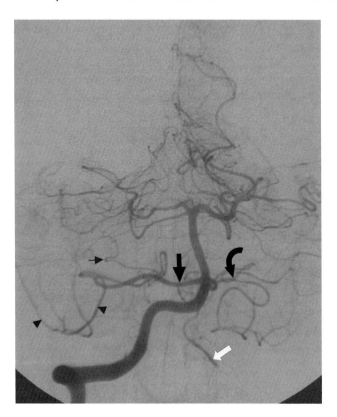

FIG. 9-17. Right vertebral angiogram, anteroposterior view, shows a prominent trunk (*large arrow*) that supplies both the anterior and posterior inferior cerebellar artery territories. The right AICA is a small branch that extends laterally in the cerebellopontine angle cistern, looping into the interior auditory canal (*small arrow*). The larger branch, the PICA (*arrowheads*), supplies the inferior part of the cerebellar hemisphere. The left VA (*white arrow*) is rudimentary. In this case the left AICA (*curved arrow*) gives rise to an accessory branch that supplements the usual PICA distribution.

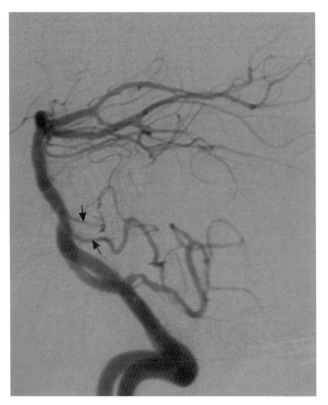

FIG. 9-18. Left vertebral angiogram, lateral view, shows the two anterior inferior cerebellar arteries (AICAs) (*arrows*). Their configuration in this view resembles the letter "M."

fied in 20% of anatomic dissections (26). *Multiple SCAs* are also common. Double (8%) or triple (2%) SCAs may be present instead of a single dominant trunk (Fig. 9-20).

Segmental *hypoplasia* of one or more vertebral–basilar components is not unusual (Fig. 9-21). If a *fetal-type PCA* is present, this vessel is not opacified when the posterior circulation is studied (see Chapter 8). If both PCAs are supplied from the anterior circulation, the BA appears to terminate by bifurcating into the SCAs (Fig. 9-22).

Anomalies

The BA is formed by fusion of the plexiform primitive longitudinal neural arteries. If these embryonic precursors fail to fuse completely, *duplication or fenestration of the BA* results. A fenestrated BA is found in 1.33% of anatomic dissections but is identified in only 0.12% of angiograms (7) (Fig. 9-23).

Persistent embryonic communications between the carotid and basilar arteries, *carotid–basilar anastomoses*, are discussed in Chapter 3.

Cerebellar branches may arise from vessels other than the BA. Reported *anomalous origin of cerebellar arteries* include origin of the AICA from the VA or cavernous ICA. SCAs arising from the ICA or PCAs also have been reported.

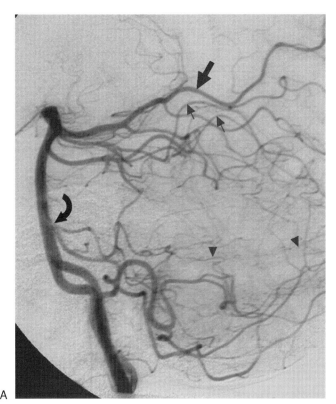
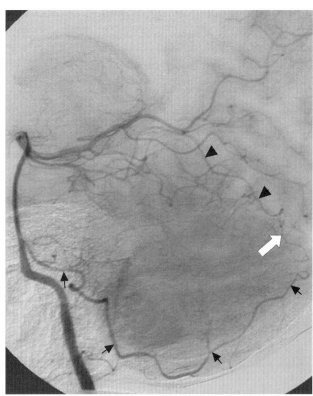

A

B

FIG. 9-19. Right vertebral angiogram, lateral view, with early **(A)** and late **(B)** arterial phase studies. **A:** As they course over the culmen, the superior vermian arteries (*small arrows*) appear close to the posterior cerebral artery (*large arrow*) in this projection. A large AICA (*curved arrow*) is present. The arrowheads demarcate the great horizontal fissure of the cerebellum. **B:** The later phase of the angiogram shows a prominent hemispheric branch (*small arrows*) that arises from the proximal AICA and supplies the inferior cerebellar hemisphere (usually part of the PICA territory). Note the watershed (*large white arrow*) where branches from the PICA and superior cerebellar artery meet.

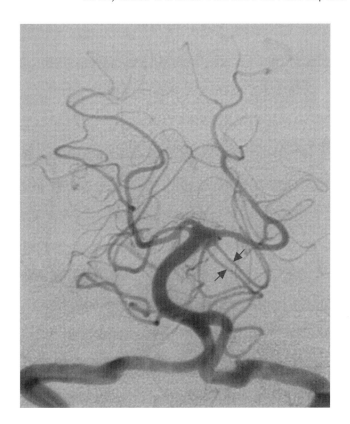

FIG. 9-20. Left vertebral angiogram, anteroposterior view, shows double superior cerebellar arteries on the left side (*arrows*). The basilar artery tortuosity is normal in this elderly patient.

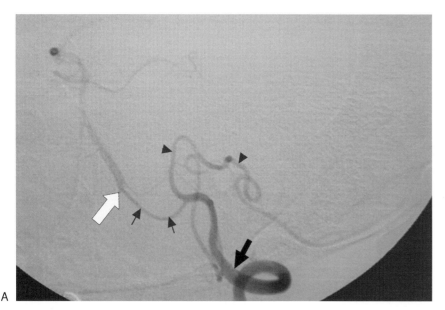

A

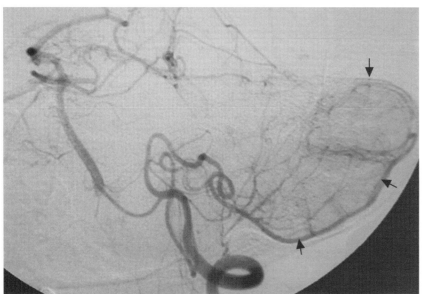

B

FIG. 9-21. Early **(A)** and late **(B)** arterial phases of a left vertebral angiogram show a normal-sized extracranial vertebral artery segment (*large black arrow*). The VA between the posterior inferior cerebellar artery (*arrowheads*) and the basilar junction (*white arrow*) is hypoplastic (*small arrows*). In this arrangement most of the VA blood flow is to the PICA (note the intense brain stain in the inferior cerebellum, indicated in **B** by the arrows).

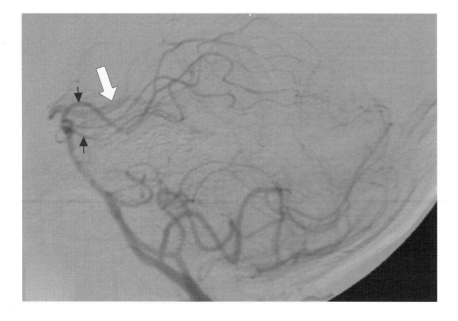

FIG. 9-22. Left vertebral angiogram, lateral view, in a patient with bilateral fetal-type posterior cerebral arteries (PCAs). The PCAs filled primarily from both internal carotid arteries (not shown). In this arrangement the basilar artery appears to end by bifurcating into the superior cerebellar arteries (*small arrows*). Transient, faint opacification of one PCA occurs (*white arrow*).

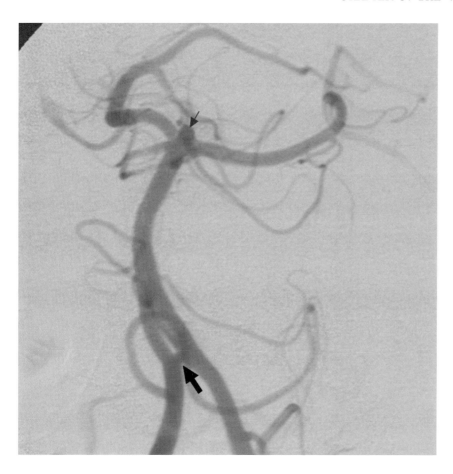

FIG. 9-23. Left vertebral angiogram, oblique view, shows a fenestrated basilar artery (*large arrow*). A small aneurysm is present at the basilar bifurcation (*small arrow*).

Associated Conditions

The most frequently reported pathology associated with BA anomalies is an *aneurysm* at the proximal end of a fenestration (see Fig. 12-7) (14).

REFERENCES

1. Parent A. The vertebral basilar system. In: *Carpenter's human neuroanatomy,* 9th ed. Media, PA: Williams and Wilkins, 1996:113–119.
2. Hashimoto H, Onishi H, Yuasa T, Kawaguchi S. Duplicate origin of the vertebral artery: report of two cases. *Neuroradiology* 1987;29:301–303.
3. Truwit CL. Embryology of the cerebral vasculature. *Neuroimaging Clin North Am* 1994;4:663–689.
4. Williams PL, ed. Subclavian system of arteries. In: *Gray's anatomy,* 38th ed. New York: Churchill Livingstone, 1995:1529–1534.
5. Farrés MT, Magometschnigg H, Grabenwöger F, et al. Stenoses of the first segment of the vertebral artery: difficulties in angiographic diagnosis. *Neuroradiology* 1996;38:6–10.
6. Trattnig S, Matula C, Karnel F, et al. Difficulties in examination of the origin of the vertebral artery by duplex and color-coded Doppler sonography: anatomical considerations. *Neuroradiology* 1993;35:296–299.
7. Newton TH, Mani RL. The verebral artery. In: Newton TH, Potts DG, eds. *Radiology of the skull and brain: angiography.* Vol. 2, Book 2. St. Louis: Mosby, 1974:1659–1709.
7a. Salas E, Ziyal IM, Bank WO, et al. Extradural origin of the posteroinferior cerebellar artery: an anatomic study with histological and radiographic correlation. *Neurosurgery* 1998;42:1326–1331.
8. Lasjaunias P, Berenstein A. The upper cervical vertebral column: the cervical arteries. In: *Surgical neuroangiography.* Vol. 1. Berlin: Springer-Verlag, 1987:155–166.
9. Akar ZC, Dujovny M, Gomez-Tortosa E, et al. Microvascular anatomy of the anterior surface of the medulla oblongata and olive. *J Neurosurg* 1995;82:97–105.
10. Friedman DP. Abnormalities of the posterior inferior cerebellar artery: MR imaging findings. *AJR* 1993;160:1257–1263.
11. Ogawa T, Fujita H, Inugami A, et al. Anomalous origin of the posterior inferior cerebellar artery from the posterior meningeal artery. *AJNR* 1991;12:186.
12. Tanohata K, Maehara T, Noda M, et al. Anomalous origin of the posterior meningeal artery from the lateral medullary segment of the posterior inferior cerebellar artery. *Neuroradiology* 1987;29:89–92.
13. Götz GF, Schumacher M. Anomalies of supraaortic vessels. *Klin Neuroradiol* 1995;5:24–34.
14. Tran-Dinh HD. Duplication of the vertebro-basilar system. *Aust Radiol* 1991;35:220–224.
15. Ahuja A, Graves VB, Crosby DL, Strother CM. Anomalous origin of the posterior inferior cerebellar artery from the internal carotid artery. *AJNR* 1992;13:1625–1626.
16. Manabe H, Oda N, Ishii M, Ishii A. The posterior inferior cerebellar artery originating from the internal carotid artery, associated with multiple aneurysms. *Neuroradiology* 1991;33:513–515.
17. Lasjaunias P. Embryology and radio anatomy of the CNS arteries. *Riv Neuroradiol* 1990;3(Suppl 2):29–34.
18. Kier EL. Development of cerebral vessels. In: Newton TH, Potts DG, eds. *Radiology of the skull and brain.* Vol. 2, Book 1. St. Louis: Mosby, 1974:1089–1141.
19. Smoker WRK, Price MK, Keyes WD, et al. High resolution computed tomography of the basilar artery. 1. Normal size and position. *AJNR* 1986;7:55–60.
20. Saeki N, Rhoton AL Jr. Microsurgical anatomy of the upper basilar artery and posterior circle of Willis. *J Neurosurg* 1977;46:563–578.
21. Schrontz C, Dujovy M, Ausman JI, et al. Surgical anatomy of the arteries of the posterior fossa. *J Neurosurg* 1986;65:540–544.
22. Brunsteins DB, Ferreri AJM. Microsurgical anatomy of VII and VIII

cranial nerves and related arteries in the cerebellopontine angle. *Surg Radiol Anat* 1990;12:259–265.

23. Takahashi M. The basilar artery. In: Newton TH, Potts DG, eds. *Radiology of the skull and brain.* Vol. 2, Book 1. St. Louis: Mosby, 1974: 1775–1795.

24. Marinkovic S, Gibo H. The surgical anatomy of the perforating branches of the basilar artery. *Neurosurgery* 1993;33:80–87.

25. Martin RG, Grant JL, Peace D, et al. Microsurgical relationships of the anterior inferior cerebellar artery and the facial-vestibulocochlear nerve complex. *Neurosurgery* 1980;6:483–507.

26. Naidich TP, Kricheff II, George AE, Lin JP. The normal anterior inferior cerebellar artery. *Radiology* 1976;119:355–373.

27. Amarenco P, Rosengart A, DeWitt LD, et al. Anterior inferior cerebellar artery territory infarcts. *Arch Neurol* 1993;50:154–161.

28. Hardy DG, Peace DA, Rhoton AL Jr. Microsurgical anatomy of the superior cerebellar artery. *Neurosurgery* 1980;6:10–28.

29. Hardy DG, Rhoton AL Jr. Microsurgical relationships of the superior cerebellar artery and the trigeminal nerve. *J Neurosurg* 1978;49: 669–678.

30. Savoiardo M, Bracchi M, Passerini A, Viscuni A. The vascular territories in the cerebellum and brainstem: CT and MR study. *AJNR* 1987;8: 199–209.

31. Smith AS, Bellon JR. Parallel and spiral flow patterns of vertebral artery contributions to the basilar artery. *AJNR* 1995;16:1587–1591.

CHAPTER 10

The Extracranial Veins and Dural Venous Sinuses

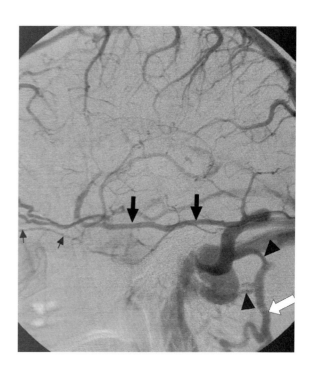

The extracranial veins and dural venous sinuses may participate directly or indirectly in a variety of pathologic processes that affect the brain. Familiarity with the normal development and gross anatomy as well as the common variations and anomalies of these structures is thus a prerequisite for correct interpretation of the complete cerebral angiographic series.

This chapter begins with an anatomic–radiographic consideration of the normal extracranial veins, including scalp and emissary veins. The diploic veins and dural sinuses are then discussed. The superficial cortical and deep cerebral veins are covered in Chapter 11, as is the normal development of the entire cranial venous system.

EXTRACRANIAL VEINS

Normal Gross Anatomy and Relationships

Scalp and Emissary Veins

Scalp veins are connected via emissary veins to the cranial dural venous sinuses (Fig. 10-1). Parietal emissary veins pass through prominent channels in the parietal bones and are located anterior to the lambda on each side of the sagittal suture. Mastoid emissary veins receive the occipital and posterior auricular veins, then pass through the mastoid foramina to drain into the sigmoid sinus. Other scalp veins communicate with the ophthalmic veins (1,2).

Orbital Veins

The orbit normally drains posteriorly via the *superior ophthalmic vein* (SOV) and the *inferior ophthalmic vein* (IOV). The SOV is by far the larger of the two vessels. Although the IOV can be identified in over 90% of anatomic specimens, it is a thinner, much less conspicuous vessel. The SOV and IOV usually form a short common venous confluence that empties directly into the anterior cavernous sinus (CS) (3).

Facial Veins

The superficial and deep veins of the face and paranasal sinuses are major tributaries of the jugular veins. The *anterior facial vein* begins near the medial palpebral angle as a direct continuation of the angular vein (Fig. 10-1). It descends obliquely across the face, crossing over the masseter muscle, then curves around

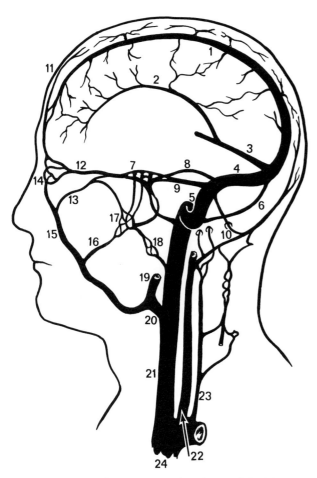

FIG. 10-1. Anatomic diagram depicts the craniofacial venous plexuses.

1, Superior sagittal sinus
2, Inferior sagittal sinus
3, Straight sinus
4, Transverse sinus
5, Sigmoid sinus
6, Occipital sinus
7, Cavernous sinus
8, Superior petrosal sinus
9, Inferior petrosal sinus
10, Emissary veins
11, Frontal scalp veins
12, Superior ophthalmic vein
13, Inferior ophthalmic vein
14, Angular vein
15, Anterior facial vein
16, Deep facial vein
17, Pterygoid venous plexus
18, Pharyngeal venous plexus
19, Posterior facial vein
20, Common facial vein
21, Internal jugular vein
22, External jugular vein
23, Vertebral vein
24, Subclavian vein

the mandible and lateral aspect of the submandibular slant (3a). During its course the anterior facial vein receives tributaries from the orbit, lips, facial muscles, and submental region. This vein has extensive interconnections with the pterygoid venous plexus via the deep facial vein and with the cavernous sinus via the angular and ophthalmic veins (4).

The *deep facial vein* connects the anterior facial vein with the pterygoid venous plexus. The *pterygoid venous plexus* is an extensive network of small vascular channels that lies partly between the temporalis and lateral pterygoid muscles and partly between the two pterygoid muscles. The pterygoid plexus receives numerous palatine, deep temporal, masseteric, buccal, dental, and orbital tributaries (1). The pterygoid plexus communicates freely with the facial veins and has extensive anastomoses with the cavernous sinus and other intracranial venous channels via sphenobasal emissary veins that pass through the foramina ovale, spinosum, and lacerum (Fig. 10-2) (4).

The pterygoid plexus drains posteriorly into a short trunk called the *maxillary vein*. Behind and just below the neck of the mandible, the maxillary vein unites with the *superficial temporal vein* to form the *retromandibular vein*. The retromandibular vein descends in the parotid gland, passing between the external carotid artery and facial nerve (cranial nerve [CN] VII). It joins the facial vein and drains into the internal jugular vein (IJV). A smaller tributary of the retromandibular vein may join the posterior auricular vein to form the external jugular vein (EJV).

Submental and anterior facial veins unite to form the *common facial vein*. After receiving lingual, submental, and thyroid tributaries, the common facial vein joins the internal jugular vein at the level of the hyoid bone (Fig. 10-1).

Neck Veins

The *external jugular vein* (EJV) is formed by segments of the retromandibular and posterior auricular veins (Fig. 10-1). The EJV begins below the mandibular angle and descends across the sternocleidomastoid muscle to end in the subclavian vein. The EJV receives tributaries from the scalp, pinna, and deep facial structures. The EJV varies considerably in size and extent and is inversely proportional to other veins in the neck.

The *internal jugular vein* (IJV) collects blood from the skull, brain, and much of the neck. The IJV begins within the pars vasacularis of the jugular fossa as the caudad continuation of the sigmoid sinus. The slight dilatation present at the origin of each IJV is termed the *jugular bulb*. The IJV courses inferiorly within the carotid space, lying posterolateral to the internal and common carotid arteries.

Each IJV terminates by uniting with its respective *subclavian vein* to form the *brachiocephalic vein*. Tributaries

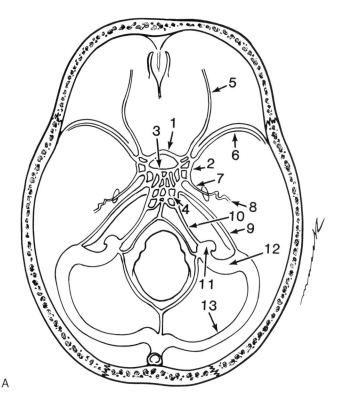

FIG. 10-2. Anatomic diagram of the basal dural venous sinuses as seen from **(A)** above and **(B)** the lateral perspective

1, Anterior intercavernous sinus
2, Cavernous sinus
3, Posterior intercavernous sinus
4, Basilar (clival) plexus
5, Superior ophthalmic vein
6, Sphenoparietal sinus
7, Foramen ovale plexus
8, Pterygoid plexus
9, Superior petrosal sinus
10, Inferior petrosal sinus
11, Internal jugular vein
12, Sigmoid sinus
13, Transverse sinus
14, Inferior ophthalmic vein

(Reprinted with permission from Osborn AG, Tong KT. *Handbook of neuroradiology,* 2nd ed. St. Louis: Mosby–Year Book, 1996.)

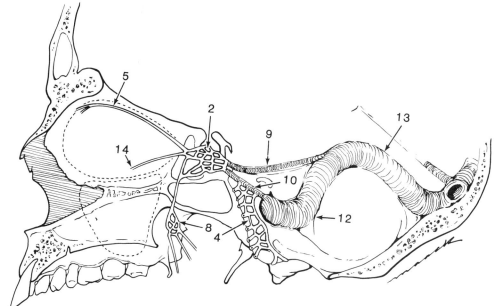

of the IJV include the inferior petrosal sinus (IPS), the common facial vein, and lingual, pharyngeal, and thyroid veins. The thoracic duct opens near the union of the left subclavian and internal jugular veins.

The *vertebral venous plexus* is formed in the suboccipital area by numerous small tributaries that arise from the cranial vertebral venous plexuses and the cervical musculature. The vertebral plexus surrounds the vertebral artery as it descends within the transverse foramina. The vertebral vein has numerous interconnections with the epidural venous plexuses. It connects with the sigmoid sinus via posterior condylar emissary veins. Prominent anastomoses with emissary and suboccipital veins can normally be seen on the late venous phase of cerebral angiograms. The vertebral venous plexus terminates in the brachiocephalic vein.

Normal Angiographic Anatomy

Scalp and Emissary Veins

Scalp veins are rarely opacified on normal internal or common carotid studies. Filling of prominent scalp or emissary veins at carotid angiography occurs with a variety of lesions such as arteriovenous malformations, scalp or skull neoplasms, sinus pericranii, increased intracranial pressure, and dural sinus occlusive disorders (Fig. 10-3).

Orbital Veins

Flow in the *superior and inferior ophthalmic veins* is normally from outside in, i.e., from the orbit into the cavernous sinus. Although faint SOV opacification is occasionally identified on the late venous phase of carotid angiograms (see Figs. 10-6 and 10-12), dense or persistent opacification of the orbital veins is always abnormal. This occurs with vascular malformations and dural sinus occlusions (Fig. 10-3). The orbital veins and basal venous

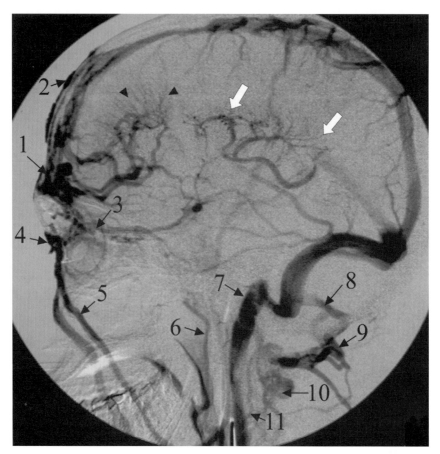

FIG. 10-3. Right internal carotid angiogram, venous phase, lateral view, in a patient with blue rubber bleb nevus syndrome, multiple venous angiomas (*arrowheads*), and sinus pericranii. Some prominent medullary veins are indicated by the open arrows. A number of veins that are not typically identified on normal angiograms are opacified (case courtesy of J. Rees).

1, Sinus pericranii
2, Scalp veins
3, Superior ophthalmic vein
4, Angular vein
5, Anterior facial vein
6, Posterior facial vein
7, Internal jugular bulb and vein
8, Emissary vein
9, Suboccipital venous plexus
10, Vertebral venous plexus
11, External jugular vein

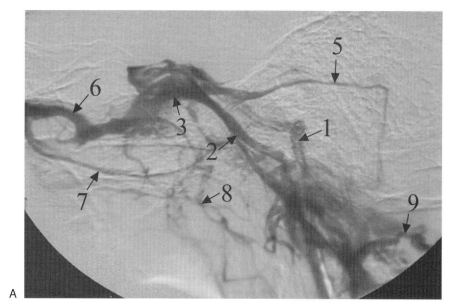

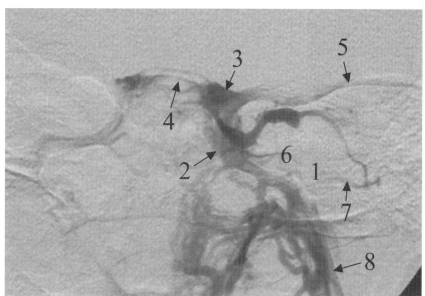

FIG. 10-4. Inferior petrosal sinus venous sampling was performed in this patient with Cushing's disease. Test injection of contrast with lateral **(A)** and anteroposterior sinus **(B)** views demonstrates filling of the basilar venous sinuses and plexi. Compare with Fig. 10-2.

1, Inferior petrosal sinus
2, Clival venous plexus
3, Cavernous sinus
4, Intercavernous sinus
5, Superior petrosal sinus
6, Superior ophthalmic vein
7, Sphenoparietal sinus
8, Pterygoid venous plexus
9, Suboccipital and vertebral plexus

sinuses are normally seen with inferior petrosal and orbital venograms (Fig. 10-4).

Face and Neck Veins

Only a few of the facial veins and their tributaries are seen routinely on the late venous phase of cerebral angiograms. The *pterygoid venous plexus* is often seen as a fine network of vessels that lies in the masticator space (Fig. 10-5; see also Fig. 10-13). If common carotid injections are performed, the *anterior facial vein* is sometimes identified as it descends obliquely and posteriorly from the orbit to the IJV. The *suboccipital veins*, tributaries of the vertebral venous plexus, occasionally appear very prominent and should not be mistaken for a vascular malformation (Fig. 10-6).

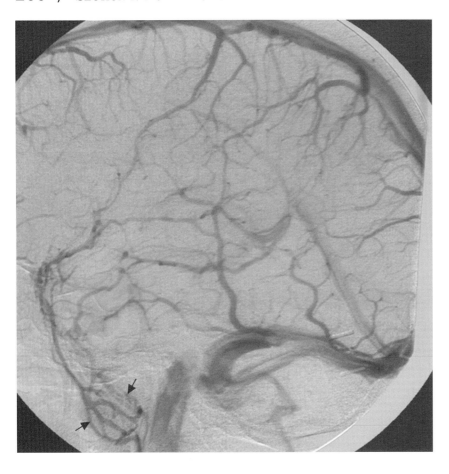

FIG. 10-5. Left common carotid angiogram, venous phase, lateral view. Note prominent drainage into the pterygoid venous plexus (*arrows*).

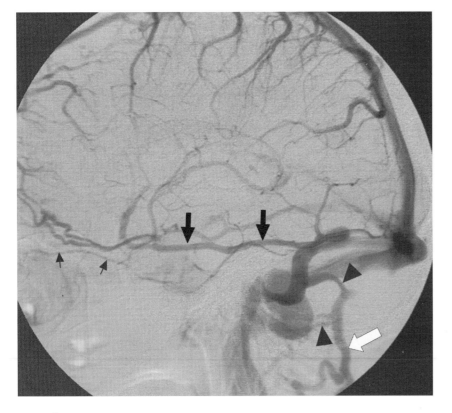

FIG. 10-6. Left internal carotid angiogram, venous phase, lateral view. Note the prominent vein of Labbé draining into the superior petrosal sinus (*large arrows*). A number of emissary veins (*large arrowheads*) drain into a large suboccipital vein (*white arrow*). The superior ophthalmic vein (*small arrows*) is opacified, a relatively unusual finding with an internal carotid injection. No abnormalities were noted on the angiogram.

DIPLOIC VEINS

Normal Gross Anatomy and Relationships

The diploic veins are large, irregular endothelial-lined vascular channels that course within the diploic spaces of the calvarium (Fig. 10-7). They do not have valves and communicate freely with meningeal veins, dural sinuses, and pericranial veins (1).

Normal Radiographic Anatomy

A number of small diploic veins may terminate in enlarged venous lakes (lacunae), forming prominent

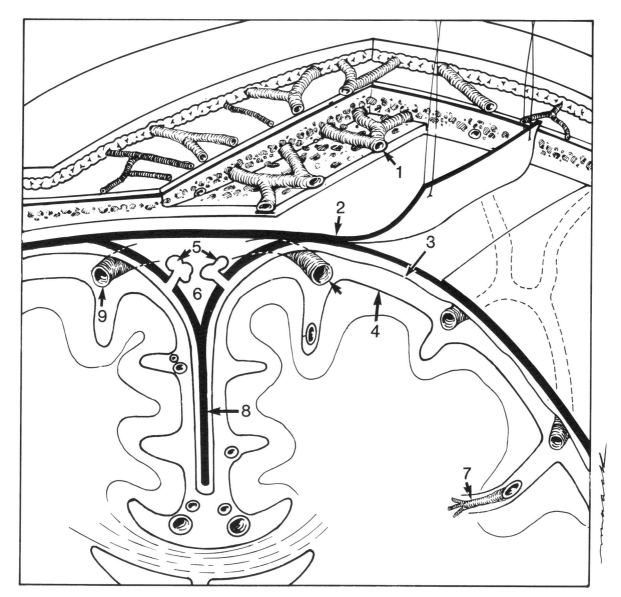

FIG. 10-7. Anatomic diagram depicts the scalp, skull, meninges, and their relationships to the dural sinuses, cortical veins, and diploic spaces. The dura is shown as the thick black line; the outer layer is reflected by sutures.

1, Diploic veins in calvarium
2, Dura (outer and inner layers are shown)
3, Arachnoid (the space between the dura and arachnoid, the subdural space, is only a potential space but is exaggerated here for purposes of illustration)
4, Pia mater (the innermost layer of the leptomeninges is closely applied to the cerebral cortex)
5, Pacchionian granulations (note projections from subarachnoid space into superior sagittal sinus)
6, Superior sagittal sinus
7, Virchow-Robin (perivascular) space surrounding a penetrating cortical artery
8, Falx cerebri
9, Cortical veins (shown as they course across the potential subdural space to enter the SSS)
(Reprinted with permission from Osborn A. *Diagnostic neuroradiology.* St. Louis: Mosby, 1994.)

sharply marginated lucencies that may be identified on plain film radiographs as well as computed tomography scans performed and displayed with bone algorithm reconstruction. Because flow in diploic veins is very slow, they are usually not visualized on cerebral angiograms.

DURAL VENOUS SINUSES

Normal Development

Embryologic development of the cranial veins and dural sinuses is discussed in detail in Chapter 11.

Gross Anatomy and Relationships

Histology

The cranial dural venous sinuses are endothelial-lined channels that are located between the periosteal (outer) and meningeal (inner) layers of the dura (Fig. 10-7). The walls of dural sinuses are composed of firm fibrous dura and do not collapse when sectioned (5). Dural sinuses do not possess valves, and their walls are devoid of muscular tissue. Occasionally small fat deposits may be identified within dural sinus walls (6). Although many texts describe dural sinuses as simple channels, most are complex trabeculated structures that have numerous crossing bands, chords, and bridges (7).

Flow Patterns

The dural sinuses collect blood from the superficial and deep cerebral veins, meninges, and calvarium. They thus form the major drainage pathway for the cranial cavity and its contents. Via a network of emissary veins that pass directly through the cranial vault and basilar foramina, the dural sinuses communicate with the extracranial venous system. These intercommunications may provide an important potential pathway for collateral venous drainage in case of cerebral venous occlusion (8) (see Chapter 15). The dural sinuses also communicate with the meningeal and diploic veins.

Gross Anatomy

The major dural venous sinuses are the superior and inferior sagittal sinuses, the cavernous and intercavernous sinuses, the superior and inferior petrosal sinuses, the occipital sinus (OS), and the straight, transverse, and sigmoid sinuses (Fig. 10-8).

The *superior sagittal sinus* (SSS) lies in a shallow midsagittal depression at the junction of the falx cerebri, with the dura lining the inner table of the calvarium (Fig. 10-7) (9). The SSS originates near the crista galli, where it communicates with facial and nasal veins. The SSS arcs posteriorly, progressively increasing in caliber as it pro-

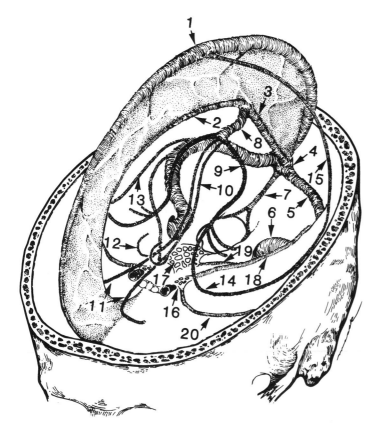

FIG. 10-8. Anatomic diagram of the cerebral venous system.

1, Superior sagittal sinus
2, Inferior sagittal sinus
3, Straight sinus
4, Torcular Herophili (sinus confluence)
5, Transverse sinus
6, Sigmoid sinus
7, Occipital sinus
8, Vein of Galen
9, Basal vein of Rosenthal
10, Internal cerebral veins
11, Septal veins
12, Thalamostriate veins
13, Vein of Labbé
14, Superficial middle cerebral vein
15, Vein of Trolard
16, Cavernous sinus
17, Clival venous plexus
18, Superior petrosal sinus
19, Inferior petrosal sinus
20, Sphenoparietal sinus

(Reprinted with permission from Osborn A. *Diagnostic neuroradiology*. St. Louis: Mosby, 1994.)

ceeds caudally and collects numerous parasagittal veins that drain the cerebral convexities.

The SSS is midline throughout most of its course. It usually terminates by joining with the straight sinus (SS) to form the torcular Herophili (sinus confluence) at the internal occipital protuberance.

The *inferior sagittal sinus* (ISS) is a relatively small channel that courses posteriorly in the inferior free edge of the falx cerebri (Fig. 10-8). The ISS begins at the junction of the anterior and middle thirds of the falx, lying above the anterior aspect of the corpus callosum body. The ISS receives tributaries from the falx, corpus callosum, cingulum, and medial cerebral hemispheres. The ISS terminates at the falcotentorial apex by joining with the great cerebral vein (vein of Galen) to form the SS.

The *straight sinus* (SS) is formed by the confluence of the ISS and vein of Galen (Figs. 10-1 and 10-8). The SS runs posteroinferiorly within the confluence of the falx cerebri and tentorium cerebelli. As it descends toward the torcular, the SS receives a number of bridging vermian and hemispheric tributaries. The SS also receives variably shaped, inconstant venous channels that originate within the tentorium cerebelli itself.

In 85% of anatomic dissections the SS is represented by a single midline tentorial channel, whereas in the remaining 15% segments of the SS is doubled or even tripled (10). The SS is approximately 5 cm in length. In two thirds of cases, its slope of inclination is tangential to the upper aspect of the corpus callosum splenium (11). The SS terminates at the internal occipital protuberance, usually by becoming the left transverse sinus (TS).

The *torcular Herophili* (confluence of sinuses) is formed by the union of the SSS, SS, and transverse sinuses. It usually has two major components, the right and left transverse sinuses, which are united by variable cross channels. The confluence is asymmetric and shows numerous variations. Its tributaries are also highly variable (12) (Fig. 10-9).

A marginal venous plexus surrounds the foramen magnum and drains into a small, variable sinus called the *occipital sinus*. The OS begins at the posterior margin of the foramen magnum and passes superiorly into the torcular (Fig. 10-2A). The OS communicates with the internal jugular vein, vertebral venous plexus, and clival venous plexus through multiple small channels (13). In approximately 2% of cases the OS forms a major draining channel for the SS or SSS (12,14).

The *transverse sinuses* (TSs), also known as the lateral sinuses, are contained within the attachments of the tentorial leaves to the calvarium. The TSs curve anterolater-

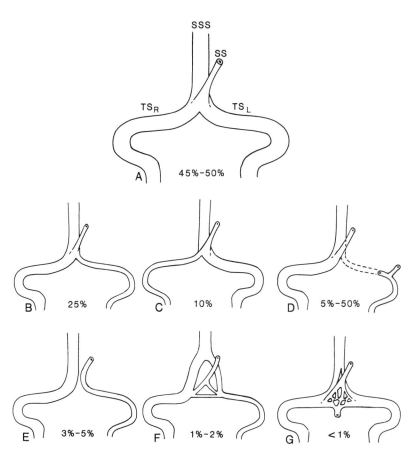

FIG. 10-9. Anteroposterior diagrams depict the great anatomic variability of the torcular Herophili (sinus confluence). The approximate prevalence of each configuration is indicated. SSS, superior sagittal sinus; SS, straight sinus; TSR, right transverse sinus; TSL, left transverse sinus; SC, sinus confluence. **A:** A typical arrangement in which both transverse sinuses are of equal size. **B:** The SSS veers off the midline and continues as the dominant right TS; the left TS is relatively small. **C:** The SSS continues as the left TS, and the right TS is relatively small. **D:** Segmental hypoplasia or aplasia of a TS is shown. Here a small TS may be reconstituted distally by a vein of Labbé or other tributaries (e.g., from the tentorial sinus), but its proximal segment is absent. This normal variant should not be mistaken for sinus occlusion. **E:** The SSS becomes the right TS; the SS becomes the left TS and there is no true sinus confluence. **F:** High-splitting SSS. **G:** Septated or fenestrated torcular Herophili, shown here with an occipital sinus. Numerous other variations also occur.

ally from the internal occipital protuberance to the petrous temporal bones (Figs. 10-2 and 10-8). At the posterior border of the petrous temporal bone, the TSs receive the superior petrosal sinus (SPS) as they turn downward and medially to become the sigmoid sinuses.

The TSs receive venous blood from the SSS and SS. Along their course, the TS almost always receive bridging venous tributaries from the cerebellum, inferolateral surfaces of the temporal and occipital lobes, and tentorium. These channels, the *tentorial sinuses*, may be quite prominent (15,15a). When it is present, the TS also receives the anastomotic cortical *vein of Labbé* (see Chapter 11). The TSs communicate with extracranial veins via mastoid emissary veins (9).

In approximately half of all cases, both TSs are well formed but asymmetric in size (Fig. 10-9). In nearly 75% of cases the right TS is the larger of the two sinuses (16). In 5% to 20% of anatomic specimens, a narrowed or atretic segment can be identified in at least one of the TSs (16,17).

The *sigmoid sinuses* represent the anteroinferior continuation of the TSs (Figs. 10-2 and 10-8). The sigmoid sinuses begin where the TS leaves the tentorial margin as they pass inferomedially in a gentle S-shaped curve to drain into the jugular bulb. The sigmoid sinuses terminate by becoming the paired *internal jugular veins*. Numerous anastomoses between sigmoid sinuses and the vertebral plexuses, suboccipital muscular and scalp veins, and condylar emissary veins are common.

The *superior petrosal sinuses* (SPSs), channels that extend from the cavernous sinus to the sigmoid sinuses, run along the attachment of the tentorium cerebelli to the dorsal ridge of the petrous temporal bones (Fig. 10-2). Tributaries of the SPSs include the petrosal veins that drain the pons and upper medulla, lateral mesencephalic vein, cerebellar veins, and veins draining the inner ear (9).

The *inferior petrosal sinuses* (IPSs) lie in a groove between the petrous apices and the clivus, extending posterolaterally along the petrooccipital fissure (Fig. 10-2). Anatomists have shown that the IPSs demonstrate marked anatomic variation, not only in size and anastomoses, but also in their relationship with the cranial nerves entering the jugular foramen and with the jugular foramen itself (18).

The IPSs usually terminate by draining into the jugular bulb. There are numerous anastomotic channels between the IPSs, basilar (clival) venous plexus, vertebral venous plexuses, pterygoid venous plexus, and epidural veins (Fig. 10-2). One or more of these may be dominant in any given patient. IPS anatomy is symmetric in nearly two thirds of patients. Absence of an anastomosis between the IPS and internal jugular vein occurs in only 1% of cases (18–20).

The *sphenoparietal sinus* is the anteroinferior continuation of the meningeal sinus and the medial extension of the superficial middle cerebral (sylvian) veins. The SPS follows the curve of the lesser sphenoid ala and has three typical drainage patterns: (a) into the cavernous sinus, (b) into the pterygoid plexus via basal emissary veins, or (c) posteriorly along the middle cranial fossa floor into the inferior petrosal or transverse sinus (9). In the latter two cases, the SPS bypasses the cavernous sinus.

The *cavernous sinuses* (CSs) lie on either side of the sphenoid body. A true cavernous sinus, i.e., a single large channel that totally surrounds the internal carotid artery, is found in less than 1% of cases. The vast majority of CSs are formed by numerous small veins, resulting in irregularly shaped, heavily trabeculated and compartmentalized venous spaces that interconnect extensively (21).

The CSs extend from the superior orbital fissure anteriorly to the petrous apex posteriorly (Fig. 10-2). The CS contains the cavernous segment of the internal carotid artery and the abducens nerve (CN VI). The oculomotor nerve (CN III), trochlear nerve (CN IV), and ophthalmic division of the trigeminal nerve (CN V₁) lie between dural leaves of the lateral cavernous sinus wall (see Fig. 4-2B).

The cavernous sinus tributaries and interconnections are complex and variable (Figs. 10-2 and 10-8). Anteriorly the CS receives the superior and inferior ophthalmic vein and also may receive the sphenoparietal sinus. Laterally they communicate with the pterygoid plexus through emissary veins that pass through the foramen ovale. Medially each CS communicates with its counterpart on the opposite side via intercavernous sinus, forming the so-called circular sinus that surrounds the sella turcica (Fig. 10-2A) (9).

Posteriorly the CSs empty into the superior and inferior petrosal sinuses, through which they drain into the transverse sinus and jugular bulb, respectively. The CSs also communicate with a network of veins that extends along the basiocciput to the foramen magnum, the *clival venous plexus* (see Fig. 10-2). The clival plexus in turn communicates with the vertebral venous plexuses.

Vascular Territory

The venous drainage of the dural sinuses is discussed together with that of the cerebral veins in Chapter 11.

Normal Angiographic Anatomy

Lateral View

Many of the dural sinuses are clearly delineated on the venous phase of cerebral angiograms. On the lateral view, the *superior sagittal sinus* appears as a curvilinear structure that hugs the inner table of the skull (Fig. 10-10). Usually the SSS originates near the crista galli and gradually increases in size as it extends posteriorly and inferiorly.

The *inferior sagittal sinus* lies within the inferior free edge of the falx cerebri and is best seen on lateral views (Fig. 10-11). Opacification of the ISS and its tributaries is

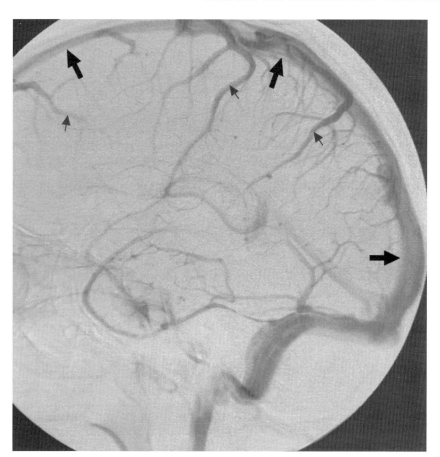

FIG. 10-10. Left internal carotid angiogram, venous phase, lateral view. The superior sagittal sinus is well shown. Note that the SSS (*large arrows*) becomes progressively larger as it courses posteriorly, collecting a number of cortical veins (*small arrows*).

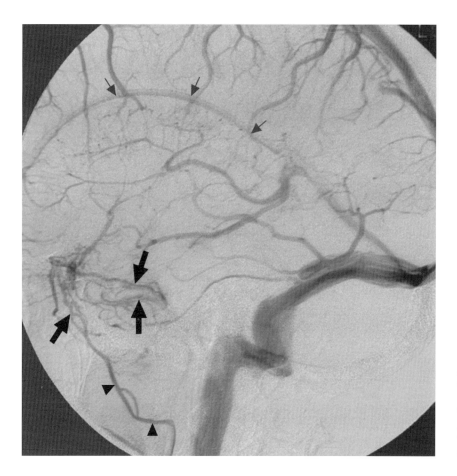

FIG. 10-11. Left internal carotid angiogram, venous phase, lateral view. A very prominent inferior sagittal sinus (*small arrows*) is present. Note filling of the septated cavernous sinus (*large arrows*). The cavernous sinus connects through the skull base with the deep extracranial venous plexi (*arrowheads*).

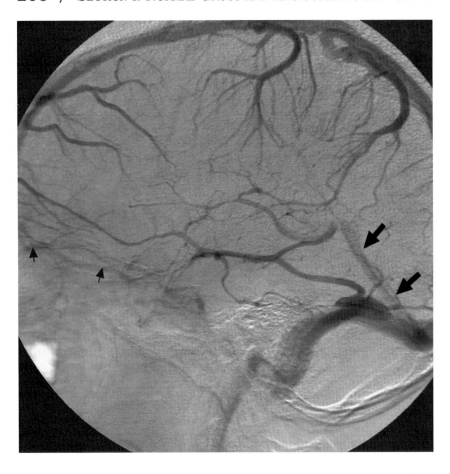

FIG. 10-12. Left common carotid angiogram, venous phase, lateral view. The straight sinus is indicated by the large arrows. Note faint opacification of the superior ophthalmic vein (*small arrows*).

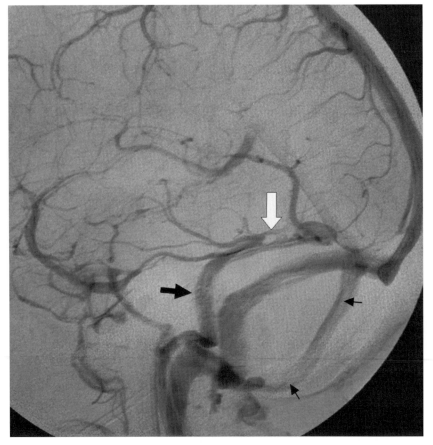

FIG. 10-13. Left internal carotid angiogram, venous phase, lateral view. Note the anteriorly convex sigmoid sinuses (*large arrow*). An unusually prominent (but normal) occipital sinus is indicated by the small arrows. The sharply delineated, rounded filling defects in one of the transverse sinuses (*white arrow*) are arachnoid granulations.

highly variable. A button-hook–shaped acute bend is sometimes present at its anterior margin, where the ISS is formed by tributaries from the falx, corpus callosum, and cingulate gyrus.

Near its origin, the ISS is closer to the inner table of the skull. As it arcs posteriorly, the ISS follows an increasingly more inferior course toward its union with the internal cerebral veins.

Formed at the confluence of the vein of Galen and the ISS, the *straight sinus* extends posteroinferiorly toward the internal occipital protuberance and is almost always well delineated on lateral cerebral angiograms (Fig. 10-12). The torcular Herophili is formed by the confluence of the SSS and SS with the *transverse sinuses* (Fig. 10-12). On lateral views the TSs often have a slight upwardly convex curve as they course anteriorly (Fig. 10-12).

The sigmoid sinuses have a short, anteriorly convex curve as they course inferomedially toward the jugular foramen (Fig. 10-13). Its inferior continuation is the jugular bulb. The bulb may have a prominent enlargement that projects slightly superiorly before it continues inferiorly through the jugular foramen to become the internal jugular vein. The IJV can be seen for some distance as it courses inferiorly within the carotid space.

Because it is usually one of the smallest major dural sinuses, the *occipital sinus* (Fig. 10-13) is rarely well

defined on carotid angiograms. When present, the OS can be seen as it extends upward from the marginal venous plexus around the foramen magnum to the torcular Herophili (see Fig. 10-16).

The skull base dural sinuses (the superior and inferior petrosal sinuses, cavernous sinus, sphenoparietal sinuses, and clival venous plexus) are variably and inconstantly visualized at carotid angiography (Fig. 10-14).

Anteroposterior View

On straight anteroposterior (AP) views, the anterior and middle portions of the SSS are superimposed (Fig. 10-15). Unless the study is slightly oblique (Fig. 10-16), the SS and ISS are also often superimposed on other prominent midline venous structures such as the SSS and therefore may be difficult to identify (Fig. 10-15).

The torcular Herophili and the transverse sinuses are easily identified on AP cerebral angiograms, although their configuration is quite variable (Fig. 10-9). Posteriorly the torcular Herophili and transverse sinuses usually form an inverted "T" with the SSS (Figs. 10-9A and 10-15). The SSS also may drain directly into the right TS. On AP views the TS sometimes slope first inferiorly, then curve slightly superiorly as they extend toward their continuation with the sigmoid sinuses (see Fig. 10-20).

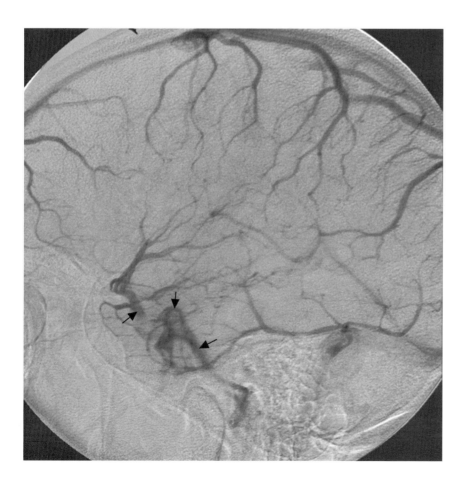

FIG. 10-14. Left internal carotid angiogram, venous phase, lateral view, shows a prominent cavernous sinus and clival venous plexus (*arrows*).

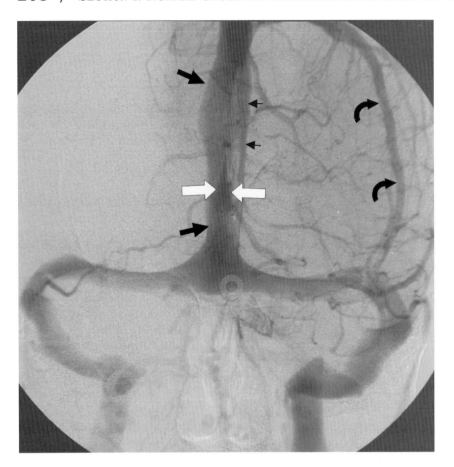

FIG. 10-15. Left internal carotid angiogram, venous phase, anteroposterior view, shows a typical configuration of the torcular Herophili (compare with Fig. 10-9A). The anterior part of the superior sagittal sinus (SSS) (*small black arrows*) is mostly superimposed on the larger, more prominent posterior part of the sinus (*large black arrows*). The straight sinus and vein of Galen are barely seen as a dense, midline contrast collection (*white arrows*) that also overlies the posterior SSS. A prominent vein of Trolard (the superior superficial anastomotic vein) is indicated by the curved arrows.

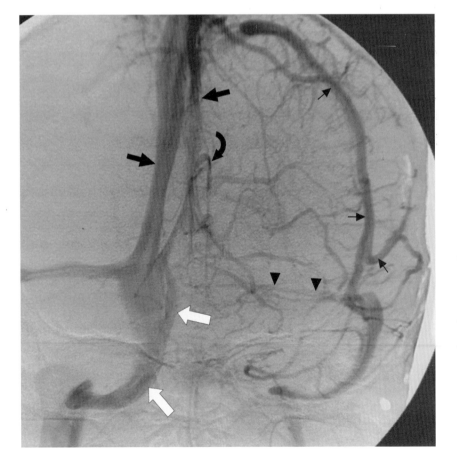

FIG. 10-16. Left internal carotid angiogram, venous phase, anteroposterior view. The inferior and straight sinuses (*curved arrow*) are visible because the superior sagittal sinus (*large black arrows*) runs off the midline to the right and the film is slightly oblique. Note hypoplasia or atresia of the left transverse sinus (*arrowheads*). The congenitally small left TS is reconstituted distally by a confluence of the superior and inferior anastomotic veins (of Trolard and Labbé), indicated by the small black arrows. A prominent occipital sinus (*white arrows*) is also present. Compare with Figure 10-9D.

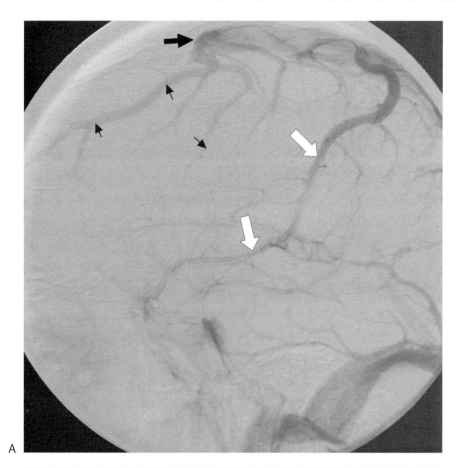

A

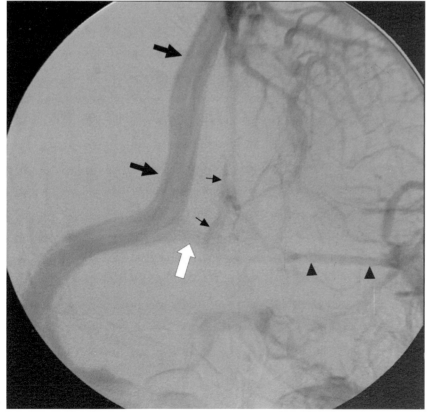

B

FIG. 10-17. Left internal carotid angiogram, venous phase. Lateral **(A)** and anteroposterior **(B)** views are shown. **A:** Lateral view shows that the anterior one third of the superior sagittal sinus (SSS) (*large arrow*) is atretic. The SSS is constituted near the coronal suture by unusually large frontal cortical veins (*small arrows*). A prominent superior anastomotic vein (of Trolard) is also present (*white arrows*). **B:** The SSS (*large arrows*) courses more than a centimeter off the midline and terminates by becoming the right transverse sinus (TSR). The straight sinus (*small arrows*) is joined to both TSs by small venous channels (*white arrow*). The left transverse sinus (TSL) (*arrowheads*) is hypoplastic. In this variant there is no true torcular Herophili (sinus confluence).

Normal Variants and Anomalies

Normal Variants

The dural sinuses are normally quite variable (Fig. 10-9). Only a few of the most important normal variants are illustrated here.

Occasionally an *absent anterior SSS* occurs. In this variant the SSS is formed more posteriorly by the union of several prominent superior cortical draining veins such as a frontal vein and a large vein of Trolard (Fig. 10-17A) The SSS often deviates slightly to the right as it descends along the occipital bone, where it ends by becoming the right transverse sinus. In 20% of normal patients, the posterior SSS deviates more than 1 cm from the midline (Figs. 10-17B and 10-18) (9).

Sometimes the *SSS terminates directly in a TS*. The opposite TS is often hypoplastic or absent (Fig. 10-18 and 10-19) (9). A common pattern is for the SSS to continue as the right TS and the SS becomes the left TS. In this arrangement the torcular Herophili is often hypoplastic or absent (Fig. 10-19). In yet another variant, a *"high-splitting"* SSS is present (Fig. 10-20).

Isolated *absence or hypoplasia of part or all of a TS* is also common (Fig. 10-21). These normal variants can usually be distinguished from dural sinus occlusion by the lack of enlarged collateral pathways and the absence of associated parenchymal hemorrhage (see Chapter 15).

Asymmetric jugular bulbs and veins are the rule, not the exception. Occasionally a *"high-riding"* jugular bulb is present. A jugular bulb also may have an upward-pointing dilatation. Both this variant, called a *jugular diverticulum*, and a high-riding bulb may cause pulsatile tinnitus and present clinically as a vascular-appearing retrotympanic mass (Fig. 10-22).

Venous lakes or lacunae are contained within the adjacent dura mater and communicate freely with the SSS. Arachnoid villi (Pacchionian granulations) project into the floor and walls of these lacunae and into the SSS and

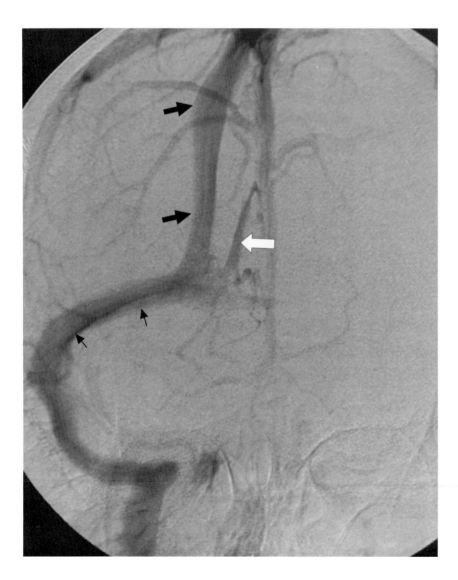

FIG. 10-18. Right internal carotid angiogram, venous phase, anteroposterior view. The superior sagittal sinus (*large black arrows*) courses off the midline and terminates by becoming the right transverse sinus (*small black arrows*). The straight sinus (*white arrow*) is easily observed. Compare with Fig. 10-9B.

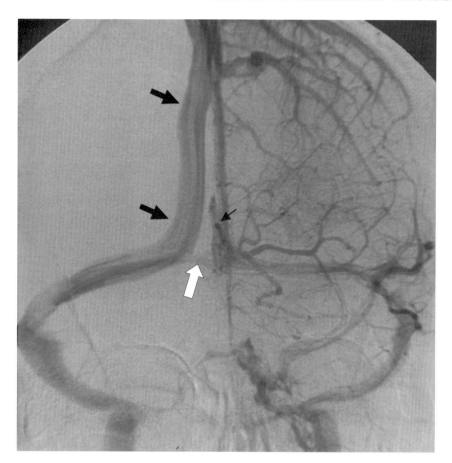

FIG. 10-19. Left internal carotid angiogram, venous phase, anteroposterior view. The superior sagittal sinus (*large arrows*) becomes the right transverse sinus; the straight sinus (*small black arrow*) becomes the smaller left transverse sinus (TS). In this case only a small venous channel (*open arrow*) connects the two TSs and there is no true torcular Herophili.

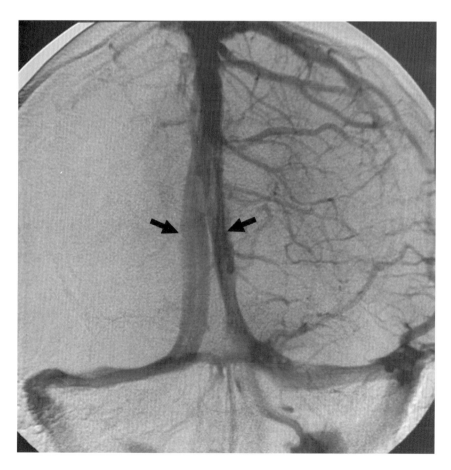

FIG. 10-20. Left internal carotid angiogram, venous phase, anteroposterior view. Note the high-splitting superior sagittal sinus (*arrows*). Compare with Fig. 10-9F.

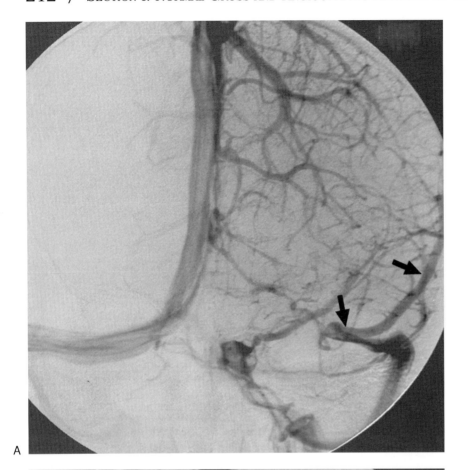

A

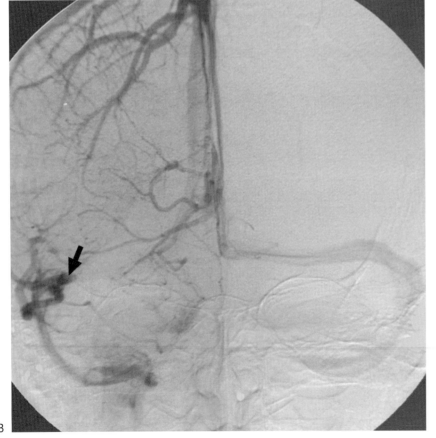

B

FIG. 10-21. Anteroposterior venous phase carotid angiograms in two different patients show congenital absence of the proximal left **(A)** and right **(B)** transverse sinuses (TSs). In both cases the TSs are formed distally (*arrows*) by large superficial inferior anastomotic veins (of Labbé). Compare with Fig. 10-9D.

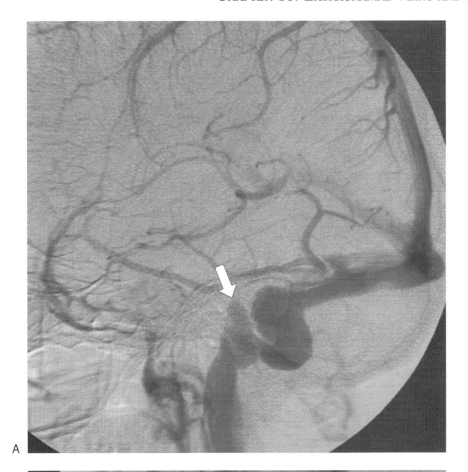

A

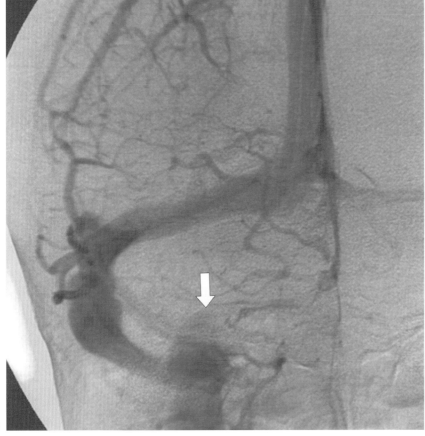

B

FIG. 10-22. Right internal carotid angiogram, venous phase, lateral **(A)** and anteroposterior **(B)** views, in a patient with pulsatile tinnitus shows a jugular bulb diverticulum (*white arrows*).

other dural sinuses such as the SS and TS. These normal structures may be quite prominent (so-called *giant arachnoid granulations*) and should not be mistaken for thrombi on cerebral angiograms (22–25) (Figs. 10-13 and 10-23). Ectopic polypoid nodules of fat, hamartomas, and other tissues may also cause intrasinus filling defects on cerebral angiograms (25a).

Anomalies

Although congenital variations in the dural sinuses are common, true anomalies of these structures are rare.

Most are associated with complex vascular (Fig. 10-3) or congenital brain malformations (26) (Fig. 10-24).

In the *Chiari II malformation* the posterior fossa is abnormally small. The transverse sinuses are low lying and the straight sinus is relatively short. The transverse and straight sinuses are inserted superiorly and posteriorly in both the *Dandy-Walker malformation* and *posterior fossa arachnoid cysts. Vein of Galen malformations* probably represent persistence of the embryonic falcine sinus and the median promesencephalic vein (see Chapter 11). Occasionally a *persistent falcine sinus* is present without other associated abnormalities.

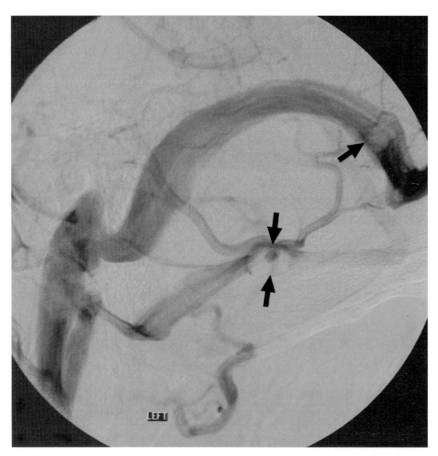

FIG. 10-23. Left internal carotid angiogram, venous phase, oblique lateral view, shows rounded filling defects (*arrows*) in both transverse sinuses. These are so-called giant arachnoid granulations, a normal variant.

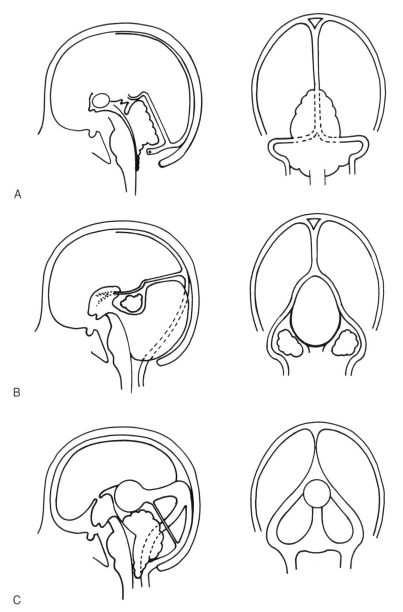

FIG. 10-24. Anatomic diagrams with lateral (*left*) and anteroposterior (*right*) views depict configuration of the dural sinuses with several congenital malformations. **A:** In Chiari II malformation, the posterior fossa is small and shallow. The straight sinus slopes sharply downward and the transverse sinuses are horizontal but very low lying. **B:** In the Dandy-Walker malformation, the posterior fossa is expanded by a large fluid-filled cyst. The torcular is elevated above the lambdoid suture, and the transverse sinuses slope downward. **C:** In the vein of Galen malformation (VOGM), the massively enlarged vein of Galen aneurysm is actually a huge primitive median promesencephalic vein with a large persistent falcine sinus. The straight sinus is often hypoplastic or absent. Severe hydrocephalus is typical.

REFERENCES

1. Williams PL, ed. Veins of the head and neck. In: *Gray's anatomy*, 38th ed. New York: Churchill Livingstone, 1995:1576–1589.
2. Hacker H. Superficial supratentorial veins and dural sinuses. In: Newton TH, Potts DG, eds. *Radiology of the skull and brain*. Vol. 2, Book 3. St. Louis: Mosby, 1974:1851–1877.
3. Spektor S, Piontek E, Umansky F. Orbital venous drainage into the anterior cavernous sinus space: microanatomic relationships. *Neurosurgery* 1997;40:532–540.
3a. Weissman JL, Carrau RL. Anterior facial vein and submandibular gland together: predicting the histology of submandibular masses with CT or MR imaging. *Radiol* 1998;208:441–446.
4. Osborn AG. Craniofacial venous plexuses: angiographic study. *AJR* 1981;136:139–143.
5. Parent A. Cerebral veins and venous sinuses. In: *Carpenter's human neuroanatomy*, 9th ed. Media, PA: Williams and Wilkins, 1996:120–128.
6. Tokiguchi S, Kurashima A, Ito J, et al. Fat in the dural sinus: CT and anatomical correlations. *Neuroradiology* 1988;30:78–80.
7. Andrews BT, Dujovny M, Mirchandani G, Ausman JI. Microsurgical anatomy of the venous drainage into the superior sagittal sinus. *Neurosurgery* 1989;24:514–520.

8. Andeweg J. The anatomy of collateral venous flow from the brain and its value in aetiological interpretation of intracranial pathology. *Neuroradiology* 1996;38:621–628.

9. Cure JK, Van Tassel P, Smith MT. Normal and variant anatomy of the dural venous sinuses. *Semin Ultrasound CT MR* 1994;15:499–519.

10. Browder J, Kaplan HA, Krieger AJ. Anatomical features of the straight sinus and its tributaries. *J Neurosurg* 1976;44:55–61.

11. Hasegawa M, Yamashita J, Yamashima T. Anatomical variations of the straight sinus on magnetic resonance imaging in the infratentorial supracerebellar approach to pineal region tumors. *Surg Neurol* 1991; 36:354–359.

12. Lang J. *Clinical anatomy of the posterior cranial fossa and its foramina.* New York: Thieme, 1991:6–9

13. Braun JP, Tournade A. Venous drainage in the craniocervical region. *Neuroradiology* 1977;13:155–158.

14. Kaplan HA, Browder J, Krieger AJ. Venous channels within the intracranial dural partitions. *Radiology* 1975;115:641–645.

15. Matsushima T, Suzuki SO, Fukui M, et al. Microsurgical anatomy of the tentorial sinuses. *J Neurosurg* 1989;71:923–928.

15A. Muthukumar N, Palaniappan P. Tentorial venous sinuses: An anatomic study. *Neurosurgery* 1998;42:363–371.

16. Zouaoui A. Cerebral venous sinuses: anatomical variants or thrombosis? *Acta Anat (Basel)* 1988;133:318–324.

17. Kaplan HA, Browder A, Browder J. Narrow and atretic transverse dural sinuses: clinical significance. *Ann Otol Rhinol Laryngol* 1973; 82:351–354.

18. Miller DL, Doppman JL, Chang R. Anatomy of the junction of the inferior petrosal sinus and the internal jugular vein. *AJNR* 1993;14: 1075–1083.

19. Miller DL, Doppman JL. Petrosal sinus sampling: technique and rationale. *Radiology* 1991;178:37–47.

20. Gebarski SS, Gebarski KS. Inferior petrosal sinus: imaging-anatomic correlation. *Radiology* 1995;194:239–247.

21. Bonneville JF, Cattin F, Racle A, et al. Dynamic CT of the laterosellar extradural venous spaces. *AJNR* 1989;10:535–542.

22. Leach JL, Jones BV, Tomsick TA, et al. Normal appearance of arachnoid granulations on contrast-enhanced CT and MR of the brain: differentiation from dural sinus disease. *AJNR* 1996;17:1523–1532.

23. Chin SC, Chen CY, Lee CC. Giant arachnoid granulation mimicking dural sinus thrombosis in a boy with headache: MRI. *Neuroradiology* 1998;40:181–183.

24. Okamoto K, Ito J, Tokiguchi S, et al. Arachnoid granulations of the posterior fossa: CT and MR findings. *Clin Imaging* 1997;21:1–5.

25. Ho VB, Rovira MJ, Borke RC, Smirniotopoulos JG. Arachnoid granulations in the transverse sinuses. *IJNR* 1997;3:482–489.

26. Heinz ER. Pathology involving the supratentorial veins and dural sinuses. In: Newton TH, Potts, DG, eds. *Radiology of the skull and brain.* Vol. 2, Book 3. St. Louis: Mosby, 1974:1878–1901.

CHAPTER 11

The Cerebral Veins

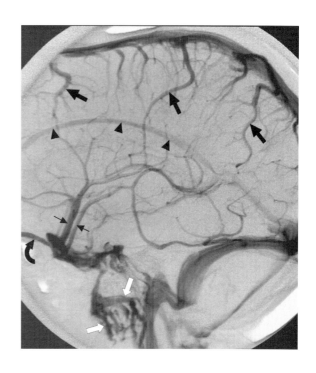

For purposes of discussion, the cerebral veins are conveniently divided into three groups: (a) superficial (cortical) veins; (b) deep (subependymal) veins, and (c) posterior fossa veins. This chapter discusses the normal development of the whole cerebral venous system, then delineates the normal gross and angiographic anatomy of the cerebral veins themselves.

SUPERFICIAL VEINS

Normal Development

Most of the definitive cerebral venous system appears during the third fetal month. It is during this stage that structures such as the superior sagittal sinus (SSS) and vein of Galen emerge. Evolution of the superficial cortical and parenchymal venous channels as well as the calvarial emissary veins also occurs at this time (1).

Focal, lobar, or hemispheric aberrations in venous development during this formative period result in a spectrum of developmental venous anomalies that range from venous angioma, sinus pericranii, and Sturge Weber syndrome, to vein of Galen malformations (see Chapter 17).

Development of some of the most important venous channels is briefly described below.

Dural Sinuses

Evolution of the dural sinuses is complex and results from fusion of multiple venous plexi that surround the developing cerebral vesicles (2). Initially, a *primary head*

sinus arises from the primary hindbrain channel. *Anterior, middle, and posterior dural plexi* drain the anterior, middle, and posterior cerebral vesicles, as well as the myelencephalon.

A pair of *primitive marginal sinuses* extends from the anterior dural plexus along both sides of the anterior cerebral vesicle (Fig. 11-1). These embryonic sinuses eventually fuse, helping to form the definitive *superior sagittal sinus* and the *transverse sinuses* (3). As the cerebellar hemispheres, vermis, and pons grow, there is concomitant lateral displacement of the transverse sinuses as they develop from the primordial dural plexi.

The *straight sinus* results from fusion and reorganization of the embryonic tentorial plexus (2). As the telencephalon develops, the straight sinus is displaced downward and becomes progressively flattened.

Veins

The precursor of the embryonic deep cerebral veins is a single transitory midline vein called the *median prosencephalic vein*. This transient vessel drains the choroid plexi, coursing backward toward a developing dorsal (interhemispheric) dural plexus called the *falcine sinus* (Fig 11-1). The median prosencephalic vein recedes as development of the basal ganglia and choroid plexus induces formation of the definitive internal cerebral veins (ICVs).

A caudal remnant of the median prosencephalic vein eventually unites with the developing *internal cerebral veins* to form the definitive *vein of Galen* (1). If the prim-

217

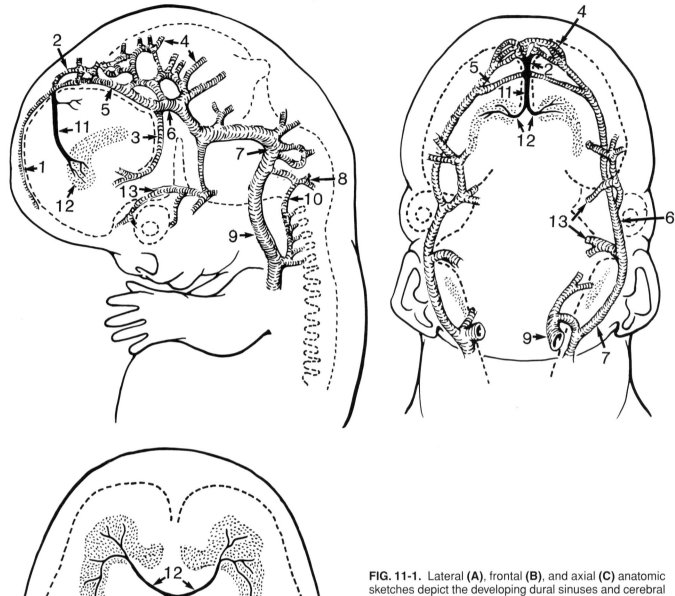

FIG. 11-1. Lateral **(A)**, frontal **(B)**, and axial **(C)** anatomic sketches depict the developing dural sinuses and cerebral veins shown at approximately 8 weeks of gestation. The choroid plexus is indicated by the dotted area. A single midline deep cerebral vein (the so-called prosencephalic vein of Markowitz or primitive internal cerebral vein) drains the choroid plexi and is indicated by the solid black lines.

1, Superior sagittal sinus
2, Primitive straight (falcine) sinus
3, Tentorial sinus
4, Tentorial plexi
5, Primitive marginal sinus
6, Primitive transverse sinus
7, Sigmoid sinus
8, Condylar, hypoglossal emissary veins
9, Internal jugular vein
10, Vertebral veins
11, Primitive internal cerebral vein (median prosencephalic vein)
12, Choroid veins
13, Primitive supraorbital, maxillary veins

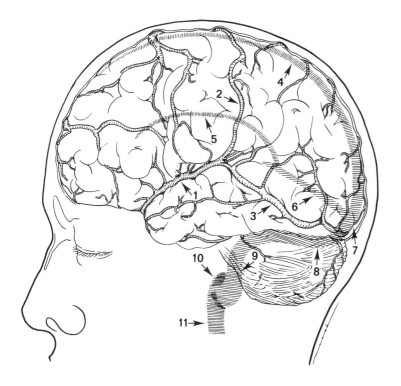

FIG. 11-2. Anatomic drawing depicts the superficial cerebral veins as seen from the lateral perspective. The major dural sinuses are shown in the shaded areas.

1, Superficial middle cerebral vein
2, Vein of Trolard
3, Vein of Labbé
4, Superior sagittal sinus
5, Inferior sagittal sinus
6, Straight sinus
7, Torcular Herophili
8, Transverse sinus
9, Sigmoid sinus
10, Jugular bulb
11, Internal jugular vein

itive median prosencephalic vein persists as an outlet for diencephalic and choroidal venous drainage, the result is aneurysmal dilatation of the vein of Galen (see Chapter 13). In such cases the straight sinus is atretic and venous drainage occurs via a persistent falcine sinus (4,5).

The *basal vein of Rosenthal* (BVR) forms from secondary anastomoses among venous tributaries that drain the caudomedial fetal brain (6). The infratentorial metencephalic and myelencephalic veins show a wide spectrum of development and prominence.

Normal Gross Anatomy

The superficial cerebral veins course along the superficial sulci, draining the cortex and some of the subjacent white matter. The cortical veins are highly variable, both in number and configuration. Abundant anastomoses between the superficial and deep cerebral veins are present but are usually inconspicuous in the absence of venoocclusive disorders.

The superficial veins are subdivided into superior, middle, and inferior groups. Because these veins are so variable, most are unnamed. However, three large cortical veins can often be identified individually. These are (a) the superficial middle cerebral vein (SMCV), (b) the superior anastomotic vein (of Trolard), and (c) the inferior anastomotic vein (of Labbé).

Superficial Middle Cerebral Vein

The superficial middle cerebral vein is a prominent but inconstant vein or group of veins that runs along the sur-

face of the sylvian fissure (Fig. 11-2). It collects a number of small tributaries that drain the opercular areas around the lateral sulcus. The SMCV then curves anteriorly around the temporal lobe tip and passes medially into the cavernous or sphenoparietal sinus (Fig. 11-3).

The SMCV anastomoses with the deep cerebral venous system (via uncal, insular, and basal veins) and with other superficial veins and dural sinuses (Fig. 11-3). The SMCV also communicates with the facial veins and pterygoid plexus through the foramen ovale (see Fig. 10-2B) (7).

Vein of Trolard

The main superior anastomotic vein, the vein of Trolard (also called the frontoparietal vein), is a large but inconstant vessel that courses posterosuperiorly from the sylvian fissure over the mid-hemispheric convexity. It connects the SMCV with the superior sagittal sinus (SSS) (Fig. 11-2).

Vein of Labbé

The inferior anastomotic vein, the vein of Labbé, is also called the occipitotemporal vein (Fig. 11-2). The vein of Labbé courses over the temporal lobe along the occipitotemporal sulcus and connects the SMCV with the transverse sinus. A vein of Labbé can be identified on one or both hemispheres in 75% of anatomic dissections (8).

Vascular Territory

The vascular territories of the entire cranial venous system are discussed in the second section of this chapter.

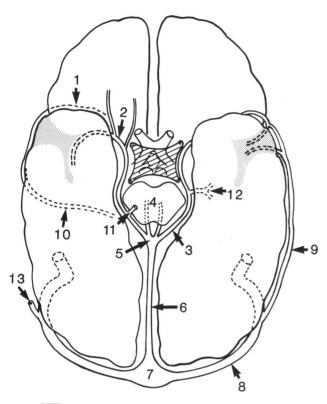

Sylvian fissure

Cavernous sinus and tributaries (cut off)

FIG. 11-3. Anatomic diagram depicts the basal vein of Rosenthal and its tributaries as seen from below. Selected superficial and deep cortical veins are also shown. The sylvian fissure is indicated by the dotted area. The cavernous sinus and its tributaries are indicated by the diagonal lines.

1, Superficial middle cerebral vein and opercular tributaries (often anastomoses with pterygoid plexus, cavernous sinus)
2, Deep middle cerebral vein with uncal, insular, and frontal tributaries
3, Basal vein of Rosenthal
4, Internal cerebral veins
5, Vein of Galen
6, Straight sinus
7, Torcular Herophili
8, Transverse sinus
9, Vein of Labbé (with frontotemporal tributaries, anastomoses with transverse sinus)
10, Vein of Trolard (with superficial middle cerebral tributaries, anastomoses with superior sagittal sinus)
11, Lateral mesencephalic vein (cut off)
12, Choroid veins (cut off)
13, Superior petrosal sinus (cut off)

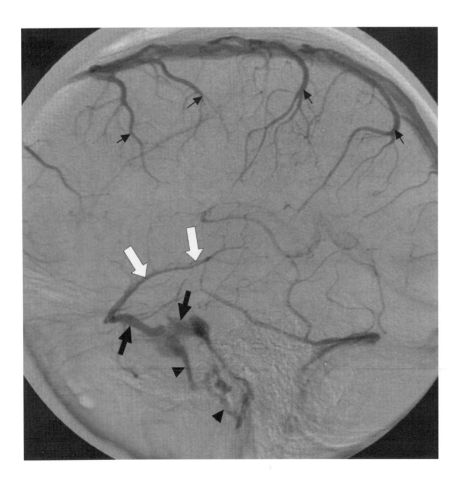

FIG. 11-4. Venous phase of an internal carotid angiogram, lateral view, shows the superior superficial cortical veins (*small arrows*). They appear to radiate outward toward the superior sagittal sinus. A prominent superficial middle cerebral vein (SMCV) (*white arrows*) is present. It drains into the cavernous sinus and clival venous plexus (*large arrows*). The SMCV also drains through the basal foramina, connecting with deep extracranial veins such as the pterygoid plexus (*arrowheads*).

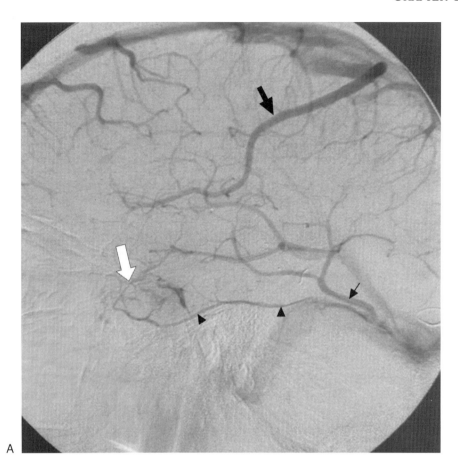

A

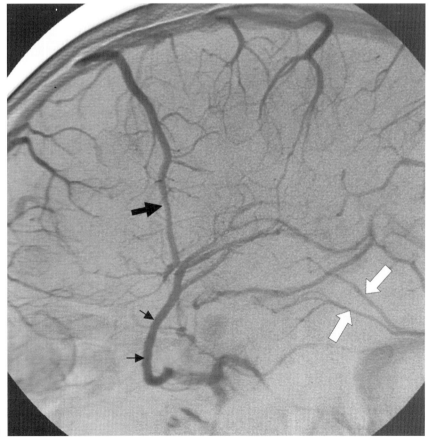

B

FIG. 11-5. A: Venous phase of a common carotid angiogram, lateral view, shows a large vein of Trolard (*large black arrow*) and a small vein of Labbé (*small black arrow*). The superficial middle cerebral vein (*white arrow*) is hypoplastic and drains into the superior petrosal sinus (*arrowheads*). **B:** In another patient, a more anteriorly located superior anastomotic vein (of Trolard) is present (*large black arrow*). In this case the SMCV (*small black arrows*) is also prominent, but the vein of Labbé and its tributaries (*white arrows*) are hypoplastic.

Normal Angiographic Anatomy

Lateral View

Eight to 12 *superior superficial cortical veins* can be identified on lateral views of cerebral angiograms. These veins are arranged in a pattern that resembles the spokes of a bicycle wheel. They appear to radiate outward toward the superior sagittal sinus (SSS), with the sylvian fissure representing the hub of the wheel (Fig. 11-4). As they approach the convexity, cortical veins cross the arachnoid and dura, draining centrifugally into the SSS (see Fig. 10-7).

In the anterior frontal region, cortical veins enter the SSS perpendicularly, but the angle becomes progressively more acute in the parietal and occipital regions. Posteriorly, the cortical veins trace a curve that is concave anteriorly, often passing a considerable distance before draining into the SSS (Fig. 11-4) (9).

Most of the superior cortical veins are 1 mm or less in diameter. If the rostral SSS is congenitally small or atretic, substitute parasagittal venous channels develop and the frontal convexity veins may become quite prominent (see Fig. 10-17A) (10).

When present, the *superficial middle cerebral vein* (SMCV) can be identified on lateral projections during the early venous phase of carotid angiography (Figs. 11-5 to 11-7). The SMCV courses anteriorly along the sylvian fissure and curves around the temporal tip, then drains either medially into the cavernous sinus or inferiorly into the pterygoid plexus.

The *vein of Trolard* is also best identified on the lateral view during the mid- to late venous phase of cerebral angiograms. It appears as a prominent channel that begins near the sylvian fissure and courses superiorly to terminate in the SSS (Fig. 11-5A). On AP projections the vein of Trolard appears to parallel the inner table of the skull as it curves upward and courses over the cerebral convexity (see Figs. 10-15 and 10-16).

On lateral venous phase angiograms the vein of Labbé appears as a posterior continuation of the SMCV. The *vein of Labbé* often has a slight posterosuperior convexity as it crosses over the temporal lobe to join the transverse sinus (Fig. 11-6). In general there is a reciprocal relationship between the veins of Labbé and Trolard. If Trolard is dominant, Labbé is usually small or absent (Fig. 11-5B).

Anteroposterior View

Although the superficial veins are optimally visualized on the lateral view, some of them can be seen on anteroposterior (AP) projections. They form a "stepladder" configuration (Fig. 11-7B).

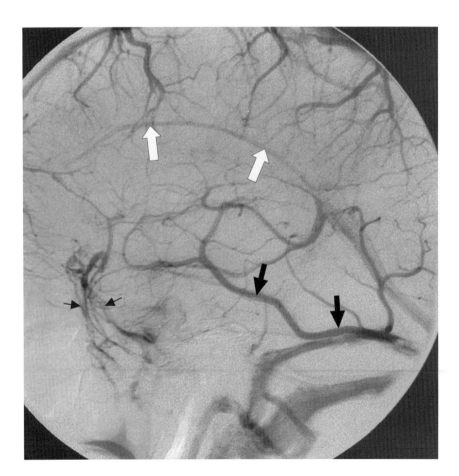

FIG. 11-6. Venous phase of an internal carotid angiogram, lateral view, shows a large vein of Labbé (*large black arrows*). A multi-channeled superficial middle cerebral vein (*small black arrows*) is present. There is no superior anastomotic vein (of Trolard) in this case, but the inferior sagittal sinus (*white arrows*) is quite prominent.

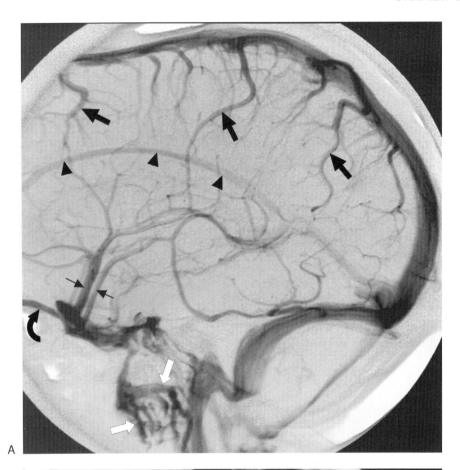

A

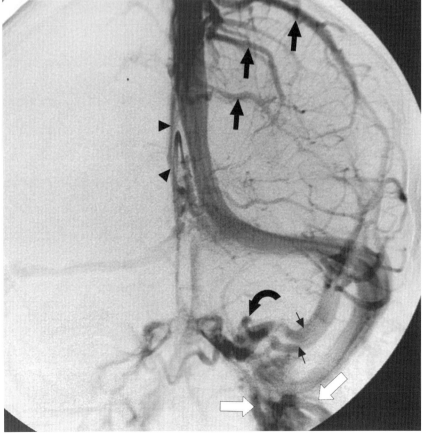

B

FIG. 11-7. Venous phase of a left internal carotid angiogram, lateral **(A)** and anteroposterior **(B)** views, shows the superior superficial cortical veins (*large black arrows*). They are easily observed in the lateral view but overlap each other somewhat in the AP projection. Here they appear to have a stepladder configuration from front to back. A very prominent multi-channeled superficial middle cerebral vein (SMCV) is also present (*small black arrows*). The SMCV drains through the foramen ovale into the pterygoid venous plexus (*white arrows*). A large inferior sagittal sinus (*arrowheads*) is identified, as is the superior ophthalmic vein (*curved arrow*).

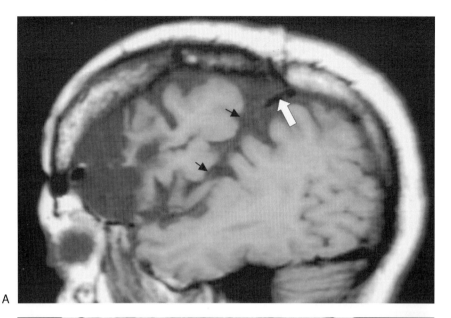

A

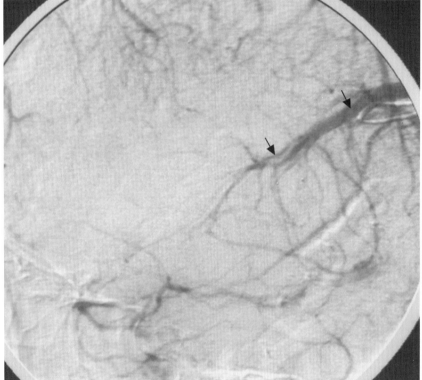

B

FIG. 11-8. Imaging studies from a 32-year-old woman with seizures since birth are shown. **A:** Sagittal T1-weighted MRI scan shows a deep schizencephalic cleft (*small black arrows*) that courses posterosuperiorly from the sylvian fissure. A prominent flow void (*white arrow*) is seen within the cleft. **B:** Venous phase from a right internal carotid angiogram shows an anomalous vein (*arrows*) in the same area as the defect. Anomalous draining veins often accompany schizencephalic clefts and foci of heterotopic gray matter.

Normal Variants and Anomalies

The superficial veins are normally quite variable. Multiple superficial middle cerebral veins are common (Fig. 11-7). If congenital anomalies such as schizencephaly and cortical dysplasia are present, The veins overlying the malformation are also often abnormal (Fig. 11-8).

DEEP VEINS

Normal Gross Anatomy and Relationships

An important exception to the generalization that the brain is drained radially in a centrifugal fashion is that the deep cerebral white matter and basal ganglia drain centrally into the subependymal veins of the lateral ventricles.

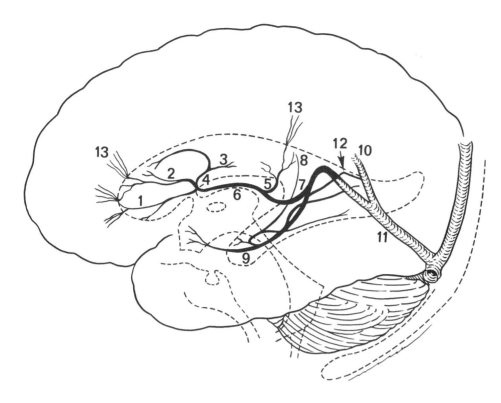

FIG. 11-9. Anatomic drawing of the medullary and subependymal veins. The medullary veins drain the deep white matter into the subependymal veins. The subependymal veins outline the lateral ventricle.

1, Septal vein
2, Anterior caudate veins
3, Terminal vein
4, Thalamostriate vein
5, Direct lateral vein
6, Internal cerebral vein
7, Vein of Galen
8, Inferior ventricular vein
9, Basal vein of Rosenthal
10, Inferior sagittal sinus (cut off)
11, Straight sinus
12, Medial atrial vein
13, Medullary veins

(Adapted with permission from Wolf BS, Huang YP. *AJR* 1964; 91:406–426.)

Medullary Veins

A number of small, deep veins originate 1 to 2 cm below the cortical gray matter. These deep *medullary veins* pass through the deep cerebral white matter and drain into subependymal veins that course along the lateral ventricular walls. The medullary veins are arranged in wedge-shaped patterns and are distributed at right angles to the subependymal veins (Fig. 11-9) (11).

Subependymal Veins

After receiving medullary veins, the subependymal veins aggregate into larger tributaries. The most important of these deep tributaries are the septal, thalamostriate, and internal cerebral veins (Fig. 11-10).

The *septal veins* begin at the lateral aspect of the frontal horns, then pass medially under the corpus callo-

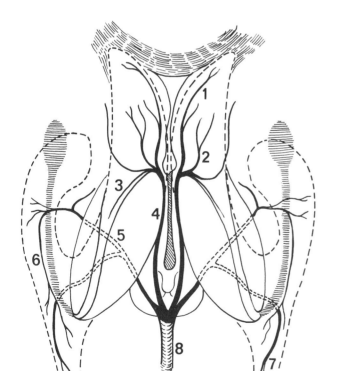

FIG. 11-10. Anatomic drawing of the subependymal veins as seen from above.

1, Septal vein
2, Anterior caudate vein
3, Terminal vein
4, Internal cerebral vein
5, Basal vein of Rosenthal
6, Inferior ventricular vein
7, Lateral atrial vein
8, Vein of Galen

(Adapted with permission from Wolf BS, Huang YP. *AJR* 1964;91:406–426.)

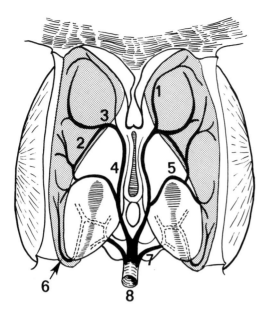

FIG. 11-11. Anatomic drawing of the subependymal veins as seen from above depicts these veins and their relationships to the caudate nuclei (*dotted areas*) and thalami.

1, Anterior caudate vein
2, Terminal vein
3, Thalamostriate vein
4, Internal cerebral vein
5, Direct lateral vein
6, Inferior ventricular vein
7, Basal vein of Rosenthal
8, Vein of Galen

(Adapted with permission from Wolf BS, Huang YP. *AJR* 1964;91:406–426.)

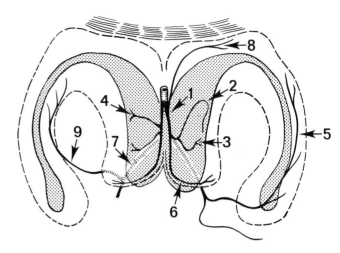

FIG. 11-12. Anatomic drawing of the subependymal veins, anteroposterior view. The lateral ventricles are indicated by the dotted lines, and the caudate nuclei are shaded.

1, Internal cerebral vein
2, Thalamostriate vein
3, Anterior caudate vein
4, Direct lateral vein
5, Inferior ventricular vein
6, Septal vein
7, Basal vein of Rosenthal
8, Medial atrial vein
9, Lateral atrial vein

(Adapted from Wolf BS, Huang YP. *AJR* 1964;91:406–426.)

sum genu. As they near the midline, the septal veins turn sharply backward to run along the septum pellucidum. Each septal vein has a slight, laterally convex curve as it passes around the pillars of the fornix to enter the internal cerebral vein behind the foramen of Monro (Fig. 11-10). In nearly half of all cases, the septal vein joins the internal cerebral vein 3-13mm posterior to the foramen of Monro (11A). The septal veins receive tributaries from the corpus callosum and deep frontal white matter.

The *thalamostriate veins* (TSVs) are among the most prominent of the subependymal veins. The TSVs are formed by the confluence of anterior caudate veins and the *terminal vein*, a vessel that runs beneath the stria terminalis and demarcates the border between the thalamus and caudate nucleus body. The TSVs unite with the septal veins to form the internal cerebral veins (Fig. 11-11).

The *internal cerebral veins* (ICVs) are the largest and most important of the deep cerebral veins. The ICVs are paired structures that originate behind the foramen of Monro. They are located near the midline in the tela choroidea of the roof of the third ventricle (the velum interpositum) (11B). As they course posteriorly, the ICVs receive a number of small subependymal tributaries before they terminate in the rostral part of the quadrigem-

inal cistern by uniting with each other and the basal veins to form the vein of Galen (Fig. 11-11 and 11-12) (12,13).

Two other important deep cerebral veins are the basal veins of Rosenthal and the great cerebral vein (of Galen).

The *basal veins of Rosenthal* (BVRs) arise deep within the sylvian fissure near the uncus of the temporal lobe (Fig. 11-2). The BVRs are formed from the confluence of anterior and deep middle cerebral veins as well as veins that drain the insula and the cerebral peduncles. After receiving these tributaries, the BVRs course posteriorly around the cerebral peduncles and across the tectum to the vein of Galen. Midway through their courses, the BVRs may receive lateral mesencephalic veins (collateral channels that join the BVRs with their respective superior petrosal sinuses).

Just under the corpus callosum splenium, the ICVs and BVRs unite to form the great cerebral *vein of Galen* (V of G). The vein of Galen is a short, U-shaped structure that curves posterosuperiorly around the splenium. It terminates near the tentorial apex, where it joins the inferior sagittal sinus to form the straight sinus (Fig. 11-2).

Vascular Territories

The venous drainage territories of the brain are much more variable and significantly less well known compared with their arterial counterparts (14). The anatomic diagrams shown in Figure 11-13 depict the most common patterns.

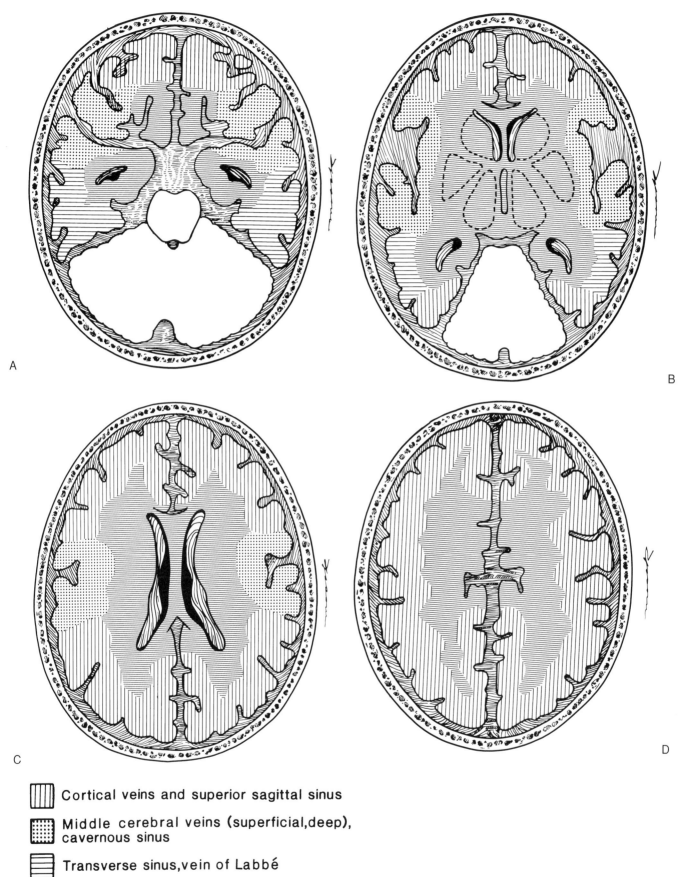

A

B

C

D

Cortical veins and superior sagittal sinus

Middle cerebral veins (superficial,deep), cavernous sinus

Transverse sinus,vein of Labbé

Internal cerebral,subependymal veins, medullary veins, vein of Galen and straight sinus

FIG. 11-13. Venous drainage territories of the supratentorial veins and dural venous sinuses. (Modified and adapted from ref. 14.)

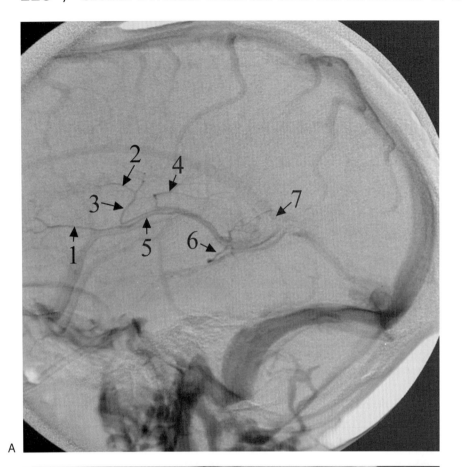

A

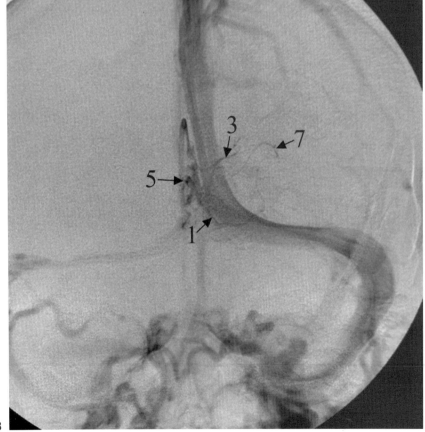

B

FIG. 11-14. Lateral **(A)** and anteroposterior **(B)** views showing the late venous phase of a left internal carotid angiogram. This is the same case as in Fig. 11-7. Note in Fig. 11-7 that the cortical veins are densely opacified in the early venous phase and most of the subependymal veins are not easily observed. On this late venous phase, study contrast has disappeared from the overlying cortical veins and the subependymal veins are now easily identified.

1, Septal vein
2, Anterior caudate veins
3, Thalamostriate vein
4, Terminal vein
5, Internal cerebral vein
6, Medial atrial vein
7, Lateral atrial vein

Normal Angiographic Appearance

In general, the medullary and subependymal veins are opacified slightly later in angiographic series compared with the superficial veins and dural sinuses. The deep veins are best identified late in the venous phase, when contrast no longer opacifies the overlying cortical veins (Fig. 11-14).

Lateral View

A few deep *medullary veins* can usually be identified on high-quality digital or film subtraction angiograms (Fig. 11-15). They are best seen on lateral views, where they appear as small, fine vessels of uniform caliber that are oriented perpendicularly to the ventricular ependyma (see Figs. 4-18D and 10-3). They are most often identified adjacent to the frontal horn and atrium and above the body of the lateral ventricle.

The various major subependymal veins are also easily observed on late venous phase angiograms. They outline the margins of the lateral ventricle, easily permitting angiographic determination of ventricular size and configuration (Fig. 11-15).

The *septal vein* follows a straight or gently undulating posterior course as seen on the lateral view (Figs. 11-14 and 11-16). The *thalamostriate vein* receives its caudate and terminal tributaries, then curves inferiorly to join the septal vein at the foramen of Monro. The *internal cerebral vein* extends from the foramen of Monro posteriorly to the vein of Galen. On lateral views, the ICV follows a somewhat sinusoidal course that is at first concave inferiorly, then convex (Figs. 11-14 and 11-16).

Near its posterior end, the ICV is joined by the *basal vein of Rosenthal*. The BVR follows an anteriorly concave course as it curves around the mid-brain, then turns posterosuperiorly within the ambient cistern to join the ipsilateral ICV (Fig. 11-17; compare with Figs. 11-2 and 11-9).

The great cerebral *vein of Galen* is also best identified on the lateral view. It forms a prominent arc, curving posterosuperiorly around the corpus callosum splenium. The vein of Galen and straight sinus confluence forms a sharp angle that demarcates the tentorial apex.

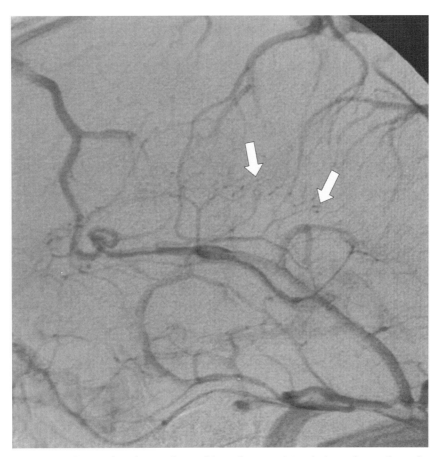

FIG. 11-15. Venous phase of an internal carotid angiogram, lateral view, shows the subependymal and medullary veins. The subependymal veins outline the roof of the lateral ventricle. The innumerable tiny contrast-filled linear structures that lie just outside the ventricle are the medullary veins (*white arrows*).

Anteroposterior View

The subependymal veins are well seen in this projection (Figs. 11-14B and 11-18). Tributaries of the *septal vein* course medially along the anterior wall of the frontal horn. As they approach the midline, the septal veins turn backward to course along the septum pellucidum toward the foramen of Monro.

On AP views the *thalamostriate vein* has a characteristic double curve that resembles an antler (Figs. 11-14B, 11-18, and 11-19). The superolateral aspect of the curve represents the outer margin of the lateral ventricle and collects a tuft of vessels, the medullary veins (Figs. 11-18 and 11-19).

The curved anterior and posterior segments of the *internal cerebral vein* are superimposed on the AP projection. In this view the ICV appears as an elliptical or vertically elongated area of increased density (Fig. 11-19). Because the ICVs are paired structures, the most medial aspect of each ICV should lie within 2 mm of the midline on AP venous phase angiograms.

The angiographic appearance of the *basal vein of Rosenthal* is quite characteristic on the AP view (Fig. 11-20). The BVR resembles the leg of a frog lying on its back with its legs pointing anterolaterally. The ankle corresponds to the most medial aspect of the uncus, whereas the "knee" corresponds to the most lateral aspect of the BVR as it courses around the cerebral peduncles (15).

Variations and Anomalies

Variations in both the superficial and deep venous drainage patterns of the brain are common, but true anomalies are rare (see Fig. 10-24).

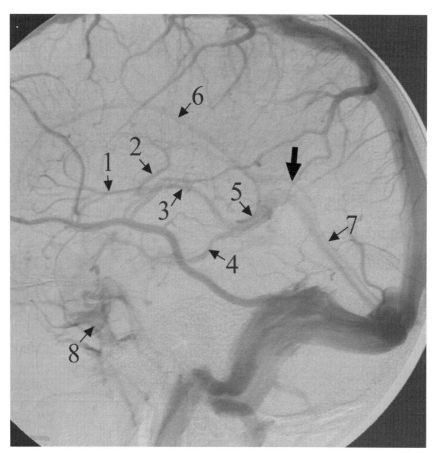

FIG. 11-16. Venous phase of an internal carotid angiogram, lateral view, shows the subependymal veins. The confluence of the vein of Galen and straight sinus demarcates the tentorial apex (*large arrow*).

    1, Septal vein
    2, Thalamostriate vein
    3, Internal cerebral vein
    4, Basal vein of Rosenthal
    5, Vein of Galen
    6, Inferior sagittal sinus
    7, Straight sinus
    8, Cavernous sinus

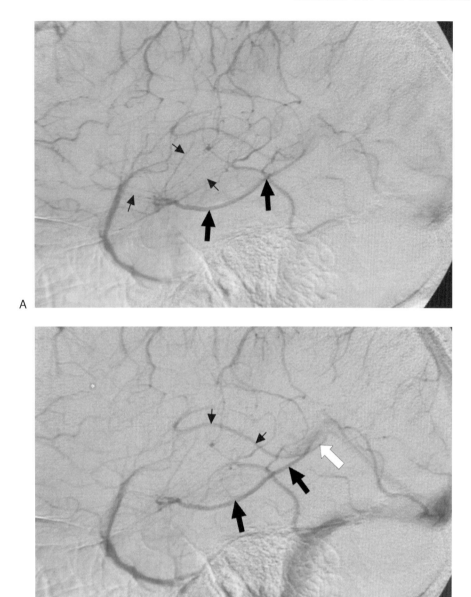

FIG. 11-17. Early **(A)** and late **(B)** venous phase films of an internal carotid angiogram show the basal vein of Rosenthal and its tributaries especially well. **A:** A group of small veins that drains the insula (*small arrows*) is collected by the BVR (*large arrows*). **B:** The BVR (*large arrows*) curves superolaterally around the mid-brain, then joins with the internal cerebral vein (*small arrows*) to form the vein of Galen (*white arrow*).

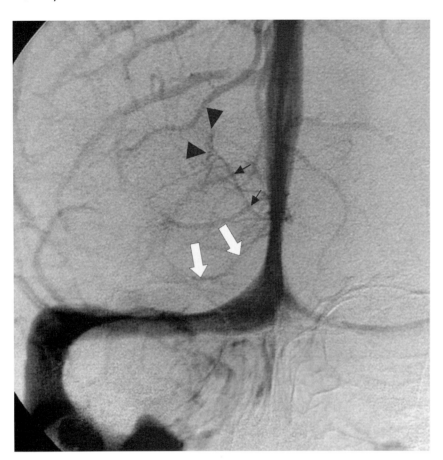

FIG. 11-18. Right internal carotid angiogram, venous phase, anteroposterior view, demonstrates the subependymal veins as they outline the frontal horn and body of the lateral ventricle. A tuft of tiny vessels (*arrowheads*) that drains into the thalamostriate vein (*small arrows*) is a collection of medullary veins. The septal vein (*open arrows*) and the thalamostriate vein converge to form the internal cerebral vein (not seen here because it overlies the densely opacified superior sagittal sinus).

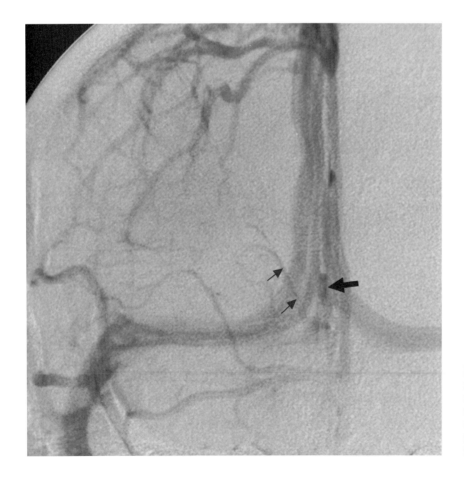

FIG. 11-19. Right internal carotid angiogram, venous phase, anteroposterior view, demonstrates the thalamostriate vein (*small arrows*). The internal cerebral vein (*large arrow*) is seen as a midline, ellipsis-shaped contrast collection.

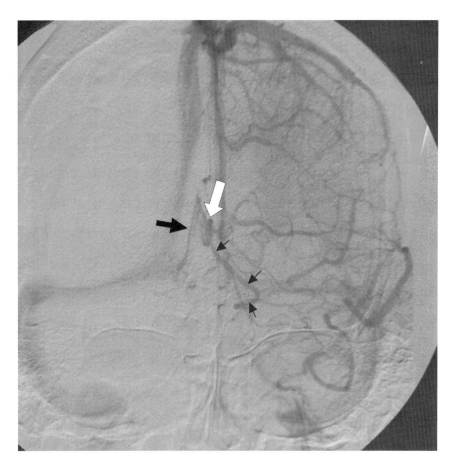

FIG. 11-20. Left internal carotid angiogram, venous phase, anteroposterior view, shows the basal vein of Rosenthal (*small arrows*). The internal cerebral vein (*white arrow*) and straight sinus (*large black arrow*) are also identified because the study is slightly off-midline.

POSTERIOR FOSSA VEINS

Normal Gross Anatomy

Three major posterior fossa venous drainage systems have been described: (a) a superior (Galenic) group; (b) an anterior (petrosal) group, and (c) a posterior (tentorial) group. Before the advent of computed tomography and magnetic resonance imaging (MRI), detailed knowledge of the numerous posterior fossa veins was essential for the angiographic diagnosis of infratentorial mass lesions. Because noninvasive studies are the primary diagnostic modality in the evaluation of posterior fossa tumors, only the most important veins are discussed here.

Superior (Galenic) Veins

Of all the superior (Galenic) group, the most important veins are the precentral cerebellar, superior vermian, and anterior pontomesencephalic veins (Fig. 11-21).

The *precentral cerebellar vein* (PCV) is a single midline vessel that originates in the fissure between the vermian lingula and central lobule. The PCV courses superiorly, paralleling the roof of the fourth ventricle. The PCV

terminates behind the inferior colliculi by draining into the vein of Galen.

The *superior vermian vein* (SVV) originates near the vermian declive, curving up and forward along the culmen. Its tributaries outline the superior surface of the vermis. The SVV terminates by entering the vein of Galen with or just anterior to the PCV.

The *anterior pontomesencephalic vein* (APMV) is not a single structure but consists of many small veins that are closely applied to the pons and demarcate its anterior surface. The APMV often curves into the interpeduncular fossa, delineating the undersurface of the cerebral peduncles.

Anterior (Petrosal) Veins

The most important of the anterior (petrosal) group of draining veins is the *petrosal vein*. Numerous venous tributaries from the cerebellum, pons, and medulla may unite in the cerebellopontine angle cistern to form its short but prominent trunk (Fig. 11-22). The petrosal vein courses anterolaterally below the trigeminal nerve (cranial nerve V) to enter the superior petrosal sinus just above the internal auditory meatus.

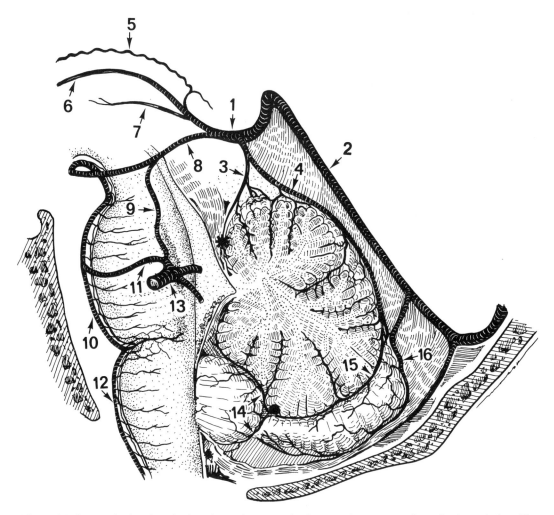

FIG. 11-21. Anatomic drawing depicts the major posterior fossa veins as seen from the lateral view. The black star represents the colliculocentral point, an angiographic landmark that should be about halfway between the tuberculum sellae and the torcular Herophili.

1, Vein of Galen
2, Straight sinus
3, Precentral cerebellar vein
4, Superior vermian vein
5, Superior choroid vein (in lateral ventricle)
6, Internal cerebral vein
7, Thalamic vein
8, Posterior mesencephalic vein (posterior part of Basal vein of Rosenthal)
9, Lateral mesencephalic vein
10, Anterior pontomesencephalic venous plexus
11, Transverse pontine vein
12, Anterior medullary venous plexus
13, Petrosal vein
14, Tonsillar veins
15, Inferior vermian vein
16, Hemispheric vein

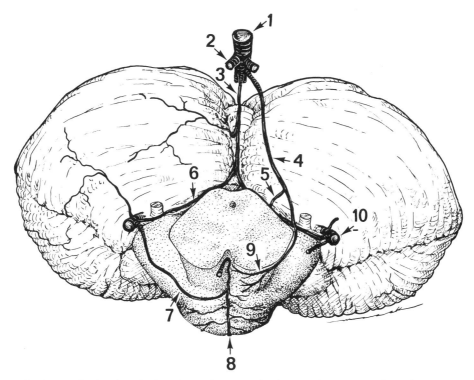

FIG. 11-22. Anatomic drawing depicts the major posterior fossa veins as seen from the anterosuperior perspective.

1, Vein of Galen
2, Internal cerebral vein (cut off)
3, Precentral cerebellar vein
4, Posterior mesencephalic vein
5, Lateral mesencephalic vein
6, Brachial vein
7, Transverse pontine vein
8, Anterior pontomesencephalic venous plexus
9, Peduncular veins
10, Petrosal vein

Posterior (Tentorial) Veins

From an angiographic point of view, the only important posterior veins are the *inferior vermian veins* (IVVs). The IVVs are paired paramedian vessels that curve posterosuperiorly along the inferior vermis. They receive hemispheric veins and usually terminate within the tentorial sinuses.

Normal Angiographic Appearance

Lateral View

Most of the posterior fossa veins are best seen in the lateral projection of vertebral angiograms (Fig. 11-23). The *precentral cerebellar vein* has an anteriorly convex curve that roughly approximates the roof of the fourth ventricle. The PCV should lie at a point about halfway between the tuberculum sellae and the torcular Herophili.

The *anterior pontomesencephalic vein* can be seen behind the clivus. The *APMV* outlines the pons and mesencephalon; in some cases even the upper cervical spinal cord is outlined by a corresponding plexus of draining veins (Fig. 11-24).

The *superior and inferior vermian veins* are also best seen on lateral projections. They outline the vermian lobules.

Anteroposterior View

Relatively few of the posterior fossa veins are visualized optimally in this projection. An exception is the *petrosal vein*. On AP Towne projections this vein is seen as a star-shaped contrast collection just above and approximately perpendicular to the petrous temporal bone (Fig. 11-25). The *vermian veins* also can be identified on AP views. They should lie near the midline.

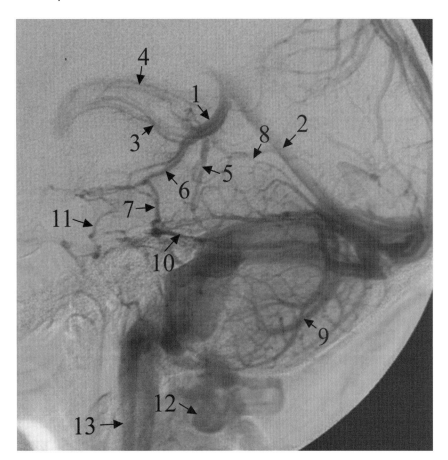

FIG. 11-23. Left vertebral angiogram, venous phase, lateral view, demonstrates many of the usual veins that are opacified on posterior fossa studies.

1, Vein of Galen
2, Straight sinus
3, Internal cerebral vein
4, Superior choroid veins
5, Precentral cerebellar vein
6, Posterior mesencephalic vein (posterior part of basal vein of Rosenthal)
7, Lateral mesencephalic vein
8, Superior vermian vein
9, Inferior vermian vein
10, Petrosal vein
11, Anterior pontomesencephalic venous plexus
12, Occipital veins
13, Internal jugular vein

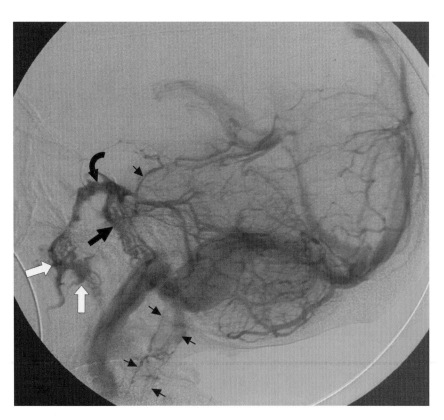

FIG. 11-24. Left vertebral angiogram, venous phase, lateral view, shows the posterior fossa veins. The venous plexus that outlines the anterior surface of the mesencephalon, pons, medulla, and spinal cord (*small arrows*) is unusually well visualized. The clival venous plexus is indicated by the large black arrow. Note that venous drainage into the posterior cavernous sinus (*curved arrow*) connects with the pterygoid venous plexus (*white arrows*).

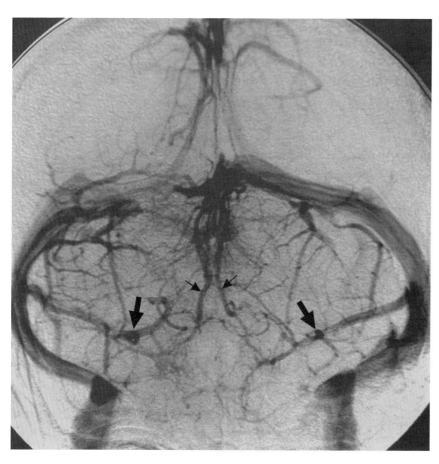

FIG. 11-25. Left vertebral angiogram, venous phase, anteroposterior view. Posterior fossa veins that are well visualized in this projection include the petrosal (*large arrows*) and inferior vermian veins (*small arrows*).

REFERENCES

1. Truitt CL. Embryology of the cerebral vasculature. *Neuroimaging Clin North Am* 1994;4:663–689.
2. Brunelle F. Arteriovenous malformation of the vein of Galen in children. *Pediatr Radiol* 1997;27:501–513.
3. Tanaka R, Miyasaka Y, Yada K, et al. Anomaly of venous system in congenital occipital dermal sinus. *Acta Neurochir (Wien)* 1994;128: 174–179.
4. Raybaud CA, Strother CM, Hald JK. Aneurysms of the vein of Galen: embryonic considerations and anatomical features related to the pathogenesis of the malformation. *Neuroradiology* 1989;31:109–129.
5. Rees JH, Smirniotopoulos JG, Mathis JM. The embryologic origins of the vein of Galen malformation. Presented at the 35th Annual Scientific Meeting, American Society of Neuroradiology, Toronto, May 18–22, 1997.
6. de Miguel MA, Maten JMD, Cusi V, Naidich TP. Embryogenesis of the veins of the posterior fossa: an overview. *IJNR* (in press)
7. Galligioni F, Bernardi R, Pellone M, et al. The superficial sylvian vein in normal and pathologic cerebral angiography. *AJR* 1969;107: 565–579.
8. Sener RN. The occipitotemporal vein: a cadaver, MRI and CT study. *Neuroradiology* 1994;36:117–120.
9. Curé JK, Van Tassel P, Smith MT. Normal and variant anatomy of the dural venous sinuses. *Semin Ultrasound CT MR* 1994;15:499–519.
10. Kaplan HA, Browder J. Atresia of the rostral superior sagittal sinus: substitute parasagittal venous channels. *J Neurosurg* 1973;38:602–607.
11. Friedman DP. Abnormalities of the deep medullary white matter veins: MR imaging findings. *AJR* 1997;168:1103–1108.
11A. Türe U, Yasargil NG, Al-Mefty O. The transcaollosal-transforaminal approach to the third ventricle with regard to the venous variations in this region. *J Neurosurg* 1997;87:706–715.
11B. Wen HT, Rhoton AL Jr, Oliveira E. Transchoroidal approach to the third ventricle: an anatomic study of the choroidal fissure and its clinical application. *Neurosurgery* 1998;42:1205–1219.
12. Parent A. Cerebral veins and venous sinuses. In: *Carpenter's human neuroanatomy*, 9th ed. Media, PA: Williams and Wilkins, 1996: 120–128.
13. Ture U, Yasargil MG, Al-Mefty O. The transcallosal-transforaminal approach to the third ventricle with regard to the venous variations in this region. *J Neurosurg* 1997;87:706–715.
14. Meder J-F, Chiros J, Roland J, et al. Venous territories of the brain. *J Neuroradiol* 1994;21:118–133.
15. Huang YB, Wolf BS. The basal vein and its tributaries. In: Newton TH, Potts DG, eds. *Radiology of the skull and brain*. Vol. 2. St. Louis: CV Mosby, 1974:2111–2154.

SECTION II

Pathology of
the Craniocervical
Vasculature

CHAPTER 12

Intracranial Aneurysms

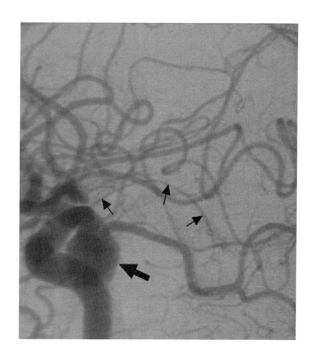

Intracranial aneurysms are classified according to their gross pathologic appearance. Three general categories are recognized: (a) saccular or "berry" aneurysms, (b) fusiform aneurysms, and (c) dissecting aneurysms. Each type has its own distinct features with differing origins, risks, and clinical presentations. In this chapter we will focus our attention on the most common group, saccular aneurysms. Fusiform aneurysms are discussed in Chapters 15 and 16. Dissecting aneurysms are considered in Chapter 17.

This chapter begins by discussing the pathology, etiology, clinical manifestations, and angiographic appearance of intracranial saccular aneurysms. In the second section keys to the complete angiographic evaluation of patients with suspected aneurysmal subarachnoid hemorrhage (SAH) are delineated. A brief consideration of diagnostic and management "dilemmas" in these challenging cases concludes the chapter.

PATHOLOGY, ETIOLOGY, AND CLINICAL CONSIDERATIONS

Pathology

Gross Pathology

Saccular aneurysms are round or lobulated focal outpouchings that usually arise from arterial bifurcations (Fig. 12-1A). Occasionally they originate directly from the lateral wall of a nonbranching artery. An aneurysmal sac may have a narrow orifice (neck), or it may arise from a more broad-based opening that connects it to the parent vessel (1).

Microscopic Pathology

Most intracranial saccular aneurysms are true aneurysms, i.e., they contain at least some layers that are normally found in arteries yet lack other components. Aneurysms are typically rounded protrusions of deficient, collagenized tunica muscularis that protrudes through a localized defect in the internal elastic lamina and tunica media (2,3).

The normal muscularis and elastic lamina usually terminate at the aneurysm neck (3a). Thus, its wall often contains only intima and adventitia (Fig. 12-1A). Acute thrombus and organized laminated clots are also frequently present within the aneurysm lumen (Fig. 12-1B) (4). Histologic changes of elastin degradation in non–aneurysm-bearing cerebral vessels are common (3,5).

Molecular Abnormalities

There is gross molecular disruption in an aneurysm wall. Type III collagen is relatively deficient compared with normal intracranial vessels. Disorganization of basement membrane proteins as well as abnormal expression of angiogenesis factors in other matrix components has been reported in patients who develop intracranial aneurysms (6).

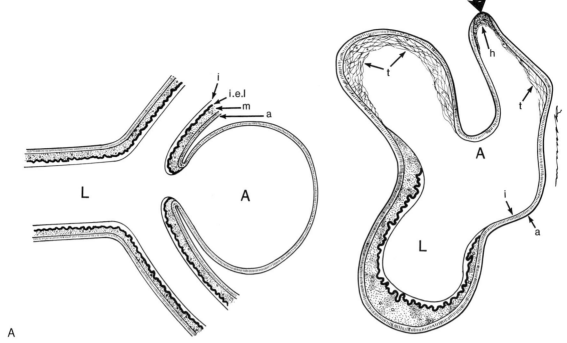

FIG. 12-1. A: Anatomic diagram depicts an intracranial saccular aneurysm arising from the middle cerebral artery bifurcation. The intima (i), internal elastic lamina (i.e.l.), media (m), adventitia (a), and lumen (L) of the normal parent vessel are indicated. The aneurysm sac (A) typically has an intima and an adventitia, but the internal elastic lamina and muscular layers are absent. **B:** Anatomic diagram, drawn from a histopathology section, shows detailed structure of an intracranial aneurysm. The collapsed sac (A) consists of intima and adventitia. Organizing thrombus (t) and other debris also may be present, constituting a potential source for distal emboli. The aneurysm has ruptured from its dome (*large black arrow*). Fresh hemorrhage (h) covers the rupture site. The lumen (L) and normal wall of the parent vessel are also shown.

Prevalence

Solitary Aneurysms

Incidental intracranial aneurysms are found in approximately 1% of autopsies and up to 7% of patients undergoing intraarterial digital subtraction angiography for indications other than subarachnoid hemorrhage (see box on page 243) (1,7).

Multiple Aneurysms

The reported frequency of multiple intracranial aneurysms varies widely, ranging from a low of 14% to nearly 45% of all cases examined. Angiographic quality, number of vessels examined, referral patterns, and experience of the angiographer all influence the detection of multiple lesions (8).

In most large referral centers with experienced angiographers, one fifth to one third of intracranial aneurysms are multiple (9). About 75% of patients have two aneurysms, 15% have three, and 10% have more than three aneurysms. There is a strong female predominance for multiple aneurysms (1,10,10a). Vasculopathies such as fibromuscu-

lar dysplasia and polycystic kidney disease are also associated with an increased incidence of multiple aneurysms.

Location

Intracranial aneurysms usually arise on the circle of Willis or at the middle cerebral artery bifurcation (Fig. 12-2). Approximately 90% are located on the anterior circulation, whereas only 10% occur in the vertebrobasilar system.

Approximately one third of all aneurysms are found on the anterior communicating artery, one third are located at the posterior communicating artery–internal carotid artery (ICA) junction, and one fifth occur at the middle cerebral artery bi- or trifurcation (10). Some series have reported a higher prevalence of middle cerebral artery aneurysms, with up to 43% found in this location (11).

Clinical Considerations

Age

Aneurysms are typically lesions of *adults.* Peak presentation is between the ages of 40 and 60 years (1). Intracranial aneurysms are rare in *children,* accounting

General Features of Intracranial Aneurysms

Pathology
Round or lobulated outpouching of intima, adventitia
Internal elastic lamina, muscular layers absent
Incidence
1% in general population
20% to 33% multiple
Location
General
90% "anterior" (carotid) circulation
10% "posterior" (vertebrobasilar) circulation
Specific sites
30% to 35% anterior communicating artery
30% to 35% internal carotid–posterior communicating artery
20% middle cerebral artery
5% basilar artery bifurcation
Age at presentation
Peak age 40 to 60 years
Rare in children (less than 2% of all cases)
Clinical presentation
85% to 95% headache (secondary to SAH)
Cranial neuropathy (cranial nerve [CN] III most common)
Rare: transient ischemic attack (TIA), seizure, symptoms of mass effect
Rupture risk
1% to 2% per year, cumulative
20% at 10 years
35% at 15 years
6.8% per year, cumulative, for multiple aneurysms
Size correlates directly with rupture risk
1% per year for lesions 6 mm or smaller
2.5% per year for lesions 7 mm or larger
Includes "giant" (more than 2.5 cm) aneurysms
Multilobed, irregular aneurysms probably more prone to rupture
Pathogenesis
Heritable connective tissue disorders with increased prevalence of intracranial aneurysm
Ehlers-Danlos type IV
Marfan's syndrome
Neurofibromatosis type 1 (NF-1)
Autosomal dominant polycystic kidney disease
Familial intracranial aneurysms (FIAs)
Two or more affected first-degree relatives
10% to 17% prevalence of unruptured aneurysms in FIA
Miscellaneous conditions
Congenital heart disease (including aortic coarctation)
Anomalous or fenestrated vessels
Vasculopathy (fibromuscular dysplasia, sickle cell disease)
Biochemical markers
Elevated plasma elastase, lipoprotein (a)
Decreased alpha 1 antitrypsin
Etiology
Not congenital
Degenerative
Flow-related
Miscellaneous
Infection
Trauma
Neoplasm
Drug abuse

for less than 2% of all cases. Several characteristics distinguish aneurysms in the pediatric age group from those in adults (Table 12-1). There is a striking (3:1) male predominance in children. Nearly 20% of aneurysms occur in either the posterior circulation or vessels distal to the circle of Willis. The terminal internal carotid artery bifurcation is the single most common location in the pediatric population, accounting for one quarter to one half of all aneurysms (12,13).

So-called "giant" aneurysms (larger than 2.5 cm) are common in children, but there is also a lower prevalence of multiple lesions. Mass effect occurs as the presenting symptom in approximately 20% of cases (13). Aneurysms in the pediatric age group are more frequently associated with trauma and infection (1,13). Children with aneurysms also have a lower mortality rate and better surgical outcome (12).

Clinical Presentation

The most common clinical manifestation of a symptomatic intracranial aneurysm is *subarachnoid hemorrhage* (SAH). In turn, headache is the most common symptom of SAH and occurs in 85% to 95% of patients (14).

Clinical manifestations other than SAH are much rarer. *Cranial neuropathy* is the second most common presentation of an intracranial aneurysm. An isolated oculomotor nerve (CN III) palsy is the most frequent finding. Both pupil-involving and pupil-sparing third nerve palsies can be caused by aneurysms (15).

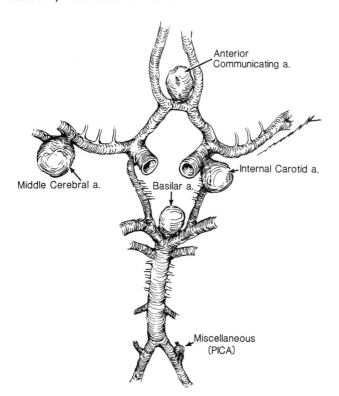

FIG. 12-2. Anatomic diagram depicts the typical location of intracranial aneurysms. The vast majority (more than 90%) arise either from the circle of Willis or the middle cerebral artery bifurcation. (Reprinted with permission from Osborn AG, Tong KT. *Handbook of neuroradiology: skull and brain,* 2nd ed. St. Louis: Mosby, 1996.)

Seizure, transient ischemic attack (TIA), and *frank cerebral infarction* are less common (1). Unruptured aneurysms are occasionally misdiagnosed clinically as optic neuritis or migraine headache, sometimes delaying diagnosis of these potentially lethal lesions for weeks to years (16).

Subarachnoid Hemorrhage

The most widely used method for *grading SAH* is the Hunt and Hess Scale. Many neurosurgeons also use the Cooperative Aneurysm Study Neurological Status Scale to assess symptom severity. Clinical signs and symptoms are used to grade the SAH and range from grade 0 (unruptured, asymptomatic aneurysm) and grade I (asymptomatic or minimal headache, nuchal rigidity) to grade V (deep coma, decerebrate, moribund appearance) on the Hunt and Hess Scale (Table 12-2) (17).

Imaging acute SAH can be performed using nonenhanced computed tomography (NECT) scans (Fig. 12-3A and B) or special magnetic resonance (MR) sequences (such as fluid-attenuated inversion recovery) that suppress the background signal from cerebrospinal fluid (Fig. 12-3C and D) (17a).

TABLE 12-1. *Intracranial aneurysms: adults versus children*

Adults	Children
Common (1% autopsy prevalence)	Rare (<2% of all aneurysms)
Females predominate	Males predominate (3:1)
Circle of Willis plus MCA	20% posterior circulation, distal vessels
Multiple aneurysms common	Multiple aneurysms rare
"Giant" aneurysms rare	"Giant" aneurysms common
Hemodynamic stresses	Trauma, infection, abnormal vessel wall matrix

TABLE 12-2. *Hunt and Hess clinical grading for intracranial aneurysm*

Grade	Clinical condition
0	Unruptured
1	Asymptomatic or minimal headache, nuchal rigidity
2	Moderate to severe headache, nuchal rigidity, no neurologic deficit other than cranial nerve palsy
3	Drowsiness, confusion, mild focal deficit
4	Stupor, moderate to severe hemiparesis, possible early decerebrate rigidity and vegetative disturbances
5	Deep coma, decerebrate rigidity, moribund appearance
+1 grade	For vasospasm or systemic disease

Data from Hunt and Hess, as reported in Ogilvy CS, Carter BS. A proposed comprehensive grading system to predict outcome for surgical management of intracranial aneurysms. *Neurosurgery* 1998;42:959–970.

The density of SAH is sometimes scored using the Fisher Scale (Table 12-3). However, the amount of SAH on NECT scans does not necessarily correlate with either clinical symptoms or aneurysm size. For example, a small aneurysm may produce massive SAH yet cause only minimal symptoms (Fig. 12-3). Clinical outcome is affected only by severe hemorrhage; patients with Fisher Scale scores of 1 or 2 do not differ from those who have no SAH (17).

Location of SAH sometimes suggests the site of a ruptured intracranial aneurysm. Focal hematomas in the sylvian fissure suggest a middle cerebral artery location. Interhemispheric SAH with relative sparing of the basal cisterns may occur with anterior communicating artery lesions (Fig. 12-4).

Hemorrhage in the fourth ventricle and cerebellopontine angle cisterns is often associated with rupture of a

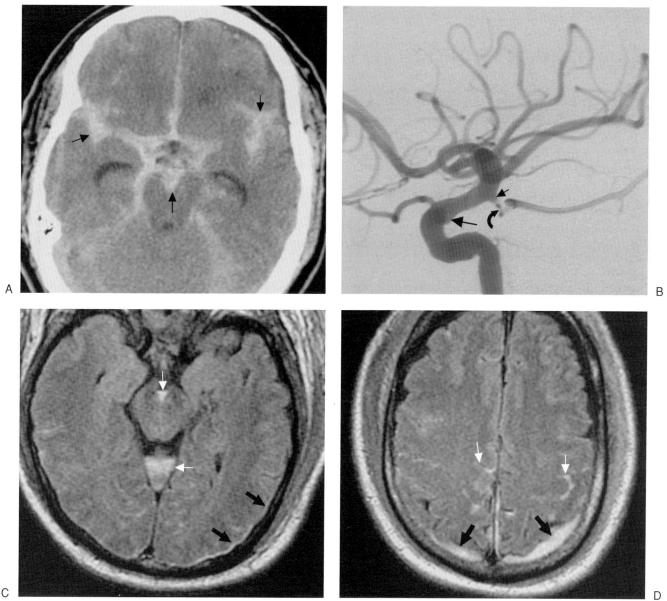

FIG. 12-3. A 34-year-old woman had complained of a mild headache for 2 days. No cognitive or neurologic deficits were present on physical examination. The patient was clinically grade I. **A:** Axial NECT scan shows a large amount of blood in the suprasellar cistern and both sylvian fissures (*arrows*). **B:** A complete cerebral angiogram was performed. The only lesion identified was a small, broad-based aneurysm arising along the posterior wall of the C6 internal carotid artery (ICA) segment (*large arrow*). A ruptured superior hypophyseal artery aneurysm was confirmed at surgery. A cone-shaped infundibulum (*small arrow*) is present at the junction of the posterior communicating artery (PCoA) with the ICA. Note that the PCoA (*curved arrow*) arises directly from the apex of the infundibulum. The infundibulum measured 2 mm in diameter. **C** and **D:** Axial fluid-attenuated inversion recovery (FLAIR) scans in another patient show subarachnoid (*white arrows*) and subdural (*black arrows*) hemorrhage.

TABLE 12-3. *Fisher Scale for scoring subarachnoid hemorrhage on nonenhanced CT scans*

Score	Description
0	Unruptured
1	No blood detected
2	Diffuse or vertical layers <1 mm thick
3	Localized clot and/or vertical layer >1 mm thick
4	Intracerebral or intraventricular clot with diffuse or no subarachnoid hemorrhage

Data from Fisher, as reported in Ogilvie CS, Carter BS. A proposed comprehensive grading system to predict outcome for surgical management of intracranial aneurysms. *Neurosurgery* 1998;42:959–970.

posterior inferior cerebellar artery (PICA) aneurysm. Vertebrobasilar circulation aneurysms may cause perimesencephalic SAH, a pattern that is also reported with nonaneurysmal hemorrhage (18).

Outcome

The *short-term outcome of* aneurysm rupture is generally dismal. Aneurysm rupture is often a devastating clinical event, with a mortality rate that may exceed 50%. Twelve percent of patients with aneurysmal SAH die without any medical attention. The typical clinicopathologic profile of sudden death in SAH includes massive intraventricular hemorrhage, pulmonary edema, and a ruptured posterior circulation aneurysm (19).

The *long-term outcome of* aneurysm rupture is variable. Permanent neurologic disability occurs in a significant number of survivors (20,21). A comprehensive grading system combining factors that are independently and strongly associated with long-term outcome recently was proposed. One point is assigned for Hunt and Hess grade IV or V, Fisher Scale score of 3 or 4, aneurysm size greater than 10 mm, patient age greater than 50 years, and if the lesion is a giant (25 mm or larger) posterior circulation lesion. Adding the total points results in a 5-point grading system (grades 0 to 5) that separates patients into groups with markedly different outcomes (17).

As the mortality and morbidity of surgery for unruptured intracranial aneurysms is quite low, patients who have aneurysms discovered incidentally may benefit from prophylactic clipping of these potentially lethal lesions (21a).

Natural History

The *risk of rupture* is approximately 1% to 2% per year for asymptomatic, as-yet-unruptured aneurysms (22–24). The cumulative hemorrhage rate is 20% at 10 years after diagnosis and 35% at 15 years. The probability of rupture is significantly higher for multiple aneurysms (24).

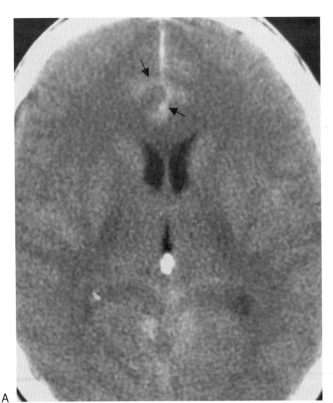

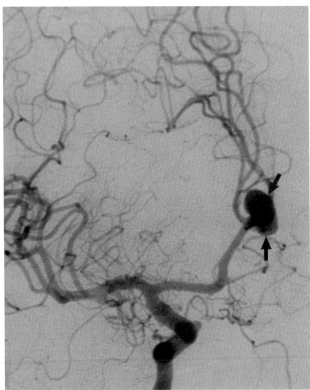

A

B

FIG. 12-4. A: Axial NECT scan in a patient with a grade III SAH shows focal hemorrhage in the anterior interhemispheric fissure (*arrows*). Almost no blood was present in the basal cisterns. **B:** Right internal carotid angiogram, arterial phase, oblique view, shows a large aneurysm (*arrows*) at the distal anterior cerebral artery (A2 segment) bifurcation.

There are several factors that have a significant effect on rupture risk. *Size* is the single most important variable that determines the risk of future rupture. Aneurysms tend to rupture at a frequency proportional to their volume (22,25). The average annual risk of rupture with a lesion diameter of 7 mm or greater is 2.5% compared with about 1% in patients with smaller aneurysms (23). The direct relationship of size with rupture risk occurs even with giant aneurysms (26,26a).

Despite substantial evidence that correlates risk of rupture with size, there is no "safe" or "critical size" below which subarachnoid hemorrhage does not occur (27,28, 28a). Even small intracranial aneurysms (i.e., those measuring less than 5 mm) are susceptible to rupture (29). Recent evidence indicates that the size of an intracranial aneurysm also varies with intracranial pressure, although the significance of this finding for rupture risk is unknown (30).

Although data from the International Study of Unruptured Intracranial Aneurysms (ISUIA) are still incomplete, aneurysm *morphology* also may help predict future rupture risk. A small, single sac with a smooth margin may be less likely to rupture than one that is the same overall size but is multilobed or has a "daughter" sac (25).

The role of *systemic hypertension* is debated. Some investigators point out that aneurysms are more common in patients with various hypertensive diseases such as aortic coarctation and polycystic kidney disease (31). Others have reported that hypertension is an independent risk factor for SAH caused by rupture of a previously intact aneurysm (20).

Pathogenesis

The pathogenesis of intracranial aneurysms is incompletely understood. Although it is generally accepted that acquired factors such as hemodynamic stresses have an important role in their development, genetic factors play an increasingly recognized role.

Heritable Disorders

A number of inherited connective tissue disorders are associated with intracranial aneurysms. As a group, these disorders account for at least 5% of all aneurysm cases (32). Many different disorders have been associated with intracranial aneurysms (see box on page 243). The most important of these are Ehlers-Danlos syndrome type IV, Marfan's syndrome, neurofibromatosis type 1 (NF-1) and autosomal dominant polycystic kidney disease (32).

Ehlers-Danlos syndrome (EDS) is a heterogenous group of nine inherited connective tissue disorders that are classified on the basis of clinical and genetic factors (33). Most of these disorders are characterized by joint hypermobility, hyperelastic or fragile skin, easy bruising, and abnormal scarring (32). *EDS type IV* is both the most

lethal and one of the least common varieties of EDS. It is caused by a deficiency of type III collagen, the major constituent of distensible tissues such as arteries and veins as well as bowel and viscera.

Complications of EDS type IV include arterial, bowel, and uterine rupture; arterial dissection and aneurysm formation; and spontaneous carotid–cavernous sinus fistulae (33). Aneurysms typically involve the large and medium-sized arteries (32).

Marfan's syndrome is characterized by skeletal and cardiovascular abnormalities as well as defects in the eye and spinal meninges. Inheritance is autosomal dominant, but family history is negative in approximately 30% of cases, and a spontaneous mutation accounts for the disorder (34).

Marfan's syndrome is caused by a mutation in the gene that encodes fibrillin-1, a glycoprotein that is a major component of elastic tissues (34). Intracranial aneurysms in patients with Marfan's syndrome may be saccular, fusiform, or dissecting, although extracranial aneurysms are more often fusiform (Fig. 12-5) (34).

Autopsy studies of the cerebral arteries in patients with Marfan's syndrome have revealed various combinations of intimal proliferation, medial degeneration, and fragmentation of the internal elastic lamina (32). Other investigators feel that the relationship between Marfan's syndrome and intracranial aneurysm is still inconclusive (35).

Neurofibromatosis type 1 (NF-1) is caused by mutations in the gene that encodes neurofibromin. Neurofibromin may have a regulatory role in the development of vascular connective tissue through its effects on microtubular function. Vascular complications of NF-1 are uncommon, but stenosis, rupture, and aneurysm or fistula formation of large and medium-sized arteries have been reported. Aneurysms in these patients may be saccular, fusiform, or dissecting (32).

Autosomal dominant polycystic kidney disease (ADKPD) is the most common monogenetic disorder in humans and is a genetically heterogeneous disease. Polycystin, the protein encoded by the PKD1 gene, is a membrane protein that may play a role in maintaining the structural integrity of connective tissues (32).

Patients with ADPKD are predisposed to develop renal and visceral cysts as well as a spectrum of vascular abnormalities (Fig. 12-6). Aortic and cephalocervical dissections and intracranial aneurysms are common. Approximately one fourth of patients with ADPKD have an intracranial aneurysm at autopsy, and these lesions are the proximate cause of death in approximately 20% of cases (32).

Ten percent of asymptomatic patients with ADPKD who are screened with magnetic resonance angiography (MRA) have an intracranial aneurysm (32). A decision analysis model has predicted that an effective MR screening strategy would increase the life expectancy of young patients with this disorder and reduce its financial impact on society significantly (36).

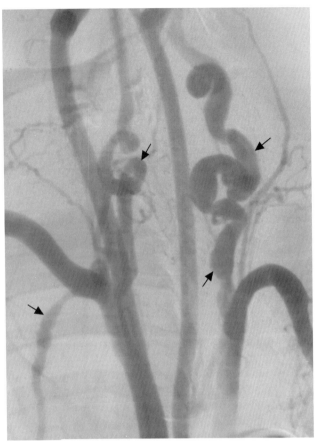

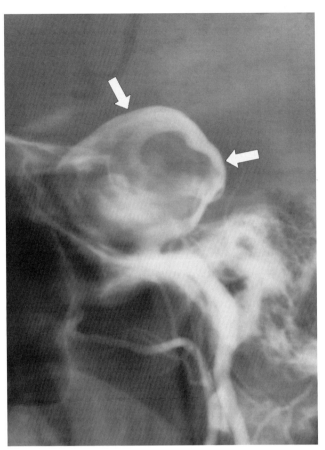

A

B

FIG. 12-5. A 38-year-old woman with cystic medial necrosis and probable Marfan's syndrome. **A:** Conventional aortic arch angiogram with film subtraction technique, left anterior oblique view, shows multiple fusiform ectasias of the great vessels (*arrows*). **B:** Unsubtracted view of the left common carotid angiogram shows a giant saccular aneurysm (*arrows*).

Familial Aggregates

So-called *familial intracranial aneurysms* (FIA) affect at least two first-degree relatives in the same family and are not associated with any known heritable connective tissue disorders. Microscopic examination of the vascular system in some FIA cases has revealed an underlying arteriopathy that involves both intra- and extracranial vessels (37).

Epidemiologic studies show that first-degree relatives of patients in FIA constitute a high-risk group and would benefit from screening MRA. An unruptured intracranial aneurysm in present in 10% to 17% of asymptomatic family members (38). The inheritance pattern of FIA is unknown.

Miscellaneous Conditions

A number of other conditions are associated with an increased prevalence of aneurysms. Individuals with a variety of *congenital heart disorders* have an increased risk for developing cephalocervical arterial dissections and intracranial aneurysms (39). These patients may have deficiencies in multiple structures that are derived from the embryonic neural crest (40).

Patients with *anomalous vessels, arterial fenestrations,* and numerous vasculopathies such as *fibromuscular dysplasia* and *sickle cell disease* also have an increased prevalence of intracranial aneurysms (Figs. 12-7 and 12-8) (41–43).

A few investigators have proposed that some *environmental risk factors* such as cigarette smoking increase the risk for multiple aneurysm formation as well as effect the outcome from subarachnoid hemorrhage once rupture occurs (10a,44). Others have noted elevated *biochemical markers* such as lipoprotein(a), serum gelatinase, and plasma elastase in patients with intracranial aneurysms (5,45,45a). Some investigators have implicated deficiency of alpha-1-antitrypsin in the development of arterial aneurysms, including intracranial aneurysms (46).

Etiology

There is no evidence to suggest that aneurysms are congenital (13). Most intracranial saccular aneurysms,

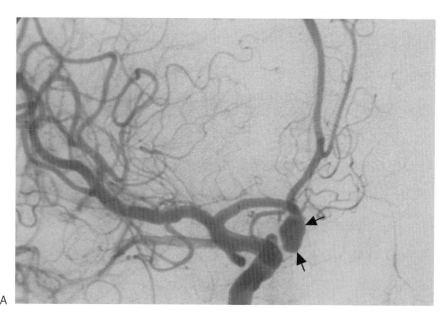

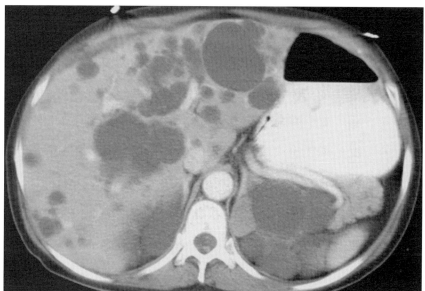

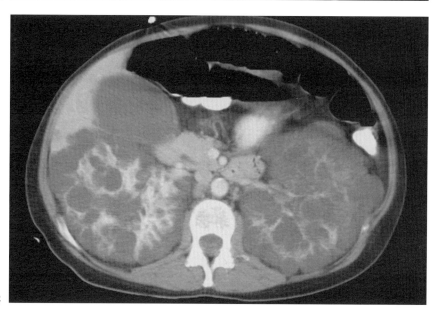

FIG. 12-6. A 28-year-old woman had complained of severe headache. Lumbar puncture at an outside emergency room showed bloody cerebrospinal fluid. An NECT scan (not shown) confirmed the presence of subarachnoid hemorrhage. The patient was referred for a cerebral angiogram. **A:** Right internal carotid angiogram, arterial phase, oblique view, shows a large lobulated aneurysm arising from the anterior communicating artery (*arrows*). Physical examination prior to surgery disclosed an abdominal mass. **B** and **C:** Axial postangiogram contrast-enhanced CT (CECT) scans show multiple cysts in the liver and both kidneys. The patient had undisclosed autosomal dominant polycystic kidney disease (ADPKD).

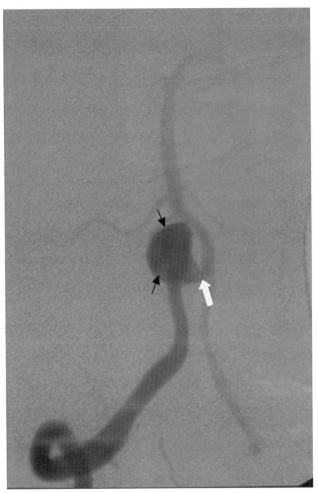

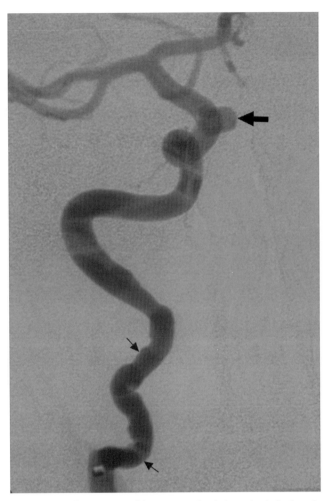

FIG. 12-7. Right vertebral angiography, early arterial phase, in a patient with acute subarachnoid hemorrhage disclosed a fenestrated basilar artery (*white arrow*) with a large lobulated aneurysm (*small black arrows*).

FIG. 12-8. A 58-year-old woman had transient ischemic attacks. A right common carotid angiogram shows typical changes of fibromuscular dysplasia in the extracranial internal carotid artery (*small black arrows*). An unruptured aneurysm (*large arrow*) is present at the origin of the ophthalmic artery.

including those in children, are acquired lesions. Although a spectrum of inherited and acquired disease processes may predispose to aneurysm formation by weakening the vessel wall matrix, most aneurysms arise from hemodynamic stresses and acquired degenerative changes within the arterial wall (48a).

Degenerative Aneurysms

These aneurysms result from hemodynamically induced vascular injury (2). Abnormal mural stresses, most pronounced at arterial bifurcations, probably account for the patterns of initiation, growth, and rupture of these lesions (4,47,48).

Flow-Related Aneurysms

The second most common cause of intracranial aneurysm is a *high-flow state* that augments mechanical stresses on vessel walls. Increased hemodynamic stress with mural thinning occurs with arteriovenous malformations and fistulae. The reported association of cerebral arteriovenous malformations (AVMs) and aneurysms varies from 3% to 23%. Most reports are in the 5% to 15% range (49). A majority of these patients have multiple aneurysms (49a).

Flow-related aneurysms are thin-walled structures that easily rupture with sudden intravascular hypertension. Among patients with AVM and hemorrhage, 80% harbor flow-related aneurysms. Both intralesional and feeding artery aneurysms are potential sources of bleeding associated with AVMs and arteriovenous fistulae (AVFs). True *intranidal aneurysms* occur in about 42% of cases, although careful superselective angiography may demonstrate flow-related aneurysms in up to 60% of AVMs. Multiple aneurysms are also common in these cases (Fig. 12-9) (see Chapter 13) (50).

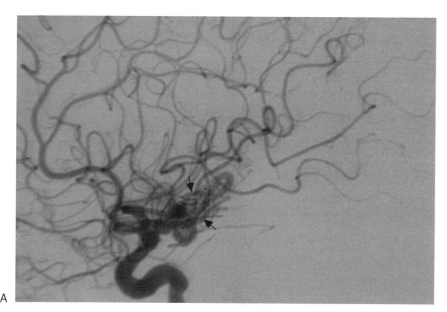

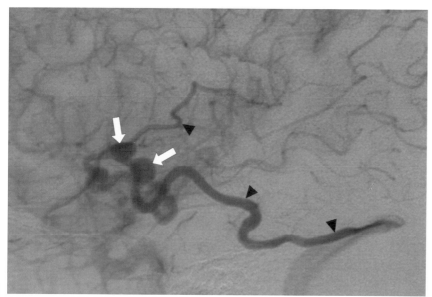

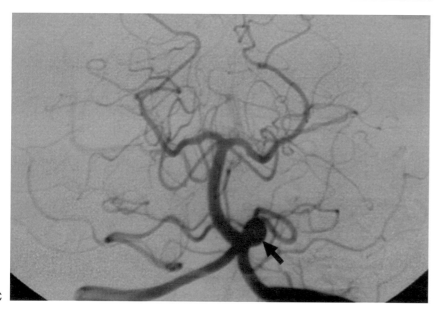

FIG. 12-9. This 24-year-old woman with long-standing seizures had an MR scan (not shown) that demonstrated multiple "flow voids" in the right anterior temporal lobe. Early **(A)** and late **(B)** arterial phase views of the right internal carotid angiogram in this patient show a pial arteriovenous malformation (AVM) (**A**, *arrows*). Early draining veins (**B**, *arrowheads*) and several dilated intranidal "aneurysms" (**B**, *white arrows*) are present. **C:** Left vertebral angiogram, arterial phase, AP view, shows a hemodynamically unrelated aneurysm (*arrow*) at the origin of the posterior inferior cerebellar artery. The vertebrobasilar circulation did not supply the AVM.

A second type of flow-related aneurysm, the so-called feeding artery or *pedicle aneurysm*, arises along the course of a vessel that supplies an AVM or AVF but is not contained within the malformation proper (Fig. 12-10) (49). Some patients with vascular malformations occasionally develop an aneurysm on a nonfeeding vessel, possibly reflecting a more generalized underlying vasculopathy (Fig. 12-9C).

Mycotic Aneurysms

Infectious or mycotic aneurysms historically have accounted for 2% to 4% of all intracerebral aneurysms but cause 5% to 15% of aneurysms in children (1,13). Mycotic aneurysms often occur in patients with infective endocarditis or a history of drug abuse (51). The most common causative bacterium is *Streptococcus viridans; Aspergillus fumigatus* is the most common agent that causes fungal aneurysms (52). These lesions have a high risk of rupture (53).

Mycotic and drug-related aneurysms typically arise on smaller vessels distal to the circle of Willis (Fig. 12-11). Most mycotic aneurysms are actually pseudoaneurysms (54). Septic emboli typically lodge at distal sites and destroy the intima or reach the adventitia through the vasa vasorum. Inflammation then disrupts the adventitia and muscularis, resulting in aneurysmal dilatation. The

sequence of infection, necrosis, and inflammation of the vessel wall is typical of these lesions (53).

Traumatic Aneurysms

Trauma causes 0.2% to 1% of all intracranial aneurysms but is responsible for 5% to 15% of aneurysms in children (1,10,13). Delayed clinical presentation (up to 3 or 4 weeks following injury) is common (13).

Traumatic aneurysms usually result from direct injury such as penetrating trauma or a contiguous skull fracture (55). Closed head injury less commonly results in a traumatic aneurysm; most are caused by shearing injury or impaction of an artery against a dural fold. Examples include forcing the distal anterior cerebral artery against the falx cerebri and the superior cerebellar artery against the tentorium (56). Most traumatic aneurysms are actually pseudoaneurysms, i.e., they do not contain components of the normal vessel wall (see Chapter 17).

Oncotic Aneurysms

Neoplastic aneurysms are rare, accounting for less than 0.1% of all aneurysms (10). They are thought to result either from direct vascular invasion by tumor or implantation of distal tumor emboli that then infiltrate and disrupt the vessel wall (57). Both primary intracranial (such as meningioma, pituitary adenoma, and high-grade astro-

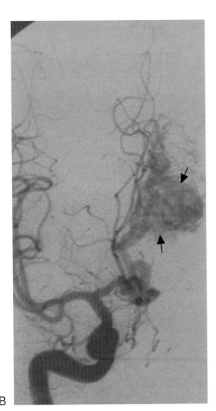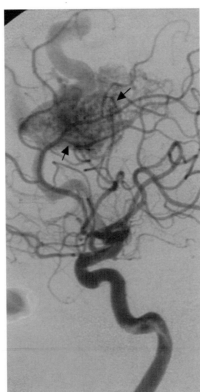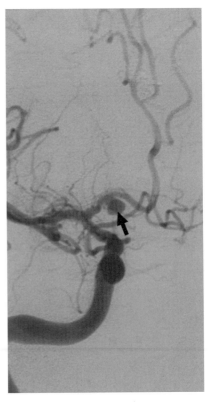

A,B   C

FIG. 12-10. AP **(A)** and lateral **(B)** views of a right internal carotid angiogram show a large arteriovenous malformation (AVM) (*arrows*). **C:** Repeat angiogram following endovascular occlusion of the AVM now clearly shows a pedicle aneurysm on the horizontal anterior cerebral artery (*arrow*).

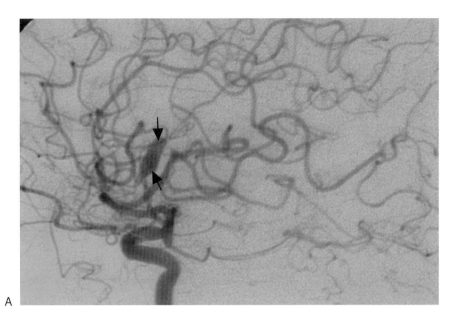

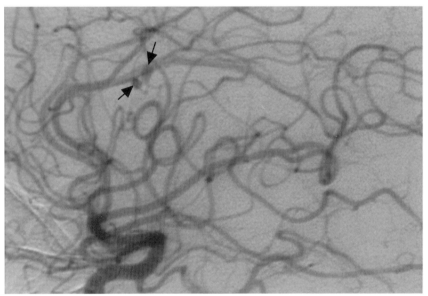

FIG. 12-11. Lateral views of the internal carotid angiograms in two different patients with infective endocarditis and suspected drug abuse show irregular-appearing mycotic aneurysms on the middle (**A**, *arrows*) and anterior cerebral arteries (**B**, *arrows*).

cytoma) (Fig. 12-12) and metastatic neoplasms (such as atrial myxoma and choriocarcinoma) (Fig. 12-13) have been reported to cause neoplastic aneurysms. Oncotic aneurysms may be either saccular or fusiform (58).

Occasionally squamous cell carcinomas invade the branches of the external carotid artery and cause an oncotic pseudoaneurysm (Fig. 12-14). The terminal event in many of these patients is often exsanguinating epistaxis.

Flow Dynamics, Aneurysm Initiation, and Growth

Initiation

Maximum hemodynamic stress occurs at the apex of vessel bifurcations (Fig. 12-1). Intimal damage caused by augmented hemodynamic stress at these vulnerable points probably initiates the aneurysm (47,48). Underlying vasculopathy with weakening of arterial walls also probably predisposes to aneurysm formation.

Flow Dynamics and Growth

Understanding intraaneurysmal flow patterns is important as these influence the growth, thrombosis, and rupture of aneurysms (59). Flow within aneurysms is complex (Fig. 12-15) (60,61). Three distinct zones have been described: (a) an "inflow zone" entering at the distal wall of the ostium; (b) an "outflow zone" that exits at the proximal ostium; and (c) a central, slow-flow vortex (60–63).

Aneurysms also tend to grow with time. Small partially or inadequately treated saccular aneurysms may become very large (64).

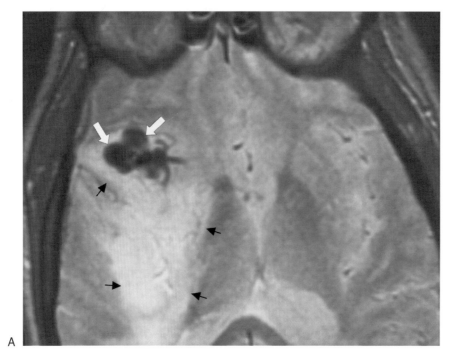

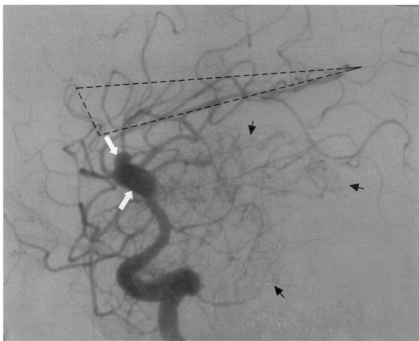

FIG. 12-12. An elderly patient presented with a first-time seizure. **A:** Long TR/short TE (proton-density weighted) MR scan shows a large mass in the right temporal lobe (*black arrows*). A multilobulated lesion with high-velocity signal loss (flow voids) appears to arise from the middle cerebral artery (MCA) (*white arrows*). **B:** Lateral view of the internal carotid angiogram shows that the mass is very vascular (*small black arrows*). An oncotic aneurysm (*white arrows*) is present. Note compression and elevation of the sylvian triangle (*dotted lines*) by the mass.

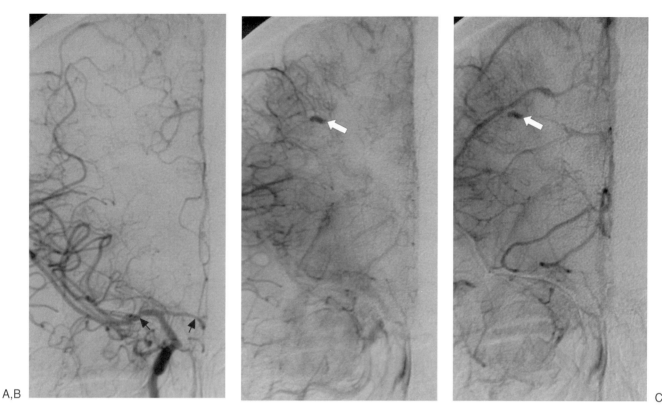

A,B

C

FIG. 12-13. A young woman with known metastatic choriocarcinoma had a seizure. Early **(A)** and late **(B)** arterial as well as venous **(C)** phase studies, anteroposterior view, of a right internal carotid angiogram show multiple irregularities in the anterior and middle cerebral arteries (**A**, *small arrows*). Multiple elongated areas of persisting contrast accumulation (**B** and **C**, *white arrows*) were noted. These findings represent neoplastic vasculitis and pseudoaneurysms from tumor emboli.

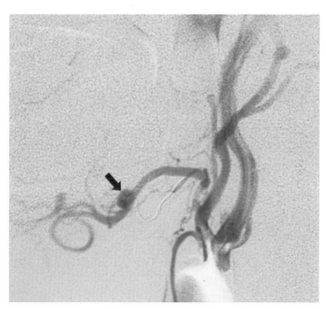

FIG. 12-14. Lateral view of a common carotid angiogram in a patient with known squamous cell carcinoma of the tongue and severe oral hemorrhage shows an oncotic pseudoaneurysm (*arrow*) arising from the lingual artery.

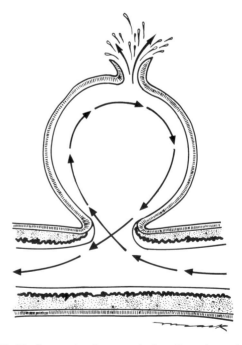

FIG. 12-15. Anatomic diagram depicts flow dynamics of a typical intracranial aneurysm. Flow usually enters the sac at the distal (downstream) aspect of the orifice and exits proximally. A central slow-flow vortex is often present, especially within large aneurysms.

Complications of Aneurysm Rupture

If a patient survives the initial hemorrhage, the delayed complications from SAH still may be devastating. These complications include vasospasm, focal hematoma, mass effect, cerebral herniation syndromes, and stroke (see list above).

Vasospasm

Vasospasm is caused by subarachnoid hemorrhage and is the leading cause of death and disability from aneurysm rupture (Fig. 12-16A) (65). The current management of aneurysmal SAH and its complications favors early surgery followed by so-called "triple H" therapy (heparinization, hypervolemia, and hypertension) to pre-

vent vasospasm. Angioplasty may be helpful in many cases (see Chapter 19) (66).

Hematoma and Mass Effect

Other complications of aneurysm rupture include a focal parenchymal hematoma and mass effect (Fig. 12-16B). Cranial neuropathy, neurologic deficit, and herniation syndromes may occur as secondary effects from this complication.

Stroke

Distal migration of thrombotic material from the aneurysm sac may cause cerebral ischemia and infarction,

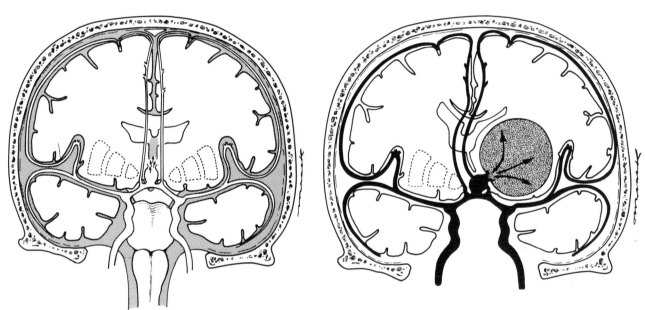

FIG. 12-16. Anatomic diagrams depict the complications of intracranial aneurysm rupture. **A:** Subarachnoid hemorrhage (SAH) (*shaded area*) with arterial constriction is the most common complication. **B:** Rupture of an intracranial aneurysm may produce a focal parenchymal hematoma (*arrows*). The secondary mass effect caused by the hematoma may in turn produce cerebral herniation. **C:** Cerebral ischemia and infarction (*shaded area*) from aneurysm rupture is usually caused by vasospasm secondary to the SAH. Occasionally debris within the aneurysm sac may cause distal emboli and subsequent infarction. (Reprinted with permission from Osborn AG, Tong KT. *Handbook of neuroradiology: skull and brain,* 2nd ed. St. Louis: Mosby, 1996.)

although vasospasm is the most common cause of cerebral infarction in patients with aneurysmal SAH (Fig. 12-16C).

Rebleeding

Untreated ruptured aneurysms have a high likelihood of rebleeding, especially within the first 24 hours following the initial hemorrhage. At least 50% of untreated aneurysms rehemorrhage within 6 months (10).

ANGIOGRAPHIC EVALUATION OF INTRACRANIAL SACCULAR ANEURYSMS

Noninvasive Angiography

Noninvasive methods of assessing the intracranial circulation for the presence of an unruptured aneurysm include MR angiography (MRA) and computed tomographic angiography (CTA) (67–71). Optimizing MRA using phased array surface coils with intensity equalization, intravenous contrast with magnetization transfer pulse sequences, high matrix size, multiple excitations, and special reconstruction techniques produce very high resolution studies with excellent visualization of the intracranial vasculature (Fig. 12-17) (72).

Conventional (Catheter) Angiography

Although noninvasive techniques are often effective in cooperative patients with unruptured aneurysms, many neurosurgeons still prefer the combination of an unenhanced CT scan followed by conventional angiography in evaluating the patient with possible aneurysmal subarachnoid hemorrhage (SAH). Catheter angiography remains the "gold standard" with which other diagnostic modalities are compared.

Performing a technically adequate cerebral angiogram in patients with a possible intracranial saccular aneurysm involves a few simple general principles (Table 12-4). These include:

1. Evaluating the complete intracranial circulation with multiple projections of each vessel studied.
2. Imaging the aneurysm in detail, including delineation of the neck and any perforating branches that may arise from the dome.
3. Using subtraction techniques (digital or film-based).
4. Assessing the potential for cross-circulation.
5. Identifying any associated abnormalities (vasospasm, mass effect, herniation).

We will discuss each of these points separately.

Evaluating the Complete Intracranial Circulation

Most saccular aneurysms arise from the circle of Willis, the middle cerebral artery (MCA) bi- or trifurcation, and the posterior inferior cerebellar artery (PICA). Sponta-

neous visualization of the entire circle of Willis (COW) on a single injection is uncommon (Fig. 12-18) (see also Chapter 5).

A technically adequate cerebral angiogram for evaluating the patient with suspected aneurysmal SAH must include visualization of all components of the circle of Willis, the MCA, and both PICAs. Multiple projections of each vessel should be obtained. At a minimum this should include standard anteroposterior (AP) and lateral as well as both 30 degree transorbital oblique views. Additional views such as the submentovertex projection are often needed for complete delineation (Fig. 12-19).

If the anterior communicating artery (ACoA) does not fill spontaneously, injection of one carotid artery during temporary cross-compression of the contralateral carotid may be required to visualize this important potential location of an intracranial aneurysm (Fig. 12-20).

The posterior communicating arteries (PCoAs) are often hypoplastic. Because most aneurysms that arise from this site originate from the PCoA origin at the C7 ICA segment, multiplanar views of the internal carotid artery usually suffice. Transient reflux of the PCoAs also may occur spontaneously during the vertebrobasilar study (Fig. 12-21). Temporary compression of the ipsilateral common carotid artery may be helpful in visualizing the PCoA (Fig. 12-20).

The origins and course of both PICAs also must be visualized completely. If contrast does not reflux from the dominant vertebral artery (VA) into the contralateral VA, separate injection of the nondominant vessel is required (Fig. 12-22).

Failure to follow these simple basic guidelines results in an incomplete angiogram and a potentially undetected aneurysm.

Imaging the Aneurysm in Detail

Delineating the aneurysm neck is important for preoperative planning. Multiple projections are often required (Fig. 12-21). Some investigators have recommended stereoscopic angiography or high-resolution endoscopic CTA, but conventional studies with multiangular views are usually sufficient.

Defining the presence of perforating branches that occasionally arise from the aneurysm dome is also essential for planning appropriate treatment (Figs. 12-23 and 12-24). Selective "aneurysmography" may be helpful in some cases (73). *Evaluating intraaneurysmal flow patterns* is also important if endovascular occlusion is contemplated (Fig. 12-25).

Using Subtraction Techniques

Because many aneurysms arise from vessels near the skull base, digital or film subtraction should be used in all cases.

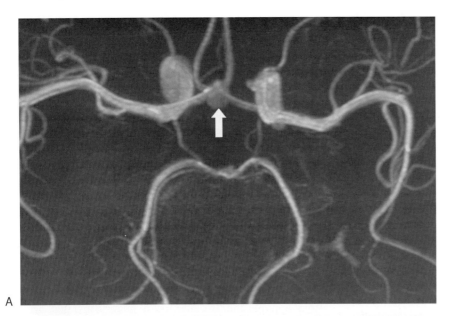

A

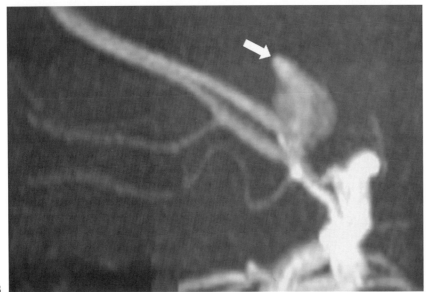

B

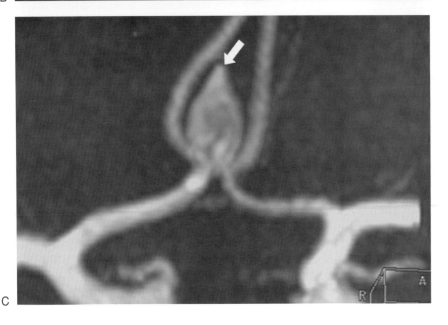

C

FIG. 12-17. An optimized three-dimensional time-of-flight screening MR angiogram (multiple overlapping thin slab acquisition) was performed in this asymptomatic but high-risk patient with a history of familial intracranial aneurysms (FIA). **A:** Submentovertex view shows an aneurysm arising from the anterior communicating artery (*arrow*). Reformatting in the oblique lateral **(B)** and anteroposterior **(C)** projections clearly delineates the lesion. Note the "tit" (*arrows*) at the aneurysm apex. The unruptured aneurysm was successfully clipped on the basis of the MR angiogram alone.

TABLE 12-4. *Complications of aneurysmal subarachnoid hemorrhage*

Vasoconstriction
Focal hematoma
Mass effect
Cerebral herniation
Cerebral ischemia and/or infarction
Rehemorrhage

Assessing the Potential for Collateral Circulation

Delineating cross-filling from one carotid to the other as well as between the carotid and vertebrobasilar circulations is helpful, especially if temporary occlusion of the parent vessel becomes necessary during surgery.

Identifying Other Lesions

Complications of aneurysm rupture include vasoconstriction, infarction and ischemia, mass effect, and contrast extravasation. Identification of multiple aneurysms is also essential.

Acute vasoconstriction following SAH is common and contributes directly to ischemic brain injury. SAH-induced vasoconstriction occurs independently of changes in intracranial pressure and cerebral perfusion pressure (74). *Vasoconstriction* is unusual with hyperacute SAH unless a prior "sentinel" bleed has occurred.

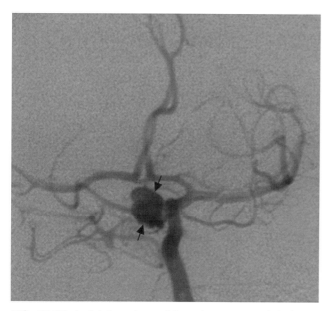

FIG. 12-18. Left internal carotid angiogram, arterial phase, AP view, in a patient with subarachnoid hemorrhage transiently opacifies almost the entire circle of Willis. A large lobulated aneurysm (*arrows*) is present.

Infarction and ischemia are therefore unusual in the setting of acute SAH but often occur as a delayed complication of aneurysm rupture (Fig. 12-26).

Mass effect can be caused by a focal hematoma adjacent to the aneurysm. Secondary mass effects such as herniation syndromes must be identified and the attending clinicians alerted to their presence (Fig. 12-27). *Contrast extravasation* is rare but can be seen if active bleeding from the aneurysm occurs during angiography (Fig. 12-28).

Diagnostic and Management Dilemmas

Difficulties in the angiographic diagnosis of intracranial aneurysms include determining which aneurysm caused the SAH when multiple lesions are present, evaluating patent giant saccular aneurysms, identifying partially or completely thrombosed aneurysms, and distinguishing aneurysms from vascular loops and infundibuli. Management issues include addressing angiogram-negative SAH and following up treated intracranial aneurysms.

Identifying the Source of SAH When More than One Aneurysm Is Present

Multiple aneurysms occur in 15% to 20% of cases (1,10). When more than one aneurysm is present, identifying which aneurysm is likely to have ruptured is essential for treatment planning. Active bleeding with contrast extravasation is the only true absolute sign of aneurysm rupture (Fig. 12-28). Helpful ancillary signs include size (the larger aneurysm is statistically more likely to have ruptured), irregularity (presence of a "tit" or multilobulated dome), and a focal mass effect (perianeurysmal hematoma) (Fig. 12-29).

"Giant" Aneurysms

Approximately 5% of all aneurysms are "giant" and by definition measure 25 mm or more in diameter (26,26a). These lesions are often multilobulated and may contain multiple layers of organized thrombus. Determining their precise origin and identifying the presence of a neck is difficult. Rapid-sequence digital subtraction studies or superselective catheterization (aneurysmography) may be required (Fig. 12-30) (73).

Partially or Completely Thrombosed Aneurysms

Patent saccular aneurysms appear as rounded or lobulated contrast-filled outpouchings that arise from major vessel bifurcations or the lateral wall of an artery. When an aneurysm is partially thrombosed, the lesion may be much larger than the patent lumen, as demonstrated with conventional angiography. An avascular mass effect that

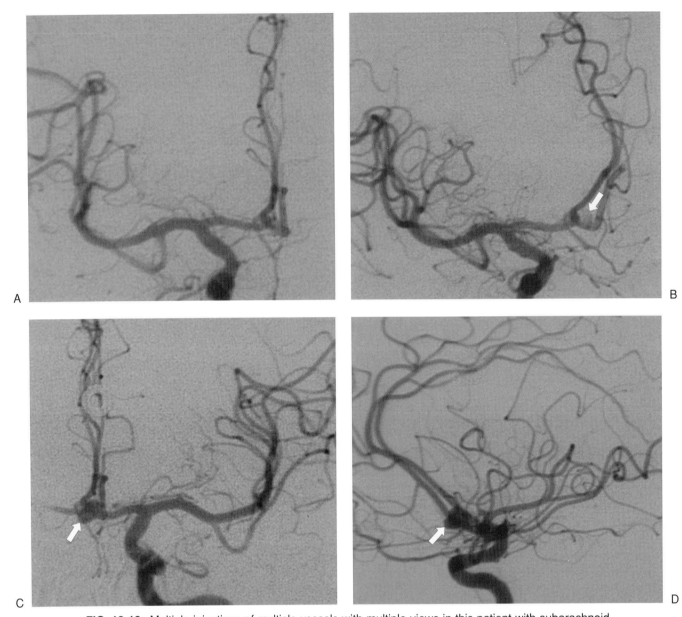

FIG. 12-19. Multiple injections of multiple vessels with multiple views in this patient with subarachnoid hemorrhage were required to delineate the small lobulated anterior communicating artery (ACoA) aneurysm. The aneurysm (*arrows*) seems to fill preferentially from the left internal carotid artery even though both horizontal ACA segments are normal sized and the ACoA is opacified from both sides. **A:** Right internal carotid angiogram, AP view. **B:** Right internal carotid angiogram, oblique view. **C:** Left internal carotid angiogram, AP view. **D:** Left internal carotid angiogram, lateral view.

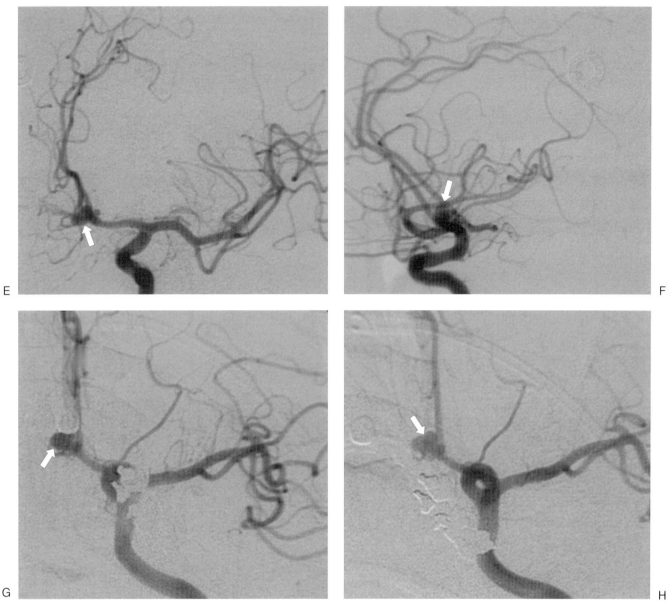

FIG. 12-19. *Continued.* **E:** Left internal carotid angiogram, standard oblique view. **F:** Left internal carotid angiogram, reverse oblique view. **G:** Left internal carotid angiogram, submentovertex view. Dental amalgam partially obscures the aneurysm. **H:** Left internal carotid angiogram, oblique submentovertex view, delineates the aneurysm nicely.

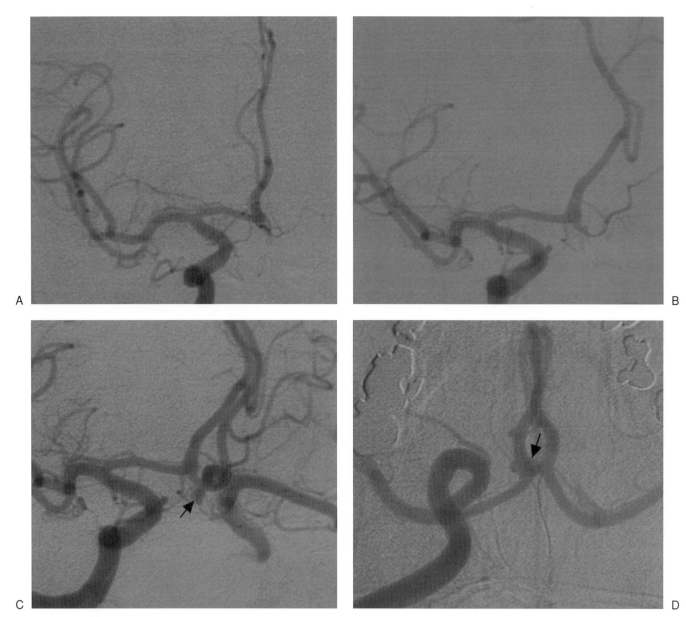

FIG. 12-20. The importance of using cross-compression in evaluating the anterior communicating artery (ACoA) is illustrated by this case. AP **(A)** and oblique **(B)** views of the standard right internal carotid angiogram do not show a lesion. When the study is repeated using manual compression of the left common carotid artery during injection of the right ICA, an ACoA aneurysm (*arrows*) is clearly seen on the oblique **(C)** and submentovertex **(D)** views.

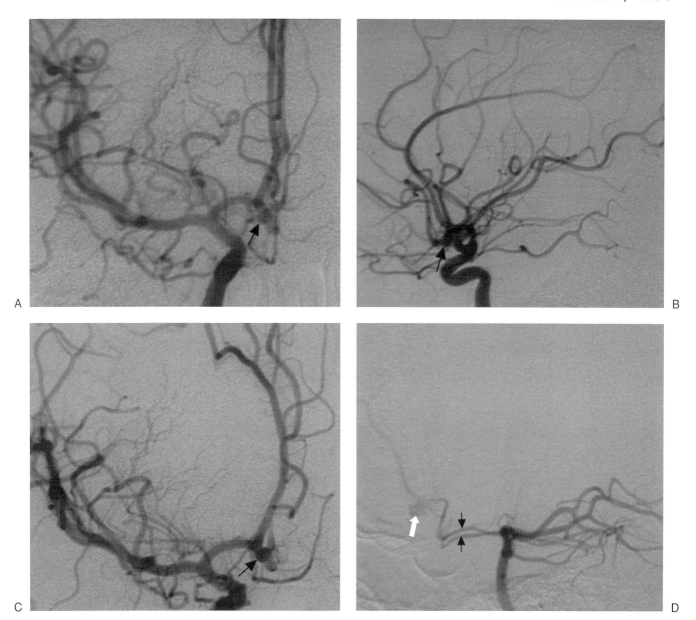

FIG. 12-21. AP **(A)**, lateral **(B)**, and oblique **(C)** views of a right internal carotid angiogram in this patient with subarachnoid hemorrhage show an extra area of contrast accumulation (*arrows*) near the anterior communicating artery (ACoA) that is suspicious for an aneurysm but is partially obscured by overlapping vessels. **D:** Left vertebral angiogram, arterial phase, lateral view, shows contrast reflux through the posterior communicating arteries (*small black arrows*). A definite aneurysm is faintly opacified (*white arrow*). A ruptured ACoA aneurysm was confirmed at surgery.

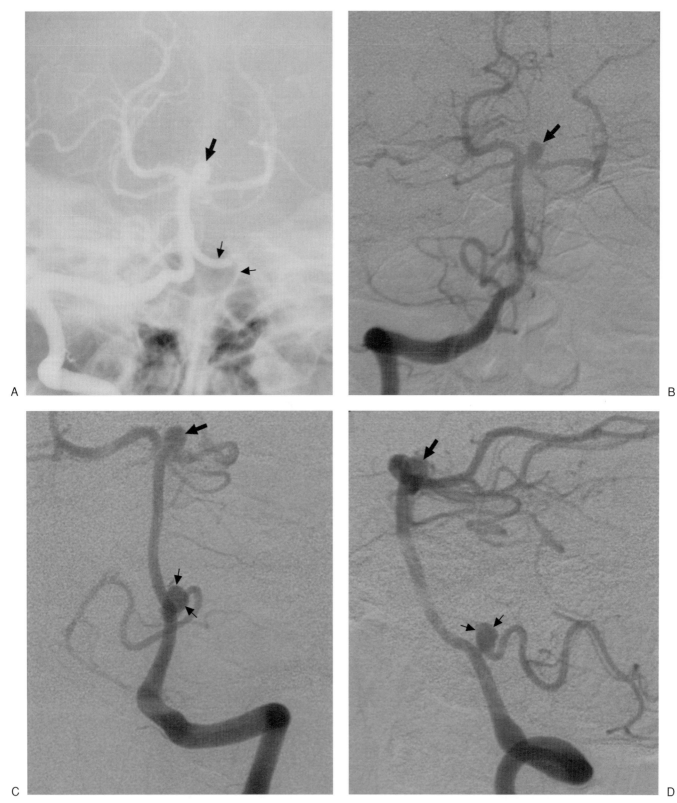

FIG. 12-22. This case illustrates the hazards of performing an incomplete angiogram in cases of suspected aneurysmal subarachnoid hemorrhage. **A:** No subtracted studies were performed on this poor-quality outside angiogram, performed via the right vertebral artery (VA). A basilar bifurcation aneurysm was identified (*large arrow*). The left vertebral artery (VA) (*small arrow*) is opacified transiently but inadequately. **B:** AP view of a repeat digital subtraction right vertebral angiogram confirms the presence of the basilar tip aneurysm (*arrow*). The left VA is not opacified. Oblique **(C)** and lateral **(D)** views of a selective left vertebral angiogram again show the basilar tip aneurysm (*large arrows*) but also opacify a larger, lobulated aneurysm (*small arrows*) that arises from the origin of the posterior inferior cerebellar artery (PICA). Surgery confirmed that the larger PICA aneurysm is the one that ruptured.

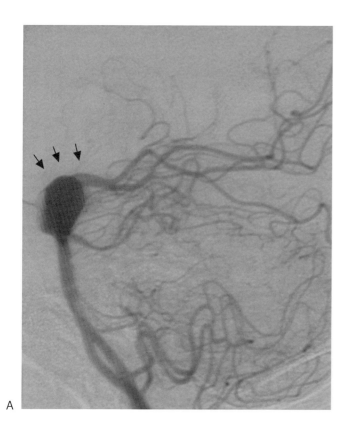

A

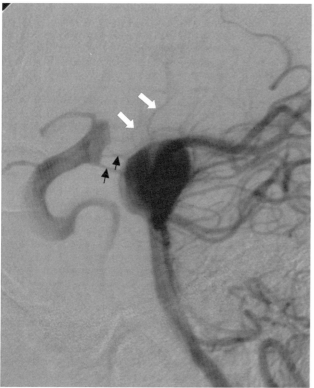

B

FIG. 12-23. A: Lateral view of a left vertebral angiogram in this patient with a large basilar artery aneurysm shows that multiple penetrating branches may be arising from the aneurysm dome (*arrows*). **B:** Magnified view, performed with temporary cross-compression of the ipsilateral common carotid artery, shows contrast refluxes into both posterior communicating arteries (*small arrows*). The penetrating branches (*white arrows*) that arise from the aneurysm are better delineated.

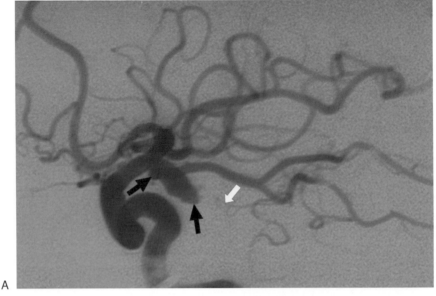

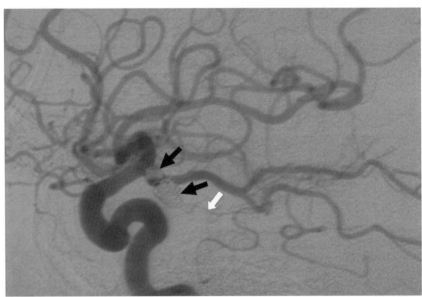

FIG. 12-24. A: Lateral view of a left internal carotid angiogram in a patient with fetal origin of the left posterior cerebral artery (PCA) show a lobulated aneurysm (*large arrows*) that arises from the internal carotid artery at the origin of the PCA. Because a prominent posterior temporal branch (*white arrow*) arises from the aneurysm dome, endovascular occlusion was performed with local anesthesia only. The patient tolerated the slow, progressive obliteration of the aneurysm well. **B:** Postprocedure study shows coils (*large arrows*) obliterate the aneurysm while preserving flow into PCA and the posterior temporal artery (*white arrow*).

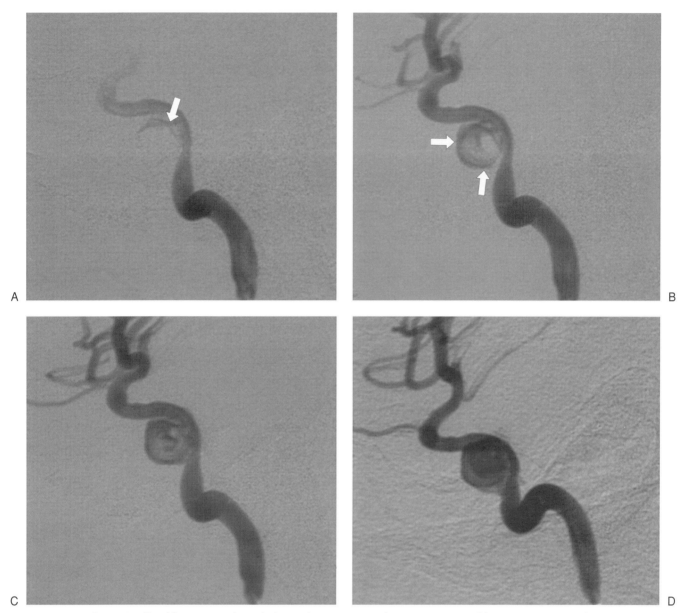

A

B

C

D

FIG. 12-25. Rapid sequence lateral views of a posttraumatic cavernous carotid artery aneurysm show the aneurysm orifice (**A**, *white arrow*) and intraaneurysmal flow patterns. Note that the contrast enters at the distal part of the orifice and circulates toward the dome (**B**, *white arrows*) before exiting proximally. **C** and **D**: A central vortex of slower flow and contrast stasis is present.

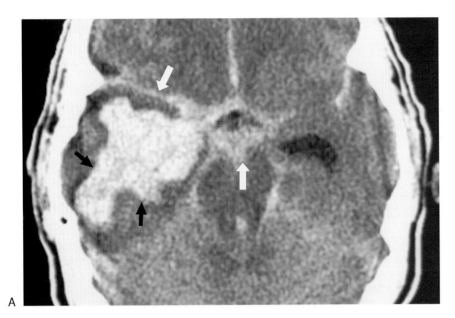

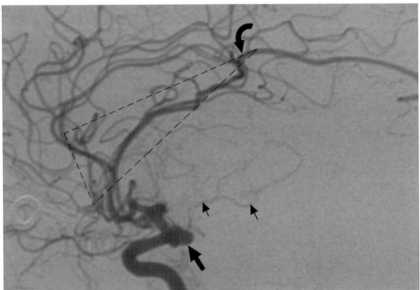

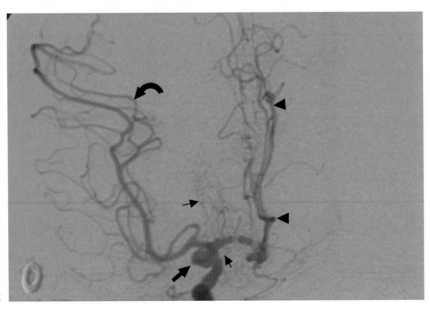

FIG. 12-26. Secondary effects of a ruptured intracranial aneurysm are illustrated in this case. **A:** Axial NECT scan shows diffuse subarachnoid hemorrhage (*white arrows*) and a large focal hematoma in the right temporal lobe (*large black arrows*). Lateral **(B)** and anteroposterior **(C)** views of the right internal carotid angiogram in this patient show a laterally projecting internal carotid artery aneurysm (*large black arrow*) and the avascular mass effect caused by the parenchymal mass. Note elevation of the sylvian triangle (**B**, *dotted lines*) and sylvian point (**C**, *curved arrow*). Medial displacement of the anterior choroidal artery (**B** and **C**, *small arrows*) indicates descending transtentorial herniation. A square shift of the anterior cerebral arteries (**C**, *arrowheads*) represents subfalcine herniation.

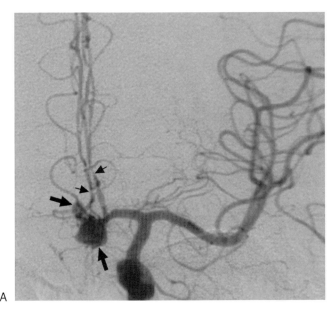

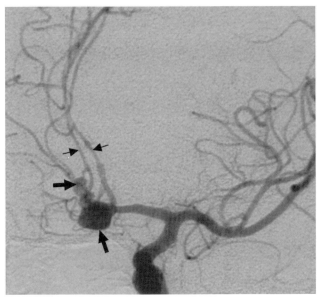

FIG. 12-27. AP **(A)** and oblique **(B)** views of the left internal carotid angiogram in this patient with a sentinel subarachnoid hemorrhage (SAH) 10 days previously show a large multilobulated anterior communicating artery aneurysm (*large arrows*). The narrowing and segmental irregularities of both distal anterior cerebral arteries (ACAs) are striking and represent vasospasm. This finding is unusual with acute SAH. When present, it should raise suspicion of a prior hemorrhage.

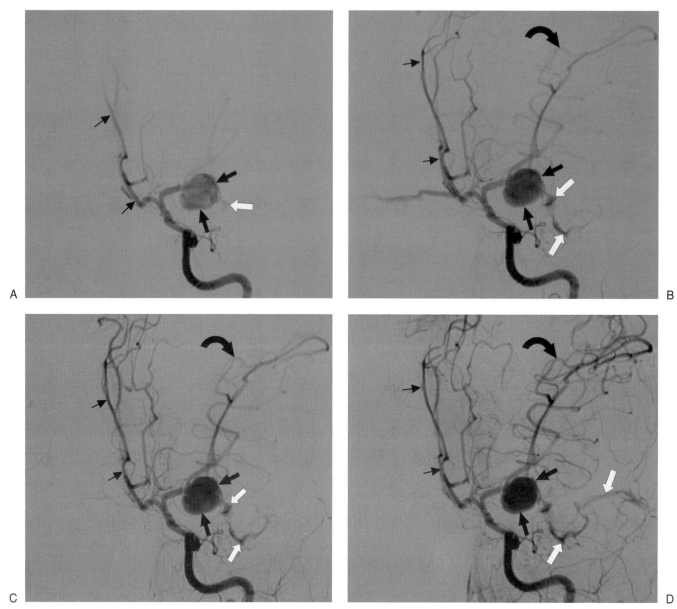

FIG. 12-28. Serial AP views of the left common carotid angiogram in this patient who initially presented with headache, drowsiness, and a pupil-involving third nerve palsy are shown. The patient suddenly lost consciousness and became decerebrate. A large irregular left middle cerebral artery aneurysm is seen (*large arrows*). Contrast extravasation is identified (*white arrows*). Severe subfalcine and descending transtentorial herniation are indicated by displacement of the anterior cerebral artery (*small arrows*) and elevation and medial displacement of the sylvian point (*curved arrows*). The patient was immediately taken to surgery. The hematoma was evacuated and the aneurysm was successfully clipped. Active arterial bleeding from the dome was noted during the operation.

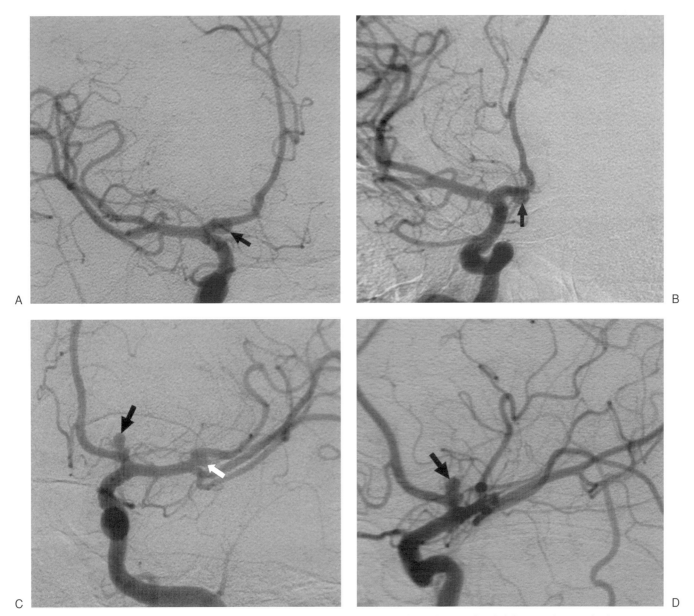

FIG. 12-29. This patient has multiple aneurysms. One arises from the proximal right anterior cerebral artery (ACA) (**A** and **B**, *small black arrows*), another arises from the proximal left ACA (**C** and **D**, *large black arrows*), and a third arises from the left middle cerebral artery trifurcation (**C**, *white arrow*). Statistically, the largest aneurysm is the one that ruptured. Rupture of the proximal left ACA aneurysm, the largest one in this case, was confirmed at surgery.

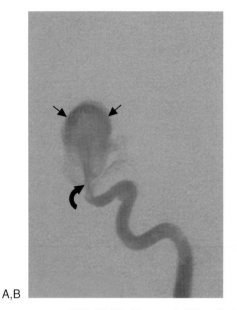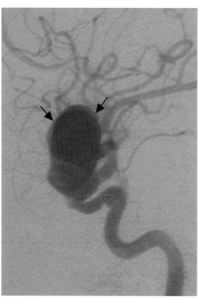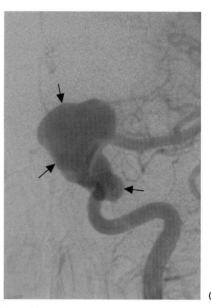

A,B

C

FIG. 12-30. Very early **(A)** and mid-arterial **(B)** phase studies, lateral view, of a rapid-sequence digital subtraction angiogram show a giant multilobulated internal carotid artery (ICA) aneurysm (*small arrows*). Note that the precise location of the aneurysm origin is obscured on the lateral **(B)** and anteroposterior **(C)** views obtained slightly later in the angiographic sequence. A jet of contrast fills the ICA, and the aneurysm neck can be identified on only one frame from the earliest phase of the study (**A**, *curved arrow*).

surrounds the patent lumen is demonstrated by stretching and draping of adjacent vessels (Fig. 12-31A). CT and MR scans are very helpful in identifying the precise extent of the thrombosed segment (Fig. 12-31B).

Small saccular aneurysms that are completely thrombosed may have normal angiographic studies.

Aneurysm Mimics

True aneurysms must be distinguished from vascular loops and infundibuli. *Infundibuli* are smooth funnel-shaped dilatations that are caused by incomplete regression of a vessel present in the developing fetus. Their

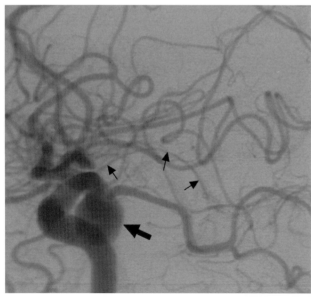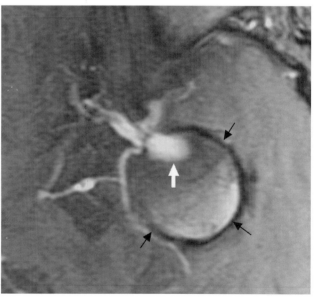

A

B

FIG. 12-31. A partially thrombosed giant aneurysm is illustrated. **A:** Left internal carotid angiogram, arterial phase, lateral view, shows a contrast-filled outpouching (*large arrow*) that arises from the internal carotid artery. Note displacement of the anterior choroidal artery (AChA) (*small arrows*). The AChA is elevated, stretched, and draped over a large avascular mass that surrounds the aneurysm. **B:** Axial source image from a contrast-enhanced MR angiogram shows flow in the patent lumen of the aneurysm (*white arrow*). The remainder of the aneurysm sac contains organized thrombus. The thin black rim represents the hemosiderin-laden aneurysm wall (*small arrows*).

most common location is at the origin of the PCoA from the ICA (see Fig. 4-13). Less commonly, an infundibulum arises at the anterior choroidal artery origin.

At angiography, infundibuli appear as round or conical dilatations that are less than 3 mm in diameter, although a few surgically proven cases have been larger (75). The distal PCoA exits from the apex of the infundibulum (see Figs. 5-14 and 12-3B). In contrast, aneurysms are usually 3 mm or larger in diameter and often appear lobulated. If the distal PCoA exits eccentrically from the dilated outpouching, an aneurysm should be suspected regardless of size (Fig. 12-32) (10,75,76).

Vascular *loops* are distinguished from aneurysms by using multiple projections to profile the vessel in question (Fig. 12-33).

Angiogram-Negative Studies in Patients with Acute SAH

The most common cause of a negative angiogram in patients with acute nontraumatic SAH is an incomplete examination (10). Other causes include microaneurysms, so-called nonaneurysmal perimesencephalic hemorrhage, and hemorrhage from lesions such as vascular malformations and neoplasms (10,18,77).

In 15% to 20% of patients with verified SAH, study results are normal, even with a complete, technically ade-

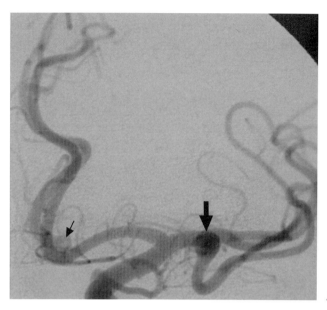

A

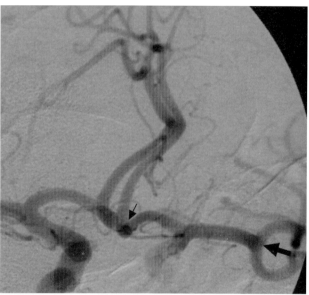

B

FIG. 12-33. The use of multiple projections to resolve the question of vascular loop versus aneurysm is illustrated by the angiogram in this case. **A:** A left internal carotid angiogram, arterial phase, anteroposterior view, shows two areas that are suspicious for aneurysm. One is at the middle cerebral artery (MCA) trifurcation (*large arrow*); the other is at the junction between the left A1 and A2 anterior cerebral artery (ACA) segments (*small arrow*). **B:** Right internal carotid angiogram, arterial phase, oblique view, performed with temporary cross-compression of the left common carotid artery, cross-fills the left circulation nicely. The study shows that the MCA bifurcation (*large arrow*) and A1–A2 junction (*small arrow*) are normal. Both suspicious areas represent vascular loops.

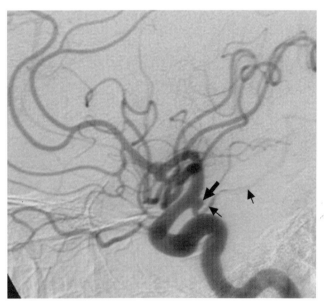

FIG. 12-32. A 43-year-old man with a seizure disorder had a cerebral angiogram prior to resection of an oligodendroglioma. Lateral view of the left internal carotid angiogram shows a 2-mm contrast-filled outpouching that arises from the junction of the internal carotid artery (ICA) and posterior communicating arteries (PCoAs) (*large arrow*). Note that the PCoA (*small arrows*) arises eccentrically from the outpouching. An unruptured aneurysm was found at surgery. Compare this case to the anatomic diagram (see Fig. 4-13) and angiograms (see Figs. 5-14 and 12-3B) of a PCoA infundibulum.

quate cerebral angiogram. Repeat angiography reveals an aneurysm in only 6% of these cases (78). Some investigators feel repeat angiography is unnecessary if the initial angiogram is both complete and adequately interpreted (79). Others recommend an MR scan and perhaps an MRA in these cases (1).

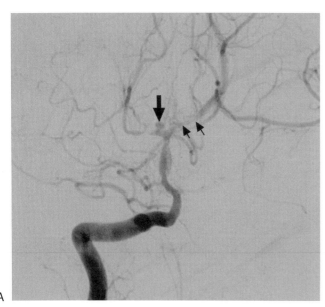
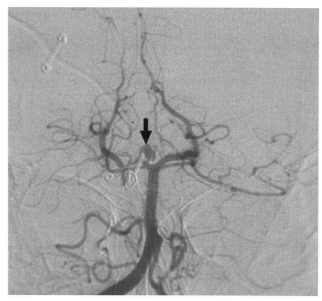

A

B

FIG. 12-34. A: Postoperative right vertebral angiogram, arterial phase, AP view, in a patient who had a basilar bifurcation aneurysm clipped. Note the residual neck (*large arrow*) and segmental narrowing of the adjacent left posterior cerebral artery (PCA) (*small arrows*). **B:** Repeat angiogram 2 months later shows interval growth of the residual aneurysm (*arrow*). The focal vasoconstriction of the PCA has resolved.

Intra- and Postoperative Angiography

A major cause of poor outcome following surgical treatment of intracranial aneurysms is distal branch occlusion or stenosis of the parent artery (80). The use of *intraoperative angiography* or color-coded duplex sonography to guide surgery is cost effective and has proved helpful in reducing perioperative morbidity, especially with large or complex aneurysms (81,82). In one study, intraoperative angiography led to clip repositioning in 27% of cases (83).

Postoperative angiography following aneurysm clipping is performed routinely in many centers. Multiple studies have shown that the frequency of significant findings such as a residual aneurysm neck approaches 10% to 20% (Fig. 12-34). However, some investigators feel that in most cases conventional angiography is unnecessary and is not cost effective (84). Others suggest that postoperative angiography is most useful in difficult cases that have an increased risk of imperfect clip placement. Deep midline aneurysm (posterior circulation, anterior communicating artery) and ophthalmic/peri-ophthalmic lesions are cited as indications for "selective" postoperative angiography (84a).

Many investigators now recommend the routine use of noninvasive techniques such as spiral CT and MRA for the postoperative evaluation of aneurysms that have been clipped with MR-compatible (nonferromagnetic) titanium clips (85).

REFERENCES

1. Osborn AG. Intracranial aneurysms. In: Brant-Zawadski M, Drayer BP, eds. *Core curriculum course in neuroradiology. Part I: Vascular lesions and degenerative diseases. American Society of Neuroradiology,* Chicago, IL, April 21–22, 1995.
2. Stehbens WE. Etiology of intracranial berry aneurysms. *J Neurosurg* 1989;70:823–831.
3. Cawley CM, Dawson RC, Shengelaia G, et al. Arterial saccular aneurysm model in the rabbit. *AJNR* 1996;17:1761–1766.
3a. Abruzzo T, Shengelaia G, Dawson RC III, et al: Histologic and morphologic comparison of experimental aneurysms with human intracranial aneurysms. *AJNR* 1998;19:1309–1314.
4. Okazaki H. Malformative vascular lesions. In: *Fundamentals of neuropathology,* 2nd ed. New York: Igaku-Shoin, 1989:70–74.
5. Connolly ES, Fiore AJ, Wingree CJ, et al. Elastin degradation in the superficial temporal arteries of patients with intracranial aneurysms reflects changes in plasma elastase. *Neurosurgery* 1997;40: 903–909.
6. Skirgaudas M, Awad IA, Kim J, et al. Expression of angiogenesis factors and selected vascular wall matrix proteins in intracranial saccular aneurysms. *Neurosurgery* 1996;39:537–547.
7. Nakagawa T, Hashi K. The incidence and treatment of asymptomatic, unruptured cerebral aneurysms. *J Neurosurg* 1994;80:217–225.
8. Rinne J, Hernesniemi J, Puranen M, Saari T. Multiple intracranial aneurysms in a defined population: prospective angiographic and clinical study. *Neurosurgery* 1994;35:803–808.
9. Pierot L, Boulin A, Castaings L, et al. The endovascular approach in the management of patients with multiple intracranial aneurysms. *Neuroradiology* 1997;39:361–366.
10. Osborn AG. Intracranial aneurysms. In: *Diagnostic neuroradiology.* St. Louis: Mosby, 1994:248–283.
10a. Qureshi AI, Suarez JI, Parekh PD, et al. Risk factors for multiple intracranial aneurysms. *Neurosurgery* 1998;43:22–27).
11. Rinne J, Hernesniemi J, Niskanen M, Vapalati M. Analysis of 561 patients with 690 middle cerebral artery aneurysms: anatomic and clinical features as correlated to management outcome. *Neurosurgery* 1996;38:2–11.

12. Kanaan I, Lasjaunias P, Coates R. The spectrum of intracranial aneurysms in pediatrics. *Minim Invas Neurosurg* 1995;38:1–9.

13. TerBrugge KG. Aneurysm in the pediatric population. *Riv Neuroradiol* 1998;11(suppl 1):54–55.

14. Kopitnik TA, Samson DS. Management of subarachnoid hemorrhage. *J Neurosurg Psychiatry* 1993;56:947–959.

15. McFadzean RM, Teasdale EM. Computerized tomography angiography in isolated third nerve palsies. *J Neurosurg* 1998;88:679–684.

16. Raps EC, Rogers JD, Galetta SL, et al. The clinical spectrum of unruptured intracranial aneurysms. *Arch Neurol* 1993;50:265–268.

17. Ogilvy CS, Carter BS. A proposed comprehensive grading system to predict outcome for surgical management of intracranial aneurysms. *Neurosurgery* 1998;42:959–970.

17a. Singer MB, Atlas SW, Drayer BP. Subarachnoid space disease: diagnosis with fluid attenuated inversion-recovery MR imaging and comparison with gadolinium-enhanced spin-echo MR imaging—blinded reader study. *Radiol* 1998;208:417–422.

18. Kallmes DF, Clark HP, Dix JE, et al. Ruptured vertebrobasilar aneurysms: frequency of the nonaneurysmal perimesencephalic pattern of hemorrhage on CT scans. *Radiology* 1996;201:657–660.

19. Schievink WI, Wijdicks EFM, Parisi JE, et al. Sudden death from aneurysmal subarachnoid hemorrhage. *Neurology* 1995;45:871–874.

20. Taylor CL, Yuan Z, Selman WR, et al. Cerebral arterial aneurysm formation and rupture in 20,767 elderly patients: hypertension and other risk factors. *J Neurosurg* 1995;83:812–819.

21. Leblanc R, Worsley KJ, Melanson D, et al. Angiographic screening and elective surgery of familial cerebral aneurysms: a decision analysis. *Neurosurgery* 1994;35:9–19.

21a. Raaymalcers TWM, Rinkel GJE, Limburg M, Algra A. Mortality and morbidity of surgery for unruptured intracranial aneurysms: a meta-analysis. *Stroke* 1998;29:1531–1538.

22. Wiebers DO, Whisnant JP, Sundt T, et al. The significance of unruptured intracranial aneurysm. *J Neurosurg* 1987;66:23–29.

23. Juvela S, Porras M, Heiskanen O. Natural history of unruptured intracranial aneurysms: a long-term follow-up study. *J Neurosurg* 1993;79:174–182.

24. Yasui N, Suzuki A, Nishimura H, et al. Long-term follow-up study of unruptured intracranial aneurysms. *Neurosurgery* 1997;40:1155–1160.

25. Forbes G, Fox AJ, Huston J, et al. Interobserver variability in angiographic measurement and morphologic characterization of intracranial aneurysms: a report from the International Study of Unruptured Intracranial Aneurysms. *AJNR* 1996;17:1407–1415.

26. Khurana VG, Piepgras DG, Whisnant JP. Ruptured giant intracranial aneurysms. Part I. A study of rebleeding. *J Neurosurg* 1998;88:425–429.

26a. Wellman BJ, Loftus CM, Noh D, et al. A combined surgical-endovascular device concept for giant aneurysm neck occlusion. *Neurosurgery* 1998;42:1364–1369.

27. Wascher TM, Golfinos J, Zabramski JM, Spetzler RF. Management of unruptured intracranial aneurysms. *BNI Q* 1992;8:2–7.

28. Schievink WI, Piepgras DG, Wirth FP. Rupture of previously documented small asymptomatic saccular intracranial aneurysms. *Neurosurgery* 1992;76:1019–1024.

28a. Rolen PB, Sze G: Small, patent cerebral aneurysms: Atypical appearance of 1.5-T. MR imaging. *Radiol* 1998;208:129–136.

29. Yasui N, Magarisawa S, Suzuki A, et al. Subarachnoid hemorrhage caused by previously diagnosed, previously unruptured intracranial aneurysms: a retrospective analysis of 25 cases. *Neurosurgery* 1996;39:1096–1101.

30. Wardlaw JM, Cannon J, Statham PFX, Price R. Does the size of intracranial aneurysms change with intracranial pressure? Observations based on color power transcranial Doppler ultrasound. *J Neurosurg* 1998;88:846–850.

31. Erbengi A, Inci S. Pheochromocytoma and multiple intracranial aneurysms: is it a coincidence? *J Neurosurg* 1997;87:764–767.

32. Schievink WI. Genetics of intracranial aneurysms. *Neurosurgery* 1997;40:651–663.

33. Pollack JS, Custer PL, Hart WM, et al. Ocular complications in Ehlers-Danlos syndrome type IV. *Arch Ophthalmol* 1997;115:416–419.

34. Schievink WI, Parisi JE, Piepgras DG, Michels VV. Intracranial aneurysms in Marfan's syndrome: an autopsy study. *Neurosurgery* 1997;41:866–871.

35. van den Berg JSP, Limburg M, Hennekam RCM. Is Marfan syndrome associated with symptomatic intracranial aneurysms? *Stroke* 1996;27:10–12.

36. Butler WE, Barker FG II, Crowell RM. Patients with polycystic kidney disease would benefit from routine magnetic resonance angiographic screening for intracerebral aneurysms: a decision analysis. *Neurosurgery* 1996;38:506–516.

37. Schievink WI, Parisi JE, Piepgras DG. Familial intracranial aneurysms: an autopsy study. *Neurosurgery* 1997;51:1247–1252.

38. Ronkainen A, Miettinen H. Karkola K, et al. Risk of harboring an unruptured intracranial aneurysm. *Stroke* 1998;29:359–362.

39. Schievink WI, Mokri B, Piepgras DG, Gittenberger-de Groot AC. Intracranial aneurysms and cephalocervical dissections associated with congenital heart disease. *Neurosurgery* 1996;39:689–690.

40. Schievink WI. Progressive intracranial aneurysmal disease: in reply [Letter]. *Neurosurgery* 1998;52:1195.

41. Cloft HJ, Kallmes DF, Kallmes MH, et al. Prevalence of cerebral aneurysms in patients with fibromuscular dysplasia: a reassessment. *J Neurosurg* 1998;88:436–440.

42. Tasker AD, Byrne JV. Basilar artery fenestration in association with aneurysms of the posterior circulation. *Neuroradiology* 1997;39:185–189.

43. Preul MC, Cendes F, Just N, Mohr G. Intracranial aneurysms and sickle cell anemia: multiplicity and propensity for the vertebrobasilar territory. *Neurosurgery* 1998;42:971–978.

44. Juvela S, Hillbom M, Numminen H, et al. Cigarette smoke and alcohol consumption as risk factors for aneurysmal subarachnoid hemorrhage. *Stroke* 1993;24:639–646.

45. Phillips J, Roberts G, Bolger C, et al. Lipoprotein (a): a potential biological marker for unruptured intracranial aneurysms. *Neurosurgery* 1997;40:1112–1117.

45a. Todor DR, Lewis I, Bruno G, Chyatte D. Identification of a serum gelatinase associated with the occurrence of cerebral aneurysms as pro-matrix metalloproteinase-2. *Stroke* 1998;29:1580–1583.

46. Schievink WI, Katzmann JA, Piepgras DG, Schaid DJ. Alpha-1-antitrypsin phenotypes among patients with intracranial aneurysms. *J Neurosurg* 1996;84:781–784.

47. Strother CM, Graves VB, Rappe A. Aneurysm hemodynamics: an experimental study. *AJNR* 1992;13:1089–1095.

48. Kerber CW, Hecht ST, Knox K, et al. Flow dynamics in a fatal aneurysm of the basilar artery. *AJNR* 1996;17:1417–1421.

48a. Stehbens WE. Aptosis and matrix vesicles in the genesis of arterial aneurysms of cerebral arteries (letter). *Stroke* 1998;29:1478–1479.

49. Gao E, Young WL, Pile-Spellman J, et al. Cerebral arteriovenous feeding artery aneurysms. *Neurosurgery* 1997;41:1345–1358.

49a. Thompson RC, Steinberg GK, Levy RP, Marks MM. The management of patients with arteriovenous malformations and associated intracranial aneurysms. *Neurosurg* 1998;43:202–212.

50. Turjman F, Massoud TF, Viñuela F, et al. Aneurysms related to cerebral arteriovenous malformations: superselective angiographic assessment in 58 patients. *AJNR* 1994;15:1601–1605.

51. Corr P, Wright M, Handler LC. Endocarditis-related cerebral aneurysms: radiologic changes with treatment. *AJNR* 1995;16:745–748.

52. Kurino M, Kuratsu J, Yamaguchi T, Ushio Y. Mycotic aneurysm accompanied by aspergillus granulomas: a case report. *Surg Neurol* 1994;42:160–164.

53. Scotti G, Li MH, Righi C, et al. Endovascular treatment of bacterial intracranial aneurysms. *Neuroradiology* 1996;38:186–189.

54. Tanaka H, Patel U, Shrier DA, Coniglio JU. Pseudoaneurysm of the petrous internal carotid artery after skull base infection and prevertebral abscess drainage. *AJNR* 1998;19:502–504.

55. Holmes B, Harbaugh RE. Traumatic intracranial aneurysms: a contemporary review. *J Trauma* 1993;35:855–860.

56. Proust F, Callonec F, Bellow F, et al. Tentorial edge traumatic aneurysm of the superior cerebellar artery. *J Neurosurg* 1997;87:950–954.

57. Maruki C, Suzukawa K, Koike J, Sato K. Cardiac malignant fibrous histiocytoma metastasizing to the brain: development of multiple neoplastic cerebral aneurysms. *Surg Neurol* 1994;41:40–44.

58. Friedman DP, Rapoport RJ. Giant fusiform oncotic aneurysms: MR and angiographic findings. *AJR* 1996;167:538–539.

59. Gonzales CF, Cho YI, Ortega HV, Moret J. Intracranial aneurysms: flow analysis of their origin and progression. *AJNR* 1992;13:181–188.

60. Chong BW, Kerber CW, Buxton RB, et al. Blood flow dynamics in the vertebrobasilar system: correlation of a transparent elastic model and MR angiography. *AJNR* 1994;15:733–745.

61. Gobin YP, Counord JL, Flaud P, Duffaux J. In vitro study of haemo-dynamics in a giant saccular aneurysm model: influence of flow dynamics in the parent vessel and effects of coil embolisation. *Neuroradiology* 1994;36:530–536.

62. Graves VG, Strother GM, Partington CR, Rappe A. Flow dynamics of lateral carotid artery aneurysms and their effects on coils and balloons: an experimental study in dogs. *AJNR* 1992;13:189–196.

63. Geremia G, Haklin M, Brennecke L. Embolization of experimentally created aneurysms with intravascular stent devices. *AJNR* 1994;15:1223–1231.

64. Barth A, deTribolet N. Growth of small saccular aneurysms to giant aneurysms. *Surg Neurol* 1994;51:277–280.

65. McCormick PW, McCormick J, Zimmerman R, et al. The pathophysiology of acute subarachnoid hemorrhage. *BNI Q* 1991;7:18–26.

66. Eskridge JM. A practical approach to the treatment of vasospasm. *AJNR* 1997;18:1653–1660.

67. Anderson GB, Findlay JM, Steinke DE, Ashforth R. Experience with computed tomographic angiography for the detection of intracranial aneurysms in the setting of acute subarachnoid hemorrhage. *Neurosurgery* 1997;41:522–528.

68. Brown JH, Lustrin ES, Lev MH, et al. Characterization of intracranial aneurysms using CT angiography. *AJR* 1997;169:889–893.

69. Imakita S, Onishi Y, Hashimoto T, et al. Subtraction CT angiography with controlled-orbit helical scanning for detection of intracranial aneurysms. *AJNR* 1998;19:291–295.

70. Harrison MJ, Johnson BA, Gardner GM, Weiling BG. Preliminary results on the management of unruptured intracranial aneurysms with magnetic resonance angiography and computed tomographic angiography. *Neurosurgery* 1997;40:947–957.

71. Ida M, Kurisu Y, Yamashita M. MR angiography of ruptured aneurysms in acute subarachnoid hemorrhage. *AJNR* 1997;18:1025–1032.

72. Tsuruda J, Parker D, Alexander A, Buswell H. Advances in MR screening for asymptomatic unruptured intracranial. *IJNR (in press)*.

73. Gailloud P, Fasel JHD, Muster M, et al. A case in favor of aneurysmographic studies: a perforating artery originating from the dome of a basilar tip aneurysm. *AJNR* 1997;18:1691–1694.

74. Bederson JB, Levy AL, Ding WH, et al. Acute vasoconstriction after subarachnoid hemorrhage. *Neurosurgery* 1998;42:352–362.

75. Zager EL, Hackney DB: clipping infundibula [Letter]. *J Neurosurg* 1992;84:538–539.

76. Endo S, Furichi S, Takaba M, et al. Clinical study of enlarged infundibular dilation of the origin of the posterior communicating artery. *J Neurosurg* 1995;83:421–425.

77. Tatter SB, Crowell RM, Ogilvy CS. Aneurysmal and microaneurysmal angiogram-negative subarachnoid hemorrhage. *Neurosurgery* 1995;37:48–55.

78. Urbach H, Zentner J, Solymosi L. The need for repeat angiography in subarachnoid hemorrhage. *Neuroradiology* 1998;40:6–10.

79. Du Mesnil de Rochemont R, Heindel W, Wesselmann C, et al. Nontraumatic subarachnoid hemorrhage: value of repeat angiography. *Radiology* 1997;202:798–800.

80. Bailes JE, Tantuwaya L, Fukushima T, et al. Intraoperative microvascular doppler sonography in aneurysm surgery. *Neurosurgery* 1997;40:965–972.

81. Leipzig J, Scott JA, Gilmor RL, DeNardo AJ. Role intraoperative angiography in the surgical treatment of cerebral aneurysms. *J Neurosurg* 1998;88:441–448.

82. Kallmes DF, Kallmes MH. Cost-effectiveness of intraoperative angiography during surgery for ruptured intracranial aneurysm. *AJNR* 1997;18:1453–1462.

83. Payner TD, Horner TG, Leipzig TJ, et al. Role of intraoperative angiography in surgical treatment of cerebral aneurysms. *J Neurosurg* 1998;88:441–448.

84. Kallmes DF, Kallmes MH, Lanzino G, et al. Routine angiography after surgery for ruptured intracranial aneurysms: a cost versus benefit analysis. *Neurosurgery* 1997;41:629–641.

84a. Rauzzino MJ, Quinn CM, Fisher WS III: Angiography after aneurysm surgery: indications for "selective" angiography. *Surg Neurol* 1998;49:32–41.

85. Van Loon JJL, Yousry TA, Fink U, et al. Postoperative spiral computed tomography and magnetic resonance angiography after aneurysm clipping with titanium clips. *Neurosurgery* 1997;51:851–857.

CHAPTER 13

Vascular Malformations

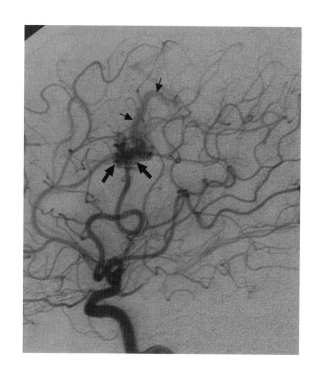

Classically, cerebral vascular malformations (CVMs) have been divided into four basic types: (a) arteriovenous malformations (AVMs); (b) venous malformations; (c) capillary telangiectasias; and (d) cavernous angiomas (see box below).

More recently, CVMs have been reclassified according to a combination of anatomic and histopathologic features, clinical presentation, biologic behavior, and imaging characteristics (1,2). The presence or absence of vascular shunting within a CVM is the fundamental distinguishing feature of these lesions and forms the primary basis on which they are now categorized (see box, on right) (1).

Although noninvasive studies such as computed tomography (CT) and magnetic resonance imaging (MRI) are usually the initial studies undertaken in patients with suspected intracranial vascular malformations, cerebral angiography remains the procedure of choice for delineating the detailed angioarchitecture of

vascular malformations and planning appropriate therapy. This chapter reviews the nature of cerebral, dural, and cutaneous vascular malformations and presents the spectrum of their angiographic findings.

This chapter discusses CVMs that exhibit arteriovenous shunting, then continues with a consideration of cutaneous venous malformations that do not have arteriovenous shunting. Dural fistulae and cutaneous vascular malformations are also discussed.

CEREBRAL VASCULAR MALFORMATIONS WITH ARTERIOVENOUS SHUNTING: OVERVIEW AND GENERAL CONSIDERATIONS

Arteriovenous shunting occurs when there is direct communication between arterial and venous channels.

These shunts can be either plexiform (AVMs) or fistulous (AVFs).

An *arteriovenous malformation* is a collection of dysplastic plexiform vessels that is supplied by one or more arterial feeders and drained by one or more venous channels (Fig. 13-1A) (3). AVMs may have a pure plexiform nidus or contain a mixed plexiform–fistulous nidus (1).

An *arteriovenous fistula* results when an arterial feeder drains directly into a venous channel without an interven-

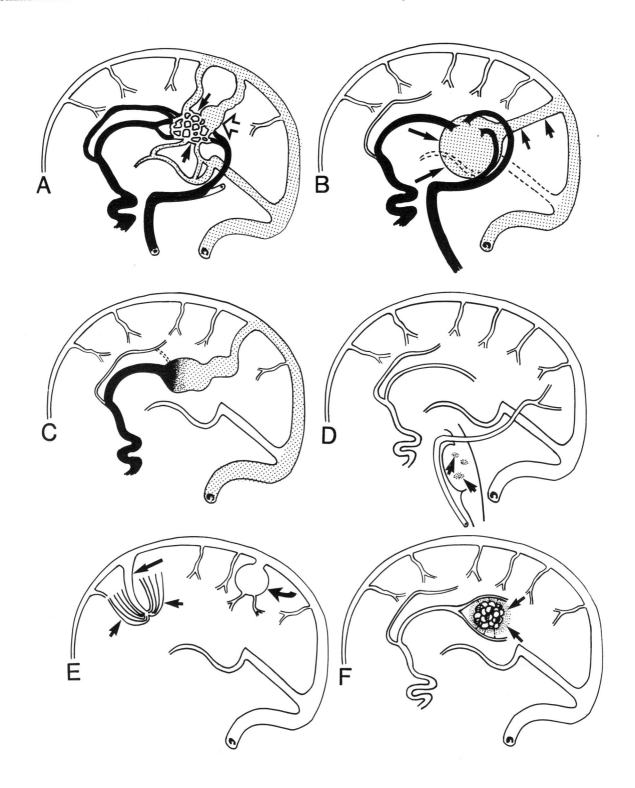

ing vascular network. Arteriovenous fistulas can be single or multiple and may be supplied by one (monopedicular) or more (multipedicular) feeding vessels (1). Examples of AVFs include neonatal vein of Galen malformations (Fig. 13-1B) and pial (parenchymal) AVFs (Fig. 13-1C).

CEREBRAL ARTERIOVENOUS MALFORMATIONS

Etiology, Molecular Biology, and Genetics

Etiology

Arteries, veins, and capillaries do not exist *per se* in the earliest stages of fetal development. Initially, all embryonic cerebral vessels are simple endothelial tubes. As heart function develops and intracranial blood flow commences, some of these primitive vascular channels normally evolve into afferent (arterial) vessels, whereas others become efferent or venous. Retention of the primordial, direct vascular connections between the future arterial and venous circulations combined with agenesis or poor development of the capillary network may result in an AVM or AVF (4).

Changes in embryonic cerebral hemodynamics induce an ongoing, extensive process of fetal vascular remodeling. New channels are constantly created as old ones regress or are resorbed (5).

Arteriovenous malformations also may be congenital lesions that are caused by developmental alterations in the embryonic vascular modeling process itself. These abnormalities are both structural and cellular. They probably involve the venous side of the primitive capillaries and may result from failure of endothelial cells to remodel the primitive embryonic vascular network (4,5a). The triggering events in the development of an AVM are unknown.

Molecular Biology

The precise molecular mechanisms that mediate the genesis and biologic behavior of AVMs are also unknown. The role of humoral angiogenic and permeability-inducing factors is increasingly recognized. A high degree of vascular endothelial growth factor (VEGF) is expressed by many AVMs (6). Collagen type IV and alpha smooth muscle actin expression are common in these lesions. Some investigators have concluded that angiogenic growth factors are expressed in all types of CVMs (7).

Genetics

The genetic mechanisms that contribute to the pathogenesis and phenotype of cerebral AVMs are unclear. Local repression of genes such as the preproendothelin-1 gene may cause absence of important vasoregulatory peptides (8).

Pathology

Gross Pathology

Arteriovenous malformations are a complex network of abnormal vascular channels that consists of one or more *arterial feeders*, a central *nidus*, and enlarged *venous outflow channels* (Fig. 13-2). Grossly, AVMs appear as tightly packed masses of abnormal vascular channels. They may contain small amounts of gliotic brain, dystrophic calcification, and blood in different stages of evolution (3).

Other gross abnormalities associated with AVMs include *flow-related aneurysms* and endothelial remodeling with resulting *angiopathy* in both the feeding arteries and draining veins (9,10). Chronic regional arterial hypoperfusion and venous hypertension may cause cere-

---

FIG. 13-1. Anatomic diagrams depict and compare several types of cerebral vascular malformations. **A:** An arteriovenous malformation (AVM) with a plexiform nidus (*small arrows*) is shown. Note numerous enlarged arterial feeders (*solid black lines*) and dilated draining veins (*dotted lines*). A venous varix (*open arrow*) in a draining vein is also illustrated. **B:** Vein of Galen malformation (VGAM) with direct mural-type fistulae from enlarged choroidal and pericallosal branches (*solid black lines*) is shown. The massively dilated vein of Galen (*dotted area, large arrows*) drains via a persistent falcine sinus (*small arrows*). The internal cerebral veins and straight sinus (*dashed lines*) are often hypoplastic or absent. Outlet stenosis is common in many VGAMs. **C:** Cerebral (pial) arteriovenous fistula (cAVF). Here an enlarged, irregular artery (*solid black line*) drains directly into a dilated cortical vein (*dotted area*). The cortical vein may become thrombosed, causing a parenchymal hematoma. **D:** Capillary malformations are shown as dotted areas (*arrows*) in the pons. Both the arterial and venous phases of cerebral angiograms in these cases are usually normal. **E:** Venous malformations are illustrated. A developmental venous anomaly (DVA) (or venous angioma) is shown as the umbrella-shaped collection of enlarged medullary veins (*small arrows*) that drain via a dilated transcortical vein (*large arrow*). An isolated venous varix (*curved arrow*) is another type of cerebral venous malformation. **F:** Cavernous malformations (CMs) are lobulated collections of sinusoidal spaces with intralesional hemorrhages in various stages of evolution, surrounded by a rim of hemosiderin-stained brain tissue (*arrows*). Arterial feeders (*dotted lines*) are very small and rarely identified at angiography. Angiograms in these cases are usually normal or show only the avascular mass effect caused by an acute hematoma. Occasionally contrast accumulation in a venous lake can be seen on the late phases of an angiogram.

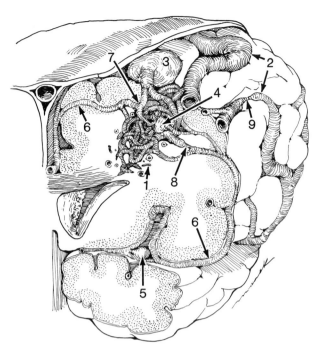

FIG. 13-2. Anatomic diagram depicts some features of a typical cerebral arteriovenous malformation (AVM). The classic AVM is a tightly packed, pyramidal or cone-shaped tangle of enlarged feeding arteries and dilated draining veins.

1, AVM nidus
2, Enlarged cortical draining veins
3, Venous varix
4, Intranidal aneurysm
5, Flow-related (pedicle) aneurysm on feeding vessel
6, Enlarged feeding arteries (anterior and middle cerebral arteries)
7, Arteriovenous fistula
8, High-flow vasculopathy with focal stenosis of feeding arteries
9, Vasculopathic change in draining vein.

(Reprinted with permission from Osborn AG. *Diagnostic neuroradiology.* St. Louis: Mosby, 1994.)

brovascular steal with resulting neuronal loss and *atrophy* in otherwise normal brain at a distance from AVMs (11,12).

Microscopic Pathology

Vascular phenotypes in AVMs vary. Some AVMs exhibit relatively differentiated mature vessels, whereas others consist of maldeveloped, less well-differentiated thick- and thin-walled vessels (8). The direct arteriovenous communications together with a high-flow, low-resistance profile predispose to further vascular recruitment and arterialization of venous structures (7).

Location and Cortical Mapping

Location

The vast majority of all AVMs are located in the cerebral hemispheres; only 15% occur in the posterior fossa. AVMs are usually round or wedge shaped. Depending on their location, cerebral AVMs are classified as *superficial* or *deep*. The ratio of superficial (convexity) to deep AVMs is approximately 2:1 to 3:1 (1,13).

Convexity lesions are further subdivided into sulcal, gyral, or mixed sulcogyral AVMs (1). A combination of high-resolution MR imaging and selective angiography is required for complete anatomic localization and delineation of these lesions.

Cortical Mapping

Because AVMs are congenital lesions that frequently involve primary cortical structures, accurate mapping of brain function is helpful in planning appropriate therapy. Primary cortical regions may have been displaced or translocated during fetal development because of inherent brain plasticity and reorganization. MR-based mapping (functional MRI) and magnetoencephalography are two techniques that are increasingly utilized to identify the true location of primary cortical structures such as the motor cortex (14).

Incidence

Solitary Arteriovenous Malformations

Large autopsy series have shown that the incidence of sporadic AVMs in the general population is 0.04% to 0.52% (15). The incidence of AVMs in syndromic CVMs such as hereditary hemorrhagic telangiectasia (HHT) is much higher (2).

Multiple Arteriovenous Malformations

Only 2% of AVMs are multiple. Multiple AVMs outside the setting of vascular neurocutaneous disorders such as HHT (also known as Osler-Weber-Rendu disease) and Wyburn-Mason syndrome are very uncommon, occurring in only 0.002% to 0.003% of all cases (16).

Clinical Features

Age and Gender

Arteriovenous malformations are the most common symptomatic CVM. Both genders are equally affected. The peak age at initial presentation is between 20 and 40 years, although about one fourth of AVMs hemorrhage within the first 15 years of life. The majority of AVMs have become symptomatic by age 50 (4).

Clinical Presentation

Approximately 50% of patients with AVMs present with symptoms caused by *hemorrhage*. Hemorrhage in AVMs is subarachnoid in 30% of cases, parenchymal in 23%, and intraventricular in another 16%. Combined hemorrhages occur in 31% of cases (17). Other than *seizure* (25%), non-hemorrhagic focal neurologic syndromes such as cerebral ischemia are relatively infrequent (18).

Risk

The overall hemorrhage risk from an AVM is estimated at 2% to 4% per year, cumulative. The combined annual morbidity and mortality is approximately 3% (15).

Arteriovenous malformations are an anatomically and clinically heterogeneous group of lesions. Some factors that reportedly predispose AVM patients to hemorrhage include history of a prior bleed, exclusively deep venous drainage, venous recruitment, presence of an intranidal aneurysm, and high feeding artery pressures (15,19,20, 20a,20b).

Some investigators report that small AVMs have an annual hemorrhage risk similar to that of the general AVM population (15), whereas others have correlated small size with an increased risk of hemorrhage (21). Hypertension is the only reported clinical factor that is positively associated with an increased risk of hemorrhage (21).

A widely used method to determine the long-term risk of an untreated AVM is the Spetzler grading system (Table 13-1). The total grade reflects the sum of points assigned for size, eloquence of adjacent brain, and pattern of venous drainage. Spetzler grades range from 1 to 5. A separate grade 6 is reserved for inoperable lesions. Prospective studies have confirmed the accuracy and utility of the Spetzler grade in guiding patient management and estimating postoperative neurologic complications (22).

Angiographic Evaluation of Arteriovenous Malformations

The angiographic evaluation of a cerebral AVM is usually performed in two steps: (a) selective angiographic investigation of the AVM itself, as well as the remainder of the cerebral vasculature, and (b) superselective angiographic investigation of the AVM nidus with microcatheters (see box below) (1).

TABLE 13-1. *Spetzler AVM Grading System*

Graded feature	Points assigned
Size of AVM	
Small (<3 cm)	1
Medium (3–6 cm)	2
Large (>6 cm)	3
Eloquence of adjacent brain	
Noneloquent	0
Eloquent	1
Venous drainage	
Superficial only	0
Deep	1

Grade is total of assigned points for size and eloquence plus venous drainage (grade 6 is reserved for inoperable lesions).

Modified from Hamilton MG, Spetzler RF. The prospective application of a grading system for arteriovenous malformations. *Neurosurgery* 1994;34:2–7.

Cerebral Angiography in Arteriovenous Malformations: Goals*

Diagnostic (selective) angiogram should delineate
Feeding arteries
  Identify individual vessels involved
  Flow-related vasculopathy (enlargements, stenoses, occlusions)
  Flow-related aneurysms
Nidus
  Size, shape
  Flow conditions
Draining veins
  Identify individual veins
  Flow-related vasculopathy (enlargements, stenoses, occlusions, varices)
  Flow patterns (drainage, collaterals, reflux into normal dural sinus)
Arterial territories involved in AVM supply
Venous drainage of brain

Superselective angiogram should delineate
Distal segments of feeding arteries (anatomy, hemodynamics)
Arterionidal junction
Nidus angioarchitecture
  Compartments
  Plexiform portion
  Presence of AVF
  Intranidal cavities (arterial aneurysm, pseudoaneurysm, venous ectasias)
Venonidal junction
Proximal segments of draining veins (stenosis, outlet obstruction, ectasias, varices)

*Modified and adapted from refs. 1 and 23.

Selective Diagnostic Angiography

A selective, technically complete diagnostic angiogram of an AVM should provide detailed information regarding the individual feeding arteries and their vascular territories as well as delineate the venous drainage. Gross assessment of the nidus as well as identification of flow-related angiopathy (both arterial and venous) and presence of an aneurysm should also be made (see list above) (1).

Arteriovenous malformations should be studied using high-resolution subtraction angiography with a high frame rate. For treatment planning, it should be performed with consistent magnification factors and calibrated markers (23).

Superselective Angiography

Delineation of the internal angioarchitecture of an AVM is often combined with endovascular treatment of these lesions and is discussed in more detail later (see Chapter 19). In general, superselective angiography with microcatheters should provide extensive, detailed information regarding AVM angioarchitecture. This includes defining angiopathic changes in the feeding arteries (such as flow-related vasculopathy or aneurysm), delineating the nidus in detail, and examining the draining veins for outlet obstruction and ectasias (see list above) (1).

Angiographic Findings

Arterial Feeders and the Arteriovenous Malformation Nidus

On standard selective cerebral angiograms an AVM appears as a tightly packed mass of *enlarged feeding arteries* that supply a central *nidus* (Fig. 13-3A and B) (1,3). Superselective angiography is essential for evaluating a cerebral AVM and delineating its angioarchitecture in detail.

Arterial feeders sometimes communicate directly with one or more *vascular cavities* within the aneurysm nidus. More often they form a *plexiform web of small vessels* that arborize around the sac before penetrating it through multiple sites (see Fig. 13-4C) (5). These intranidal vascular cavities may be single or multiple and may represent intranidal arterial aneurysms, posthemorrhagic arterial or venous pseudoaneurysms, or intranidal venous ectasias (1).

Draining Veins

One or more *dilated veins* drain the AVM nidus. *Arteriovenous (AV) shunting* is present when contrast appears in draining veins abnormally early in the angiographic sequence (Fig. 13-3). Although AV shunting is characteristic of AVMs, it may occur with other lesions such as cerebral ischemia and neoplasms. Draining veins are often tortuous, ectatic, and sometimes even appear aneurysmal (Figs. 13-4 and 13-5). So-called venous varices are also common, especially with superficial AVMs.

Associated Abnormalities

Because AVMs are congenital lesions that replace rather than displace normal brain parenchyma, they exhibit *little or no mass effect*. If acute hemorrhage has occurred, adjacent vessels may appear stretched and displaced around the avascular clot.

Flow-induced angiopathy secondary to endothelial hyperplasia is common in AVMs. These changes include arterial stenoses in the feeding arteries, found in up to 20% of cases, as well as venous stenoses and ectasias (1).

Two types of aneurysms occur in AVMs (23a). The first type, *flow-related aneurysms*, represent one third to two thirds of all aneurysms that are associated with AVMs. These aneurysms may be located within the nidus itself (intranidal aneurysm) or on a feeding vessel (pedicle aneurysm) (Fig. 13-6; see also Fig. 12-10C). The second type of aneurysm occurs on remote vessels that are not hemodynamically related to the vascular malformation (see Fig. 12-9C).

Unusual Arteriovenous Malformations

Diffuse Arteriovenous Malformations

Occasionally an AVM is infiltrating and involves an entire lobe or hemisphere of the brain. Histopathology in these unusual cases shows innumerable enlarged, abnormal vessels interspersed among relatively normal-appearing neurons and white matter (24).

On cerebral angiograms the AVM appears as a diffuse collection of multiple arterial feeders and draining veins without an identifiable compact nidus. These diffuse AVMs may be very large, yet cause almost no discernible mass effect (Fig. 13-7). These lesions often present clinically with intractable seizures rather than symptoms of hemorrhage. Diffuse AVMs may exhibit a "proliferative angiopathy," continuing to recruit additional feeding vessels (10).

Hemodynamically Mixed Arteriovenous Malformations

If a pial (parenchymal) AVM attains sufficient size, it may recruit vascular supply from dural vessels such as the middle meningeal artery or meningohypophyseal

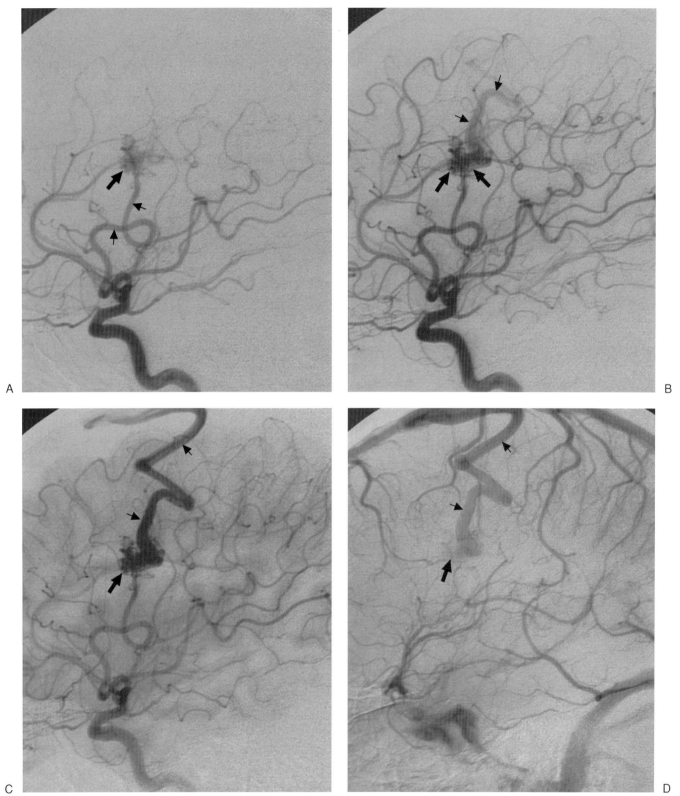

FIG. 13-3. Left internal carotid angiogram, lateral view, in a patient with Osler-Weber-Rendu disease shows a classic solitary monopedicular AVM. **A:** Early arterial phase study shows the nidus (*large arrow*) and feeding artery (*small arrows*). **B:** Slightly later frame again shows the nidus (*large arrows*). Contrast is now beginning to opacify an enlarged early draining vein (*small arrows*). **C:** Late arterial phase study shows the nidus (*large arrow*) and dense opacification of the single draining vein (*small arrows*). Because the study is still in the arterial phase, no other cortical veins are seen. **D:** Venous phase study shows that contrast is disappearing from the nidus (*large arrow*) into the draining vein (*small arrows*). The vein drains freely into the superior sagittal sinus. There is no outlet stenosis or venous ectasia in this case.

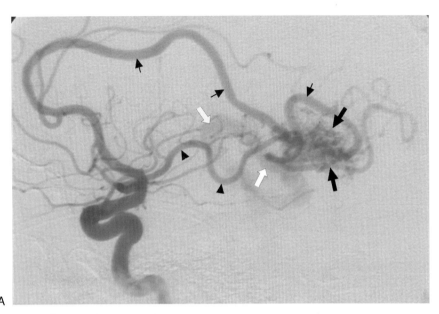

A

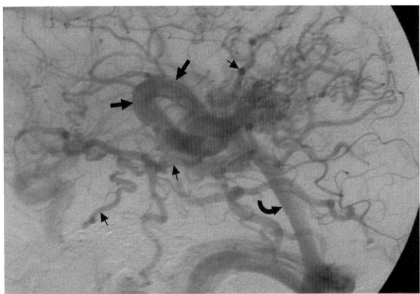

B

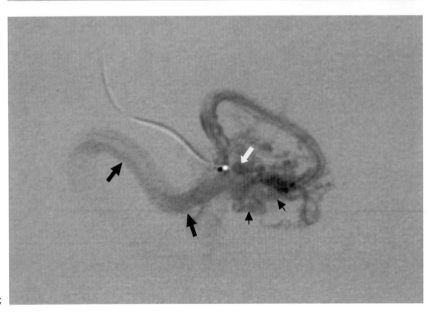

C

FIG. 13-4. A: Left internal carotid angiogram, early arterial phase, lateral view, shows an AVM that is supplied by enlarged pericallosal (*small arrows*) and angular (*arrowheads*) arteries. The nidus is indicated by the large arrows. Note early draining deep veins (*white arrows*). **B:** Late arterial phase study shows very poor filling of the superior sagittal sinus. Instead, the AVM is drained by multiple tortuous, ectatic cortical veins (*small arrows*). The major drainage is deep, via a dilated subependymal vein (*large arrows*) and straight sinus (*curved arrow*). **C:** Superselective injection of the distal pericallosal artery clearly delineates the plexus of vessels within the nidus (*small arrows*). An intranidal aneurysm is indicated by the white arrow. Note early opacification of the massively enlarged deep subependymal vein (*large arrows*).

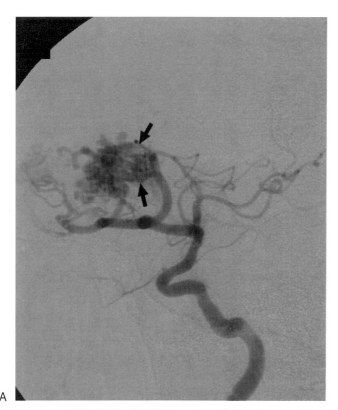
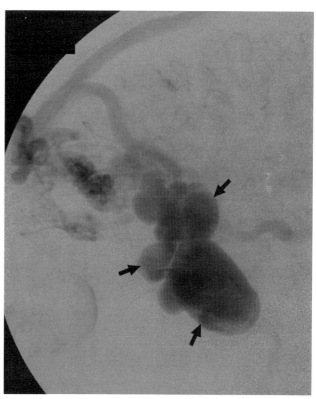

A   B

FIG. 13-5. Right internal carotid angiogram, lateral view, with early arterial **(A)** and capillary **(B)** phase studies shows an AVM **(A**, *arrows*) that is associated with enormous venous varices **(B**, *arrows*).

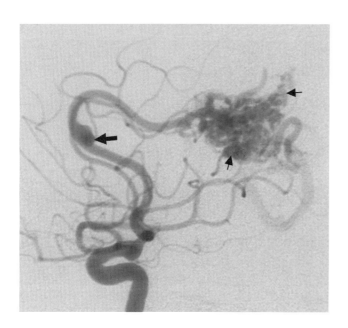

FIG. 13-6. Right internal carotid angiogram, arterial phase, lateral view, shows an AVM (*small arrows*) supplied by an enlarged pericallosal artery. A broad-based pedicle aneurysm is present (*large arrow*).

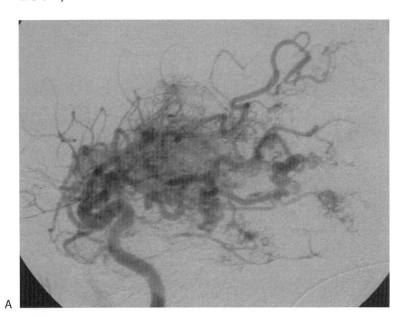

A

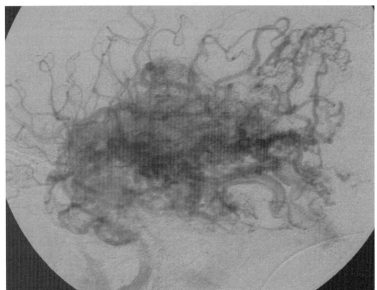

B

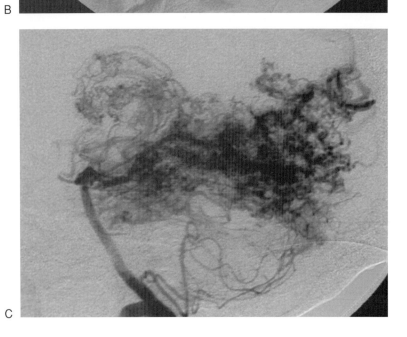

C

FIG. 13-7. A 15-year-old girl presented with intractable seizures. MR scan (not shown) showed innumerable areas of high-velocity signal loss (flow voids) involving nearly all of the right hemisphere. Angiography disclosed a "diffuse" AVM with proliferative angiopathy, seen here as innumerable small, corkscrewlike branches that resemble the collateral vessels in moyamoya disease. Early **(A)** and late **(B)** arterial phase studies from a right internal carotid angiogram show that the extensive malformation essentially replaces most of the temporal and parietal lobes. **C:** The vertebrobasilar angiogram shows the lesion also involves the occipital lobe.

trunk (Fig. 13-8). These lesions are sometimes termed *"mixed" pial–dural AVMs*.

Pathologically Mixed Arteriovenous Malformations

Histologically mixed CVMs are common. The most frequent combination is a mixed cavernous–venous malformation. AVMs are rarely mixed (25–27). However, the combination of an AVM with a DVA (or venous angioma) does occur (25). These *mixed AVM–DVAs* are sometimes called arterialized venous malformations (26). *Mixed AVM–capillary telangiectasias* have been reported but are rare (27).

Thrombosed Arteriovenous Malformations

An AVM may hemorrhage and thrombose spontaneously (Fig. 13-9). Thrombosis also may be induced deliberately with stereotaxic neurosurgery. This subset of

AVMs is sometimes erroneously referred to as *cryptic AVMs*. A more accurate term is "angiographically occult AVM" (28).

Angiograms in patients with completely thrombosed AVMs may appear normal, show an avascular mass effect, or demonstrate only subtle arteriovenous shunting. An early draining vein without identifiable feeding vessels or nidus is sometimes observed. Occasionally irregular-appearing arteries are present with slow blood flow that persists into the late arterial or capillary phase. These abnormal vessels, termed "stagnating arteries," are sometimes identified on the postoperative angiograms of excised AVMs (Fig. 13-10). They are also seen following stereotactic radiosurgery (3).

Differential Diagnosis

The angiographic differential diagnosis of a patent AVM is limited. Occasionally, highly vascular malignant primary brain tumors such as glioblastoma multiforme can mimic an AVM (3).

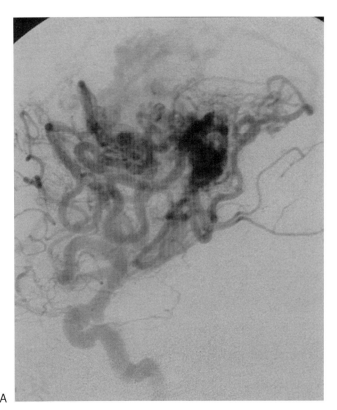
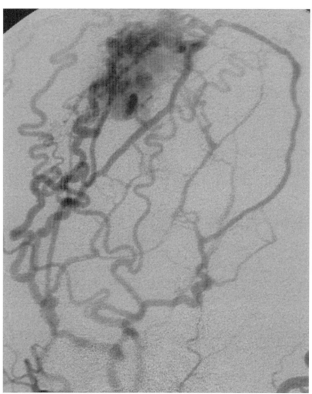

A   B

FIG. 13-8. A hemodynamically mixed (i.e., pial–dural) AVM is illustrated by this case. Vascular supply is from both pial and dural feeders. **A:** Left internal carotid angiogram, arterial phase, lateral view, shows a large parenchymal AVM that is supplied by several enlarged middle cerebral artery branches. **B:** Left external carotid angiogram, late arterial view, shows that the AVM is also supplied via dural vessels (branches of the middle meningeal and superficial temporal arteries).

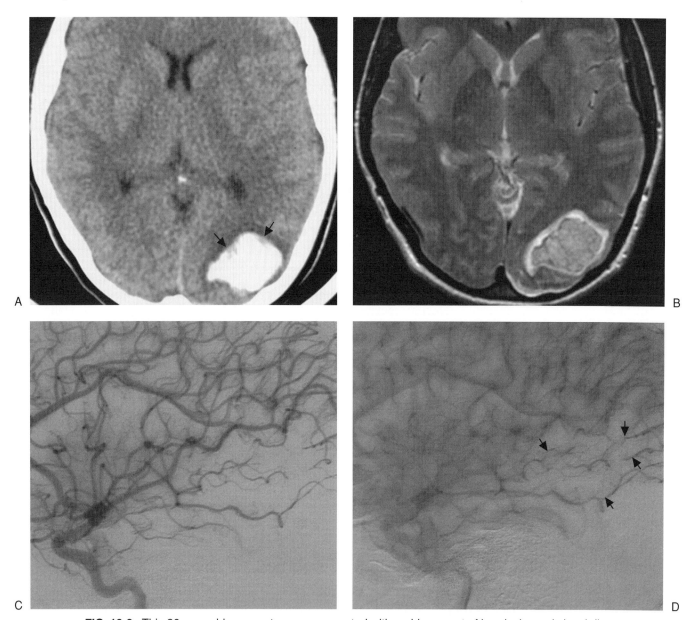

FIG. 13-9. This 26-year-old pregnant woman presented with sudden onset of headache and visual disturbance. **A:** Axial NECT scan shows a focal hematoma in the left occipital lobe (*arrows*). **B:** Axial T2-weighted MR scan shows the acute clot with surrounding edema. No abnormal vessels are seen. Lateral views of an early **(C)** and late **(D)** arterial phase carotid angiogram show no enlarged arteries or draining veins. The study shows an avascular mass effect with stretching and draping of the parietooccipital branches around the mass. Note slow-flow, irregular appearance and occlusion with retrograde filling in some of the arteries (**D**, *arrows*).

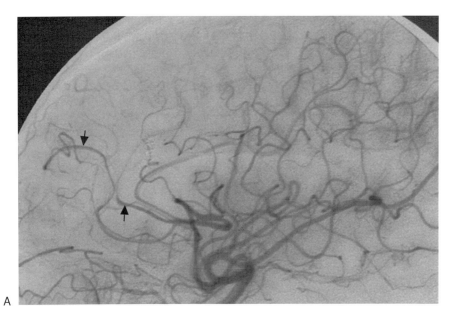

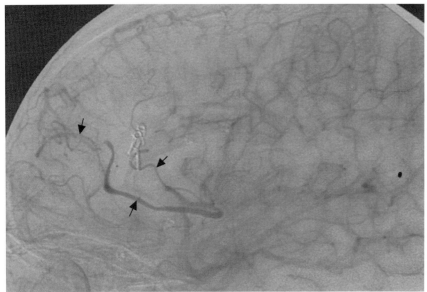

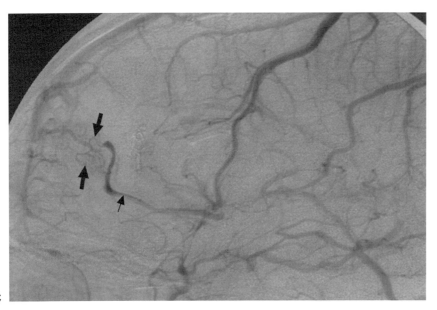

FIG. 13-10. This 33-year-old man had a left frontal sulcal–gyral AVM resected. Mid- **(A)** and late **(B)** arterial as well as venous **(C)** phase views of a left internal carotid angiogram performed 3 months after surgery show somewhat irregular, stagnating arteries (**A–C**, *small arrows*). Note the small persistent vascular blush (**C**, *large arrows*), which probably represents residual malformation.

CEREBRAL ARTERIOVENOUS FISTULAE

Arteriovenous malformations are the most common type of CVM that exhibits arteriovenous shunting. Arteriovenous fistulae (AVFs) are much less common. Cerebral AVFs (cAVFs) are characterized by direct shunts between pial arteries and venous channels. Two major forms occur: (a) the vein of Galen aneurysmal malformations (VGAMs) that occur predominately in neonates and infants and (b) pial or subependymal AVFs (1).

Vein of Galen Aneurysmal Malformation

Classification

Berenstein and Lasjaunias have classified anomalous arteriovenous shunts involving the vein of Galen into two groups: (a) true *vein of Galen aneurysmal malformations* (VGAMs) and (b) *vein of Galen dilatations* that occur secondary to high-flow parenchymal AVMs draining into this vessel (10,29,30).

Two subtypes of VGAMs recently have been identified on the basis of their angioarchitecture: (a) a *mural* form and (b) a *choroid* form (10). The so-called choroidal form is the most common type. Choroidal VGAMs classically demonstrate an abundance of bilateral arataerial supply from choroidal arteries, pericallosal arteries, and subependymal branches of the thalamoperforating vessels. These vascular connections are extracerebral, subarachnoid, and communicate with the anterior aspect of the median prosencephalic vein (see below) (30a).

Mural-type VGAMs represent approximately one-third of VGAMs. They receive uni- or bilateral arterial supply from the collicular and posterior choroidal vessels and drain into a persistent median prosencephalic vein. Outlet obstruction is common (10).

Etiology

Vein of Galen aneurysmal malformations probably represent an arteriovenous fistula (AVF) in the wall of a persistent embryonic vascular channel called the *median prosencephalic vein* (see Chapter 11) (10,31). This dorsal vein lies in the roof of the diencephalon and drains the developing choroid plexus (32). In turn, the median prosencephalic vein drains into a primitive accessory sinus called the *falcine sinus*.

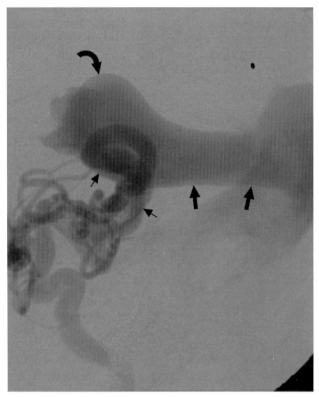 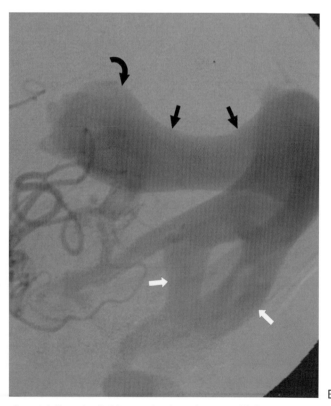

A   B

FIG. 13-11. A newborn infant with florid congestive heart failure had this cerebral angiogram. Right internal carotid angiogram with early **(A)** and mid- **(B)** arterial phase studies, lateral view, shows massively enlarged anterior choroidal arteries (*small arrows*) with early opacification of a dilated vein of Galen (*curved arrow*) and horizontally oriented venous channel (*large arrows*), which probably represents a persistent prosencephalic vein and falcine sinus. Note filling of massively enlarged marginal and occipital sinuses (**B**, *white arrows*).

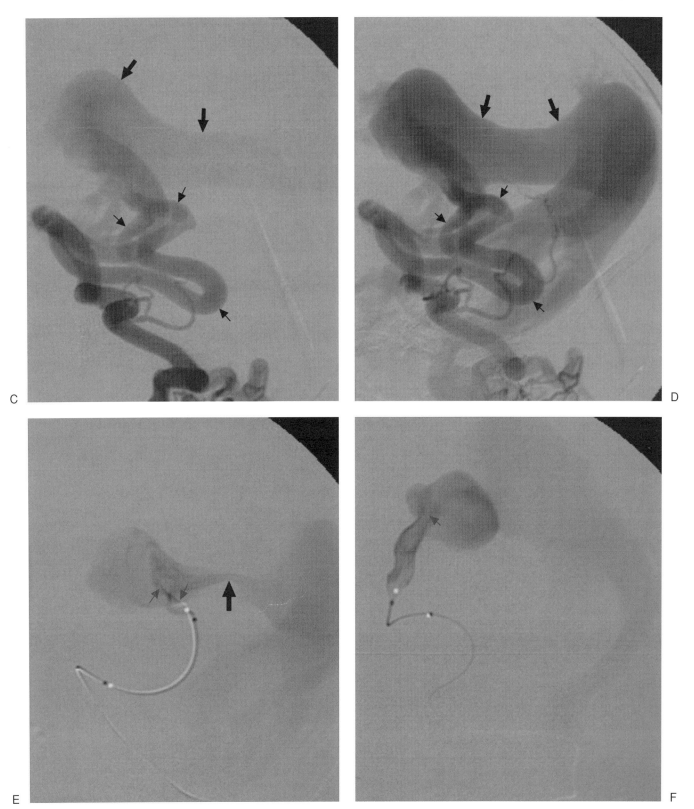

FIG. 13-11. *Continued.* The straight sinus is not visualized. Left vertebral angiogram with early **(C)** and mid- **(D)** arterial phase studies, lateral view, shows that markedly enlarged PChAs (*small arrows*) fill the venous channel (*large arrows*). Lateral **(E)** and anteroposterior (AP) **(F)** views from a superselective angiogram of the left medial posterior choroidal artery show the fistulous connection (*small arrows*) with the vein of Galen. Note stenosis between the vein of Galen and falcine sinus (**E**, *large arrows*), well visualized here but obscured on the nonselective study (compare with **C** and **D**).

By week 10 of fetal development the median prosencephalic vein regresses as the definitive internal cerebral veins appear. A caudal remnant remains as the vein of Galen (33). If the median prosencephalic vein does not regress normally, a fistulous connection with the primitive *choroidal arteries* may persist. A VGAM is the result (34).

Clinical Presentation

Neonatal VGAMs present with high-output congestive heart failure, tachycardia, respiratory distress, and cyanosis (32).

Angiographic Findings

The typical VGAM consists of one or more enlarged arteries that empty directly into a massively enlarged vein of Galen (Fig. 13-11).

The arterial supply to a VGAM usually involves all the choroidal arteries (Fig. 13-12) (10). The medial and lateral *posterior choroidal arteries* (PChAs) are the most common arteries that supply these lesions, followed by the *anterior choroidal arteries*. In one series, the PChAs were involved in all VGAMs (32). Branches from the pericallosal artery also supplied the lesion in nearly 70% of cases. In many cases an arterioarterial maze is interposed between the arterial feeders and the vein (35).

Venous drainage patterns of VGAMS include *aneurysmal dilatation of the vein of Galen* (a venous varix), with or without distal (outlet) *venous stenosis*. Drainage into an accessory *falcine sinus* with thrombosis or *absence of the straight sinus* is also common, seen in the majority of cases (32). The falcine sinus is a primitive channel that connects the vein of Galen to the superior sagittal sinus, coursing posterosuperiorly within the falx cerebri.

Dilated *choroidal veins* are often present in VAGMs, usually draining anteroinferiorly into the cavernous sinus. The internal cerebral veins are visualized in only 50% of VAGMs. When present, they are rarely involved as part of the malformation (35). The cortical veins are also usually normal in size unless occlusion of the sigmoid sinuses or jugular veins has occurred (32).

Complications

Complications of VAGMs include obstructive hydrocephalus, atrophy of adjacent structures due to compression, venous thrombosis, and hemorrhage. Periventricular leukomalacia, cortical laminar necrosis, and atrophy secondary to ischemia and steal phenomenon or congestive heart failure are common (32).

Cerebral Arteriovenous Fistula

In contrast to dural AVFs, cerebral arteriovenous fistulae (cAVFs) are rare. One or more dilated, often bizarre-looking pial arteries drains directly into a venous channel (Fig. 13-1C). Stenosis of the draining vein with sudden thrombosis and hemorrhage is common (Fig. 13-13).

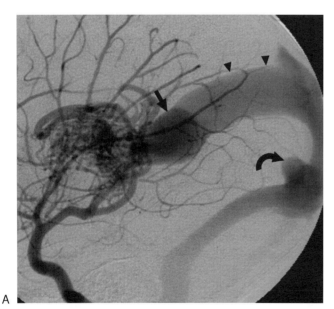 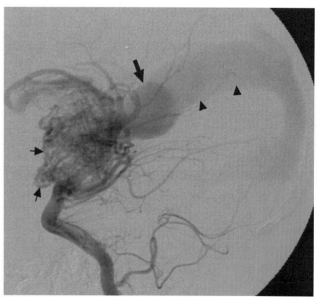

A B

FIG. 13-12. A 4-month-old girl had a cranial bruit auscultated. CT scan (not shown) showed a vein of Galen vascular malformation. Left internal carotid (**A**) and vertebral (**B**) angiograms, arterial phase, lateral view, show a midline vascular malformation (**B**, *small arrows*) with supply mostly from the choroidal arteries. Note opacification of the vein of Galen (*large arrows*) and a superiorly oriented channel, a falcine sinus (*arrowheads*). The straight sinus (**A**, *curved arrow*) is occluded. Superselective angiography prior to embolization (not shown) showed a thalamic AVM with at least four areas of direct arteriovenous fistulae in the nidus.

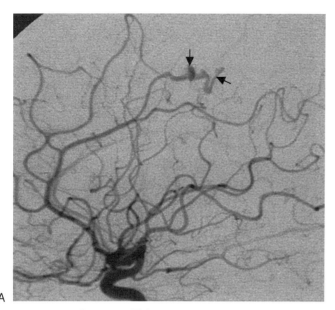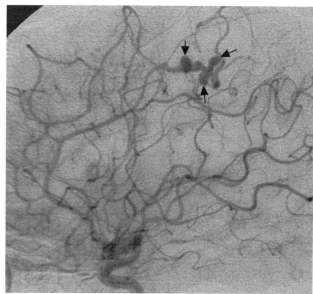

A   B

FIG. 13-13. This 24-year-old woman had sudden onset of severe headache and right upper extremity weakness. There was no evidence for drug abuse or infection. Laboratory studies were normal. A nonenhanced CT scan (not shown) showed a focal hematoma in the high posterior frontal region. Mid- **(A)** and late **(B)** arterial phase films, lateral view, of a left internal carotid angiogram show bizarre, fusiform enlargement of the distal anterior cerebral artery (*arrows*) with stretching and draping of adjacent vessels around an avascular mass effect. No definite arteriovenous shunting is identified. Surgery disclosed a single feeder pial arteriovenous fistula (pAVF) with a thrombosed draining vein and acute hematoma.

CEREBRAL VASCULAR MALFORMATIONS WITHOUT ARTERIOVENOUS SHUNTING: OVERVIEW AND GENERAL CONSIDERATIONS

Cerebral vascular formations without evidence of arteriovenous shunting arise from postarteriolar vascular channels. Three basic types are recognized: capillary, venous, and cavernous malformations (3). Some investigators include cavernous malformations as a subcategory of venous malformations while others have suggested that capillary telangiectasias and cavernous malformations are part of a single histologic spectrum (1,36,36a).

Capillary malformations (telangiectasias) contain focal collections of dilated capillaries. Brain capillary telangiectasias are typically quite small and are usually invisible on cerebral angiograms (Fig. 13-1D). Capillary malformations of the scalp and mucosa are seen in Osler-Weber-Rendu disease. These lesions can be identified on external carotid angiograms.

Venous malformations comprise a spectrum of vascular malformations. The most common is a developmental venous anomaly (DVA), formerly called a venous angioma. These lesions are actually nonmalformative developmental anomalies of the medullary (white matter) veins (Fig. 13-1E). Other types of venous CVMs include venous varices (Fig. 13-1E).

Cavernous malformations are morphologically, histopathologically, and clinically distinct from venous malformations of the central nervous system. Cavernous

malformations exhibit a propensity to evolve and enlarge through repetitive intralesional hemorrhages (2).

Because cerebral angiograms in patients with uncomplicated capillary telangiectasias and cavernous angiomas are usually normal, these lesions are sometimes called cryptic vascular malformations (36). A more accurate term is "angiographically occult vascular malformations" because most lesions can usually be identified on MR scans (37).

CAPILLARY MALFORMATIONS

Pathology and Pathogenesis

Pathology

Capillary malformations or telangiectasias are small nests of dilated capillaries that are interspersed with normal brain (Fig. 13-1D). The walls of capillary malformations are histologically similar to normal capillaries, lacking both smooth muscle and elastic fibers (2).

Pathogenesis

Whether capillary telangiectasias are congenital or acquired lesions is debatable (38). Vascular telangiectasias that closely resemble capillary telangiectasias have been reported as a long-term complication of radiation therapy (36a,39).

Location and Incidence

Location

Capillary telangiectasias most often occur in the pons, cerebellum, and spinal cord, although they can be found anywhere in the brain, including the cerebral hemispheres.

Incidence

Capillary telangiectasias are usually incidental findings at autopsy, and multiple lesions are common. Capillary telangiectasias are second only to developmental venous anomalies as the most common vascular malformation identified at postmortem examination, representing 16% to 20% of all CVMs (2).

Imaging Findings

Cerebral Angiography

Cerebral angiograms in patients with capillary telangectasias of the brain usually appear normal unless a mixed capillary–venous malformation is present. Extracranial mucocutaneous telangiectasias occur in Osler-Weber-Rendu disease and can be identified on external carotid angiograms.

Magnetic Resonance Imaging

T2-weighted MR scans often appear normal, although solitary or multifocal areas of decreased signal intensity may be identified on gradient-echo sequences. Contrast-enhanced T1-weighted scans may show faintly enhancing lesions with brushlike, poorly delineated borders (38,40).

Mixed Capillary Malformations

Capillary telangiectasias may be histologically mixed, occurring with either cavernous or venous malformations (41). Capillary telangiectasias are usually asymptomatic, but a coexisting cavernous or venous angioma may hemorrhage (42).

VENOUS MALFORMATIONS

There are several varieties of cerebral venous malformations, including developmental venous angiomas and isolated venous varices. Although some investigators also include cavernous malformations as part of the spectrum of venous malformations, we will consider each of these entities separately (1).

Developmental Venous Anomaly

Pathology

Grossly, developmental venous anomalies (DVAs, formerly known as venous angiomas) are composed of radially arranged, dilated medullary (white matter) veins that converge in an enlarged transcortical or subependymal draining vein (Fig. 13-1E). Microscopically, venous angiomas consist of dilated venous channels that are sometimes thickened and hyalinized. The enlarged veins are separated by, and provide the main venous drainage for, intervening normal brain.

Developmental venous anomalies can be histologically heterogeneous. They are commonly associated with other vascular malformations, especially cavernous angioma (43–45). When they become symptomatic, most investigators consider the associated abnormality, not the coincident DVA, as the causative lesion (43).

Etiology

Venous angiomas represent extreme anatomic variants of medullary (white matter) venous drainage. Their precise etiology is unknown, although some investigators propose that DVAs result from arrested embryonic medullary vein development at a time when normal arterial development is nearly complete. This results in retention of primitive venous channels in the white matter that empty into a single, large draining vein. Others have suggested that venous angiomas are only one part of a spectrum of focal developmental abnormalities (46,47).

Incidence and Clinical Presentation

Developmental venous anomalies are the most common of all intracranial vascular malformations, representing 60% of CVMs at autopsy. Most venous angiomas are solitary, asymptomatic lesions that are discovered incidentally on imaging studies (2). The hemorrhage rate of CVMs is similar to cavernous malformations without previous hemorrhage (47a). Multiple CVMs are detected in 2.5% to 9% of cases when contrast-enhanced MR is used (48).

Angiographic Findings

The arterial phase of a cerebral angiogram is normal in nearly all cases of DVA. Although a late capillary blush may be present, the pathognomonic angiographic appearance appears during the venous phase of cerebral angiograms (3). A wedge- or umbrella-shaped collection of dilated medullary veins, the so-called *caput medusae*, converges in an enlarged transcortical or subependymal collector vein (Fig. 13-14) (47,49). Occasionally there is focal stenosis of the draining vein as it enters the adjacent dural sinus. Developmental venous anomalies with venous restrictive disease or a coexisting cavernous malformation may cause parenchymal hemorrhage with location-specific symptoms.

Atypical Developmental Venous Anomalies

A few DVAs do not fit into the description of a typical mixed malformation. Some of these lesions probably represent venous–arteriovenous malformation transition

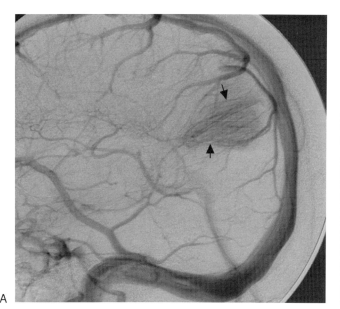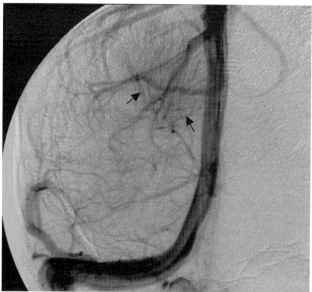

A   B

FIG. 13-14. This 35-year-old man with headaches and a normal neurologic examination had a "suspicious" area noted on an MR scan (not shown). A right carotid angiogram, venous phase, with lateral **(A)** and anteroposterior **(B)** views shows the classic caput medusae of a venous angioma or developmental venous anomaly (*arrows*). The arterial phase (not shown) was normal.

forms (50). An angiographically identifiable arterial component is present in about 5% of these atypical cases (51,52). Multiple tiny, slightly dilated arterial feeders drain directly into medullary veins, with each vessel acting as a single miniature arteriovenous fistula. On the venous side, the vessels are organized into a classic caput medusae (Fig. 13-15) (51).

Associated Lesions

Focal *cortical dysplasias* and other sulcation–gyration disorders such as schizencephaly have been reported with DVAs. *Blue rubber bleb nevus syndrome* is an unusual neurocutaneous syndrome with cutaneous vascular nevi and multiple intracranial DVAs (53).

Sinus pericranii is a rare vascular anomaly of the cranial vault. It presents clinically as a round, soft, tumorlike lesion that is nonpulsatile and easily compressible. The distinguishing feature of sinus pericranii is presence of abnormal communications between a blood-filled extracranial sac and intracranial venous sinus through fenestrations in the cranial vault that contain emissary veins (Fig. 13-16) (54).

Pathologically, sinus pericranii is an extracranial collection of nonmuscular veins or a slow-flow venous hemangioma that adheres tightly to the skull and communicates directly with an intracranial venous sinus by an enlarged diploic vein (55).

Sinus pericranii is often associated with other vascular anomalies such as cerebral aneurysmal venous malformations, DVAs, systemic angiomas, and cavernous

hemangiomas (54). When present, the DVAs are often unusually large or multiple.

Differential Diagnosis

Because the angiographic appearance of DVAs is so typical, the differential diagnosis of a classic venous angioma is limited. An angiographic appearance similar to that of a DVA can be seen in some cases of chronic, long-standing dural sinus occlusion. Here the deep medullary veins enlarge as a collateral route for venous drainage. Patients with Sturge-Weber syndrome lack normal cortical veins and also may develop striking enlargement of deep medullary, subependymal, and choroidal veins (2).

Venous Varices

Varicose dilatation of cerebral veins usually occurs in association with VGAMs and other high-flow vascular shunts. Occasionally cerebral varices coexist with venous angiomas (52). Isolated saccular or fusiform enlargement of cortical veins does occur but is uncommon (56) (Figs. 13-1E and 13-17).

Cavernous Malformations

Pathology

On gross examination, cavernous malformations (CMs, sometimes called cavernous angiomas) appear as discrete, well-circumscribed, multilobulated lesions that

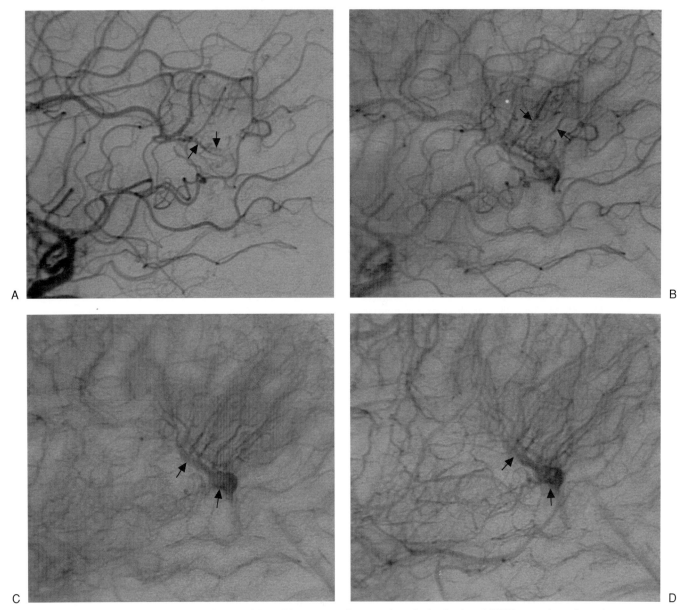

FIG. 13-15. A 31-year-old man with sudden onset of severe headache had an NECT scan (not shown) that showed high density in the left lateral ventricle that was interpreted as hemorrhage. A cerebral angiogram was obtained. Left internal carotid angiogram, lateral view, with mid- **(A)** and late- **(B)** arterial phase, **(C)** capillary phase, and **(D)** early venous phase studies shows a bizarre-appearing vascular malformation adjacent to the lateral ventricle. A cluster of tiny, slightly dilated arteries (**A**, *arrows*) drains into a collection of enlarged medullary veins (**B**, *arrows*). Early opacification of these veins in the late arterial phase indicates arteriovenous shunting. The capillary **(C)** and venous phase **(D)** studies show opacification of a subependymal collector vein (*arrows*). This is a transitional form of venous–arteriovenous malformation. Each arterial feeder acts as a single miniature arteriovenous fistula. The venous side of the malformation is a classic caput medusae.

contain blood-filled cysts with hemorrhage in various stages of evolution (Fig. 13-1F). Cavernous malformations (CMs) are benign hamartomas that do not contain normal brain tissue.

Microscopically, cavernous angiomas consist of a honeycomb network of endothelial-lined sinusoidal spaces separated by fibrous septa. Cavernous malformations are surrounded by a variably thick transition zone of gliotic, hemosiderin-stained brain (2). Calcification and even ossification are common (57).

Cavernous malformations are often histologically heterogeneous, coexisting with other vascular malformations.

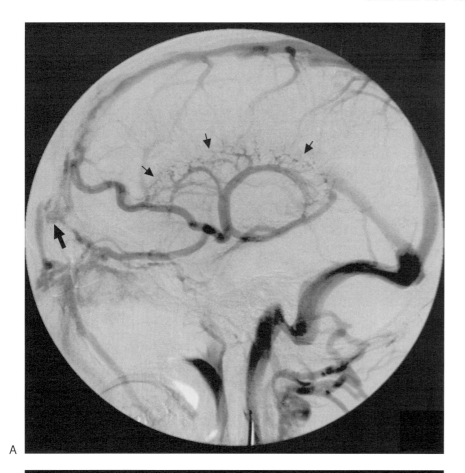

A

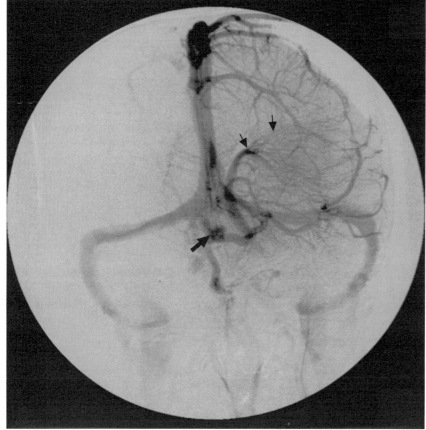

B

FIG. 13-16. A 22-year-old man had a compressible, bluish discolored lesion on his forehead that enlarged with Valsalva maneuver. Lateral **(A)** and anteroposterior **(B)** venous phase views of a left carotid angiogram show an extensive developmental venous anomaly (venous angioma, *small arrows*) with a sinus pericranii (*large arrow*), a transosseous channel that connects the intra- and extracranial venous systems. (Case courtesy of J. Rees.)

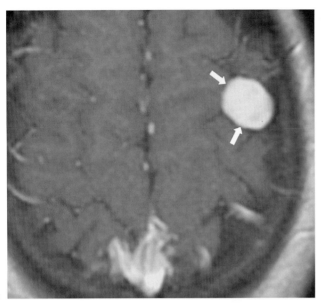 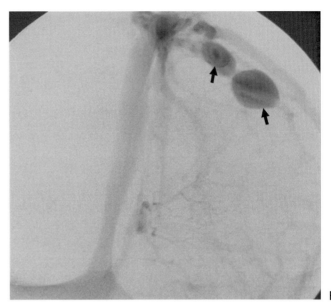

A

B

FIG. 13-17. A: Axial contrast-enhanced T1-weighted MR scan shows a well-delineated, strongly enhancing extraaxial mass (*arrows*). **B:** Left internal carotid angiogram, venous phase, anteroposterior view, shows an isolated venous varix (*arrows*). The arterial phase (not shown) was normal, and there was no evidence for associated developmental venous anomaly.

A mixed *cavernous–venous malformation* is the most common combination (10% to 30% of cases) (2,41).

Etiology and Pathogenesis

The precise etiology of CMs is unknown. Immunohistochemically, they exhibit characteristics of immature or new blood vessels, and lesions do appear to arise *de novo* (2).

Incidence and Inheritance

Cavernous angiomas are found in 0.02% to 0.13% of autopsies. Most are sporadic, although 10% to 30% of cases occur as part of a familial syndrome (57). *Familial cavernous angioma syndrome* is inherited in an autosomal-dominant pattern with variable penetrance. The defective gene has been mapped to chromosome 7q (58).

Location

Cavernous malformations can be found in any part of the brain or spinal cord. About 80% are supratentorial; the pons is the most common posterior fossa site. Approximately one third of sporadic CMs are multiple. In contrast, multiple lesions occur in more than 70% of familial cases (2).

Clinical Presentation

The most frequent symptoms are headache, seizure, and focal neurologic deficit. Between 7% and 29% of CMs are asymptomatic and are discovered incidentally during MR examination (2).

Natural History

Cavernous malformations are clinically and histopathologically dynamic lesions. They exhibit a propensity to evolve, enlarging through repetitive intralesional hemorrhages as well as by "pseudotumoral" growth of the cavernous matrix itself (58a). The risk of symptomatic hemorrhage in sporadic cases is estimated at 0.25% to 0.7% per person-year and 0.10% per person-year for each lesion. The risk is much higher in familial cavernomas, estimated at 1% per lesion per year and 6.5% per patient per year (57).

Angiographic Findings

Because CMs are slow-flow lesions with no large arterial feeders, no arterialized veins, and no large venous outflow vessels, cerebral angiography is usually normal (57). Cavernous angiomas have therefore been called cryptic or angiographically occult vascular malformations.

Occasionally an avascular mass effect is present secondary to a large intralesional hemorrhage. Rarely, angiograms demonstrate a faint vascular blush, abnormally draining veins, or pooling of contrast in small venous lakes (Fig. 13-18).

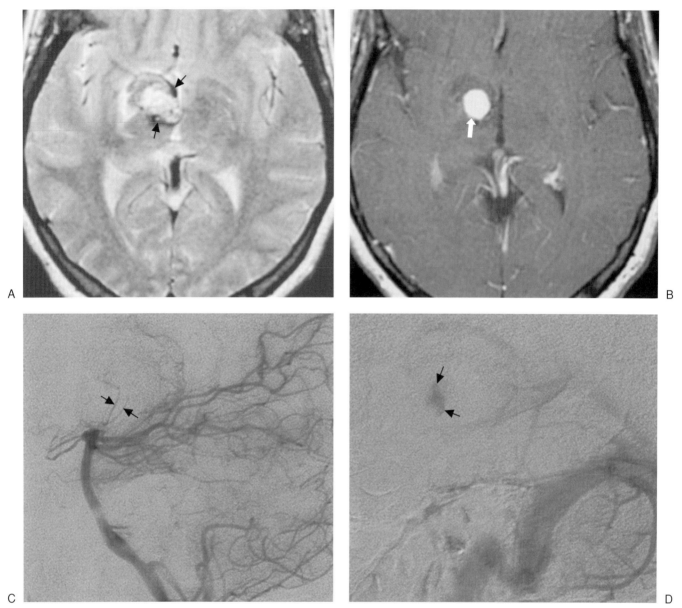

FIG. 13-18. This previously healthy, normotensive 42-year-old woman had a spontaneous intracranial hemorrhage. **A:** Axial T2-weighted MR scan shows a mixed-signal lesion in the right thalamus and midbrain (*arrows*). The popcornlike appearance suggests cavernous angioma. No additional lesions were identified on gradient-refocused sequences. **B:** Axial contrast-enhanced T1-weighted scan shows a well-delineated, strongly enhancing area in the center of the lesion (*white arrow*). A cerebral angiogram was performed. The left internal carotid study (not shown) was normal. **C:** The early arterial phase from a vertebrobasilar angiogram shows some stretching and straightening of the thalamoperforating arteries (*arrows*), but there is no evidence of arteriovenous shunting. **D:** The late venous phase shows pooling of contrast (*arrows*) in a venous lake or pseudoaneurysm. The differential diagnosis was a thrombosed AVM with a venous sac versus a cavernous malformation with a sinusoidal sac. Surgery three months later confirmed the presence of a cavernous angioma.

DURAL ARTERIOVENOUS SHUNTS

Arteriovenous lesions that involve the dura and the epidural space are called dural arteriovenous shunts (DAVS). These lesions are much more common than cAVFs but are only one tenth as common as brain AVMs. DAVS can be either congenital or acquired.

The most common types of DAVS also vary between different age groups. In general, three types are recognized: (a) dural sinus malformation with arteriovenous shunt; (b) infantile DAVS; and (c) adult-type DAVS (10,59). Adult-type DAVS with multiple dural arteriovenous microfistulae are the most common type of dural vascular malformation. Adult-type DAVS also occur in children (10).

Dural Sinus Malformation with Arteriovenous Shunt

These uncommon lesions are found in neonates or infants. They are usually seen as giant pouches or dural lakes that have slow-flow communications with other sinuses and cerebral veins (Fig. 13-19) (59). Although

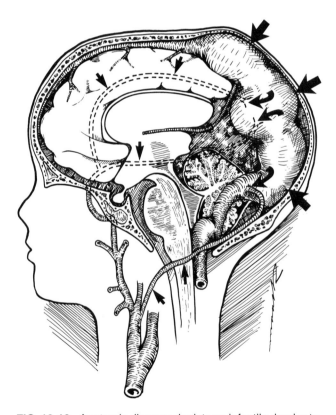

FIG. 13-19. Anatomic diagram depicts an infantile dural arteriovenous shunt (DAVS). Here the posterior aspect of the superior sagittal sinus (*large arrows*) is massively enlarged by direct arteriovenous shunts (*curved arrows*) from multiple dural and transosseous perforating branches (*small arrows*). Obstructive hydrocephalus is present. The straight sinus is often absent in these cases. Note thinning and expansion of the calvarium.

they may occur laterally, most of these unusual lesions involve the superior sagittal sinus with thrombosis, occlusion, or hypogenesis of one jugular bulb. Dural arteriovenous shunts are demonstrated within the wall of the venous lake (10).

Infantile Dural Arteriovenous Shunts

Infantile DAVS are also rare. In contrast to typical adult lesions, most infantile DAVS have high flow rates and volumes (60). Infantile DAVS are often multifocal. They typically have large sinuses with multiple local arteriovenous shunts and large feeding vessels (Fig. 13-19). Secondary induced corticopial shunts are common. Spontaneous thrombosis or occlusion of the venous outlets may lead to increased intracranial pressure, hydrocephalus, cerebral venous ischemia, and "melting brain" syndrome (10,59).

Adult-Type Dural Arteriovenous Shunts

Pathology

In contrast to AVMs, there is no true nidus in a DAVS. Instead, a DAVS consists of numerous abnormal direct communications (so-called cracklike vessels) between dural arteries and dilated dural veins without an intervening capillary bed (61).

Etiology and Pathogenesis

Although the precise etiology of dural arteriovenous shunts is debated, many seem to be acquired lesions that are preceded by hemodynamic compromise (stenosis, thrombosis, or occlusion) of a dural venous sinus. When the lumen recanalizes, microscopic arteriovenous shunts that are normally present in the sinus wall may enlarge and form numerous small artery-to-sinus communications (microfistulae). The result is a DAVS (5,62).

Because sinus thrombosis is not invariably associated with DAVS, other investigators have proposed that various initiating events lead to a common pathway, i.e., activating or stimulating angiogenesis within the dura. Budding and proliferation of microarterial or capillary vessels within the dura then result in formation of a DAVS (2,63) (see Fig. 17-8).

Location

Dural arteriovenous shunts are located in the dural wall of a venous sinus, not within the sinus itself. The transverse and sigmoid sinuses are the most common sites (61,63). The cavernous sinus is also a frequent location for a DAVS. Most DAVS are solitary lesions. With the exception of bilateral cavernous sinus DAVS, multiple lesions are uncommon and account for only 7% of DAVS (3).

Incidence

Dural arteriovenous shunts account for 10% to 15% of all intracranial arteriovenous malformations. However, one third of posterior fossa AVMs are purely dural (2,3).

Age and Clinical Presentation

Dural arteriovenous shunts may occur at any age and are not uncommon in children. However, most become symptomatic between the ages of 40 and 60 years (3).

Clinical presentation varies both with location and venous drainage pattern. Bruit and headache are the most common symptoms of DAVS that involve the transverse or sigmoid sinuses, whereas proptosis, chemosis, retroorbital pain, and ophthalmoplegia are associated with cavernous sinus lesions. Pulse-synchronous tinnitus and cranial neuropathy are less common manifestations (3). DAVS with venous hypertensive encephalopathy may cause a potentially reversible vascular dementia (63a).

Natural History

Most DAVS behave benignly, sometimes even involuting spontaneously. However, others present with an aggressive neurologic course or a fatal cerebral hemorrhage (64). *Venous drainage patterns* are the single most important determinant of clinical presentation, neurologic status, and long-term prognosis of DAVS (65,66). Dural arteriovenous shunts are classified by venous drainage patterns into several types that correlate well with clinical outcome (Table 13-2).

Type I DAVS are located in the main sinus wall and have normal antegrade flow. These lesions typically have a benign course. Type II lesions are located in the main sinus and have reflux into either the sinus (IIa), cortical veins (IIb), or both (IIa-b). In one series, reflux into the sinus

induced intracranial hypertension in 20% of cases, whereas cortical vein reflux caused hemorrhage in 10% (66).

Type III DAVS have direct cortical venous drainage without venous ectasia. Hemorrhage occurs in 40% of these cases. Type IV lesions have direct cortical venous drainage with venous ectasia. Nearly two thirds of type IV DAVS hemorrhage. Type V DAVS have spinal venous drainage; progressive myelopathy occurs in half of these cases (67). Retrograde leptomeningeal (i.e., cortical) venous drainage is also associated with venous congestive encephalopathy (68). Stenosis or thrombosis of venous drainage also portends a worse prognosis (69).

Cerebral Angiography

Most DAVS have *multiple dural feeders*. Because these lesions usually occur in or around the skull base and posterior fossa, the most commonly involved vessels that supply DAVS are the occipital artery and meningeal branches of the external carotid artery. Tentorial and dural branches of the internal carotid and vertebral arteries are also frequent sources of supply (Fig. 13-20).

Dural arteriovenous shunts do not have a nidus *per se*. Instead, numerous arteriovenous microfistulae form a fine vascular network in the wall of the affected dural sinus (Fig. 13-21).

Determining the DAVS type (I to V) depends on accurate assessment of the *venous drainage pattern* and *hemodynamics*. Angiography should delineate the dural sinus(es) involved as well as determine whether the flow is ante- or retrograde. *Reflux into cortical or spinal perimedullary veins* must be noted (Fig. 13-22). *Venous ectasias* portend a worse prognosis (Fig. 13-23). *Dural sinus stenosis or occlusion* is a common but not invariable finding in DAVS (70).

TABLE 13-2. *Classification of intracranial dural arteriovenous shunts: venous drainage patterns and correlation with clinical course*

Borden classification[a]	Cognard classification[b]	Aggressive clinical course[c]
Type I: DVS/MV outflow only	Type I:DVS/MV outflow only	Benign (2% or less)
	Type IIA: DVS/MV outflow only (retrograde)	
Type II:DVS/MV outflow and RLVD	Type IIB: DVS/MV outflow (anterograde) and RLVD	40% hemorrhage
	Type IIA+B: DVS/MV outflow (retrograde) and RLVD	
Type III: RLVD only	Type III: RLVD only (no ectasia)	80–100% hemorrhage
	Type IV: RLVD only (ectasia)	
	Type V: RLVD only (into spinal perimedullary veins)	

[a]Borden JA et al. A proposed classification for spinal and cranial dural arteriovenous fistulous malformations and implications for treatment. *J Neurosurg* 1995;82:166–179.

[b]Cognard C et al. Cerebral dural arteriovenous fistulas: clinical and angiographic correlation with a revised classification of venous drainage. *Radiology* 1995;194:671–680.

[c]Davies MA et al. The validity of classification for the clinical presentation of intracranial dural arteriovenous fistulas. *J Neurosurg* 1996;85:830–837.

DVS, dural venous sinus; RLVD, retrograde leptomeningeal (cortical) venous draining.

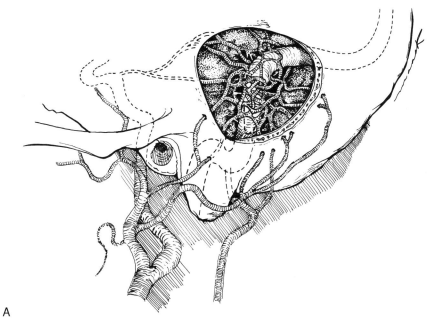

A

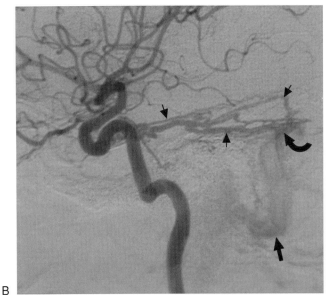

B

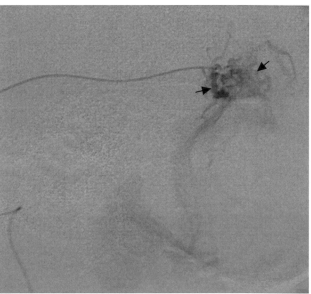

C

FIG. 13-20. A: Anatomic diagram depicts a dural arteriovenous shunt (DAVS) at the transverse–sigmoid sinus junction. This lesion is supplied by numerous dural branches of the external carotid artery as well as the meningohypophyseal trunk, a branch of the internal carotid artery. The DAVS is a collection of numerous microfistulae within the dural wall of the sinus, not the sinus itself. **B:** Left internal carotid angiogram, arterial phase, lateral view, in a patient with pulsatile tinnitus shows multiple enlarged branches of the meningohypophyseal trunk (*small arrows*) that supply a DAVS (*curved arrow*) at the transverse–sigmoid sinus junction. The DAVS drains in an anterograde direction through a patent sigmoid sinus (*large arrow*). **C:** Superselective catheterization of the DAVS via the middle meningeal artery is shown in this magnified view. Note the weblike collection of innumerable microfistulae in the dura of the sinus wall (*arrows*) (compare with Fig. 13-20A). This is a type I DAVS. (Part **A** reprinted with permission from Osborn AG. *Diagnostic neuroradiology.* St. Louis: Mosby, 1994.)

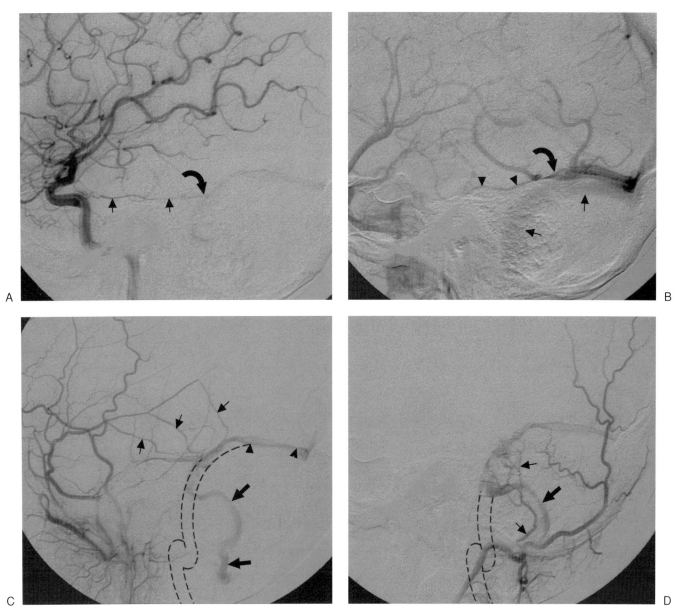

FIG. 13-21. A: A 43-year-old woman had a 3-month history of left-sided pulsatile tinnitus and occipital headaches. Left internal carotid angiogram, arterial phase, lateral view, shows that an enlarged tentorial branch of the meningohypophyseal trunk (*small arrows*) has formed a fistula at the transverse–sigmoid sinus junction (*curved arrow*). Note retrograde filling of the proximal transverse sinus (*arrowheads*). **B:** Venous phase from the same study shows occlusion at the left transverse–sigmoid sinus junction (*curved arrow*). Note collateral venous drainage via the superior petrosal sinus (*arrowheads*) and the faintly opacified normal right transverse sinus (*small arrows*). **C:** Left external carotid angiogram, arterial phase, lateral view, shows several branches of the middle meningeal artery (*small arrows*) feed the dural arteriovenous shunt. There is retrograde filling of the left transverse sinus (*arrowheads*). The distal transverse and sigmoid sinuses are occluded distal to the fistula (approximate location is shown by the dotted lines). Collateral venous drainage is present through mastoid emissary veins to the suboccipital venous plexus (*large arrows*). **D:** Superselective injection of the occipital artery shows that transosseous perforating branches (*small arrows*) supply the fistula. The occluded distal sigmoid sinus is indicated by the dotted lines. Note opacification of collateral mastoid emissary veins (*large arrow*). This is a type IIa DAVS.

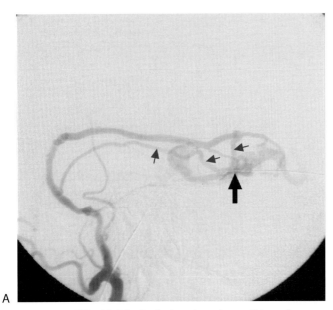
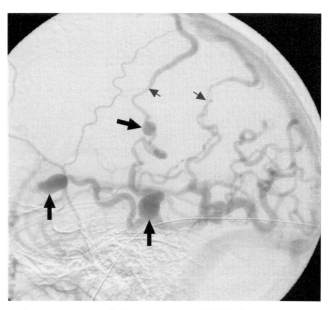

A

B

FIG. 13-22. A: Left external carotid angiogram, arterial phase, lateral view, shows a DAVS (*large arrow*) that is supplied by several enlarged posterior branches of the middle meningeal artery (*small arrows*). **B:** Venous phase view shows that the DAVS drains via numerous ectatic cortical veins. Note aneurysmal-like ectasias (*large arrows*) and focal areas of stenosis (*small arrows*) in the draining veins.

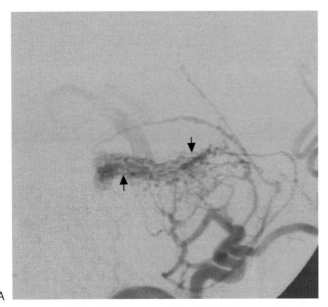
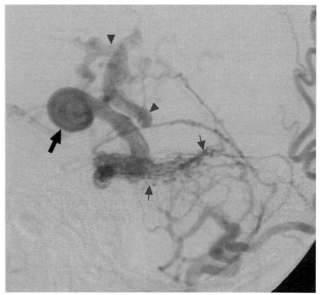

A

B

FIG. 13-23. A type IV DAVS is illustrated. Superselective injection of the left occipital artery with early **(A)** and later **(B)** arterial phase films, lateral view, shows innumerable transosseous dural feeders to a DAVS of the tentorium cerebelli (*small arrows*). Note the striking deep venous drainage (*arrowheads*) and venous varix (*large arrow*).**C:** AP view of the arterial phase shows the extensive DAVS (*arrows*). **D:** AP view of the venous phase shows that drainage is via dilated deep veins (**D,** *small arrows*). The venous varix is indicated by the large arrow. **E–H:** Lateral views of a left internal carotid angiogram performed after embolization of the occipital artery feeders show that numerous dilated meningohypophyseal branches also supply the DAVS (*small arrows*). Note early opacification of the large deep draining vein (*large arrow*). Capillary and venous phase studies show nonfilling of the internal cerebral veins, vein of Galen, and straight sinus.

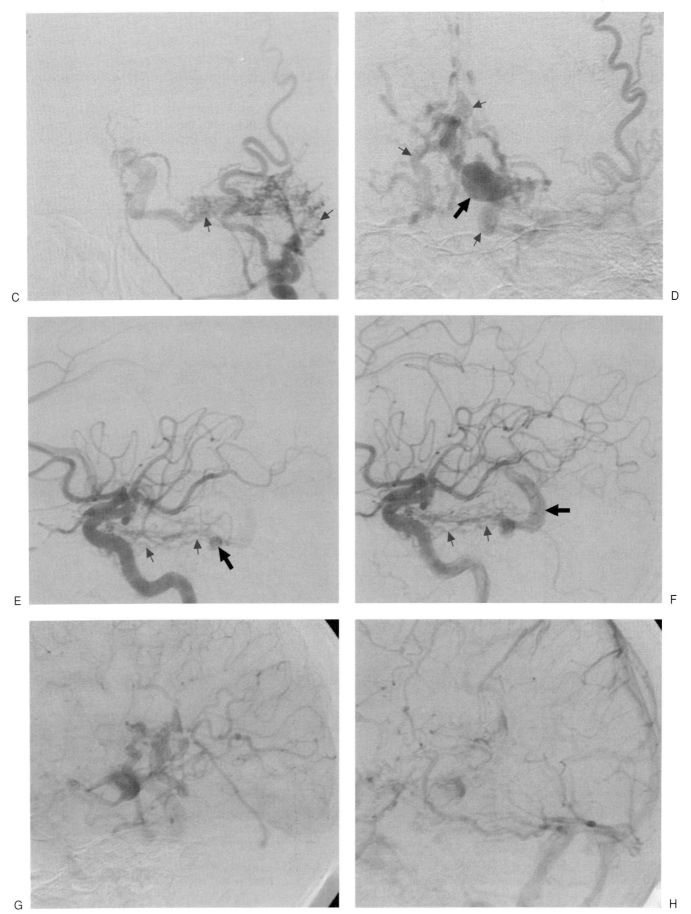

C

D

E

F

G

H

FIG. 13-23. *Continued.*

Location

The most common site for a DAVS is at the *transverse–sigmoid sinus junction* (Figs. 13-20 and 13-21). The next most common location is the cavernous sinus.

Cavernous sinus DAVS typically affect middle-aged women. Presenting symptoms depend on venous drainage. Arterialized venous drainage often reverses flow direction within the ophthalmic vein, causing proptosis, chemosis, and conjunctival edema. Blood supply is usually derived from dural branches of both the internal and external carotid arteries (Fig. 13-24) (62).

Less commonly, adult-type DAVS involve the *superior sagittal sinus* or anterior skull base (so-called *ethmoid DAVS*) (62).

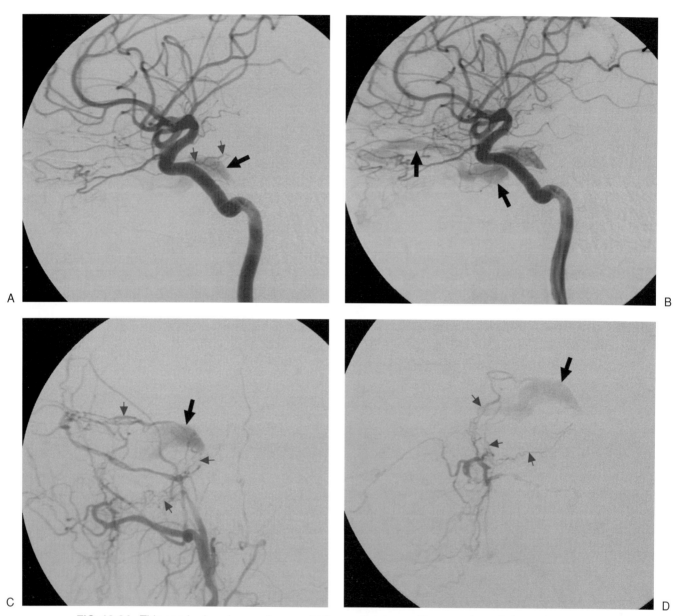

FIG. 13-24. This cerebral angiogram from a middle-aged woman with proptosis and chemosis shows a cavernous sinus dural arteriovenous shunt. **A:** Left internal carotid angiogram, early arterial phase, lateral view, shows prominent branches of an enlarged meningohypophyseal trunk (*small arrows*). Note early opacification of the cavernous sinus (*large arrow*). **B:** Later arterial phase study shows the enlarged cavernous sinus with reversal of flow into a dilated superior ophthalmic vein (*large arrows*). **C:** External carotid angiogram, arterial phase, lateral view, shows early opacification of the cavernous sinus (*large arrow*) by numerous enlarged branches from the internal maxillary and middle meningeal arteries (*small arrows*). **D:** Superselective injection of the distal maxillary artery shows that enlarged arteries of the foramen rotundum and pterygoid (vidian) canal (*small arrows*) shunt directly into the cavernous sinus (*large arrow*).

CUTANEOUS VASCULAR MALFORMATIONS

Much confusion exists over the nomenclature of cutaneous vascular lesions. These lesions are classified into two basic groups: (a) hemangiomas, which demonstrate endothelial hyperplasia, and (b) malformations, which in general are nonproliferating lesions with normal endothelial turnover (Table 13-3).

Hemangiomas

Pathology

Hemangiomas are true neoplasms, so-called vasoformative tumors with increased proliferation and turnover of endothelial cells, mast cells, fibroblasts, and macrophages (71). Hemangiomas are classified pathologically by the predominant type of vascular channel seen at histologic examination. Hemangiomas can be capillary, cavernous, arteriovenous or venous. Nonvascular components also can be identified in angiomatous lesions (72).

Age, Incidence, and Biologic Behavior

Hemangiomas are the most common tumor of infancy. Approximately 60% are located in the head and neck. They may involve the bones or soft tissues. Multiple lesions occur in 20% of cases.

Biological Behavior and Clinical Presentation

Infantile hemangiomas are characterized by a phase of initial growth and angiogenesis, a plateau phase of inactivity, slow resolution of angiogenesis, and regression of both the size and vascularity of the tumors (72a). About 70% of hemangiomas have resolved by age 7 (71).

TABLE 13-3. *Cutaneous vascular lesions*

Hemangiomas	Vascular malformations
True neoplasm	Malformation
Proliferative	Generally nonproliferative
Regress spontaneously	Do not regress
Infants, young children	Any age
High-flow	Variable flow
	Arterial high
	Venous low
	Lymphatic none
Examples	Examples
Capillary hemangioma of the face	Capillary telangiectasias (Osler-Weber-Rendu disease)
	Venous malformation
Association with intracranial CVMs	Association with intracranial CVMs
None (but is associated with cutaneous hemangioma-vascular complex syndrome)	AVM (Osler-Weber-Rendu disease)
	DVA (sinus pericranii, blue rubber bleb nevus)

The clinical severity of hemangiomas varies widely. These benign vascular lesions range from an asymptomatic, discolored spot on the skin to large, disfiguring masses that can be life-threatening when they occur near vital structures (e.g., the airway). Their high vascularity may cause high output heart failure. Sequestration of platelets within the lesion may lead to thrombocytopenia (Kasabach-Merritt syndrome) (72a).

Imaging Characteristics

Hemangiomas typically are high signal intensity on T2-weighted MR scans and enhance following contrast administration. High vessel density and high peak arterial Doppler shift are useful findings that help distinguish hemangiomas from other soft-tissue masses (72a).

Because most hemangiomas require no intervention, angiograms are rarely performed. When angiography is obtained, hemangiomas appear well-circumscribed with a lobular pattern of intense, persistent tissue staining. They are relatively high-flow lesions and often exhibit arteriovenous shunting (Table 13-3) (71).

Associated Conditions

Many cutaneous hemangiomas of the head, neck, and chest are associated with anomalies that affect the intra- and extracranial arteries, cerebellum, and sometimes the cerebral hemispheres and aortic arch. This neurocutaneous syndrome is called the *cutaneous hemangioma–vascular complex syndrome* (73). Progressive aneurysmal and occlusive changes that may cause cerebral ischemia and infarction also have been reported (74).

Vascular Malformations

Cutaneous vascular malformations are congenital lesions. They are true vascular malformations that contain nonproliferating endothelial cells (71,75). These lesions are subdivided into high-flow malformations and low-flow lesions (Table 13-3) (71). In contrast to hemangiomas, cutaneous vascular malformations do not involute spontaneously.

High-Flow Lesions

High-flow cutaneous vascular malformations include arterial, arteriovenous, and arteriolymphovenous malformations. *AVMs* and *AVFs* are included in this category. These lesions are usually noted at birth and continue to grow proportionally with the child. They may be associated with a thrill or bruit, pain, ulceration, and congestive heart failure (71). They may involve the facial bones and mandible, causing bony erosion.

Angiographically, arterial malformations are characterized by rapid flow with enlarged, tortuous arteries and dilated draining veins. Shunts and fistulae are common (Fig. 13-25).

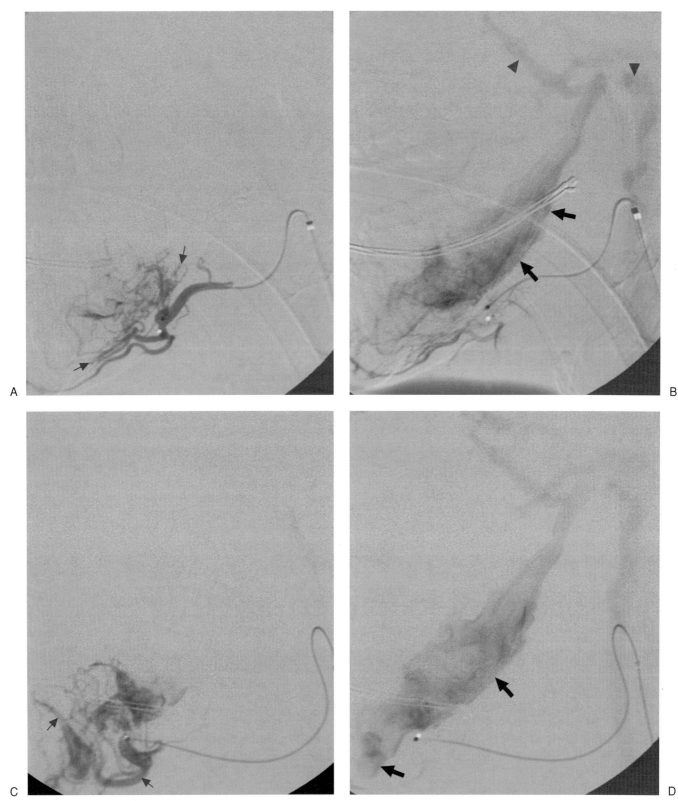

FIG. 13-25. A 9-year-old child with loose teeth in the lower jaw and known facial vascular malformation had a diagnostic angiogram prior to embolization. Superselective injection of the facial artery with early **(A)** and late **(B)** arterial phase films, lateral view, shows a high-flow arteriovenous malformation of the mandible (**A**, *small arrows*) with drainage into a massively enlarged inferior alveolar vein (**B**, *large arrows*). Note retrograde filling of deep facial and external jugular veins (*arrowheads*). Superselective catheterization of the lingual artery with early **(C)** and late **(D)** arterial phase films, lateral view, shows additional feeding vessels (**C**, *small arrows*) and venous ectasias (**D**, *large arrows*).

Low-Flow Lesions

Low-flow cutaneous vascular malformations include capillary, venous, and lymphatic malformations.

A *port-wine stain* is the most common type of cutaneous capillary malformation. Port-wine stains are often associated with neurocutaneous syndromes such as Wyburn-Mason, Cobb, and Sturge-Weber syndromes.

Capillary telangiectasias are associated with hereditary syndromes such as ataxia–telangiectasia (Louis-Bar syndrome) and Osler-Weber-Rendu disease. Osler-Weber-Rendu disease, also known as hereditary hemorrhagic telangiectasia (HHT), is an autosomal dominant vascular dysplasia that is linked to chromosomes 9q and 12q.

Approximately 25% of patients with Osler-Weber-Rendu disease have at least one episode of epistaxis per year. External carotid angiograms in these patients disclose multiple nests of dilated capillaries with prolonged vascular staining (Fig. 13-26).

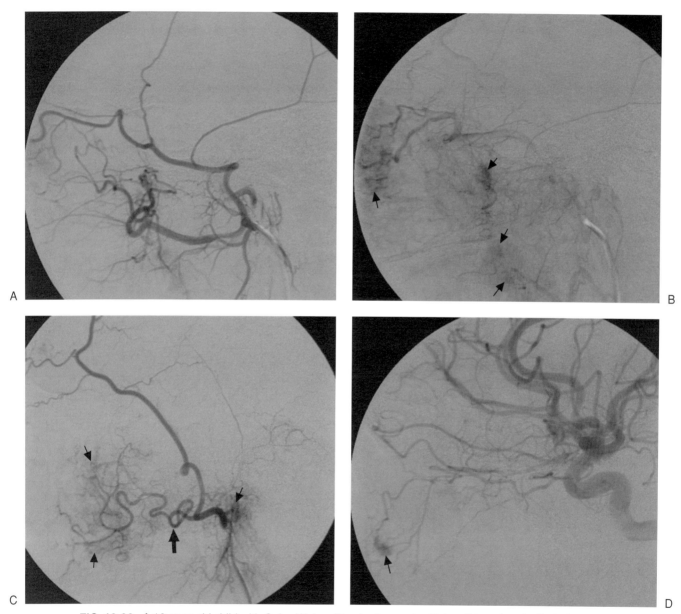

FIG. 13-26. A 10-year-old child with Osler-Weber-Rendu disease had intractible epistaxis. Early **(A)** and late **(B)** arterial phase views of a selective left internal maxillary angiogram, lateral view, show multiple nests of dilated capillaries with prolonged vascular staining in the orbital, nasopharyngeal, and oral mucosa (*arrows*). **C:** Selective left superficial temporal angiogram, mid-arterial phase, lateral view, shows that the transverse facial artery (*large arrow*) also opacifies numerous sinonasal capillary telangiectasias (*small arrows*). **D:** Left internal carotid angiogram, late arterial phase, lateral view, shows that extraocular branches of the ophthalmic artery supply a telangiectatic nest in the orbital mucosa (*arrow*).

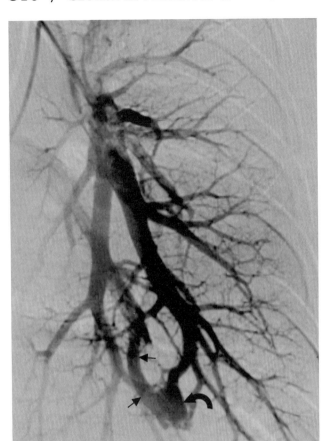

FIG. 13-27. A young woman with known Osler-Weber-Rendu disease and multiple intracranial AVMs (not shown) had a stroke. Pulmonary angiogram disclosed a pulmonary AVF (*curved arrow*) with arteriovenous shunting into the left pulmonary vein (*small arrows*).

Cerebrovascular malformations occur in 23% of patients with Osler-Weber-Rendu disease. These are not capillary telangiectasias; most are AVMS, venous angiomas, or an "indeterminate" type of CVM (76). Among patients with neurologic deficits, 61% are due to embolic complications of pulmonary vascular malformations (Fig. 13-27), whereas 28% result from intracerebral hemorrhages secondary to CVMs (2,76).

Cutaneous *venous malformations* of the head and neck are slow-flow lesions that manifest as soft-tissue swellings under normal or bluish skin. They increase in size with a Valsalva maneuver. Cerebral DVAS are found in 20% of cases with extensive cutaneous venous malformations (77).

REFERENCES

1. Valavanis A. The role of angiography in the evaluation of cerebral vascular malformations. *Neuroimag Clin North Am* 1996;6:679–704.
2. Chaloupka JC, Huddle DC. Classification of vascular malformations of the central nervous system. *Neuroimag Clin North Am* 1998;8: 295–321.
3. Osborn AG. Intracranial vascular malformations. In: *Diagnostic neuroradiology*. St. Louis: Mosby, 1994:284–329.
4. Lasjaunias P. A revised concept of the congenital nature of cerebral arteriovenous malformations. *Interv Neuroradiol* 1997;3:275–281.
5. Mullan S, Mojtahedi S, Johnson DL, Macdonald RL. Embryological basis of some aspects of cerebral vascular fistulas and malformations. *J Neurosurg* 1996;85:1–8.
5a. Nussbaum ES, Heros RC, Madison MT, et al. The pathogenesis of arteriovenous malformations: insights provided by a case of multiple arteriovenous malformations developing in relation to developmental venous anomaly. *Neurosurg* 1998;43:347–352.
6. Sonstein WJ, Kader A, Michelsen WJ, et al. Expression of vascular endothelial growth factor in pediatric and adult cerebral arteriovenous malformations: an immunocytochemical study. *J Neurosurg* 1996;85: 838–845.
7. Rothbart D, Awad IA, Lee J, et al. Expression of angiogenic factors and structural proteins in central nervous system vascular malformations. *Neurosurgery* 1996;38:915–925.
8. Rhoten RLP, Comair YG, Shedid D, et al. Specific repression of the preproendothelin-1 gene in intracranial arteriovenous malformations. *J Neurosurg* 1997;86:101–108.
9. Lasjaunias P, Redesch G, TerBrugge K, Taylor W. Arterial and venous angioarchitecture of cerebral AVM in adults. *Riv Neuroradiol* 1994; 7(suppl 4):35–39.
10. Lasjaunias P. *Vascular diseases in neonates, infants and children*. New York: Springer-Verlag, 1997.
11. Fogarty-Mack P, Pile-Spellman J, Hacein-Bey L, et al. The effect of arteriovenous malformations on the distribution of intracranial arterial pressures. *AJNR* 1996;17:1443–1449.
12. Sekhon LHS, Morgan MK, Spence I, Weber NC. Chronic cerebral hypoperfusion: pathological and behavioral consequences. *Neurosurgery* 1997;40:548–556.
13. Müller-Forell W, Valavanis A. How angioarchitecture of cerebral arteriovenous malformations should influence the therapeutic considerations. *Minim Invasive Neurosurg* 1995;38:32–40.
14. Turski PA, Cordes D, Mock B, et al. Basic concepts of functional magnetic resonance imaging and arteriovenous malformations. *Neuroimag Clin North Am* 1998;8:371–381.
15. Pollock BE, Flickinger JC, Lundsford LD, et al. Factors that predict the bleeding risk of cerebral arteriovenous malformations. *Stroke* 1996;27:1–6.
16. Ericson K, Söderman M, Karlsson B, et al. Multiple intracranial arteriovenous malformations: a case report. *Neuroradiology* 1994;36: 157–159.
17. Hartmann A, Mast H, Mohr JP, et al. Morbidity of intracranial hemorrhage in patients with cerebral arteriovenous malformations. *Stroke* 1998;29:931–934.
18. Mast H, Mohr JP, Osipov A, et al. "Steal" is an unestablished mechanism for the clinical presentation of cerebral arteriovenous malformations. *Stroke* 1995;26:1215–1220.
19. Turjman F, Massoud TF, Viñuela F, et al. Correlation of the angioarchitectural features of cerebral arteriovenous malformations with clinical presentation of hemorrhage. *Neurosurgery* 1995;37:856–862.
20. Nataf F, Meder JF, Roux FX, et al. Angioarchitecture associated with haemorrhage in cerebral arteriovenous malformations: a prognostic statistical model. *Neuroradiology* 1997;39:52–58.
20a. Duong DH, Young WL, Vang MC, et al. Feeding artery pressure and venous drainage pattern are primary determinants of hemorrhage from cerebral arteriovenous malformations. *Stroke* 1998;29: 1167–1176.
20b. Nurayama Y. Massoud TF, Viñuela F. Hemodynamic changes in arterial feeders and draining veins during embolotherapy of arteriovenous malformations: an experimental study in a swine model. *Neurosurg* 1998;43:96–106.
21. Langer DJ, Lasner TM, Hurst RW, et al. Hypertension, small size, and deep venous drainage are associated with risk of hemorrhagic presentation of cerebral arteriovenous malformations. *Neurosurgery* 1998; 42:481–489.
22. Hamilton MG, Spetzler RF. The prospective application of a grading system for arteriovenous malformations. *Neurosurgery* 1994;34:2–7.
23. Wallace RC, Bourekas EC. Brain arteriovenous malformations. *Neuroimag Clin North Am* 1998;8:383–399.

23a. Thompson, et al. The management of patients with arteriovenous malformations and associated intracranial aneurysms. *Neurosurgery* 1998;43 (in press).

24. Chin LS, Raffel C, Gonzalez-Gomez I, et al. Diffuse arteriovenous malformations: a clinical, radiological, and pathological description. *Neurosurgery* 1992;31:863–868.

25. Akai T, Kuwayama N, Kubo M, et al. Treatment of an arteriovenous shunt draining into a venous angioma by selective embolisation. *Interv Neuroradiol* 1997;3:329–332.

26. Meyer B, Stangl AP, Schramm J. Association of venous and true arteriovenous malformation: a rare entity among mixed vascular malformations of the brain. *J Neurosurg* 1997;86:699–703.

27. Chang SD, Steinberg GK, Rosario M, et al. Mixed arteriovenous malformation and capillary telangiectasia: a rare subset of mixed vascular malformations. *J Neurosurg* 1997;86:699–703.

28. Hallam DK, Russell EJ. Imaging of angiographically occult cerebral vascular malformations. *Neuroimag Clin North Am* 1998;8:323–347.

29. Berenstein A, Lasjaunias P. Arteriovenous fistulas of the brain. In: *Surgical neuroangiography. 4: Endovascular treatment of cerebral lesions.* New York: Springer-Verlag, 1991:268–319.

30. Lasjaunias P, Alvarez H, Rodesch G, et al. Aneurysmal malformations of the vein of Galen. *Interv Neuroradiol* 1996;2:15–26.

30a. Halbach VV, Dowd CF, Higashida RT, et al. Endovascular treatment of mural-type vein of Galen malformations. *J Neurosurg* 1998;89:74–80.

31. Tomsick TA, Ernst RJ, Twe JM, et al. Adult choroidal vein of Galen malformation. *AJNR* 1995;16:861–865.

32. Brunelle F. Arteriovenous malformation of the vein of Galen in children. *Pediatr Radiol* 1997;27:501–513.

33. Horowitz MB, Jungreis CA, Quisling RG, Pollock I. Vein of Galen aneurysms: a review and current perspective. *AJNR* 1994;15:1486–1496.

34. Mickle JP, Quisling RG. Vein of Galen fistulas. *Neurosurg Clin North Am* 1994;5:529–540.

35. Raybaud CA, Strother CM, Hald JK. Aneurysms of the vein of Galen: embryonic considerations and anatomical features relating to the pathogenesis of the malformation. *Neuroradiology* 1989;31:109–128.

36. Dillon WP. Cryptic vascular malformations: controversies in terminology, diagnosis, pathophysiology, and treatment. *AJNR* 1997;18:1839–1846.

36a. Detwiler PA, Porter RW, Zabramski JM, Spetzler RF. Radiation-induced cavernous malformation (letter). *J Neurosurg* 1998;89:167–168.

37. Gewirtz RJ, Steinberg GK, Crowley R, Levy RP. Pathological changes in surgically resected angiographically occult vascular malformations after radiation. *Neurosurgery* 1998;42:738–743.

38. Guillaud L, Pelizzari M, Guilbal AL, Pracos JP. Slow-flow vascular malformation of the pons: congenital or acquired capillary telangiectasia? *AJNR* 1996;17:1798–1800.

39. Gaensler EHL, Dillon WP, Edwards MSB, et al. Radiation-induced telangiectasia in the brain simulates cryptic vascular malformations at MR imaging. *Radiology* 1994;193:629–636.

40. Barr RM, Dillon WP, Wilson C. Slow-flow vascular malformations of the pons: capillary telangiectasias? *AJNR* 1996;17:71–78.

41. Robinson JR Jr, Awad IA, Masaryk TJ, Estes ML. Pathological heterogeneity of angiographically occult vascular malformations of the brain. *Neurosurgery* 1993;33:547–555.

42. McCormick PW, Spetzler RF, Johnson PC, Drayer BP. Cerebellar hemorrhage associated with capillary telangiectsia and venous angioma: a case report. *Surg Neurol* 1993;39:451–457.

43. Wilms G, Demaerel P, Robberecht W, et al. Coincidence of developmental venous anomalies and other brain lesions: a clinical study. *Eur Radiol* 1995;5:495–500.

44. Huber G, Henkes H, Hermes M, et al. Regional association of developmental venous anomalies with angiographically occult vascular malformations. *Eur Radiol* 1996;6:30–37.

45. Abe T, Singer RJ, Marks MP, et al. Coexistence of occult vascular malformations and developmental venous anomalies in the central nervous system: MR evaluation. *AJNR* 1998;19:51–57.

46. Friedman DP. Abnormalities of the deep medullary white matter veins: MR findings. *AJR* 1997;168:1103–1108.

47. Saba PR. The caput medusae sign. *Radiology* 1998;207:599–600.

47a. McLaughlin MR, Kondziolka D, Flickinger JC, et al. The prospective natural history of cerebral venous malformations. *Neurosurgery* 1998;43:195–201.

48. Uchino A, Hasuo K, Matsumoto S, et al. Varix occurring with cerebral venous angiomas: a case report and review of the literature. *Neuroradiology* 1995;37:29–31.

49. Lee C, Pennington MA, Henney CM III. MR evaluation of developmental venous anomalies: medullary venous anatomy of venous angiomas. *AJNR* 1996;17:61–70.

50. Mullan S, Mojtahedi S, Johnson DL, Macdonald RL. Cerebral venous malformation-arteriovenous malformation transition forms. *J Neurosurg* 1996;85:9–13.

51. Bergui M, Bradae GB. Uncommon symptomatic cerebral vascular malformations. *AJNR* 1997;18:779–783.

52. Uchino A, Hasuo K, Matsumoto S, Masuda K. Double cerebral venous angiomas: MRI. *Neuroradiology* 1995;37:25–28.

53. Sherry RG, White ML, Olds MV. Sinus pericranii and venous angioma with the blue-rubber bleb nevus syndrome. *AJNR* 1984;5:832–834.

54. Spektor S, Weinberger G, Constantini S, et al. Giant lateral sinus pericranii. *J Neurosurg* 1998;88:145–147.

55. Bollar A, Allut AG, Prieto A, et al. Sinus pericranii: radiological and etiopathological considerations. *J Neurosurg* 1992;77:469–472.

56. Kelly KJ, Rockwell BH, Raji R, et al. Isolated cerebral intraaxial varix. *AJNR* 1995;16:1633–1635.

57. Bellon RJ, Seeger JF. Cavernous angiomas: a radiologic review. *IJNR* 1997;3:343–355.

58. Gunel M, Awad IA, Anson JA, et al. Cavernous malformation in Hispanic-Americans is due to a single mutation with low penetrance inherited from a common ancestor. *J Neurosurg* 1996;84:365A.

58a. Houtteville J-P. Brain cavernoma: a dynamic lesion. *Surg Neurol* 1997;48:610–614.

59. Lasjaunias P, Magufis G, Goulao A, et al. Anatomoclinical aspects of dural arteriovenous shunts in children. *Interv Neuroradiol* 1996;2:179–191.

60. Borden NM, Dean BL, Flom RA, et al. High-flow dural arteriovenous malformations in children. *BNI Q* 1996;12:12–17.

61. Hamada Y, Goto K, Inoue T, et al. Histopathological aspects of dural arteriovenous fistulas in the transverse-sigmoid sinus region in nine patients. *Neurosurgery* 1997;40:452–458.

62. Malek AM, Halbach VV, Dowd CF, Higashida RT. Diagnosis and treatment of dural arteriovenous fistulas. *Neuroimag Clin North Am* 1998;8:445–468.

63. Lawton MT, Jacobowitz R, Spetzler RF. Redefined role of angiogenesis in the pathogenesis of dural arteriovenous malformations. *J Neurosurg* 1997;87:267–274.

63a. Hurst RW, Bagley LJ, Galetta S, et al: Dementia resulting from dural arteriovenous fistulas: The pathologic findings of venous hypertensive encephalopathy. *AJNR* 1998;19:1267–1273.

64. Lucas CP, Azbramski JM, Spetzler RF, Jacobwitz R. Treatment for intracranial dural arteriovenous malformations: a meta-analysis from the English language literature. *Neurosurgery* 1997;40:1119–1132.

65. Davies MA, TerBrugge K, Willinsky R, et al. The validity of classification for the clinical presentation of intracranial dural arteriovenous fistulas. *J Neurosurg* 1996;85:830–837.

66. Davies MA, Saleh J, TerBrugge K, et al. The natural history and management of intracranial dural arteriovenous fistulae. Part 1: Benign lesions. *Interv Neuroradiol* 1997;3:299–302.

67. Cognard C, Gobin YP, Pierot L, et al. Cerebral dural arteriovenous fistulas: clinical and angiographic correlation with a revised classification of venous drainage. *Radiology* 1995;194:671–680.

68. Willinsky R, TerBrugge K, Monanera W, et al. Venous congestion: an MR finding in dural arteriovenous malformations with cortical venous drainage. *AJNR* 1994;15:1501–1507.

69. Cognard C, Houdart E, Casasco A, et al. Long-term changes in intracranial dural arteriovenous fistulae leading to worsening on the type of venous drainage. *Neuroradiology* 1997;39:59–66.

70. Arnautovic KI, Al-Mefty O, Angtuaco E, Phares LJ. Dural arteriovenous malformations of the transverse/sigmoid sinus acquired from dominant sinus occlusion by a tumor: report of two cases. *Neurosurgery* 1998;42:383–388.

71. Chen JW, Spetzler RF, Reiff J, Beals SP. Hemangiomas and vascular malformations. *BNI Q* 1994;10:19–25.

72. Murphey MD, Fairbairn KJ, Parman LM, et al. Musculoskeletal angiomatous lesions: radiologic-pathologic correlation. *Radiographics* 1995;15:893–917.

72a. Dubois J, Patriquin HB, Garel L, et al. Soft-tissue hemangiomas in infants and children: diagnosis using Doppler sonography. *AJR* 1998;171:247–252.

73. Pascual-Castroviejo I, Viaño J, Moreno F, et al. Hemangiomas of the head, neck, and chest with associated vascular and brain anomalies: a complex neurocutaneous syndrome. *AJNR* 1996;17:461–471.

74. Burrows PE, Robertson RL, Mulliken JB, et al. Cerebral vasculopathy and neurologic sequelae in infants with cervicofacial hemangioma: report of eight patients. *Radiology* 1998;207:601–607.

75. Yang WT, Ahuja A, Metreweli C. Sonographic features of head and neck hemangiomas and vascular malformations: review of 23 patients. *J Ultrasound Med* 1997;16:39–44.

76. Fulbright RK, Chaloupka JC, Putman CM, et al. MR of hereditary hemorrhagic telangiectasia: prevalence and spectrum of cerebrovascular malformations. *AJNR* 1998;19:477–484.

77. Boukobza M, Enjolras O, Guichard J-P, et al. Cerebral developmental venous anomalies associated with head and neck venous malformations. *AJNR* 1996;17:987–994.

CHAPTER 14

Neoplasms and Mass Effects

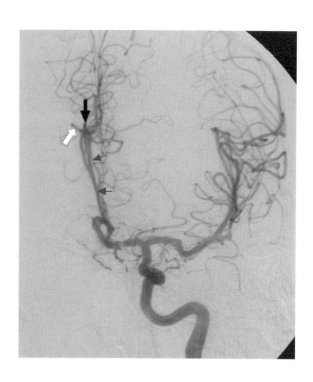

Noninvasive studies have replaced conventional angiography in the initial evaluation of patients with suspected extra- and intracranial masses (1). Magnetic resonance angiography (MRA) nicely demonstrates gross brain displacements and depicts involvement of large vessels such as the anterior cerebral artery (ACA) and middle cerebral artery (MCA) (2). However, diagnostic cerebral angiograms are sometimes obtained to guide management decisions in difficult cases. Angiography provides a high-resolution method for directly assessing the vascular abnormalities associated with tumors for purposes of both surgical planning and neurointerventional procedures. Involvement of important structures such as the dural venous sinuses and detecting secondary effects such as herniation syndromes also can be achieved. Evaluating the potential for collateral blood flow and performing functional testing for eloquent brain can be incorporated into the diagnostic paradigm if desired (1).

This chapter begins by examining the general angiographic findings with intracranial masses. Characteristic vascular displacement patterns are discussed using schematic diagrams paired with illustrative case examples. Then angiographic findings with some frequently encountered intracranial neoplasms are described. The chapter concludes with a brief consideration of common vascular tumors of the head and neck.

GENERAL ANGIOGRAPHIC FEATURES OF INTRACRANIAL MASSES

The angiographic findings of intracranial masses reflect both their indirect and direct effects on the cerebral vasculature. Focal and generalized mass effect, including herniation syndromes, are indirect manifestations of intracranial space-occupying lesions. The direct effects of brain tumors include angiogenesis with neovascularity, tumor "blush," blood–brain barrier disruption, and arteriovenous shunting.

Focal Mass Effects

Intraaxial Masses

Diffusely infiltrating parenchymal tumors usually have normal cerebral angiograms. When small, avascular neoplasms and other intraaxial masses also may produce no discernible effect on the cerebral vasculature. As they enlarge, parenchymal masses cause focal displacement of arterial branches and adjacent cortical or subependymal veins (Fig. 14-1).

Extraaxial Masses

Both non-neoplastic extraaxial masses such as subdural hematomas (Fig. 14-2) and neoplasms such as

313

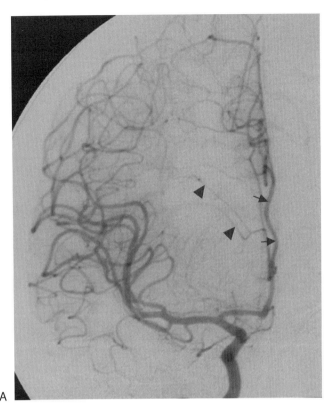 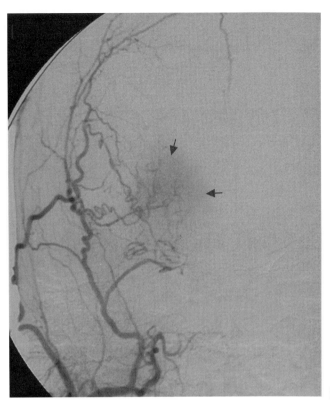

A   B

FIG. 14-1. A: Internal carotid angiogram, arterial phase, AP view, shows angiographic features of a small avascular intracranial mass (arrows). Note slight right-to-left subfalcine herniation of the anterior cerebral artery (small arrows) with focal stretching and draping of cortical branches (arrowheads) around an avascular-appearing mass. B: Selective external carotid angiogram, arterial phase, AP view, shows that enlarged branches from the middle meningeal and superficial temporal arteries supplies a vascular mass. Typical meningioma was found at surgery.

meningioma (see Figs. 14-15C and 14-16C) may cause either localized or more diffuse arterial displacements.

Generalized Mass Effects

Anatomic Considerations

After the sutures close, the skull becomes a rigidly enclosed space. Dural folds and bony ridges functionally divide the intracranial cavity into three major compartments: (a) the supratentorial compartment (with right and left sides) and (b) the infratentorial compartment (posterior fossa) (3,4).

The *falx cerebri* is a vertical midline dural fold that extends from the crista galli anteriorly to the tentorial confluence. The falx divides the supratentorial compartment into two halves. The *tentorium cerebelli* is a more horizontal, tentlike dural fold that extends from the clinoid processes to the torcular Herophili. It is attached to the superior border of the petrous temporal bone and posterolaterally to the transverse sinuses. It has a variably shaped opening, the *tentorial incisura*, that transmits the mid-brain and other accompanying structures such as the basilar artery.

Physiologic Considerations

The Monro-Kellie doctrine holds that the total volume of the intracranial compartments with its vascular, cerebrospinal fluid (CSF), and tissue constituents is constant because these components are essentially incompressible over physiologic pressure ranges. Therefore, change in the volume of one must be accompanied by an equal and opposite change in the others (5).

Because the intracranial contents exhibit the viscoelastic properties of a solid, adding extra tissue (e.g., tumor cells) or fluid (e.g., hemorrhage) causes abnormal pressure gradients to develop (5). At first, it is mostly interstitial fluid and CSF that are displaced. With increasing mass effect, the brain and its accompanying vessels are displaced from one compartment into another.

Cerebral Herniations

Classification

Cerebral herniations are caused by gross mechanical displacement of brain, CSF, and blood vessels from one cranial compartment to another. Patterns of herniation are

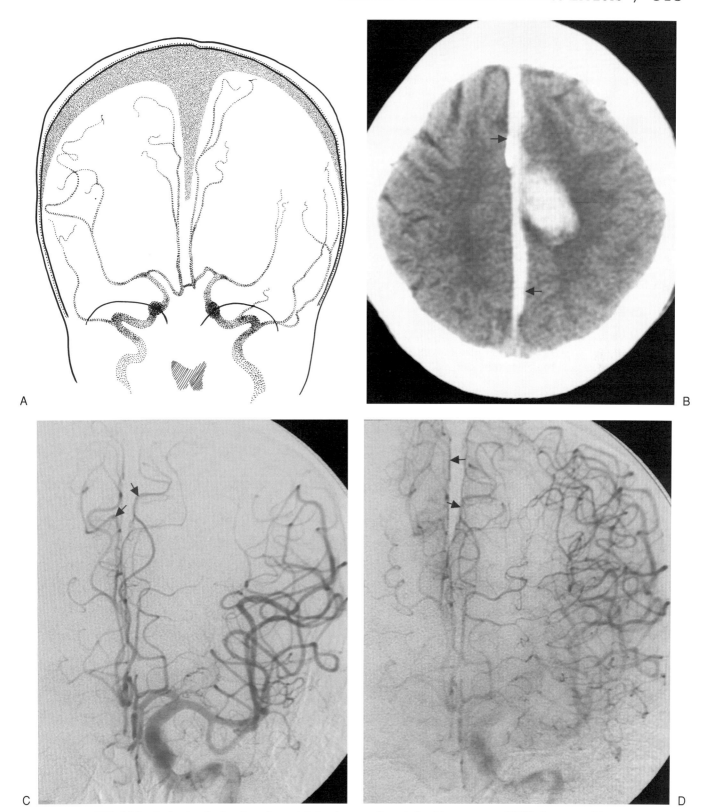

FIG. 14-2. A: Anatomic drawing shows bilateral convexity subdural hematomas (SDH) that extend into the interhemispheric fissure. **B:** Axial NECT scan shows an acute left posterior frontal clot and an adjacent interhemispheric SDH (*arrows*). Early **(C)** and late **(D)** arterial phase films of a left internal carotid angiogram, AP view, show a mass effect extending into the interhemispheric fissure. Note lateral displacement of both anterior cerebral arteries (*arrows*). The subdural hematoma was evacuated at surgery.

TABLE 14-1. *Intracranial herniations*

Type	Dural fold/ bony ridge	What herniates
Subfalcine	Falx cerebri	ACA, cingulate gyrus, lateral ventricles
Transtentorial	Tentorial incisura	
Descending		Uncus, hippocampal gyrus, AChA, PCA
Ascending		Vermis, superior cerebellar arteries
Transalar	Greater sphenoid wing	
Ascending		Temporal lobe, MCA
Descending		Frontal lobe
Tonsillar	Foramen magnum	Tonsils, PICA

ACA, anterior cerebral artery; AChA, anterior choroidal artery; MCA, middle cerebral artery; PCA, posterior cerebral artery; PICA, posterior inferior cerebellar artery.

classified according to which anatomic boundary the herniating structures cross (3). The four major types of cerebral herniations are subfalcine, transtentorial, transalar, and tonsillar herniation (Table 14-1). Each of these herniation syndromes and their angiographic manifestations separately, although combinations of two or more patterns are common, especially with larger masses.

Subfalcine Herniation

Subfalcine herniation (also known as cingulate, supracallosal, and transfalcial herniation) is the most common of all the cranial herniations. Part or all of the cingulate (supracallosal) gyrus is displaced across the midline under the inferior free margin of the falx cerebri (5a). This side-to-side herniation displaces the ipsilateral anterior cerebral artery (ACA) and internal cerebral vein (ICV) across the midline.

The initial vascular displacements caused by subfalcine herniation may be relatively minor, with only minimal displacement of the ACA and ICV (Fig. 14-1A). With larger herniations, gross shifts of the A2 and A3 ACA segments under the falx take place. Even with very large herniations, the displaced ACA returns to the midline as it passes posterosuperiorly and angles back under the falx (see Figs. 14-4B and 14-5B).

Anterior cerebral artery displacement patterns as seen on anteroposterior (AP) carotid angiograms suggest the general location of the mass effect (computed tomography [CT] and MR are more accurate indicators). A *proximal ACA shift* occurs with anteriorly located masses, such as an inferofrontal or anterior temporal lesion (Fig. 14-3). A *distal ACA shift* is seen with more posterior masses. These are usually found in the parietal and occipital lobes, as well as the posterior temporal lobes (Fig. 14-4). A *"square" ACA shift* suggests a mass in the temporal lobe (Fig. 14-5),

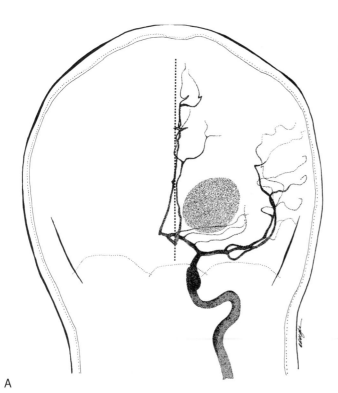

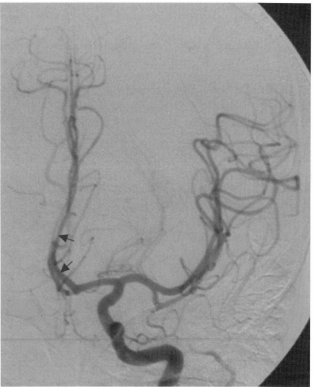

A   B

FIG. 14-3. Anatomic drawing **(A)** and left internal carotid angiogram, AP view **(B)**, show a proximal shift of the anterior cerebral artery across the midline **(B**, *arrows*). This appearance is usually caused by a mass **(A**, *dotted area*) located in the anterior frontal or temporal lobes.

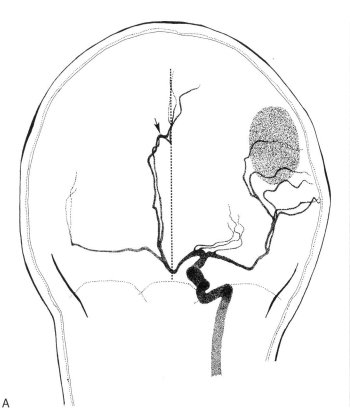
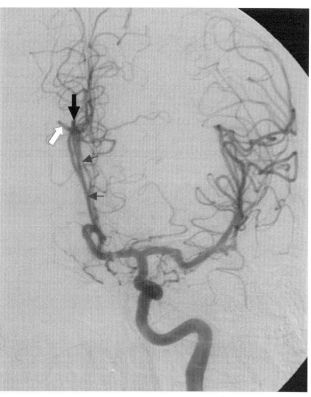

A

B

FIG. 14-4. Anatomic diagram **(A)** and left internal carotid angiogram, AP view **(B)**, show a distal ACA shift **(B**, *small arrows*). This appearance is usually caused by a mass **(A**, *dotted area)* located in the posterior parietal or temporal lobe. Note abrupt angulation of the ACA as it returns to midline under the falx cerebri (*large arrows*). The vascular blush of the pericallosal pial plexus is tilted and displaced by the herniating cingulate gyrus **(B**, *open arrow)*.

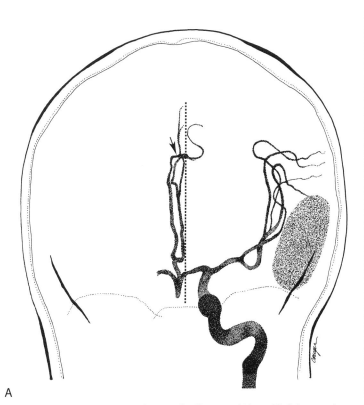
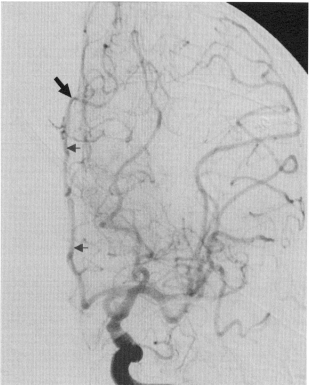

A

B

FIG. 14-5. Anatomic diagram **(A)** and left internal carotid angiogram, AP view **(B)**, show a "square" ACA shift **(B**, *small arrows)*. This appearance is usually caused by a holotemporal lobe mass **(A**, *dotted area)*. Note abrupt ACA angulation as it returns to midline under the falx (*large arrow)*.

whereas a *"round" ACA shift* occurs with deep frontal (often insular and basal ganglionic) masses (Fig. 14-6).

Side-to-side *ICV displacement* is another angiographic sign of subfalcine herniation. With small or anteriorly located masses, there may be no discernible ICV displacement. Larger mass effects cause distinct ICV displacement (Fig. 14-7A). Very large masses displace both the thalamostriate vein (TSV) and ICV across the midline. As the ICV courses posteriorly toward the falcotentorial junction, it must return toward the midline. This large TSV–ICV displacement pattern is sometimes called the *alpha sign* because it resembles the Greek letter alpha.

Pseudoshifts or *negative mass effects* are ACA and ICV displacements that are caused by volume loss in the opposite hemisphere instead of a mass effect on the same side (Fig. 14-8). Slight rotation of the patient's head also may produce a spurious appearance of subfalcial ACA shift.

Transtentorial Herniation

Two types of herniations occur across the tentorial incisura: descending and ascending tentorial herniation.

Descending transtentorial herniation (DTH) is the second most common intracranial herniation. The uncus and parahippocampal gyrus are initially displaced medially and protrude over the medial edge of the tentorium. The anterior choroidal, posterior communicating, and posterior cerebral arteries are all displaced inferomedially in severe descending herniations (Fig. 14-9; see also Fig. 12-26B and C). As the temporal lobes protrude downward through the tentorial incisura, they also displace the superior cerebellar arteries inferiorly (see Fig. 14-13A).

Ascending transtentorial herniation is much less common than descending displacement of the temporal lobe through the tentorial notch. The central lobule, culmen, and superior surface of the cerebellum are displaced upward through the incisura (6). Angiographic findings are those of a large posterior fossa mass effect with upward displacement of the superior cerebellar arteries (Fig. 14-10A) (7). With very severe herniations, the proximal posterior cerebral arteries (PCAs) are also displaced superiorly as the cerebellum is forced upward through the incisura (Fig. 14-10B).

Transalar Herniation

Transalar herniation, also known as transsphenoidal herniation, is less common than either subfalcine or transtentorial displacements. Two types of herniations

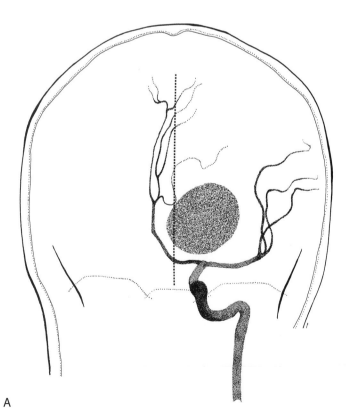
A

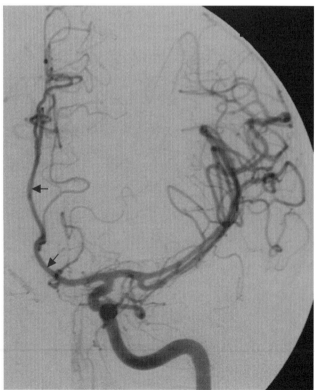
B

FIG. 14-6. Anatomic diagram **(A)** and left internal carotid angiogram, AP view **(B)**, show a "round" ACA shift **(B**, *small arrows*). This appearance is usually caused by a deep frontal or basal ganglionic mass **(A**, *dotted area*).

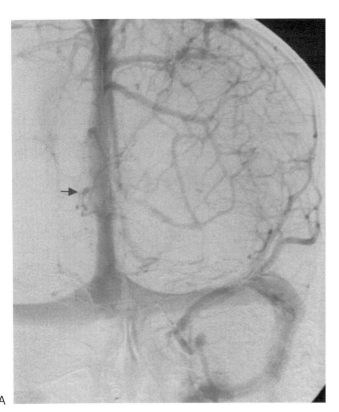

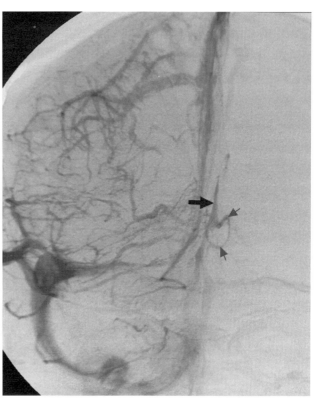

A   B

FIG. 14-7. Anteroposterior venous phase studies in two different patients show side-to-side internal cerebral vein (ICV) displacements. **A:** A relatively small left-sided mass effect displaces the ICV (*arrow*) across the midline (same case as seen in Fig. 14-4B). **B:** Alpha sign with a larger mass. The thalamostriate (TSV) and internal cerebral veins (*small arrows*) are both displaced across the midline. The ICV returns to the midline to join the straight sinus (*large arrow*). The loop formed by the TSV and ICV resembles the Greek letter alpha.

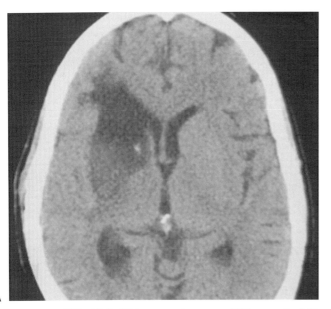

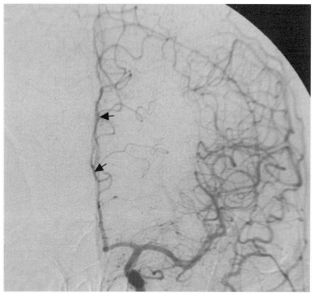

A   B

FIG. 14-8. This case shows an ACA pseudoshift caused by atrophy. **A:** NECT scan shows postinfarction encephalomalacia of the basal ganglia. **B:** Left internal carotid angiogram, arterial phase, AP view, shows slight left-to-right subfalcine ACA displacement (*small arrows*) caused by volume loss in the right hemisphere instead of a mass effect on the left side.

occur across the sphenoid wing: descending and ascending transalar herniation.

Descending transalar herniation is less common than the ascending variety. The frontal lobe is forced posteriorly over the greater sphenoid ala, causing posterior displacement of the middle cerebral artery (MCA) and sylvian triangle (Fig. 14-11).

Ascending transalar herniation is caused by large temporal lobe masses. The MCA is displaced upward and over the sphenoid ridge. The sylvian triangle is compressed, rotated, and elevated (Fig. 14-12; see also Fig. 14-9A for a more severe example of ascending transalar herniation).

Tonsillar Herniation

Two thirds of patients with upward and one half of those with downward transtentorial shift have concurrent tonsillar herniation (6). With large posterior fossa mass effects of any etiology, the cerebellar tonsils are displaced inferiorly through the foramen magnum (4). Angiographic signs include downward displacement of the posterior inferior cerebellar artery (PICA) and its tonsillar branches through the foramen magnum (Fig. 14-13A). Venous phase studies may demonstrate angulation of the inferior vermian and tonsillar veins over the rim of the foramen magnum (Fig. 14-13B).

Clinical Symptoms of Cerebral Herniations

A pupil-involving *oculomotor palsy* is often the earliest focal sign of descending transtentorial herniation. The oculomotor nerve (cranial nerve [CN] III) is compressed as the uncus herniates medially into the incisura.

As herniation progresses and the mid-brain is forced against the opposite side of the tentorium, the uncrossed contralateral corticospinal and corticobulbar pathways may become ischemic. This results in paresis or paralysis that is ipsilateral to the mass effect, a phenomenon sometimes called a *false localizing sign* (3). The visible grooving produced by mid-brain compression against the tentorium is known as *Kernohan's notch.*

Complications of Cerebral Herniations

Hydrocephalus as well as *coma* and *respiratory arrest* may occur with severe cerebral herniations. Compression and stretching of arteries and veins with gross brain displacements may cause circulatory disturbances in the cerebral hemispheres and brainstem. Because the positions of arteries as they cross dural folds differ from patient to patient, the precise location of vascular disturbances and subsequent symptoms of herniation syndromes are also somewhat variable (8).

Occipital infarction is the most common ischemic complication. It occurs when the PCA is compressed against the tentorial incisura by a herniating temporal lobe (4).

Less common ischemic complications of brain herniations include *superomedial hemisphere (ACA territory) infarcts.* Here subfalcine herniation of the cingulate gyrus compresses the callosomarginal artery against the inferior (free) margin of the falx cerebri. *Basal ganglionic infarcts*

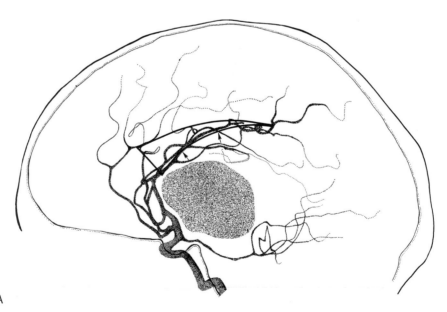

A

FIG. 14-9. Anatomic diagram **(A)** and right cerebral angiogram, lateral view **(B–D)**, show descending transtentorial (DTH) and ascending transalar (ATH) herniation caused by a large temporal lobe hematoma secondary to partially thrombosed AVM. **A:** A large mass (*dotted area*) elevates the sylvian triangle (*arrows*) up and over the greater sphenoid wing (ATH). Note inferior displacement of a fetal posterior cerebral artery (DTH).

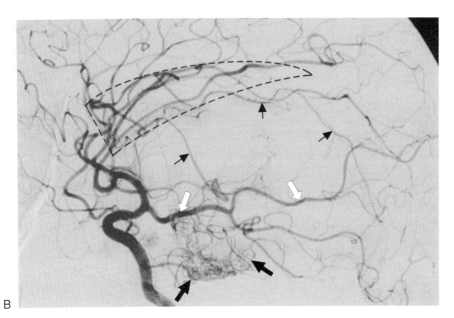

B

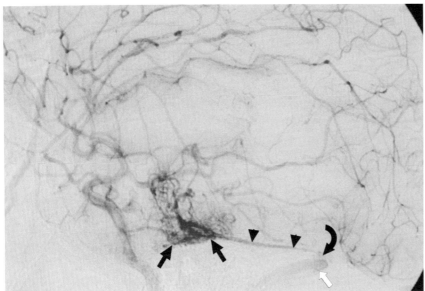

C

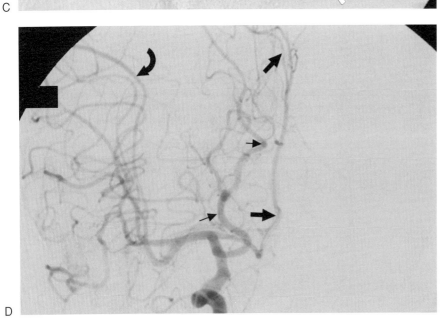

D

FIG. 14-9. *Continued.* Mid- (**B**) and late (**C**) arterial phase films of the carotid angiogram, lateral view, show a large mass effect with elevation of the sylvian triangle (**B**, *dotted lines*) and stretching and draping of MCA temporal lobe branches (*small arrows*). A cluster of abnormal vessels is seen (**B** and **C**, *large arrows*). The PCA is displaced downward (*open arrows*). Early opacification of the superior petrosal sinus (SPS) (**C**, *arrowheads*) is seen. The SPS is narrowed, irregular, and partially thrombosed (**C**, *curved arrow*) at its junction with the faintly opacified sigmoid sinus (**C**, *curved arrow*). **D:** AP view shows square ACA shift (subfalcine herniation) (*large arrows*) and medial displacement of the PCA (*small arrows*) secondary to DTH. The sylvian point (*curved arrow*) is elevated by the temporal lobe hematoma.

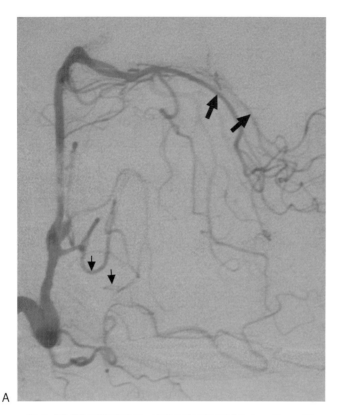

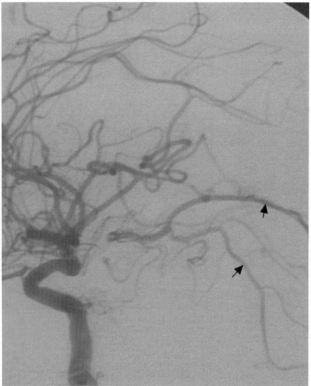

FIG. 14-10. Ascending transtentorial herniation secondary to marked posterior fossa mass effect is shown. **A:** Vertebral angiogram, lateral view, shows striking upward displacement of the superior cerebellar and posterior cerebral arteries (*large arrows*) and anteroinferior displacement of the posterior inferior cerebellar artery (PICA) and its branches (*small arrows*). **B:** Internal carotid angiogram, lateral view, with transient filling of the posterior cerebellar arteries (PCAs), shows elevation, stretching, and draping of the PCA and its branches (*arrows*) caused by ascending herniation of the cerebellum through the tentorial incisura.

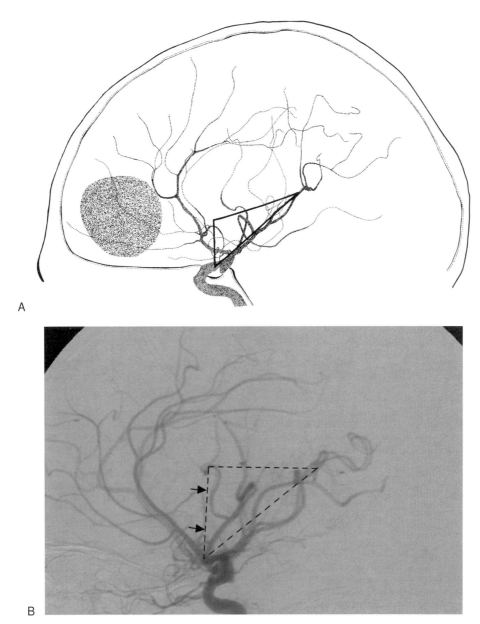

FIG. 14-11. A: Anatomic diagram depicts descending transalar herniation caused by a large frontal mass (*dotted area*). Note posterior and inferior displacement of the sylvian triangle, shown with the solid lines. **B:** Internal carotid angiogram, arterial phase, lateral view, shows posterior displacement of the sylvian triangle (*dotted lines*) (same case as seen in Fig. 14-3B).

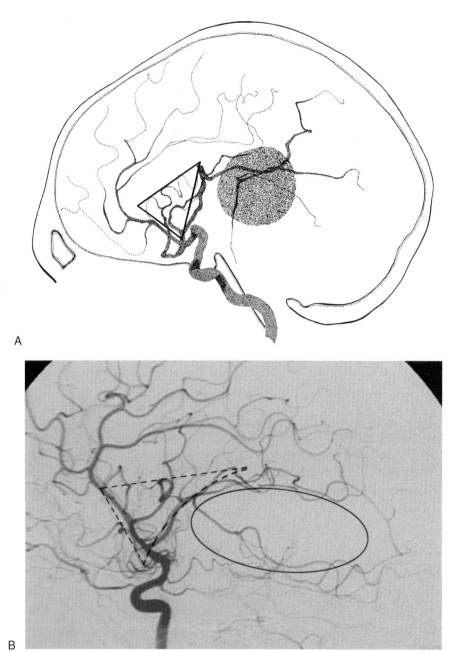

FIG. 14-12. A: Anatomic diagram depicts ascending transalar herniation caused by a large posterior temporal lobe mass (*dotted area*). The sylvian triangle, shown with the solid lines, is displaced antero-superiorly over the sphenoid wing. **B:** Left internal carotid angiogram, arterial phase, lateral view, shows an avascular temporal lobe mass (*circle*) with elevation and anterior displacement of the sylvian triangle (*dotted lines*).

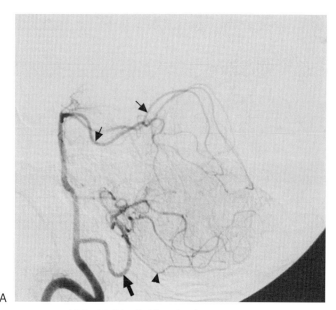
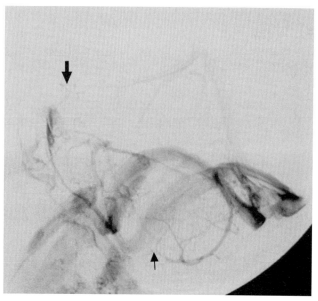

FIG. 14-13. A: Vertebral angiogram, arterial phase, lateral view, in a patient with DTH and secondary tonsillar herniation (same case as seen in Fig. 14-9). The temporal lobe has herniated inferiorly through the tentorial incisura (see Fig. 14-9B–D), displacing the superior cerebellar arteries downward (*arrows*). Inferior displacement of the lateral medullary loop of the PICA (*large arrow*) and its tonsillar branches (*arrowhead*) indicates tonsillar herniation. **B:** Venous phase of the angiogram shows inferior displacement and kinking of the pontomedullary venous plexus (*large arrow*). Note angulation of the inferior vermian veins over the rim of the foramen magnum (*small arrow*).

occur with severe descending transtentorial herniation. Perforating branches from the circle of Willis are occluded as they are kinked or occluded against the skull base (9,10).

INTRACRANIAL NEOPLASMS

Intracranial tumors have both direct and indirect angiographic findings. Direct abnormalities include enlargement of arteries that supply a vascular neoplasm, visualization of abnormal vessels within the tumor (tumor blush and neovascularity), arteriovenous shunting, oncotic pseudoaneurysms, and vascular encasement and occlusion. Indirect abnormalities are primarily those of vascular displacement.

Direct Abnormalities

Arterial Enlargement

Vessels that supply vascular neoplasms may enlarge, reflecting increased blood flow to the tumor (see Figs. 14-15A, 14-18A, and 14-21A). The increase in size is rarely as striking as occurs with arteriovenous malformations and fistulae.

Blush

An accumulation of contrast called a blush or stain is sometimes observed on the late arterial or early capillary phase of cerebral angiograms. *An angiographic blush is not pathognomonic for neoplasm.* It occurs normally in some relatively vascular areas such as the basal ganglia (see Fig. 7-16B) and simply reflects increased capillary density.

An abnormal vascular blush is a nonspecific angiographic finding and may occur with trauma, infection, cerebral ischemia, and increased metabolic activity accompanying prolonged seizures (see Chapter 16).

Tumor blush also may represent increased vessel density secondary to neoplastic vascular proliferation. A spectrum of both benign and malignant intracranial neoplasms demonstrate a uniform, prolonged vascular blush on cerebral angiograms. Examples of tumors for which angiograms are sometimes obtained prior to surgery or neurointerventional procedures include meningioma, invasive pituitary adenoma, choroid plexus papilloma, and hemangioblastoma.

Meningioma is the most common nonglial primary brain tumor. Grossly, meningiomas are usually sharply circumscribed lesions that have a distinct tumor–brain interface. A cleft of arachnoid with trapped CSF and prominent vessels often surrounds these tumors (Fig. 14-14). Microscopically, meningiomas are histologically heterogeneous lesions that are divided into three basic categories: (a) meningioma (i.e., the common "benign" meningioma), (b) atypical meningioma, and (c) anaplastic (malignant) meningioma.

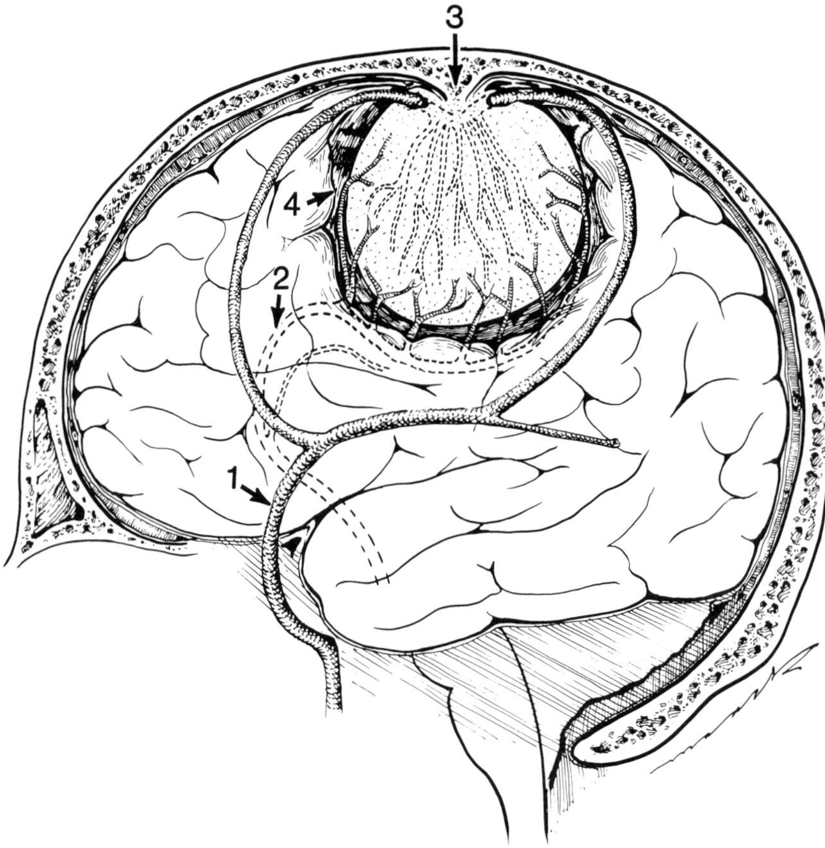

FIG. 14-14. Anatomic drawing, lateral view, shows a large convexity meningioma invaginating into the brain. The overlying skull has been removed for purposes of illustration, leaving the middle meningeal artery (MMA) intact. The dual vascular supply that is characteristic for a large meningioma is depicted. The major vascular supply is via the enlarged MMA. As shown here, dural vessels typically supply the *center* of a meningioma. Note the sunburst of vessels (*small dotted lines*) that radiates outwards from the central vascular pedicle at the enostotic spur. Pial branches, shown here as arising from the anterior cerebral artery (*large dotted lines*), typically supply the *periphery* of meningiomas. A characteristic cleft of trapped cerebrospinal fluid (CSF) and vessels is present between the tumor and the displaced cortex.

1, Enlarged middle meningeal artery
2, Displaced anterior cerebral artery
3, Enostotic spur with central vascular pedicle at attachment of the meningioma
4, CSF-vascular cleft

Angiographically, most meningiomas are very vascular tumors that are initially supplied by a "sunburst" of vessels from hypertrophied meningeal arteries (Fig. 14-15A). Late arterial and capillary phase films often show a prolonged homogeneous vascular blush (Fig. 14-15B). The internal carotid or vertebral angiogram may show only an avascular mass effect (Fig. 14-15C and D). The periphery of larger tumors can be supplied by parasitized pial vessels (Figs. 14-14 and 14-16).

The angiographic patterns of meningioma vary widely and are not well correlated with tumor grade. Some histologically typical meningiomas exhibit neovascularity with arteriovenous shunting. Benign meningiomas may grow into, and subsequently occlude, an adjacent dural sinus (Fig. 14-17).

Pituitary adenomas are common extraaxial neoplasms. Angiography is now performed only when these tumors are invasive and radical skull base surgery is planned. Angiographic findings with pituitary adenomas include vascular displacement and a prolonged, relatively uniform vascular blush (Fig. 14-18; see also Fig. 14-22).

Hemangioblastomas are uncommon tumors of unknown origin. They account for approximately 7% of

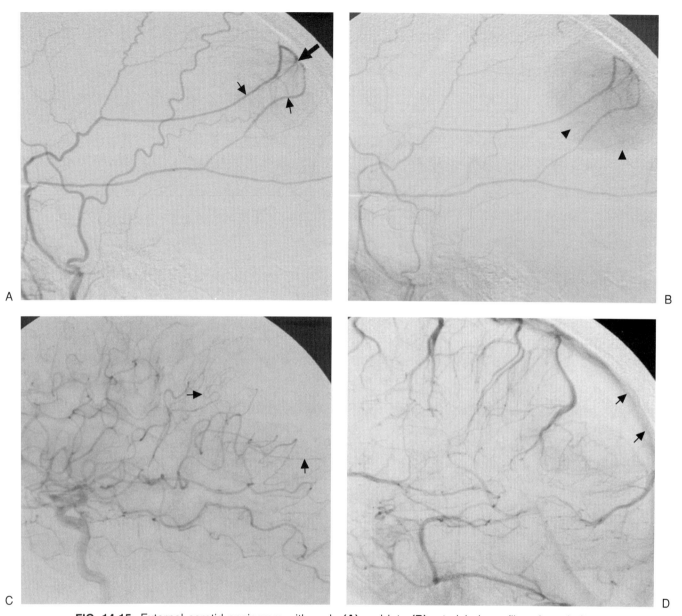

FIG. 14-15. External carotid angiogram with early **(A)** and late **(B)** arterial phase films, lateral view, shows that enlarged branches of the middle meningeal artery (*small arrows*) supply a dural-based vascular tumor (**A**, *large arrow*). Note prolonged contrast accumulation (**B**, *arrowheads*). **C:** Internal carotid angiogram, late arterial phase, lateral view, shows an avascular mass effect with focal stretching and draping of distal pial branches (*small arrows*). **D:** Venous phase shows that the mass has slightly compressed the superior sagittal sinus (*arrows*), but it is still patent. A typical meningioma was surgically removed.

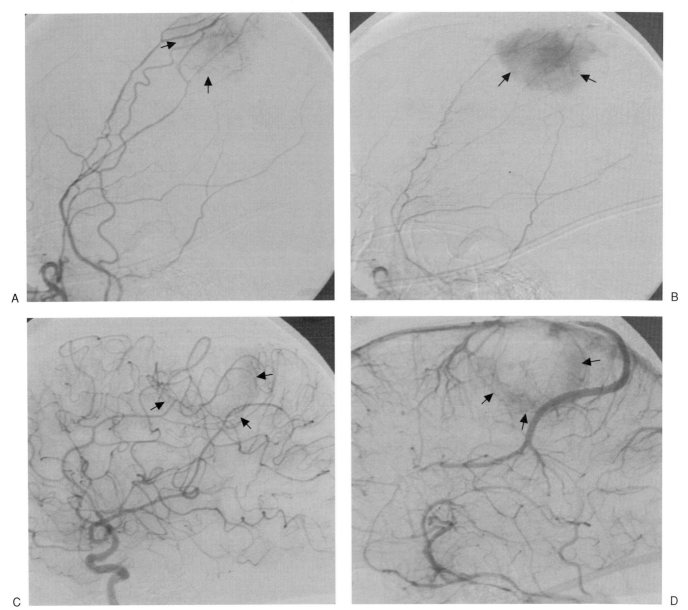

FIG. 14-16. This typical meningioma shows dual external and internal carotid artery supply. External carotid angiogram with early **(A)** and late **(B)** arterial phase films, lateral view, shows that enlarged middle meningeal arteries supply the center of a convexity meningioma (*arrows*). Internal carotid angiogram with arterial **(C)** and venous **(D)** phase films, lateral view, shows pial supply (*arrows*) to the rim of the tumor.

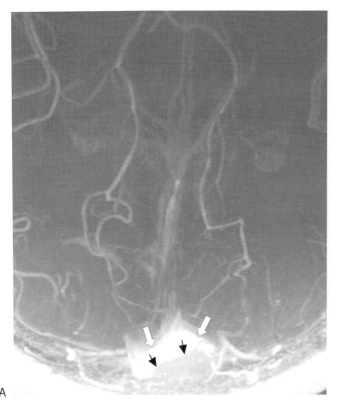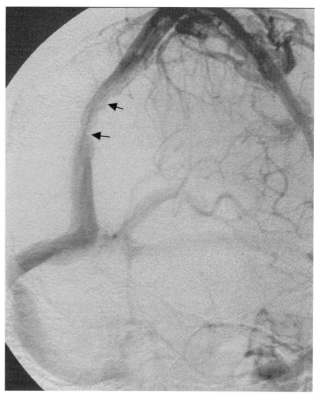

A   B

FIG. 14-17. A small falcine meningioma with invasion of the superior sagittal sinus (SSS) is illustrated. **A:** Axial view of a high-resolution contrast-enhanced MR angiogram shows that the tumor (*small black arrows*) invades, but does not occlude, the SSS (*large white arrows*). **B:** Left internal carotid angiogram, venous phase, oblique view, shows the SSS invasion (*arrows*).

primary posterior fossa tumors in adults. Although 10% to 20% are associated with von Hippel-Lindau syndrome (VHL), most occur sporadically. Multiple hemangiomas may occur and are diagnostic of VHL. About 60% of hemangioblastomas are cystic masses with a mural nodule that abuts a pial surface; 40% are solid (4).

Angiographic findings are those of a cystic (or solid) posterior fossa mass with a very vascular mural nodule. Intense, prolonged contrast accumulation that persists into the capillary phase is typical (Fig. 14-19).

Neovascularity

Microvascular proliferation in tumors can be induced by angiogenic growth factors. Neoplastic angioarchitectural changes include formation of new blood vessels (neovascularity), development of microaneurysms, venous ectasia, and vessel distention. Neovascularity often occurs in conjunction with physio-

logic or ultrastructural disruptions in the blood–brain barrier (1).

The angiographic manifestations of neovascularity include an increase in vascular density within the tumor bed, irregular and bizarre-appearing vessels, laking and pooling of contrast, pseudoaneurysms, and arteriovenous shunting. These angiographic findings occur with highly malignant primary brain tumors such as *glioblastoma multiforme* and *anaplastic oligodendroglioma* (see Figs. 12-12 and 12-13). Identical findings can be seen with metastases from vascular extracranial primary tumors (Fig. 14-20).

Arteriovenous Shunting

Arteriovenous shunting is characterized angiographically by abnormally early venous opacification (*early draining veins*). Although it is often seen with *high-grade astrocytomas* and *metastases* (Fig. 14-20), arteriovenous shunting is not pathognomonic for neoplasm. It often

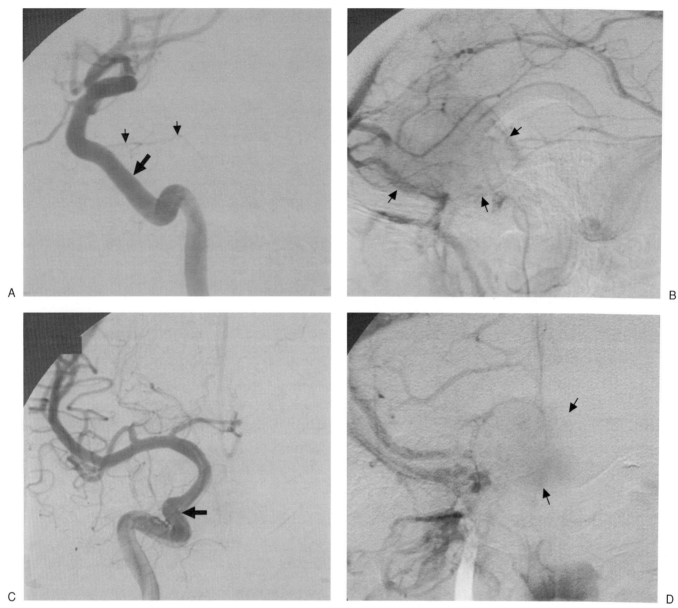

FIG. 14-18. Invasive pituitary adenoma. Early arterial **(A)** and venous phase **(B)** films of a right internal carotid angiogram, lateral view, show that an enlarged meningohypophyseal artery (**A**, *arrows*) supplies a mass that has a uniform vascular blush persisting into the early venous phase (**B**, *arrows*). Arterial **(C)** and venous phase **(D)** films, AP view, show the vascular mass (**D**, *small arrows*). Note lateral (**C**, *large arrow*) and inferior (**A**, *large arrow*) displacement of the internal carotid artery by the mass. An invasive pituitary adenoma was resected.

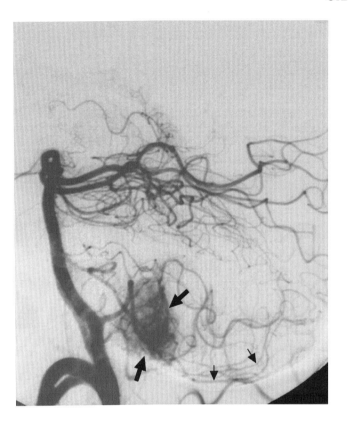

FIG. 14-19. Left vertebral angiogram, arterial phase, lateral view, shows a very vascular mass (*large arrows*) that is supplied by branches from the posterior inferior cerebellar artery (PICA). Note stretching and draping of PICA hemispheric branches by an avascular mass effect (*small arrows*). A typical cystic cerebellar hemangioblastoma with mural nodule was resected.

occurs with benign lesions such as arteriovenous malformations and fistulae. Other causes for so-called early draining veins include cerebral ischemia, contusion, and prolonged seizures (see box below).

Neoplastic arteriovenous shunting results from two distinct processes: (a) the development of abnormal arteriovenous connections secondary to tumor angiogenesis and (b) physiologic changes resulting from tumor elaboration of various vasoactive factors as well as necrosis, hemorrhage, and local effects (e.g., metabolic changes and alterations in pH) (1).

Vascular Displacement, Encasement, and Occlusion

Intracranial tumors often displace and encase adjacent arteries. Classic examples are changes in the internal carotid and vertebrobasilar arteries that occur with large skull base tumors such as pituitary adenoma, meningioma, and chordoma (Figs. 14-21 and 14-22).

Frank arterial occlusions and strokes are uncommon manifestations of intracranial neoplasms. In contrast, cortical vein occlusions and dural sinus invasion do occur.

Early Draining Veins on Cerebral Angiograms

Nonneoplastic etiology	Neoplasm
Common	Common
Cerebral ischemia with "luxury perfusion"	Glioblastoma multiforme
Arteriovenous malformation or fistula	Vascular metastasis
Rare	Uncommon
Metabolic (postictal)	Meningioma
Infection (abscess, encephalitis)	Hemangioblastoma
Trauma (contusion)	Paraganglioma

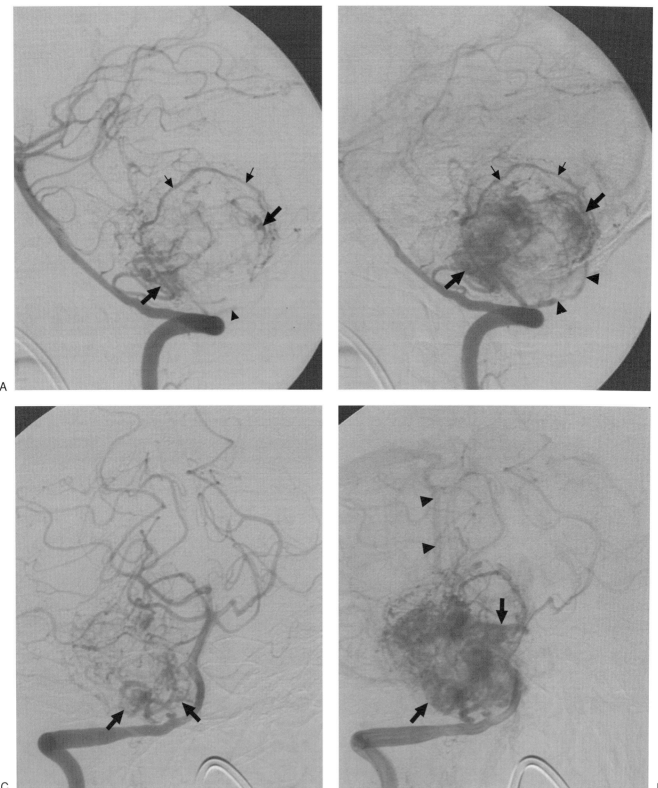

FIG. 14-20. Neovascularity is illustrated by this case of a posterior fossa metastasis. Right vertebral angiogram with early **(A)** and late **(B)** arterial phase films shows that an enlarged posterior inferior cerebellar artery (*small arrows*) supplies a vascular mass with bizarre-appearing vessels and laking and pooling of contrast (*large arrows*). Arteriovenous shunting is present (*arrowheads*). Early **(C)** and late **(D)** arterial phase films, AP view, show the mass (*large arrows*) with early opacification of draining veins (*arrowheads*).

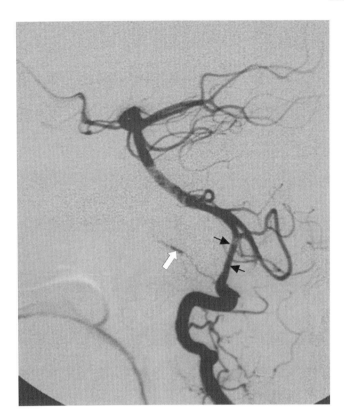

FIG. 14-21. Left vertebral angiogram, arterial phase, lateral view, in a patient with a large skull base tumor shows posterior displacement and encasement of the vertebral artery (*black arrows*). A small branch (*white arrow*) supplies the hypovascular mass.

A

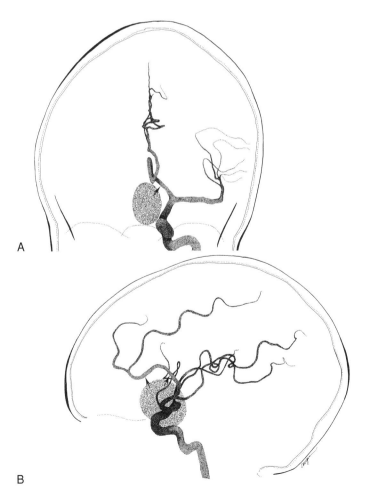

B

FIG. 14-22. AP **(A)** and lateral **(B)** anatomic diagrams depict a pituitary adenoma (*dotted area*) with suprasellar extension. Note elevation and displacement of the anterior cerebral artery (ACA) (*arrows*).

(Continued)

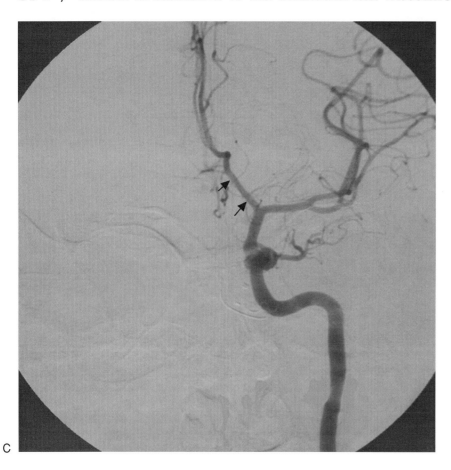

C

FIG. 14-22. *Continued.* **C:** Left internal carotid angiogram, arterial phase, AP view, shows elevation of the horizontal (A1) ACA segment (*arrows*) by an avascular mass. A large pituitary adenoma was resected.

Venous stenosis and occlusion are more common with extraaxial tumors such as meningiomas and dural metastases (Fig. 14-17).

EXTRACRANIAL NEOPLASMS

Diagnostic angiography in patients with extracranial neoplasms is often obtained when initial imaging studies show the lesion is highly vascular, may have difficult surgical access, invades the skull base, or is intimately related to important vessels such as the carotid artery (11). Delineating vascular supply and identifying potentially dangerous collateral blood flow patterns is also an essential part of neurointerventional procedures in these patients.

Benign Extracranial Tumors

Angiography is often performed for evaluating and treating juvenile nasopharyngeal angiofibromas (JNAs), glomus tumors, and meningiomas.

Juvenile Nasopharyngeal Angiofibroma

Juvenile nasopharyngeal angiofibroma is a highly vascular benign neoplasm that occurs almost exclusively in adolescent boys, although rare cases in females have been well documented. Juvenile nasopharyngeal angiofibroma is rare in the United States and Europe but is more common in the Near and Far east and accounts for only 0.5% of all head and neck tumors. Nasal obstruction and epistaxis are the most common presenting symptoms (12).

Juvenile nasopharyngeal angiofibromas originate near the sphenopalatine foramen and spread via natural foramina and fissures into the nose, pterygopalatine fossa, orbit, sphenoid sinus, and cavernous sinus.

Angiographic findings in JNA include an enlarged, displaced internal maxillary artery that supplies a lobulated vascular mass within the pterygopalatine fossa. An intense, prolonged vascular stain is typical, although early draining veins are uncommon (Fig. 14-23). Other vessels such as the ascending pharyngeal and the vidian arteries may supply JNAs (Fig. 14-24). Preoperative embolization of these very vascular lesions is often performed to decrease blood loss during surgery (12).

Paraganglioma

Paragangliomas, also known as glomus tumors and chemodectomas, arise from neural crest derivatives. They are neuroendocrine tumors that are histologically similar to adrenal pheochromocytoma and paraaortic sympa-

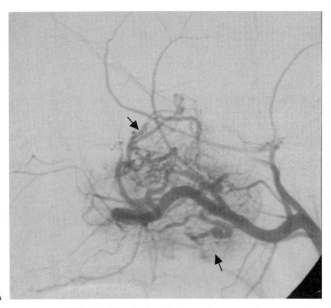
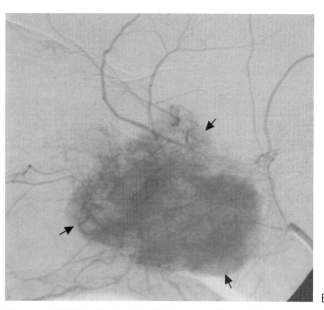

A   B

FIG. 14-23. A classic juvenile nasopharyngeal angiofibroma (JNA) is illustrated. A left external carotid angiogram with early **(A)** and late **(B)** arterial phase films, lateral view, shows the lobulated vascular mass (*arrows*). Note prolonged, relatively uniform contrast accumulation.

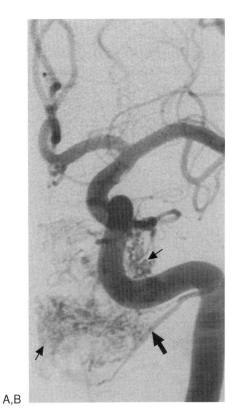
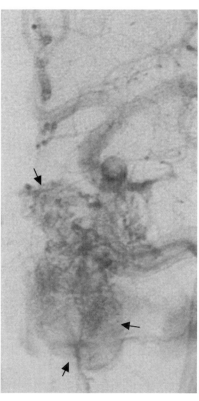
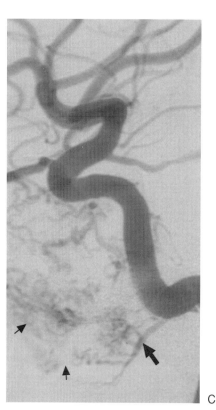

A,B   C

FIG. 14-24. A large juvenile nasopharyngeal angiofibroma is shown that has significant vascular supply from the vidian artery, a branch of the petrous internal carotid artery. Left internal carotid angiogram with early **(A)** and late arterial **(B)** phase films, AP view, shows that the enlarged vidian artery **(A**, *large arrow*) supplies the vascular mass **(A** and **B**, *small arrows*). **C:** Lateral view shows that the vidian artery (*large arrow*) supplies the vascular mass (*small arrows*).

thetic paragangliomas. There is no known association with neurofibromatosis or multiple endocrine neoplasia syndromes.

Paragangliomas usually become symptomatic between the ages of 40 and 60. Most present with cranial neuropathy or a slowly enlarging neck mass. Secretory activity is rare, with less than 5% demonstrating catecholamine or serotonin production. Although angiography can precipitate hypertensive crisis, the risk is relatively small (11).

Paragangliomas are found in many locations and are named by site. *Glomus tympanicum* tumors are middle ear paragangliomas that arise from Jacobson's nerve. They typically—but not invariably—occur on the cochlear promontory and may cause pulsatile tinnitus. *Glomus jugulare* tumors arise advintinia of the jugular fossa and thus often present with CN IX to XI neuropathy. The term *glomus jugulotympanicum* is used when a large glomus jugulare tumor grows into the middle ear (12a).

A *carotid body tumor*, another form of glomus tumor, occurs at the carotid bifurcation and represents one third of head and neck paragangliomas. *Glomus vagale* and *juxtavagale* tumors account for about 10%; all other sites

are rare. Multifocal tumors occur in about 10% of cases. A familial form has been described that has an increased incidence of multiple tumors (30% of cases) (11).

Glomus tumors have striking angiographic findings. Paragangliomas appear similar regardless of location. A round or lobulated, well-delineated vascular mass with dense, prolonged contrast accumulation is typical (Fig. 14-25). Vessel encasement and narrowing may occur with larger tumors (Fig. 14-26). Arteriovenous shunting with early draining veins also occurs (Fig. 14-27). Glomus jugulare tumors often occlude the jugular vein (Fig. 14-27B).

Meningiomas and Schwannomas

Inferior extension from a skull base or intracranial *meningioma* is common. However, only 1% of meningiomas occur outside the CNS dura. The most common extracranial, extraspinal site is the paranasal sinuses.

Schwannomas arise from the neural sheath of peripheral, spinal, or cranial nerves. They are relatively uncommon lesions; the head and neck, including the CNS, is by far their most common location. Almost two thirds of schwannomas occur in the CNS; the vestibulocochlear

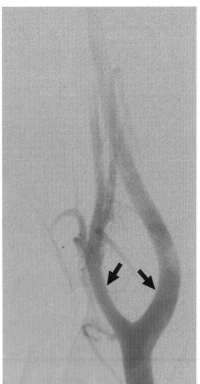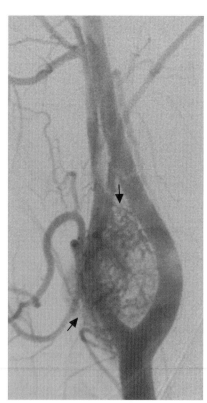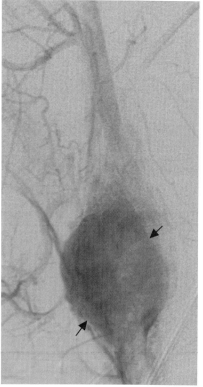

A,B

C

FIG. 14-25. A common carotid angiogram with early **(A)**, mid- **(B)**, and late **(C)** arterial phase films, lateral view, shows a classic carotid body tumor. Note splaying apart of the external and internal carotid arteries (**A**, *arrows*) by the mass. Contrast accumulates in the tumor (**B and C**, *small arrows*), as shown by the prolonged, intense vascular stain.

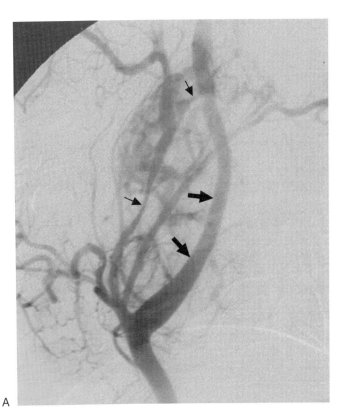
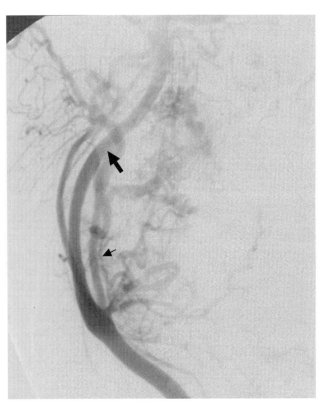

A

B

FIG. 14-26. Lateral **(A)** and anteroposterior **(B)** views of a right common carotid angiogram show a very vascular tumor with marked displacement of the internal carotid artery (*large arrows*). Note stretched, draped, and encased external carotid artery branches (*small arrows*). A paraganglioma, probably arising from the carotid body, was resected.

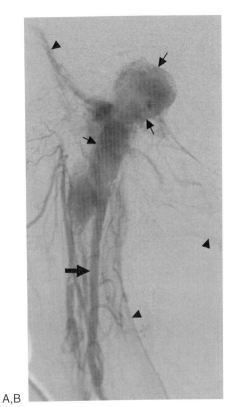
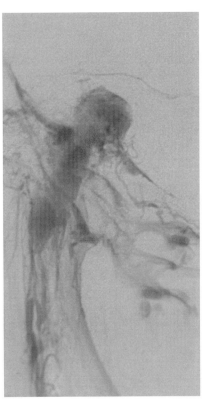
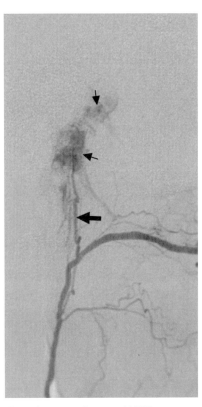

A,B

C

FIG. 14-27. A classic glomus jugulare tumor is illustrated. Selective ascending pharyngeal artery (APA) angiogram with mid- **(A)** and late **(B)** arterial phase films, lateral view, shows that an enlarged APA **(A,** *large arrow*) supplies a very vascular tumor **(A,** *small arrows*). The sigmoid sinus is occluded by the tumor, and contrast appears early in the internal jugular vein, clival venous plexus, and occipital venous plexus **(A,** *arrowheads*). The collateral venous drainage is particularly striking on the late arterial phase **(B)**. **C:** Selective injection of the occipital artery shows that an enlarged stylomastoid branch (*large arrow*) also supplies the tumor (*small arrows*).

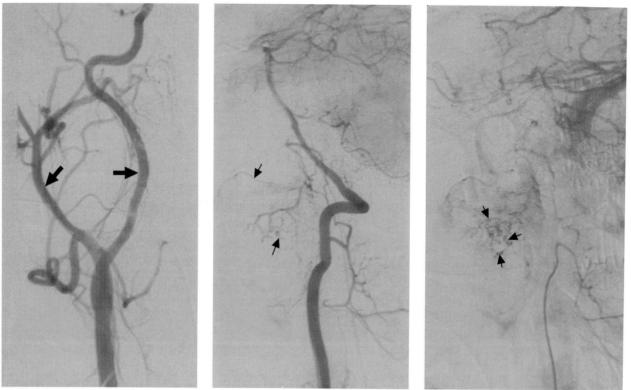

FIG. 14-28. A: Anteroposterior view of a right common carotid angiogram, early arterial phase, shows anteromedial internal carotid artery and lateral external carotid artery displacement around an avascular mass (*arrows*). Right vertebral angiogram, with mid- **(B)** and late **(C)** arterial phase films, lateral view, shows vascular supply to the mass (**B**, *arrows*) and scattered clusters of contrast puddles (**C**, *arrows*). A vagal schwannoma was found at surgery.

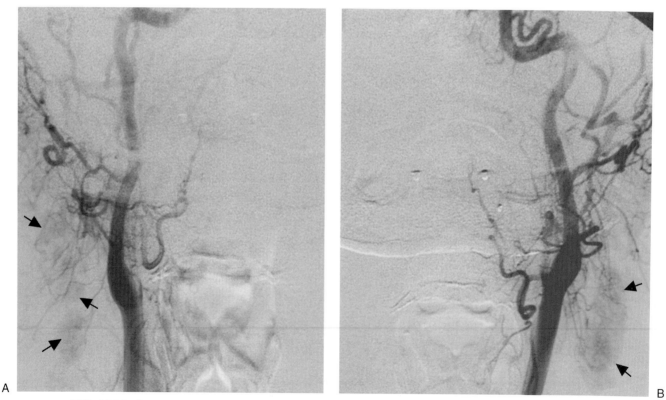

FIG. 14-29. Anteroposterior views of right **(A)** and left **(B)** common carotid angiograms show multiple bilateral foci of contrast accumulation (*arrows*). Non-neoplastic reactive adenopathy.

nerve (CN VIII) is the most common site. They can occur at any anatomic site in the head and neck.

Angiographic findings disclose a moderately vascular or hypovascular mass that displaces adjacent vessels. Tortuous tumor vessels with nonshunting, scattered clusters of contrast "puddles" are seen in many cases (Fig. 14-28) (13).

Tumor Mimics

Reactive adenopathy may occasionally appear vascular on carotid angiograms. Contrast accumulation in these cases produces a mild, prolonged vascular stain. Reactive adenopathy often involves multiple nodes and is frequently bilateral (Fig. 14-29).

Malignant Extracranial Tumors

Malignant head and neck tumors, especially *squamous cell carcinoma*, may encase and invade the carotid arteries (Fig. 14-30). Although this occurs in only 5% to 20%

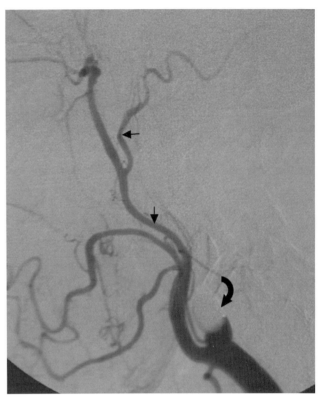

FIG. 14-31. A patient with an extensive squamous cell carcinoma had a balloon test occlusion (*curved arrow*) prior to radical neck dissection. The external carotid artery and some of its branches appear encased and displaced (*arrows*). The patient tolerated the test occlusion well but had a cerebral infarct after carotid ligation during surgery.

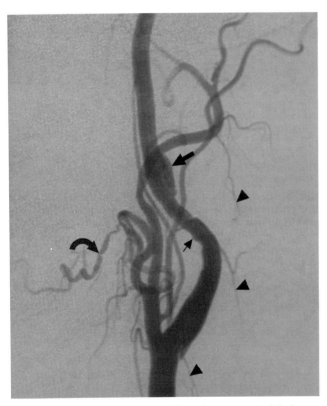

FIG. 14-30. Left common carotid angiogram, arterial phase, oblique view, in a patient with carotid fixation from an extensive, invasive adenoid cystic carcinoma of the tongue. Note encasement and irregularity of the internal carotid artery (*small arrow*) with a pseudoaneurysm (*large arrow*). The lingual artery (*curved arrow*) also appears narrow, irregular, and encased by tumor. Other external carotid artery branches are stretched and draped around the extensive avascular mass (*arrowheads*).

of patients undergoing radical neck dissection, the prognosis in such cases is dismal and the surgical complications are very high (14).

Because angiography is less helpful than CT, ultrasonography, or MR imaging in determining carotid artery invasion, it is used mostly to perform temporary balloon occlusion and predict neurologic complications should carotid ligation become necessary (Fig. 14-31) (15). Transcranial Doppler sonographic monitoring may increase the accuracy of balloon test occlusions in such cases (14).

Angiographic findings in these patients include vessel displacement, encasement, and invasion. Oncotic pseudoaneurysms may cause focal mass effect, transient ischemic attacks, and exsanguinating hemorrhage (Fig. 14-30; see also Fig. 12-14).

REFERENCES

1. Masters LT, Pryor JC, Nelson PK. Angiographic findings associated with intra-axial intracranial tumors. *Neuroimag Clin North Am* 1996;6:739–749.
2. Wilms G, Bosmans H, Marchal D, et al. Magnetic resonance angiog-

raphy of supratentorial tumors: comparison with digital subtraction angiography. *Neuroradiology* 1995;37:42–47.

3. Laine FJ, Shedden AI, Dunn MM, Ghatak NR. Acquired intracranial herniations: MR imaging findings. *AJR* 1995;165:967–973.

4. Osborn AG. Secondary effects of craniocerebral trauma. In: *Diagnostic neuroradiology*. St. Louis: Mosby, 1994:222–229.

5. Neff S, Subramaniam RP. Monro-Kellie doctrine [Letter]. *J Neurosurg* 1996;85:1195.

5a. Bruner JM, Tien RD, Thorstad WL. Structural changes produced by intracranial tumors and by various forms of antineoplastic therapy. In: Bigner DD, McLenden RE, Bruner JM (eds). *Russell and Rubinstein's pathology of tumors of the nervous system, 6th ed.* New York: Oxford University Press, 1998:451–484.

6. Reich JB, Sierra J, Camp W, et al. Magnetic resonance imaging measurements and clinical changes accompanying transtentorial and foramen magnum brain herniation. *Ann Neurol* 1993;33:159–170.

7. Wackenheim A, Braun JP, Babin E, et al. The herniation of the superior cerebellar vermis. *Neuroradiology* 1974;7:221–227.

8. Blinkov SM, Gabibov GA, Tanyashin SV. Variations in location of the arteries coursing between the brainstem and the free edge of the tentorium. *J Neurosurg* 1992;76:973–978.

9. Nguyen JP, Djindjian M, Brugieres P, et al. Correlations anatamo-scanographiques dans les engagements cerebraux transtentoriels. *J Radiol* 1990;71:671–679.

10. Endo M, Ichikawa F, Miyasaka Y, et al. Capsular and thalamic infarction caused by tentorial herniation subsequent to head trauma. *Neuroradiology* 1991;33:296–299.

11. Hu WY, TerBrugge KG. The role of angiography in the evaluation of vascular and neoplastic disease in the external carotid artery circulation. *Neuroimag Clin North Am* 1996;3:625–644.

12. Ungkanont K, Byers RM, Weber RS, et al. Juvenile nasopharyngeal angiofibroma: an update of therapeutic management. *Head Neck* 1996;18:60–66.

12a. Weissman JL, Hirsch BE. Beyond the promontory: the multifocal origin of glomus tympanicum tumors. *AJNR* 1998;19:119–122

13. Abramowitz J, Dion JE, Jensen ME, et al. Angiographic diagnosis and management of head and neck schwannomas. *AJNR* 1991;12:977–984.

14. Yousem DM, Hatabu H, Hurst RW, et al. Carotid artery invasion by head and neck masses: prediction with MR imaging. *Radiology* 1995;195:715–720.

15. Eckert B, Thie A, Carvajal M, et al. Predicting hemodynamic ischemia by transcranial Doppler monitoring during therapeutic balloon occlusion of the internal carotid artery. *AJNR* 1998;19:577–582.

CHAPTER 15

Nonatheromatous Vasculopathy

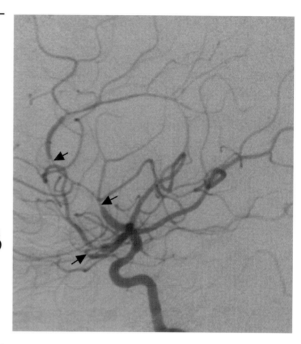

Atherosclerosis is the most common cause of both generalized arterial narrowing and a vasculitislike angiographic pattern. However, a number of nonatheromatous disorders also affect the craniocerebral vessels. In this chapter, the initial focus is on nonatheromatous diseases that cause extracranial vasculopathy, then disorders that affect the intracranial vessels are considered. Atherosclerosis and carotid stenosis are discussed in Chapter 16.

EXTRACRANIAL VASCULOPATHY

Vasculopathy causes both arterial stenosis and enlargement. Nonatheromatous causes of extracranial vascular narrowing span the gamut from congenital abnormalities to neoplastic encasement. Consequently, the angiographic finding of a small great vessel has an extensive differential diagnosis (Fig. 15-1 and Table 15-1) (1). The opposite appearance, i.e., ectasia and fusiform enlargement, is a less common manifestation of nonatheromatous vasculopathy, but this finding has an equally broad differential diagnosis (Table 15-2).

Congenital Abnormalities

Aplasia and Hypoplasia

Congenital absence of an internal carotid artery (ICA) is a rare anomaly that should be diagnosed only if

the bony carotid canal is absent (see Chapter 3). True *ICA hypoplasia* is also uncommon. In contrast, absence or hypoplasia of a vertebral artery is a common normal variant. *Fenestration* or *duplication* of a great vessel is an uncommon cause of vascular narrowing (see Fig. 9-12).

Neurocutaneous Syndromes

Most of the phakomatoses that have vasculopathy as a recognized part of their disease spectrum affect the intracranial vessels; extracranial involvement is comparatively rare. *Neurofibromatosis type 1* (NF-1) may be complicated by arteriovenous fistulae. Tortuosity and fusiform ectasias are less common manifestations of NF-1 (2).

Other Inherited Disorders

Most heritable disorders with craniocervical vasculopathy involve the intracranial vessels. An exception is *Marfan's syndrome*. Cystic medial necrosis (CMN) is the most common characteristic arterial lesion of Marfan's syndrome (see Fig. 12-5). However, CMN is also associated with other disorders and is found in 2% of general autopsy cases (3).

The most common cardiovascular complication of Marfan's syndrome is aortic dissection. It is also the most

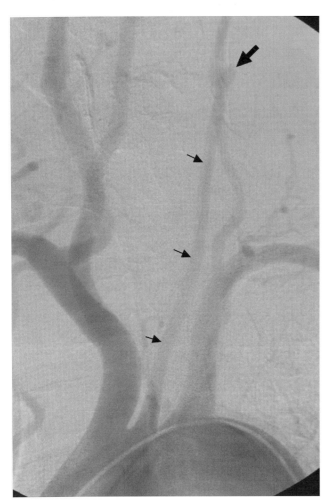

FIG. 15-1. Aortic arch angiogram, arterial phase, LAO view, in a patient with radiation therapy for invasive squamous cell carcinoma of the neck. The left internal carotid artery is occluded just distal to the bulb (*large arrow*). Note diminished caliber of the entire common carotid artery (*small arrows*) secondary to reduced distal flow.

TABLE 15-1. *"Small" great vessel: differential diagnosis*

Etiology	Internal Carotid Artery	Vertebral Artery
Congenital hypoplasia	Rare	Common
Acquired flow reduction	Common	Rare
Dissection	Common	Common
Acute		
Chronic/healed		
Post CEA	Rare	N/A
Vasospasm (catheter, SAH)	Common	Common
Tumor encasement	Common	Rare
Fibromuscular dysplasia	Rare	Rare

CEA, carotid endarterectomy; SAH, subarachnoid hemorrhage.

genic disorders such as catheter-induced vasospasm and stationary "arterial waves" to extracranial vasculitides such as Takayasu's arteritis.

Iatrogenic Narrowing

Catheter-induced vasospasm is a relatively common but transient complication of cerebral angiography. Findings range from smooth or fusiform constrictions to alternating areas of stenosis and dilatation that resemble fibromuscular dysplasia (FMD) (Figs. 15-4 to 15-6). Catheter- or guidewire-induced vasospasm may be severe, causing contrast stasis in the affected vessel that persists into the late venous phase of the angiographic sequence (Fig. 15-7). Most cases rapidly resolve as soon as the catheter is removed. Cerebral ischemia or frank infarction is rare.

Stationary arterial waves, a form of so-called *circular spastic contractions*, are regular, evenly spaced transient

frequent cause of death in adults. Spontaneous dissections that involve the craniocephalic arteries occur but are less common (Fig. 15-2). Ectasia and tortuosity of the extracranial carotid and vertebral arteries are also observed in some cases (see Fig. 12-5A) (4).

Other heritable connective tissue disorders that are associated with spontaneous arterial dissections include *Ehlers-Danlos syndrome type IV* and *autosomal-dominant polycystic kidney disease* (2). Patients with *congenital heart disease* are also at increased risk for both intra- and extracranial arterial dissections (5).

Acquired Disorders

A number of acquired diseases may cause narrowing of the great vessels (Fig. 15-3). These range from iatro-

TABLE 15-2. *Enlarged great vessel: differential diagnosis*

Etiology	Internal Carotid Artery	Vertebral Artery
Age-related	Common	Common (VBD)
Atherosclerosis	Common	Common
Flow-related (AVM/AVF)	Common	Common
Pseudoaneurysm	Common	Rare
Collagen vascular disease (SLE)	Rare	Rare
Takayasu arteritis	Rare	Rare
NF-1	Rare	Rare
Marfan's syndrome	Rare	Rare
Menkes' kinky hair disease	Rare	Rare
Mucocutaneous lymph node (Kawasaki) disease	Rare	Rare

VBD, vertebrobasilar dolichoectasia.

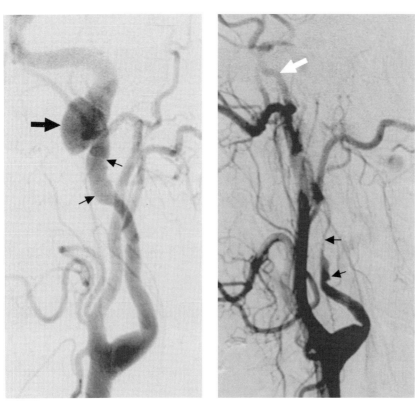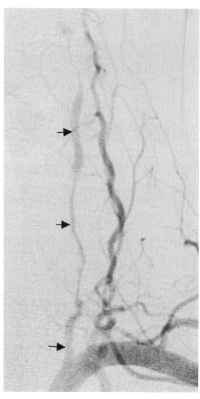

A,B   C

FIG. 15-2. A 34-year-old woman had endured several days of dull headache and neck pain. **A:** Right common carotid angiogram, arterial phase, lateral view, shows a dilated, irregular mid-cervical internal carotid artery (ICA) segment (*small arrows*) with a pseudoaneurysm (*large arrow*). **B:** Left common carotid angiogram, arterial phase, lateral view, shows marked narrowing of the ICA distal to the carotid bulb. Slow antegrade flow with a "string sign" (*small arrows*) is seen. The cavernous ICA (*white arrow*) appears small because of the flow reduction. **C:** Left subclavian angiogram, arterial phase, AP view, shows long segments of alternating constrictions and dilatations (*arrows*). The patient has Marfan's syndrome with multiple dissections and right carotid pseudoaneurysm.

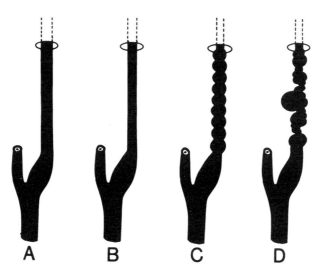

    A   B   C   D

FIG. 15-3. Anatomic drawings, lateral view, depict the common carotid bifurcation and cervical internal carotid artery in health and disease. **A:** Normal. **B:** Mild but long segment ICA narrowing spares the bulb and petrous segment. This appearance is nonspecific and can be seen with acute spontaneous or healed dissection as well as the tubular form of fibromuscular dysplasia. Diminished vessel caliber secondary to simple flow reduction can also produce a similar appearance on cerebral angiograms but usually also reduces caliber of the common carotid artery and bulb (see Fig. 15-15). **C:** Arterial "standing waves" are temporary circular spastic contractions that appear symmetric and uniform, involve both sides of the vessel wall equally, and do not cause stenosis. The regularly spaced waves are exaggerated for the purposes of illustration. **D:** Fibromuscular dysplasia with the typical string-of-beads appearance is shown. Note irregular areas of outpouching alternating with stenoses. Vessel wall involvement is asymmetric.

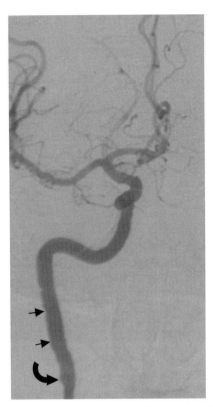

FIG. 15-4. Right internal carotid angiogram, arterial phase, AP view, shows catheter spasm. Note area of constriction (*large curved arrow*) with distal contractions of the ICA (*small black arrows*).

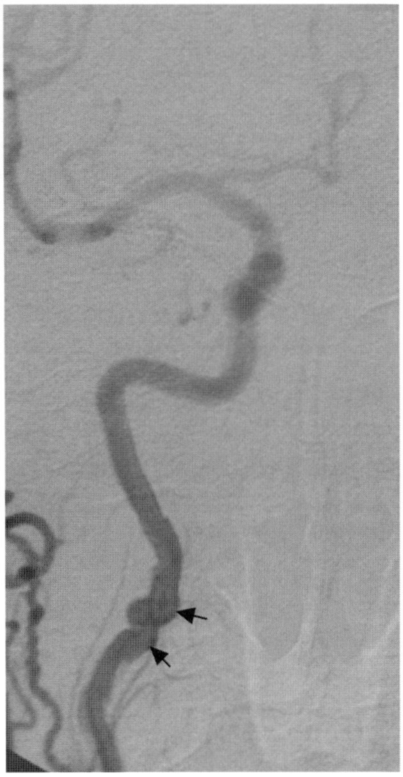

FIG. 15-5. Right common carotid angiogram, arterial phase, AP view. The guidewire was inadvertently passed up the internal carotid artery (ICA), causing vasospasm with temporary stenoses and dilatations that resemble fibromuscular dysplasia (*arrows*). The results of repeat angiogram (not shown) were normal.

constrictions that are sometimes observed during cerebral angiograms (Figs. 15-3C and 15-8). The differential diagnosis of stationary waves is FMD. In contrast to the alternating constrictions and dilatations that characterize FMD, the vessel caliber between circular contractions is normal (6).

Delayed complications from *endarterectomy* or *endovascular stenting* may cause iatrogenic narrowing of the carotid artery. Recurrent stenosis sometimes occurs secondary to progressive intimal hyperplasia (see Chapter 16).

Fibromuscular Dysplasia

Fibromuscular dysplasia (FMD) is an arteriopathy that affects medium-sized arteries in many locations. Although its precise origin is unknown, FMD is reportedly associated with α_1-antitrypsine deficiency (6a). The most common site is the renal artery. The ICA is affected in nearly three quarters of all cases involving the cephalocervical vessels; the vertebral artery is affected in 15% to 25%. Multiple vessels are involved in 60% to 75% of cases (1).

Fibromuscular dysplasia is most often found in 30- to 50-year old women. Asymptomatic cases of FMD may be discovered incidentally, although transient ischemic attacks, cerebral infarction, or subarachnoid hemorrhage (SAH) from an associated aneurysm are common presentations (7).

Fibromuscular dysplasia is classified into three histologic types, according to which layer of the arterial wall is affected. *Medial FMD* with thickened concentric rings of fibrous proliferation and smooth muscle hyperplasia is the most common type, accounting for 90% to 95% of cases. *Intimal FMD* with intimal thickening and internal elastic lamina fragmentation accounts for about 5% of cases. The least common type is *adventitial FMD* with fibrosis and thickening of the adventitia and periarterial tissues (7).

The angiographic findings in FMD depend on histologic type. The most common finding is multifocal stenoses that alternate with areas of mural dilatation, the so-called *"string of beads"* appearance (Figs. 15-3D and

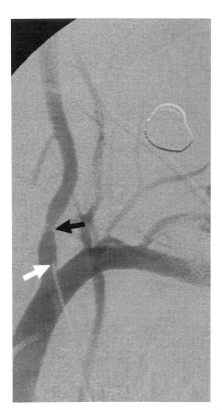

FIG. 15-6. Left subclavian angiogram, arterial phase, AP view. The catheter tip (*white arrow*) was passed into the proximal vertebral artery (VA) and then withdrawn to its orifice. Note smooth narrowing of the VA (*black arrow*), representing temporary vasospasm.

15-9). Septae, diverticulae, or aneurysmal-like outpouchings may occur in severe cases. Fibromuscular dysplasia is usually located around the C2–3 level, sparing the great vessel origins, carotid bifurcations, and bulbs.

A long area of *multisegmental tubular stenosis* is observed in 6% to 12% of cases (Fig. 15-3B). Diffuse thickening of the arterial wall, usually the intima, causes concentric cylindrical narrowing of the affected vessels in this uncommon form of FMD (7).

Complications of FMD include *dissection, saccular aneurysm,* and *arteriovenous fistulae* (Fig. 15-10) (7). Angiographic changes of FMD have been reported in 10% to 20% of patients with spontaneous cervical artery dissections (3). The prevalence of intracranial aneurysms in patients with FMD is approximately 7% (see Fig. 12-5B) (8).

Dissection

Extracranial ICA dissections are increasingly recognized as causes of stroke, accounting for up to 20% of ischemic strokes in young adults. Pathologically, dissections result from penetration of blood into the arterial wall, with narrowing or occlusion of the arterial lumen and an enlarged external diameter of the affected vessel (see Figs. 18-1 and 18-2A and B) (9).

Cephalocervical dissections can be traumatic or nontraumatic. Traumatic dissection is discussed in Chapter

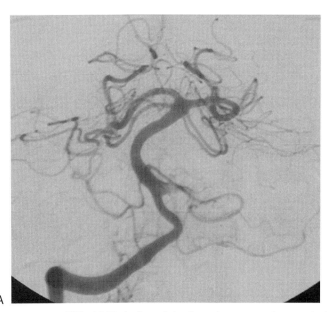

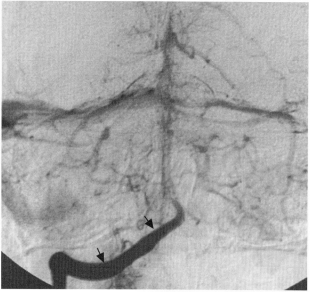

FIG. 15-7. Left vertebral angiogram, anteroposterior view, with early arterial **(A)** and late venous **(B)** phase films. Catheter-induced vasospasm in the proximal vertebral artery (not shown) resulted in persisting contrast stasis (**B**, *arrows*). The vasospasm resolved when the catheter was promptly removed.

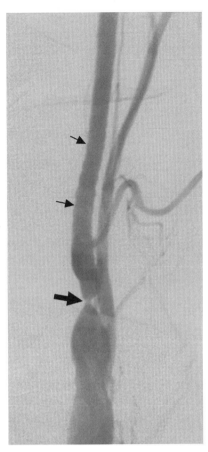

FIG. 15-8. Right common carotid angiogram, arterial phase, oblique view, shows a high-grade stenosis (*large arrow*) with regularly spaced arterial standing waves in the internal carotid artery (*small arrows*). Compare with Fig. 15-3C.

18. Nontraumatic dissections can be either spontaneous or occur in association with an underlying vasculopathy such as FMD. Other reported conditions that predispose to dissection include hypertension, migraine headaches, vigorous physical activity, sympathomimetic drugs, pharyngeal infections, and oral contraceptives (1). Environmental events such as weather- or infectious disease-related factors may account for the peculiar seasonal patterns of spontaneous cervical artery dissection (the peak occurs in October) (9a).

The clinical presentation of spontaneous ICA dissection is highly variable. Some are asymptomatic. Others cause headache, neck, or suboccipital pain. Dissections may cause cerebral ischemia and infarction, either from flow reduction or thromboembolic complications. Some patients develop a postganglionic Horner's syndrome (10). Lower cranial nerve palsies (CNs IX to XII) are less common manifestations of ICA dissection (11).

The angiographic appearance of extracranial ICA dissection is variable. The most common finding is a relatively smooth or slightly irregular tapered mid-cervical narrowing (Figs. 15-3B and 15-11) (12). Dissections that occlude the ICA may terminate in a rat-tail–shaped tapered occlusion (Fig. 15-12). Internal carotid artery dissections typically spare the carotid bulb and terminate near the skull base. Angiographic demonstration of an intimal flap, false lumen, or pseudoaneurysm is relatively uncommon (Fig. 15-13). Coexisting ICA kinking or coiling is seen in approximately 30% of cases (13).

Vertebral and vertebrobasilar (VB) dissections are an underrecognized cause of subarachnoid hemorrhage or brainstem ischemia (14). Vertebrobasilar dissections are usually located between the skull base and C1 or between C1 and C2 (1).

Arteritis

The two forms of arteritis that primarily affect the extracranial vessels are Takayasu's arteritis and temporal arteritis. Both are forms of giant cell arteritis and are distinguished by their quite different clinical presentations. A third type of arteritis, Kawasaki disease, is a pediatric febrile vasculitis that is probably caused by super-antigens.

Takayasu's arteritis is a primary panarteritis of unknown etiology that usually affects females between the ages of 15 and 45 years. Takayasu's arteritis involves medium- and large-sized arteries, particularly the aorta and its branches. The abdominal aorta, brachiocephalic (especially subclavian), and renal arteries are the most common sites.

Angiography discloses smooth tapered stenoses or occlusions that involve the origins of the subclavian, innominate, and common carotid arteries (14). Marked dilatations and aneurysms are less common and involve mainly the ascending aorta and brachiocephalic arteries (15).

Temporal arteritis involves medium and large cranial branches of the great vessels. Females over the age of 50 are typically affected; 95% are over the age of 50. Headache and scalp tenderness may be associated with a thickened, nodular superficial temporal artery. The diagnosis is usually made with biopsy of this vessel. When angiography is performed, it is either normal or shows segments of smooth, tapering stenosis or frank vessel occlusion (14).

Kawasaki disease, also known as acute infantile febrile mucocutaneous lymph node syndrome, affects young children of all races. It produces histologic changes of a systemic vasculitis and is most likely caused by super-antigens. There is a predilection for the coronary arteries although the great vessels, especially the axillary segment of the subclavian artery, may be involved. Stenosis, thrombosis, and aneurysm formation are the major

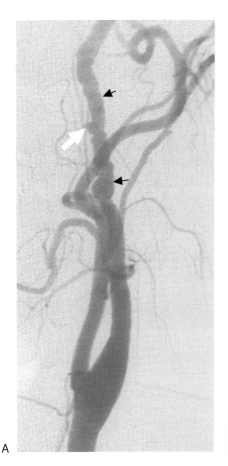

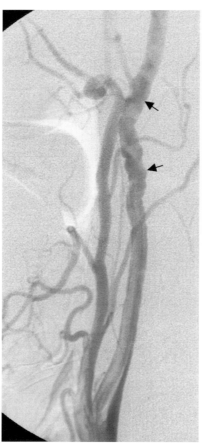

A

B

FIG. 15-9. Right **(A)** and left **(B)** common carotid angiograms, arterial phase, lateral view, in a patient with bilateral fibromuscular dysplasia (FMD) (*arrows*). Note the irregularly spaced areas of alternating dilatations and stenoses in the mid-cervical internal carotid artery (ICA). This is the typical string-of-beads appearance of FMD (compare with Fig. 15-3D). A protrusion from the right ICA (**A**, *white arrow*) represents a small pseudoaneurysm. The carotid bulbs and petrous ICA segments are normal.

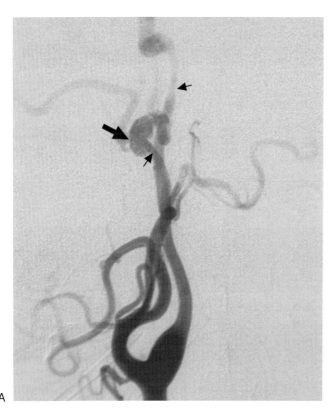

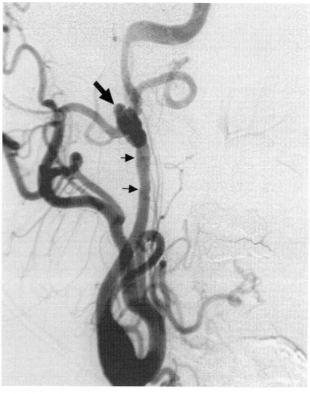

A

B

FIG. 15-10. A 28-year-old hypertensive man presented with a right Horner's syndrome. MR scan (not shown) disclosed a paravascular hematoma in the carotid space with suspected dissection of the internal carotid artery (ICA). Lateral **(A)** and oblique **(B)** views of the right common carotid angiogram in this patient show narrowing and irregularity of the distal internal carotid artery (*small arrows*) with a pseudoaneurysm (*large arrows*). Renal angiogram (not shown) showed typical findings of fibromuscular disease.

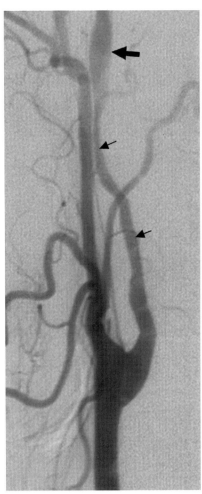

FIG. 15-11. This patient presented with sudden onset of severe headache and left-sided neck pain. A left common carotid angiogram, arterial phase, lateral view, shows tapered narrowing of the internal carotid artery (ICA) (*arrows*). Note that the bulb is spared and the distal ICA assumes a more normal caliber (*large arrow*). Spontaneous carotid dissection was diagnosed.

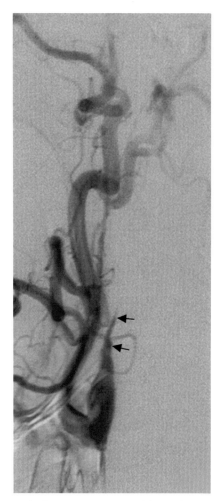

FIG. 15-12. Left common carotid angiogram, arterial phase, lateral view, shows a carotid dissection with irregular tapering (*arrows*) and distal occlusion. The bulb is spared.

abnormalities. Neurologic complications occur in 1% of children with Kawasaki disease and include facial nerve palsy, seizures, ataxia, encephalopathy, hemiplegia, and cerebral hypoperfusion infarction (15a,15b).

Miscellaneous Causes of Extracranial Stenosis

Neoplasms may displace, encase, invade, and eventually occlude cervical vessels (Fig. 15-14; see also Figs. 12-14, 14-26, and 14-30). *Radiation* may injure both the extra- and the intracranial vasculature. Accelerated atherosclerosis, fibrinoid necrosis, and endothelial damage with stroke are late complications of radiation therapy. Angiographic findings range from stenosis or

occlusion of the affected vessels (see Fig. 15-1) to an acquired moyamoya pattern with slowly progressive supraclinoid carotid stenosis (16).

Infection, either via septic emboli or contiguous spread from a retropharyngeal or peritonsillar abscess, may involve the cervical carotid arteries. Pyogenic, fungal, and syphilitic infections all occur in this location. Abnormalities include vascular displacement, narrowing, and mycotic pseudoaneurysm (6,17,18).

Flow reduction causes a passive decrease in vessel size. Distal flow reduction occurs when intracranial "runoff" is reduced. Severe vasospasm, increased intracranial pressure, and hemodynamically significant proximal stenosis can all diminish flow in the cervical carotid arteries (see Fig. 15-15B) (18a).

Angiography in cases with reduced distal run-off discloses a smoothly tapered vessel that may be dif-

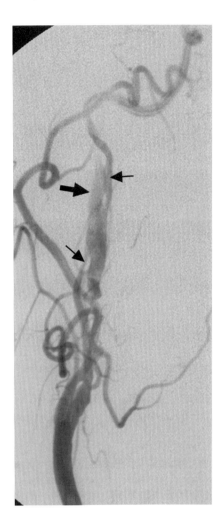

FIG. 15-13. Right common carotid angiogram, arterial phase, oblique view, shows marked narrowing of the internal carotid artery (*small arrows*) with a prominent elongated contrast-filled outpouching (*large arrow*). The patient has a carotid dissection with pseudoaneurysm.

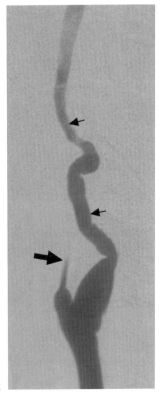

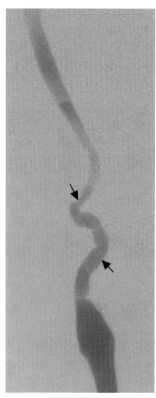

FIG. 15-14. Lateral **(A)** and anteroposterior **(B)** views of the right common carotid angiogram in a 56-year-old man with invasive squamous cell carcinoma show irregular encasement of the internal carotid artery (*small arrows*). The external carotid artery is occluded (**A**, *large arrow*).

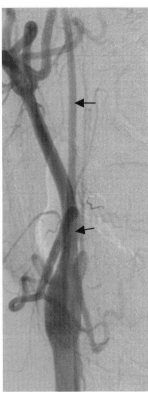
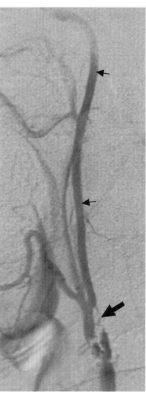

A   B

FIG. 15-15. Two different cases illustrate passive diminution in internal carotid artery (ICA) caliber secondary to reduced blood flow. **A:** Right common carotid angiogram, arterial phase, AP view, shows a small cervical ICA (*arrows*). Distal run-off is markedly reduced in this case, causing the proximal vessel to diminish in caliber (see Fig. 15-16 for the cause of this flow-related reduction). **B:** Left common carotid angiogram, arterial phase, lateral view, in a patient with very high grade stenosis of the proximal ICA (*large arrow*). Note diminished size of the entire carotid system, including the bulb (*small arrows*).

ficult to distinguish from dissection (Figs. 15-3B and 15-15A). All carotid segments, including the bulb, usually appear small when ICA flow is reduced. Proximal flow reduction occurs when a high-grade stenosis limits flow distal to the lesion (Fig. 15-15B; see also Fig. 16-12).

INTRACRANIAL VASCULITIS AND VASCULOPATHY

Atherosclerosis is by far the most common cause of a vasculitislike angiographic pattern in adults (see Chapter 16). However, a number of both congenital and acquired nonatheromatous disorders can produce cerebral vasculitis and noninflammatory vasculopathy. Some of the more important causes are discussed below.

Congenital and Inherited Disorders

Neurocutaneous Syndromes

Neurofibromatosis type 1 and *tuberous sclerosis* (TS) are the two phakomatoses that most often involve the intracranial vessels (19). NF-1 is the most common neurocutaneous syndrome with vascular manifestations. Nearly 90% of the lesions in NF-1 are stenotic or occlusive. Slowly progressive stenosis of the supraclinoid carotid arteries may cause a moyamoya pattern to develop (20).

Less common vascular complications of NF-1 include aneurysm, vessel ectasias, or fistula formation involving large- and medium-sized arteries (2). Intracranial aneurysms in patients with NF-1 may be saccular, fusiform, or dissecting.

Miscellaneous Inherited Arteriopathies

A number of other inherited disorders may affect the craniocerebral vasculature. *Menkes' kinky hair disease* causes severely elongated, tortuous abdominal, visceral, and cranial arteries.

Ehlers-Danlos syndrome (type IV) is characterized by vascular complications that include spontaneous rupture, dissection, or aneurysm formation of large- and medium-sized arteries. Most aneurysms in this disorder are intracranial, commonly located in the cavernous sinus (see Chapter 12). Spontaneous direct carotid–cavernous sinus fistulae also may develop in these patients (2).

Sickle-cell disease (SCD) is the most common inherited hemoglobinopathy. Most complications of SCD are caused by vascular occlusion with sickled red cells and subsequent tissue infarction. Sickled erythrocytes damage the vascular endothelium, producing arterial wall injury and noninflammatory intimal hyperplasia (21).

Neurologic complications are common in SCD, occurring in approximately 25% of patients. Frank cerebral infarction is the most serious of these complications, although magnetic resonance (MR) imaging demonstrates ischemic change in 13% of SCD patients without a clinically recognized stroke (21).

Angiography discloses narrowing of the supraclinoid ICA as well as the proximal anterior and middle cerebral artery segments. A moyamoya pattern with extensive basal collateral circulation may develop (22). Multiple intracranial aneurysms with a predilection for the vertebrobasilar territory also have been reported with SCD (23).

Idiopathic Progressive Arteriopathy of Childhood

Sometimes called *moyamoya disease*, idiopathic progressive arteriopathy of childhood is a disorder of unknown etiology. In Japan and the Pacific rim countries,

Moyamoya has two peak ages of presentation: one in childhood (early onset) and the other in adulthood (late onset). The initial symptoms in children are usually ischemic, whereas intracranial hemorrhage is also a common presentation in adults (24,24a). The prognosis in idiopathic progressive arteriopathy of childhood depends on the rapidity and extent of the vascular occlusions as well as the development of effective collateral circulation.

Angiographic findings are stenosis or occlusion of the distal ICAs with collateral circulation from multiple enlarged lenticulostriate and thalamoperforating arteries (Fig. 15-16A–C). Basal collaterals may become so extensive that they resemble a vascular malformation, the "puff of smoke" appearance for which the disease is named (Fig. 15-16B and D–F). Widespread dural, leptomeningeal, and pial collaterals also may develop.

Moyamoya is an angiographic pattern, not a specific disease, and may be acquired as well as inherited. Any slowly progressive occlusion of the supraclinoid ICAs may develop so-called telangiectatic basal collaterals. Moyamoya vessels have been reported in a number of disorders ranging from idiopathic progressive arteriopathy of childhood and neurofibromatosis to atherosclerosis and radiation therapy (25). There is also a relatively high association of moyamoya with other arterial anomalies, including aneurysms, arteriovenous malformations, ectasia or fenestration of the cerebral arteries, and congenital heart disease (26,27).

Acquired Disorders

Terminology

"Vasculitis" and "angiitis" are synonymous terms that denote inflammation and necrosis of either arteries or veins. "Arteritis" refers specifically to arterial inflammation. "Vasculopathy" is a more general term that indicates any vascular pathology. Here we use "vasculopathy" to indicate nonvasculitic, noninflammatory disorders or vasculopathies of indeterminate nature (28).

Classification

A number of classifications have been proposed for intracranial vasculitis. The simplest is one that distinguishes between true vasculitis (angiitis) and noninflammatory vasculopathy (see box on right). The modification shown here subdivides vasculitis into primary (isolated) angiitis of the central nervous system (PACNS) and systemic vasculitides that involve the CNS.

General Imaging Appearance

The imaging appearance of the intracranial vasculitides is similar regardless of specific etiology. Multifocal

Intracranial Vasculopathy

Vasculitis
  Primary (isolated) angiitis of the central nervous system (CNS)
  Systemic vasculitis with CNS involvement
    Systemic necrotizing vasculitis
      Polyarteritis nodosa (PAN)
      Hypersensitivity granulomatosis (Churg and Strauss)
    Wegener granulomatosis
    Behçet's disease
    Giant cell arteritis (its two variants, Takayasu and temporal arteritis, rarely affect the intracranial vessels)
  Systemic diseases that may cause secondary CNS angiitis
    Systemic lupus erythematosus (SLE)
    Antiphospholipid syndrome (APS)
    Scleroderma
    Rheumatoid disease
    Sjogren's syndrome
  CNS disorders with secondary vasculitis
    Meningitis
      Pyogenic
      Tuberculous
      Fungal
      Parasitic
      Syphilitic
    Septic emboli
    Nongranulomatous inflammations
    Sarcoid
Vasculopathy (noninflammatory)
  Inherited disorders
    Neurocutaneous syndromes
      Neurofibromatosis type 1 (NF-1)
      Tuberous sclerosis
    Menkes' kinky hair disease
    Ehlers-Danlos type IV
    Sickle-cell disease
  Idiopathic progressive arteriopathy of childhood
  Drug-related vasculopathy
  Oncotic vasculopathy
    Tumor emboli
    Pseudoaneurysm
    Intravascular lymphoma
  Radiation-induced vasculopathy
  Vasomotor disorders
    Severe systemic hypertension
    Posterior reversible encephalopathy syndromes
      Eclampsia
      Hemolytic uremic syndrome/thrombotic thrombocytopenic purpura
      Chemotherapy

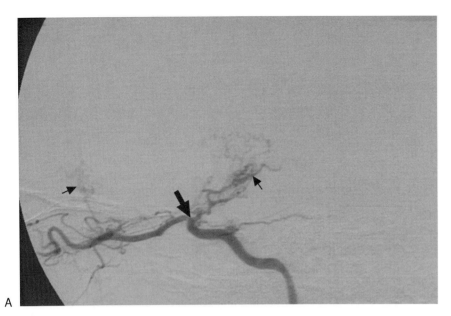

A

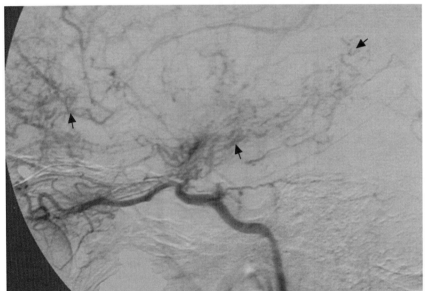

B

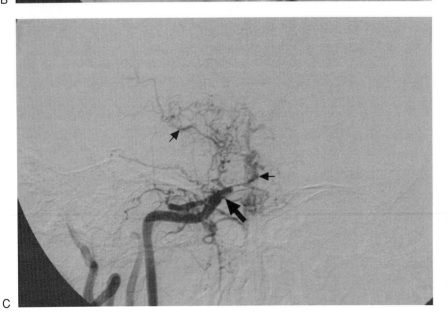

C

FIG. 15-16. A series of angiograms in this 18-year-old patient with idiopathic progressive arteriopathy of childhood shows the typical moyamoya pattern. Occlusion of the supraclinoid internal carotid artery (*large arrows*) is seen with innumerable small basal collaterals that give the characteristic puff-of-smoke appearance (*small arrows*). **A:** Right internal carotid angiogram, early arterial phase, lateral view. **B:** Right internal carotid angiogram, late arterial phase, lateral view. **C:** Right internal carotid angiogram, early arterial phase, AP view (contrast reflux into the external carotid artery is present).

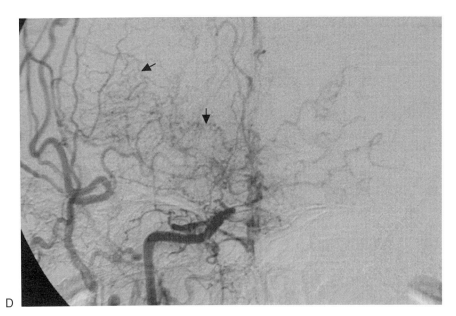

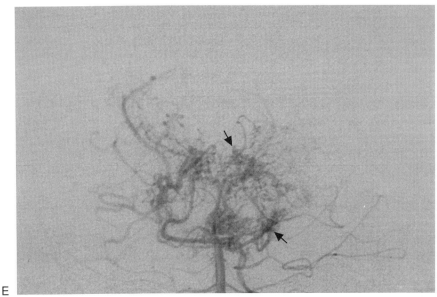

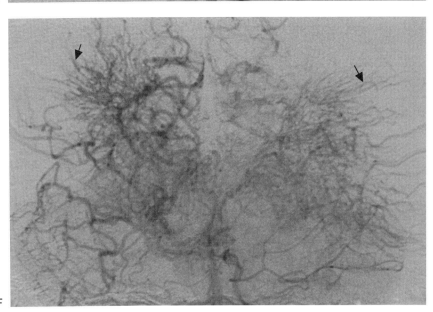

FIG. 15-16. *Continued.* **D:** Right internal carotid angiogram, late arterial phase, AP view. **E:** Right vertebral angiogram, mid-arterial phase, AP view. **F:** Right vertebral angiogram, late arterial phase, AP view.

areas of smooth or slightly irregularly shaped stenosis alternating with dilated segments is typical (Fig. 15-17).

Primary Angiitis of the Central Nervous System

Primary angiitis of the central nervous system (PACNS) is characterized pathologically by inflammation of the media and adventitia of small leptomeningeal arteries and veins, but vessels of any size can be affected. The presence of granulomas is variable (28).

Some investigators have suggested that the diagnosis of PACNS should be established only if (a) the patient presents with headache and a combination of focal and diffuse neurologic deficits of at least 6 months' duration (except in cases of "devastating onset"); (b) several areas of segmental arterial narrowing are demonstrated on cerebral angiography; (c) systemic inflammation or infection has been ruled out; and (d) a leptomeningeal/parenchymal biopsy result demonstrates vascular inflammation but no signs of infection, atherosclerosis, or neoplastic disease (29).

Systemic Vasculitis with CNS Involvement

There are several types of necrotizing vasculitides that may involve the cerebral vessels. Polyarteritis nodosa (PAN) is a widespread necrotizing arteritis that involves small- and medium-sized arteries. It is one of three closely related systemic necrotizing vasculitides. The second is *hypersensitivity (allergic) angiitis* and granulomatosis (Churg-Strauss variant). The third variant is polyangiitis *overlap syndrome*, a vasculitis that has features of both PAN and allergic angiitis (30).

The few cases with angiographic findings in PAN have reported either frank occlusions or alternating segments of narrowing and widening in the small- and medium-sized intracranial arteries. These findings are indistinguishable from other forms of intracranial vasculitis (30).

Systemic Diseases that May Have Secondary CNS Angiitis

Although neurologic involvement is common in *systemic lupus erythomatous* (SLE), true cerebral vasculitis is rare (31). The most common angiographic finding in patients with SLE is a normal examination results (Fig. 15-18), followed by nonspecific vascular occlusion and stroke (Fig. 15-19).

The causes of stroke in SLE are numerous and include thrombosis secondary to hypercoaguability from antiphospholipid antibodies, emboli from Libman-Sacks endocarditis, accelerated atherosclerosis (perhaps secondary to hypertension or long-term corticosteroid therapy), and cerebral vasculitis (either primary lupus vasculitis or secondary to CNS infection) (31).

Antiphospholipid antibodies are circulating immunoglobulins that are associated with a hypercoagulable state and ischemic cerebrovascular disease. Primary *antiphospholipid syndrome* (APS) occurs in patients with elevated APAs who do not have SLE or other connective tissue diseases. A secondary form of APS occurs in individuals who meet the diagnostic criteria for SLE (32).

Antiphospholipid syndrome is characterized clinically by strokes that occur at an unusually early age, recurrent arterial or venous thromboses, infertility and spontaneous fetal loss, and thrombocytopenia. The most common intracranial arterial abnormalities are solitary stem or dis-

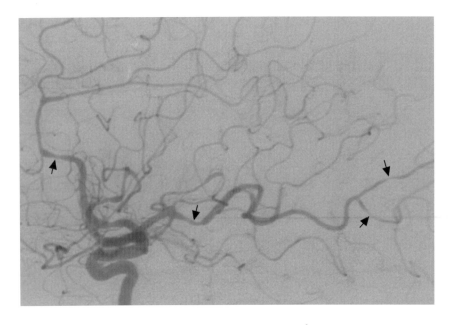

FIG. 15-17. This 20-year-old woman presented with sudden onset of severe headache. There was no evidence for subarachnoid hemorrhage on NECT scan and lumbar puncture. Right internal carotid angiogram, arterial phase, lateral view, disclosed multiple areas of alternating constrictions and dilatations in the middle and anterior cerebral arteries (*arrows*). There was no evidence of drug abuse or infection. The symptoms resolved with steroids, and results of a repeat angiogram 2 months later were normal. No specific diagnosis was established. The angiographic picture is typical for vasculitis.

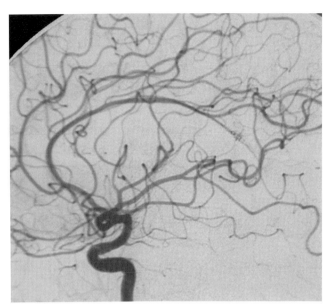

FIG. 15-18. This 19-year-old man with documented systemic lupus erythomatosus (SLE) presented with rapidly decreasing mental status. MR scan showed multiple abnormalities, prompting an angiogram to evaluate the cerebral vasculature for possible lupus vasculitis. A right internal carotid angiogram, arterial phase, lateral view, is shown. No abnormalities are identified.

tal branch occlusions. A pattern suggestive of vasculitis also occurs, as does nonatherosclerotic stenosis at the great vessel origins (Fig. 15-20) (33).

Other systemic diseases that may cause CNS angiitis include *scleroderma, rheumatoid disease,* and *Sjogren's syndrome* (28,34).

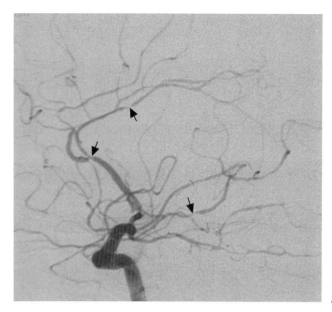

A

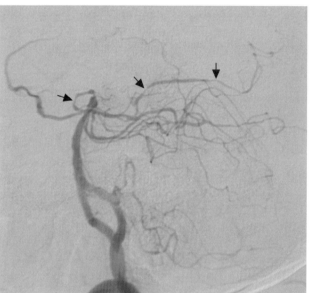

B

FIG. 15-20. A 38-year-old woman with antiphospholipid antibody syndrome had a cerebral angiogram. Lateral views of the right internal carotid **(A)** and left vertebral **(B)** angiograms show multifocal areas of irregular stenosis (*arrows*).

CNS Disorders with Secondary Vasculitis

A number of infectious and noninfectious inflammatory vasculopathies occur in the CNS. Pyogenic, granulomatous, fungal, and parasitic *meningitis*, as well as nongranulomatous processes such as sarcoidosis, all have a predilection for the basal cisterns. Most intracranial infections and inflammations narrow the terminal ICA segment as well as involve the proximal anterior and middle cerebral arteries (35). Cysticercosis, Lyme disease, human immunodeficiency virus infection, and meningovascular syphilis are other infectious causes of intracra-

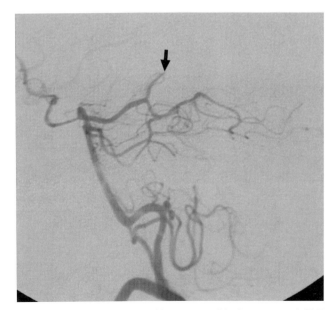

FIG. 15-19. This 31-year-old woman with documented SLE had sudden onset of a right homonymous hemianopsia. A vertebral angiogram, arterial phase, lateral view, disclosed occlusion of the left posterior cerebral artery (*arrow*).

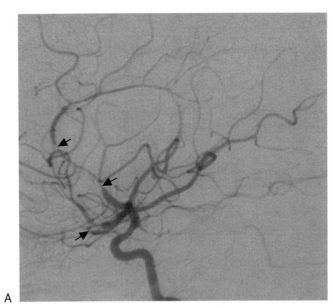 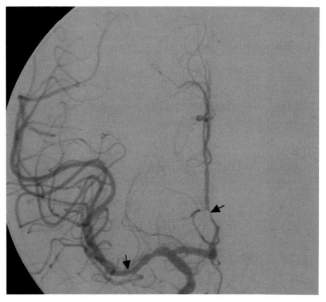

A   B

FIG. 15-21. This 22-year-old woman was taking monoamine oxidase inhibitors but was not following her recommended dietary restrictions. A cerebral angiogram was performed when she presented with a 5-day history of increasingly severe headaches. Lateral **(A)** and anteroposterior **(B)** views of a right internal carotid angiogram, arterial phase, show multifocal vascular stenoses (*arrows*). Drug-related vasculitis was

nial vasculopathy (36). Both stenoses and ectasias have been reported (28).

Some prescription and "street" *drugs* may cause a vasculiticlike pattern on cerebral angiograms (Fig. 15-21). Cocaine, methamphetamines, and a spectrum of sympathomimetic drugs have all been implicated in causing cerebral hemorrhages, vasospasm, and vasculitis (Fig. 15-22) (37). A less common drug-related angiopathy is multifocal arterial ectasias (38).

Neoplasms with tumor emboli may cause pseudo-aneurysms and stenoses of the intracranial vessels (see Figs. 12-12 and 12-13). Vasculitis may be the initial presentation of some lymphoproliferative diseases such as angiocentric large cell lymphoma (39).

Miscellaneous Disorders

Behçet's disease is an idiopathic multisystem inflammatory disorder that is classically characterized by the triad of recurrent oral and genital ulcers and uveitis. Arthritis, thrombophlebitis, neurologic abnormalities, and skin lesions are also common. The dominant histo-

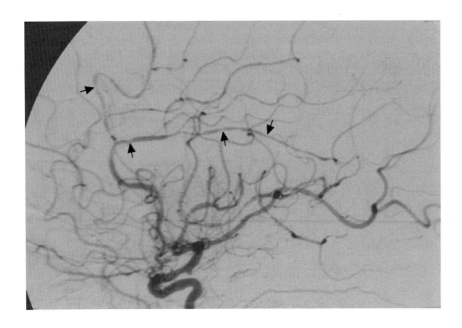

FIG. 15-22. This 50-year-old woman was taking heavy doses of caffeine and ergotamine for migraine headaches. Visual symptoms prompted an MR scan that disclosed a left occipital hematoma. A common carotid angiogram, lateral view, disclosed typical vasculitic changes (*arrows*).

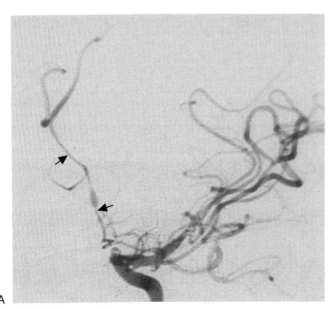
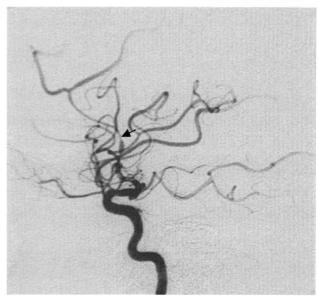

A   B

FIG. 15-23. This 47-year-old woman with a 5-day history of severe headache and subarachnoid hemorrhage (SAH) on NECT scan had a cerebral angiogram. Oblique **(A)** and lateral **(B)** views of the left internal carotid angiogram show multiple foci of segmental narrowing in the anterior cerebral artery (*arrows*). No aneurysm was demonstrated. Follow-up angiogram 3 weeks later was normal.

pathologic lesion is a vasculitis that involves small- and medium-size vessels. Parenchymal lesions in the brainstem, cerebellum, and basal ganglia often can be detected on MR scans (40). Cerebral venous thrombosis and meningitis are also features of Behçet's disease (41).

Differential Diagnosis

The most common cause of a vasculitislike pattern on cerebral angiograms is *atherosclerosis* (see Chapter 16). Acute vasoconstriction after *subarachnoid hemorrhage* (SAH) may cause extensive global ischemic damage. Control of cerebrovascular tone involves a balance between opposing vasoconstrictive and vasodilatory influences, both of which are pathologically altered after SAH (42). Angiography in patients with SAH who develop ischemic symptoms often discloses severe vasospasm. Alternating areas of stenosis may mimic vasculitis (Fig. 15-23).

REFERENCES

1. Osborn AG. Nonartheromatous causes of arterial narrowing and occlusion. In: *Diagnostic neuroradiology*. St. Louis: Mosby, 1994: 369–382.
2. Schievink WI. Genetics of intracranial aneurysm. *Neurosurgery* 1997; 40:651–663.
3. Schievink WI, Björnsson J, Piepgras DG. Coexistence of fibromuscular dysplasia and cystic medial necrosis in a patient with Marfan's syndrome and bilateral carotid artery dissections. *Stroke* 1994;25: 2492–2496.
4. Schievink WI, Mokri B, Piepgras DG, Michels VV. Intracranial aneurysms with Marfan's syndrome: an autopsy study. *Neurosurgery* 1997;41:866–871.

5. Schievink WI, Modri B, Piepgras DG, Gittenberger-de Grato AC. Intracranial aneurysms and cervicocephalic arterial dissection associated with congenital heart disease. *Neurosurgery* 1996;39:685–690.
6. Russo CP, Smoker WRK. Nonatheromatous carotid artery disease. *Neuroimag Clin North Am* 1998;4:773–797.
6a. Schievink WI, Meyer FB, Parisi JE, Wijdicks EFM. Fibromuscular dysplasia of the internal carotid artery associated with α_1-antitrypsin deficiency. *Neurosurgery* 1998;43:229–234.
7. Furie DM, Tien RD. Fibromuscular dysplasia of the arteries of the head and neck: imaging finding. *AJR* 1994;162:1205–1209.
8. Cloft HJ, Kallmes DF, Kallmes MR, et al. Prevalence of cerebral aneurysms in patients with fibromuscular dysplasia: a reassessment. *J Neurosurg* 1998;88:436–440.
9. Leclerc X, Lucas C, Godfrey O, et al. Helical CT for the follow-up of cervical internal carotid artery dissections. *AJNR* 1998;19:831–837.
9a. Schievink WI, Wijdicks EFM, Kuiper JD. Seasonal pattern of spontaneous cervical artery dissection. *J Neurosurg* 1998;89:101–103.
10. Digre KB, Smoker WRK, Johnston P, et al. Selective MR imaging approach for evaluation of patients with Horner's syndrome. *AJNR* 1992;13:223–227.
11. Sturzenegger M, Huber P. Cranial nerve palsies in spontaneous carotid artery dissection. *J Neurol Neurosurg Psychiatry* 1993;46:1191–1199.
12. Provenzale JW. Dissection of the internal carotid and vertebral arteries: imaging features. *AJR* 1995;165:1099–1104.
13. Ozdoba C, Sturzenegger M, Schroth G. Internal carotid artery dissection: MR imaging features and clinical-radiologic correlation. *Radiology* 1996;199:191–198.
14. Hurst RW. Angiography of non-atherosclerotic occlusive cerebrovascular disease. *Neuroimag Clin North Am* 1996;6:651–678.
15. Kumer S, Radhakrishnan S, Radke RV, et al. Takayasu's arterites: evaluation with three-dimensional time-of-flight MR angiography. *Eur Radiol* 1997;7:44–50.
15a. Chung CJ, Stein L. Kawasaki disease: A review. *Radiology* 1998;208: 29–33.
15b. Ichiyama T, Nishikawa M, Hayashi T, et al. Cerebral hypoperfusion during acute Kawasaki disease. *Stroke* 1998;29:1320–1321.
16. Bowen J, Paulsen CA. Stroke after pituitary irradiation. *Stroke* 1992;23:908–911.
17. Ide C, Bodart E, Remacle M, et al. An early MR observation of carotid involvement by retropharyngeal abscess. *AJNR* 1998;19:499–501.

18. Tanaka H, Patel V, Shrier DA, Coniglio JU. Pseudoaneurysm of the petrous internal carotid artery after skull base infection and prevertebral abscess drainage. *AJNR* 1998;19:502–504.
18a. Dix JE, McNulty BJ, Kallmes DF. Frequency and significance of a small distal ICA in carotid artery stenosis. *AJNR* 1998;19:1215–1218.
19. Spangler WJ, Cosgrove GR, Moumdjian RA, Montes JL. Cerebral arterial ectasia and tuberous sclerosis: case report. *Neurosurgery* 1997;40:191–194.
20. Rizzo JR III, Lessell S. Cerebrovascular abnormalities in neurofibromatosis type 1. *Neurology* 1994;44:1000–1002.
21. Moser FG, Miller ST, Bello JA, et al. The spectrum of brain MR abnormalities in sickle-cell disease: a report from the cooperative study of sickle cell disease. *AJNR* 1996;16:965–972.
22. Howlett DC, Hatrick AG, Jarosz AG, Jarosz JM, et al. Pictorial review: the role of CT and MR in imaging the complications of sickle cell disease. *Clin Radiol* 1997:52:821–829.
23. Preul MC, Cendes F, Just N, Mohr G. Intracranial aneurysms and sickle cell anemia: multiplicity and propensity for the vertebrobasilar territory. *Neurosurgery* 1998;42:971–978.
24. Okada Y, Shima T, Nishida M, et al. Effectiveness of STA-MCA anastomosis in adult moyamoya disease. *Stroke* 1998;29:625–630.
24a. Chiu D. Shedden P, Bratina P, Grotta JC. Clinical features of Moyamoya disease in the United States. *Stroke* 1998:29:1347–1351.
25. Bitzer M, Topka H. Progressive cerebral occlusive disease after radiation therapy. *Stroke* 1998;26:131–136.
26. Vörös E, Kiss M, Hankó J, Nagy E. Moyamoya with arterial anomalies: relevance to pathogeneiss. *Neuroradiology* 1997;39:842–856.
27. Llutterman J, Scott M, Nass R, Gera T. Moyamoya syndrome associated with congenital heart disease. *Pediatrics* 1998;101:57–60.
28. Harris KG, Yuh WTC. Intracranial vasculitis. *Neuroimag Clin North Am* 1998;4:773–797.
29. Mishikawa M, Sakamoto H, Katsuyama J, et al. Multiple appearing and vanishing aneurysms: primary angiitis of the central nervous system. *J Neurosurg* 1998;88:133–137.
30. Provenzale JM, Allen NB. Neuroradiologic findings in polyarteritis nervosa. *AJNR* 1996;17:1119–1126.
31. Liem MD, Gzesh DJ, Flanders AE. MRI and angiographic diagnosis of lupus cerebral vasculitis. *Neuroradiology* 1996;38:134–136.
32. Insko EK, Haskal ZJ. Antiphospholipid syndrome: patterns of life-threatening and severe recurrent vascular complications. *Radiology* 1997;202:319–326.
33. Provenzale JM, Barboriak DP, Allen NB, Ortel TL. Antiphospholipid antibodies: findings at arterography. *AJNR* 1998;19:611–616.
34. Nagahiro S, Montani A, Yamada K, Ushlo Y. Multiple cerebral arterial occlusions in a young patient with Sjögren's syndrome: case report. *Neurosurgery* 1996;38:592–595.
35. Gupta RK, Gupta S, Singh D, et al. MR imaging and angiography in tuberculous meningitis. *Neuroradiology* 1994;36:87–92.
36. Barinagarrementeria F, Cantu C. Frequency of cerebral arteritis in subarachnoid cysticercosis: an angiography study. *Stroke* 1998;29:123–125.
37. Konzen JP, Levine SR, Garcia JH. Vasospasm and thrombus formation as possible mechanisms of stroke related to alkaloidal cocaine. *Stroke* 1995;26:1114–1118.
38. Lazar EB, Russell EJ, Cohel BA, et al. Contrast-enhanced MR of cerebral arteritis: intravascular enhancement related to flow stasis within areas of focal arterial ectasia. *AJNR* 1992;13:271–276.
39. Wooten MD, Jasin HE. Vasculitis and lymphoproliferative disease. *Sum Artheritis Rheum* 1996;26:564–574.
40. Tah ET, Atilla S, Keskin T, et al. MR in neuro-Behcet's disease. *Neuroradiology* 1997;39:2–6.
41. Gerber S, Biondi A, Dormont D, et al. Long-term MR follow-up of cerebral lesions in neuro-Behcet's disease. *Neuroradiology* 1996;38:761–768.
42. Bederson JB, Levy AL, Ding WH, et al. Acute vasoconstriction after subarachnoid hemorrhage. *Neurosurgery* 1998;42:352–362.

CHAPTER 16

Atherosclerosis and Carotid Stenosis

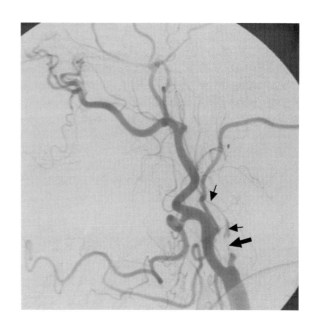

Cardiovascular disease is the leading cause of death in the United States and many other industrialized nations. Nearly half of all deaths in these countries are caused by diseases of the heart and blood vessels. Most of these diseases can be attributed to atherosclerosis and its complications (1).

Stroke is the major cause of disability among adult Americans and is the third leading cause of death after noncerebral cardiovascular disease and cancer. Atherosclerosis is the underlying cause for over 90% of cerebral thromboembolic events in the United States and Europe; carotid artery disease is the primary source of these embolic strokes (2).

This chapter begins with a brief consideration of atherosclerosis itself, followed by a discussion of the general angiographic features of atherosclerotic vascular disease (ASVD) in the head and neck. The important issue of carotid stenosis, its measurement, and the implications of recent multicenter trials for its treatment are discussed in the concluding section.

ATHEROSCLEROSIS

Definition

Atherosclerosis is the principal pathologic process affecting large elastic arteries (e.g., the aorta and the iliac arteries) and medium-sized muscular arteries (e.g., the

coronary and carotid arteries). It is a degenerative process that is characterized by accumulation of plasma lipids, connective tissue fibers, and local and circulating cells in the tunica intima of these vessels. Atherosclerosis has many manifestations, including plaque formation with stenosis, ulceration with thrombosis, distal emboli, and arterial dilatations and fusiform aneurysms (3).

Pathophysiology and Etiology

Lipid Metabolism

There is strong epidemiologic and experimental evidence that increased dietary lipid, particularly cholesterol and saturated fats, correlates with the development of atherosclerotic lesions. Ingested cholesterol, phospholipids, and triglycerides are solubilized with apolipoproteins and released from the liver. These very low density lipoproteins (VLDLs) are transformed into low-density lipoproteins (LDLs) that bind to receptors in arterial intima and smooth muscle cells in the walls of large- and medium-sized cervical and cerebral arteries (4).

Pathology

The principal feature of atherosclerosis is the deposition of plasma lipids in arterial walls. Development of an atherosclerotic plaque occurs in several stages.

The initial lesion in atherosclerosis is *lipid deposition* in the tunica intima and the cellular reaction associated with such deposits. Intimal *fatty streaks* are the earliest macroscopically visible lesions. Other than fatty streaks and slight intimal thickening, the histologic changes at this stage are minimal (Fig. 16-1A) (3).

Fibrous atheromatous plaques are the basic lesion of atherosclerosis. Uncomplicated fibrous plaques are smooth, eccentric lesions that are covered with intact endothelium. These plaques have three major components: (a) cells, including smooth muscle cells, monocytes or macrophages, and other leukocytes; (b) connective tissue, including collagen, elastic fibers, and proteoglycans; and (c) intracellular and extracellular lipid deposits (Fig. 16-1B).

A necrotic core of lipid material, cholesterol, cellular debris, lipid-laden foam cells, fibrin, and other plasma proteins may form deep within the plaque (Figs. 16-1C). Proliferating small blood vessels (so-called neovascularization) are common at the periphery of these plaques. These abnormal vessels may rupture, causing *intraplaque hemorrhage* and *ulceration* (Fig. 16-1D). *Calcification* is also a prominent feature of complicated plaques and may be extensive, involving both the superficial and deeper regions of the lesion (3).

Carotid *plaque rupture* occurs when the overlying fibrous cap weakens and fractures, releasing necrotic tissue that may occlude distal intracranial vessels via arterioarterial embolization (Fig. 16-1E). A rupture site also may act as a nidus for platelet and fibrin aggrega-

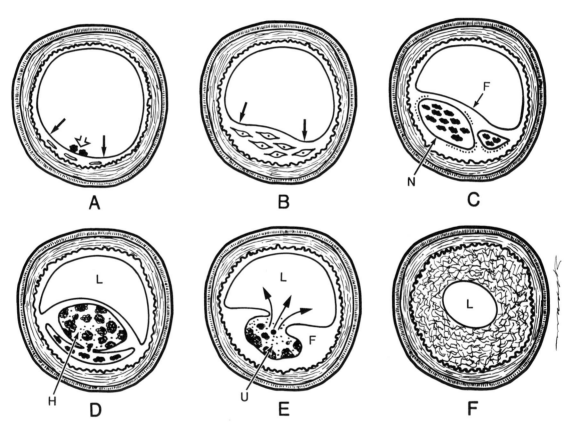

FIG. 16-1. Anatomic diagrams in the axial plane depict development of an atherosclerotic plaque. **A:** The vessel appears nearly normal. Slight eccentric thickening of the intima with a few fatty streaks is present (*solid arrows*). Some platelet adhesion to the intima has occurred (*open arrow*). **B:** Subintimal proliferation of monocyte-derived macrophages and smooth muscle cells causes a smooth, eccentric fibrotic thickening of the intima (*arrows*). Some of these cells become lipid-filled "foam" cells. **C:** A necrotic core (N) of foam cells, cellular debris, and cholesterol accumulates under the fibrous cap (F). The intima remains intact. Some neovascularity develops around the necrotic core, shown here as dotted lines. **D:** Subintimal hemorrhage (H) from the "new vessels" further narrows the lumen (L). **E:** Ulceration (U) with rupture of the fibrous cap and intima releases necrotic debris and platelet aggregates (*arrows*) into the vessel lumen. **F:** Concentric subintimal fibrosis without ulceration is shown. This may narrow the vessel lumen (L) and cause hemodynamically significant stenosis. Stenotic vessels such as this one are also prone to ulceration and thrombosis.

tion, leading to arterial thrombosis (5). Slowly swirling fluid within an ulcerated plaque allows platelets to aggregate; an intermittent Bernoulli effect then pulls the aggregates into the rapidly flowing main artery slipstream (6).

Etiology

Atherosclerotic vascular disease probably has no single cause, no universal initiating event, and no exclusive pathogenetic mechanism (7). Three main hypotheses have been proposed to explain the development of atherosclerotic lesions in arterial walls. These are (a) the lipid hypothesis; (b) the response to injury hypothesis; and (c) the so-called unifying theory (4).

The *lipid hypothesis* relates ASVD to high plasma LDL levels causing LDL-cholesterol deposits in the arterial intima. The *response to injury hypothesis* suggests that ASVD is initiated by focal endothelial change or subtle intimal injury that initiates platelet aggregation and plaque formation.

The *unifying theory* combines elements of both the lipid and response to injury hypotheses, positing that endothelial injury is accompanied by increased permeability to macromolecules such as LDL (8). The two most significant mechanisms by which plaques grow seem to be formation of thrombi on the plaque surface and transendothelial leakage of plasma lipids (3).

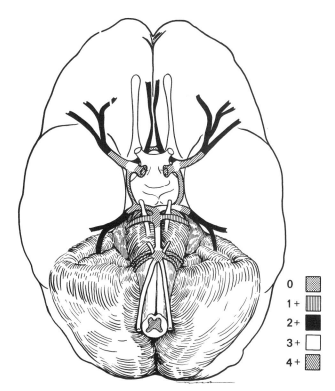

0
1+
2+
3+
4+

FIG. 16-2. Anatomic diagram depicts the location of intracranial atherosclerosis. Involvement of the carotid siphon and large vessel bifurcations predominates. Drawn and adapted from 1,175 consecutive autopsies. (Originally reported by Baker AB, Iannone A. *Neurology* 1961;11: 23–32.)

Location

The pattern of plaque formation at sites where arteries bifurcate suggests that local hemodynamic effects contribute to plaque formation. In the neck, plaques have a predilection for the great vessel origins, common carotid bifurcation, and proximal internal carotid artery (ICA). The unique anatomy of the *carotid bulb* with its flow separation, flow stasis, increased particle residence time, and shear stress oscillations accounts at least in part for the high prevalence of atheromata at this location (3).

Intracranial ASVD typically involves the cavernous ICA segment (*carotid siphon*) (see 16-25,16-26b) and major *vessel bifurcations* (such as the basilary artery bifurcation) (Fig. 16-2). The distal vessels are less commonly affected, but *arteriolosclerosis* and an atheromatous *vasculitis-like pattern* of alternating foci of stenosis and dilatation may develop (see Fig. 16-20).

Clinicopathologic Correlation

Atherosclerotic lesions are often asymptomatic. They become symptomatic in several ways. Ulceration and

intraplaque hemorrhage are prominent histologic features of symptomatic carotid plaques (3). Thrombotic occlusion of the lumen may occur.

If a plaque causes critical (i.e., hemodynamically significant) stenosis, perfusion pressure distal to the stenosis is reduced accordingly and a low-flow infarction may occur (9). Critical stenosis, defined as greater than 70% diameter narrowing, also has an increased incidence of ulceration, thrombosis, and luminal irregularity when compared with nonstenotic atherosclerotic plaques (3).

ANGIOGRAPHY OF ATHEROSCLEROSIS

Noninvasive imaging modalities are widely used to screen patients for extracranial atherosclerosis and its complications. Each technique has its own distinct advantages as well as drawbacks (10). High-resolution magnetic resonance (MR) imaging, MR angiography, carotid duplex ultrasonography (US) with color Doppler flow imaging, and intravascular US all have been proposed as primary diagnostic studies for suspected craniocervical ASVD (2,5,9,11,12).

Although conventional angiography is no longer used as the initial screening procedure in these patients, it remains the standard for evaluating carotid stenosis and planning subsequent therapy, whether surgical or neurointerventional (13). Angiography is still the most precise technique for evaluating the aortic arch and assessing the intracranial circulation. So-called tandem stenosis (see Fig. 16-26), patterns of collateral circulation (see Chapter 17), and incidental nonatheromatous lesions (see Fig. 16-6) such as aneurysms are all nicely evaluated with conventional angiography.

Technical Considerations

Goals

The most important goals of angiography in patients with craniocervical ASVD are to (8,14):

1. Determine the degree of carotid stenosis precisely (measuring carotid stenosis is considered in detail later in this chapter).
2. Identify tandem lesions (e.g., in the carotid siphon or intracranial circulation).
3. Evaluate existing and potential pathways for collateral circulation.
4. Identify coexisting pathology (aortic arch and great vessels, intracranial vessels) that may be difficult to detect on noninvasive studies.

The Angiographic Examination

Because proximal aortic atheromas are an independent risk factor for cerebral ischemia, an angiographic examination for craniocervical ASVD should begin at the *aortic arch* (Fig. 16-3) (15,15a). A single left anterior oblique (LAO) view is usually sufficient for evaluating the *great vessel origins* (Fig. 16-3A). Other views or selective catheterization of the innominate and sub-

clavian arteries may be necessary to depict the vertebral artery origins completely (Fig. 16-3B) (see Chapters 1 and 9). Occasionally an aortic arch appears normal while the distal carotid arteries are diseased (Fig. 16-4).

The *carotid bifurcations* must be profiled in a minimum of at least two projections, usually the lateral and anteroposterior (AP) views (see Fig. 16-4). Both oblique views are often necessary to display plaques in their entirety and detect the maximum area of stenosis (Fig. 16-5). Common carotid injections with digital or film subtraction are usually sufficient.

Demonstrating the carotid bifurcations alone is not sufficient. The *carotid siphon and intracranial circulation* also must be imaged in at least two planes. Detection of an unsuspected tandem stenosis or an incidental lesion such as an aneurysm or vascular malformation is very important for patient management (Fig. 16-6). Up to 20% of examinations performed for carotid bifurcation disease may yield such findings (16).

If cervical or intracranial vascular occlusion or hemodynamically significant stenosis is present, determining the presence and adequacy of *collateral circulation* becomes very important for planning appropriate therapy (see Chapter 17).

Angiographic Findings

The most common angiographic findings in ASVD are luminal irregularities, varying degrees of vessel stenosis, occlusion, and thrombosis. Elongation and ectasia, fusiform enlargement, and giant (serpentine) aneurysms are less common manifestations (8).

Irregularity

Nonstenotic luminal irregularities are the most common finding with ASVD (Fig. 16-4B and C). Because detecting plaque ulceration accurately on cerebral

FIG. 16-3. This 67-year-old man with transient ischemic attacks and diffuse atherosclerotic vascular disease (ASVD) had a previous coronary artery bypass graft (CABG). **A:** Aortic arch angiogram, LAO view, shows the sternal wires (*white arrows*). The left common carotid artery is occluded at its origin (*large straight arrow*). Atherosclerosis narrows the left subclavian artery origin (*curved arrow*). The origins of both vertebral arteries (VAs) also appear compromised (*small arrows*). **B:** Selective left subclavian artery injection confirms stenosis of the left VA at its origin (*large arrow*). Note contrast collection within a shallow atherosclerotic plaque (*small arrow*). **C:** Right common carotid angiogram, arterial phase, oblique view, shows hemodynamically significant narrowing of the internal carotid artery at its origin (*arrow*). **D:** Right common carotid angiogram, arterial phase, lateral view, shows coexisting ASVD in the carotid siphon (*arrow*). The cervical ICA stenosis is hemodynamically significant; the siphon stenosis is not yet flow reducing. Further ASVD progression in the cavernous ICA would result in tandem stenosis.

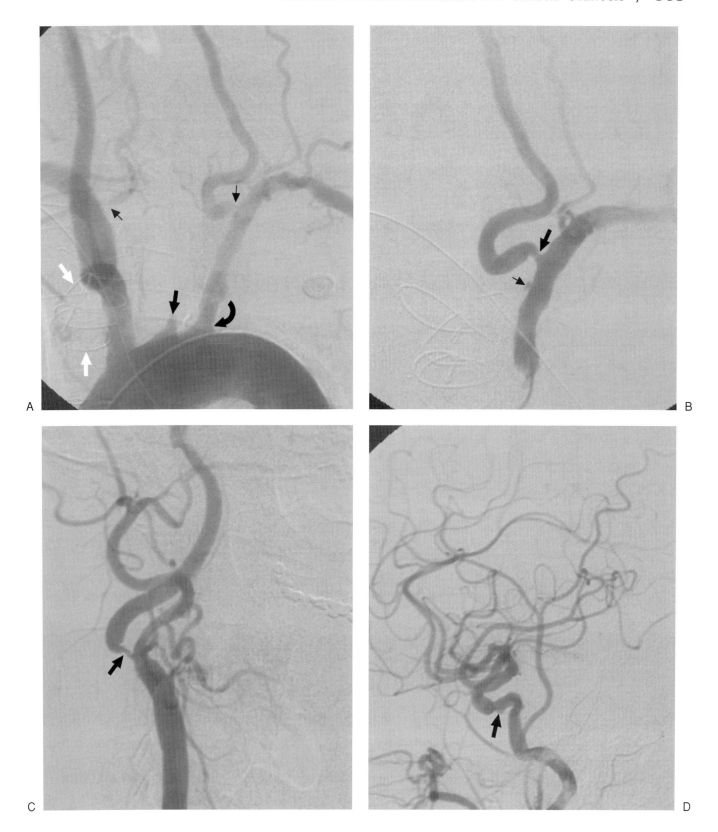

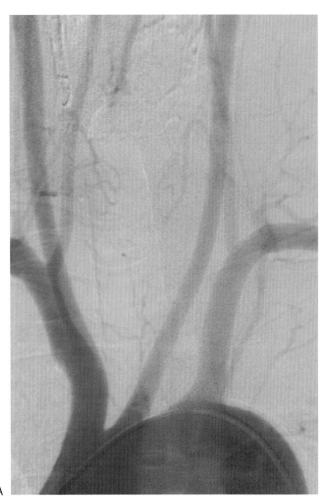
A

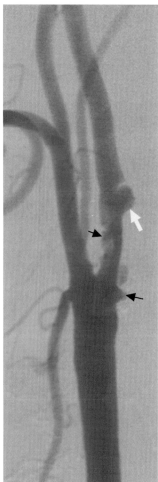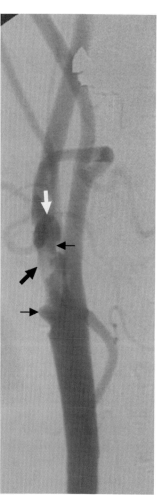
B,C

FIG. 16-4. **A:** Aortic arch angiogram, arterial phase, LAO view, in a 70-year-old man with transient ischemic attacks is normal. Lateral **(B)** and anteroposterior **(C)** views of the right common carotid angiogram show extensive changes of atherosclerosis involving the common carotid bifurcation and proximal internal carotid artery (ICA). Note multiple irregularities along the vessel wall (**B,C,**small black arrows). A double density of contrast accumulation is seen on the AP view (**C**, white arrow). This corresponds to the outpouching seen on the lateral view (**B**, white arrow) and is sometimes called an ulcer niche, but the correlation between angiography and direct surgical observation is poor. Note filling defect in lumen, probably a thrombus (**C**, large black arrow).

angiograms is difficult, the significance of these findings is debatable.

Stenosis

Narrowing of the contrast-filled vessel lumen is a commonly identified lesion in patients with craniocervical ASVD. Stenoses vary widely in both configuration and extent. A smooth subintimal mass effect with asymmetric vessel wall involvement often correlates with *intraplaque hemorrhage* (Fig. 16-7). Generalized circumferential stenosis without luminal irregularity may occur with *fibrotic plaques* (Fig. 16-8; compare with Fig. 16-1F). *Stenosis calculation* is discussed in the concluding section of this chapter.

Ulceration

Plaque ulceration and lumen thrombus are the main sources of cerebral microemboli in high-grade ICA stenosis (17). However, the accuracy of diagnosing plaque ulceration is disputed. The reported sensitivity of detecting plaque ulceration on carotid angiograms varies from 53% to 86% in single-center studies (18).

Determining the presence or absence of ulceration in stenotic (30% to 99%) plaques was initially used as one factor in stratifying patients for the ongoing North American Symptomatic Carotid Endarterectomy Trial (NASCET). Findings suggesting possible ulceration included an "ulcer niche," presence of a *double density*, and *luminal irregularity* (Figs. 16-9 and 16-10) (19). Recent multicenter studies have shown unacceptably high

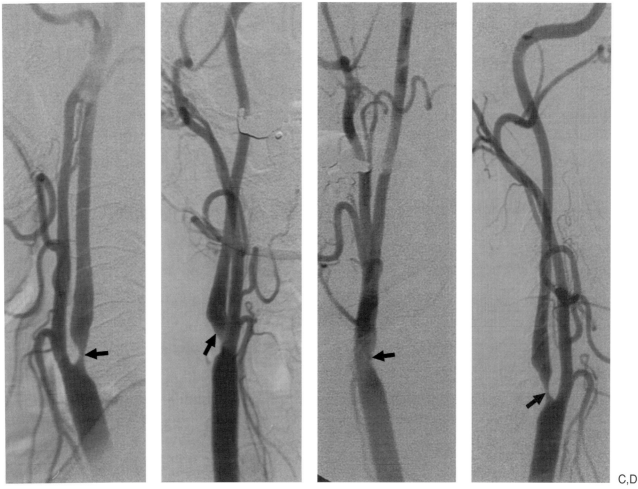

FIG. 16-5. The use of multiple projections to profile an atherosclerotic plaque is illustrated. Lateral **(A)**, anteroposterior **(B)**, and both oblique **(C** and **D)** projections are shown. Note that the hemodynamically significant stenosis (*arrows*) is partially obscured on some views but well seen in others.

false-positive and false-negative results (25.9% and 54.1%, respectively) for the angiographic detection of plaque ulceration compared with direct surgical observation (18). Preliminary studies suggest high-resolution MR imaging and intravascular ultrasound may provide important information regarding both plaque content and morphology (2,12).

Occlusion

Stenosis secondary to ASVD is often progressive and may eventually result in vessel occlusion. The differences between hemodynamically significant stenosis (more than 70% to 99%), true occlusion, and carotid pseudoocclusion are important distinctions for patient management. Regardless of etiology, an *occluded artery* appears to end blindly in a blunted, rounded, or pointed pouch (Fig. 16-11).

Very high grade stenosis may cause very slow antegrade flow with delayed contrast wash-out (Fig. 16-12). The so-called *string sign,* also called the *carotid slim sign, carotid pseudoocclusion,* and *99% stenosis* or *preocclusion* occurs when there is only a trickle of antegrade flow detected at angiography or with color-flow Doppler imaging (20). In such cases it is necessary to examine late phases of the angiogram to document subtle arterial patency (Fig. 16-13).

Thrombosis

Fissuring or rupture of an atherosclerotic plaque may be complicated by platelet adhesion and vessel thrombosis (Fig. 16-14). Both extra- and intracranial thrombotic occlusions usually occur at the site of greatest luminal compromise or just distal to it (21).

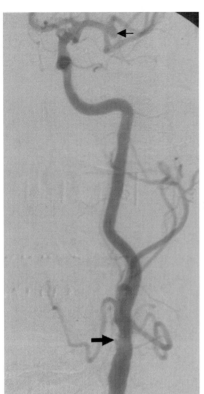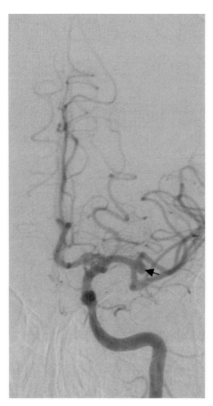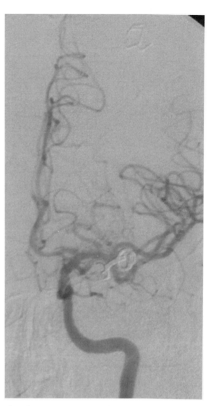

A,B   C

FIG. 16-6. The answer to "Why bother to examine the intracranial circulation in patients with TIAs?" is illustrated in this case. **A:** Standard left common carotid angiogram, arterial phase, AP view, shows a shallow, irregular plaque at the internal carotid origin (*small arrow*). An unruptured aneurysm (*large arrow*) at the left middle cerebral artery bifurcation was found incidentally. **B:** Multiple views including this left common carotid angiogram, arterial phase, AP view, confirmed the presence of a small aneurysm (*arrow*). **C:** Postoperative angiogram shows surgical obliteration of the aneurysm.

Ectasia, Tortuosity, and Fusiform Enlargement

Enlargement, elongation, tortuosity, and some degree of vessel *ectasia* without stenosis or irregularity are part of the aging process and may affect both the extra- (Fig. 16-15) and intracranial vessels (Fig. 16-16) (see Chapter 3). Lumenal enlargement with accompanying arterial wall thickening is also associated with several risk factors, including hypertension and high lipid levels (22).

The difference between uncomplicated age-related ectasia and *atherosclerotic fusiform enlargement* of these vessels is sometimes difficult to determine. The presence of ancillary ASVD in small- and medium-sized vessels may be helpful (Fig. 16-17).

A very elongated, ectatic basilar artery (*vertebrobasilar dolichoectasia* [VBD]) is a relatively common finding on MR scans in elderly patients. The significance of VBD relative to causing vertebrobasilar insufficiency and other symptoms such as lower cranial nerve palsy is debated because the pathophysiologic mechanisms of transient ischemic attacks (TIAs) in the vertebrobasilar territory are more variable and complex than are those in the carotid system (23,24).

Aneurysms

Most atherosclerotic aneurysms are *fusiform aneurysms*. These lesions are exaggerated arterial ectasias due to a severe and unusual form of atherosclerosis (25). Damage to the media results in arterial stretching and elongation. The ectatic vessels may develop more focal areas of fusiform or even saccular enlargement (Fig. 16-18).

Both the cervical and the intracranial circulations may be affected, although *extracranial aneurysms* are uncommon. Most involve the ICA and can rupture, thrombose, or cause distal emboli. Ischemic symptoms and mass effect are the typical clinical presentations. Although atherosclerosis is the single most common cause of an extracranial ICA aneurysm, nearly two thirds of these

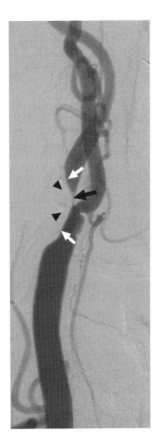

FIG. 16-7. Right common carotid angiogram, arterial phase, oblique view, shows a smooth eccentric atherosclerotic plaque involving the distal common and proximal internal carotid arteries (ICA) (*white arrows*). Note subtraction artifact from plaque calcification (*arrowheads*) and high-grade stenosis (*large black arrow*) of the ICA. Atherosclerotic plaque with hematoma under an intact intima was confirmed at surgery.

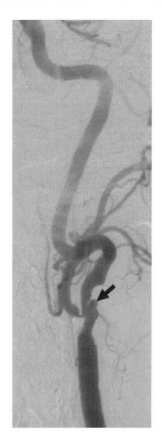

FIG. 16-9. Left common carotid angiogram, arterial phase, AP view, in this patient with transient ischemic attacks (TIAs) shows narrowing of the common carotid bifurcation, external carotid artery origin, and carotid bulb. Note niche of contrast that has collected in a smooth excavation (*arrow*). The correlation between the angiographic diagnosis of plaque ulceration and surgical–pathologic observations is poor.

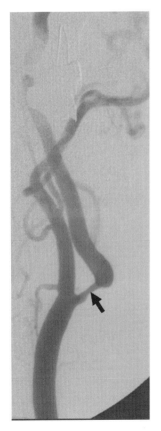

FIG. 16-8. An asymptomatic carotid bruit with high-grade stenosis on ultrasound examination prompted this angiogram. Left common carotid angiogram, arterial phase, AP view, shows smooth concentric stenosis of the proximal internal carotid artery (*arrow*). Fibrotic atherosclerotic narrowing without intimal ulceration was confirmed at endarterectomy (compare with Fig. 16-1D).

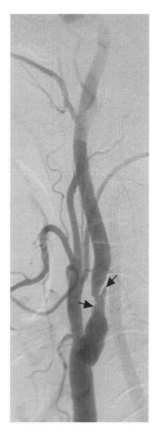

FIG. 16-10. Right common carotid angiogram, arterial phase, lateral view, shows a hemodynamically significant, irregular plaque (*arrows*).

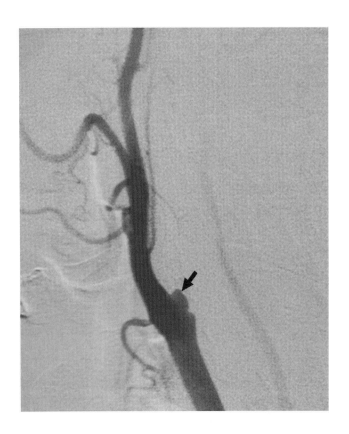

FIG. 16-11. Right common carotid angiogram, arterial phase, oblique view, shows an occluded internal carotid artery (ICA). The ICA ends in a rounded, blind outpouching (*arrow*). No antegrade flow was identified on later phases of the angiogram.

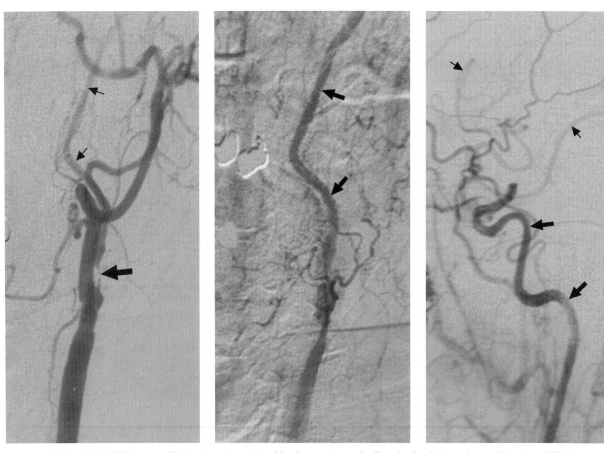

A,B   C

FIG. 16-12. This case illustrates stenosis with slow antegrade flow in the internal carotid artery (ICA). Early **(A)** and very late **(B)** arterial phase films, AP view, show an atherosclerotic plaque with very high grade stenosis (**A**, *large arrow*). Note delayed contrast washout with very slow antegrade flow in the cervical ICA (**A** and **B**, *small arrows*). **C:** Lateral view of the intracranial circulation in the same patient shows that the distal ICA (*large arrows*) retains contrast late into the angiographic sequence and fills some intracranial branches very slowly (*small arrows*).

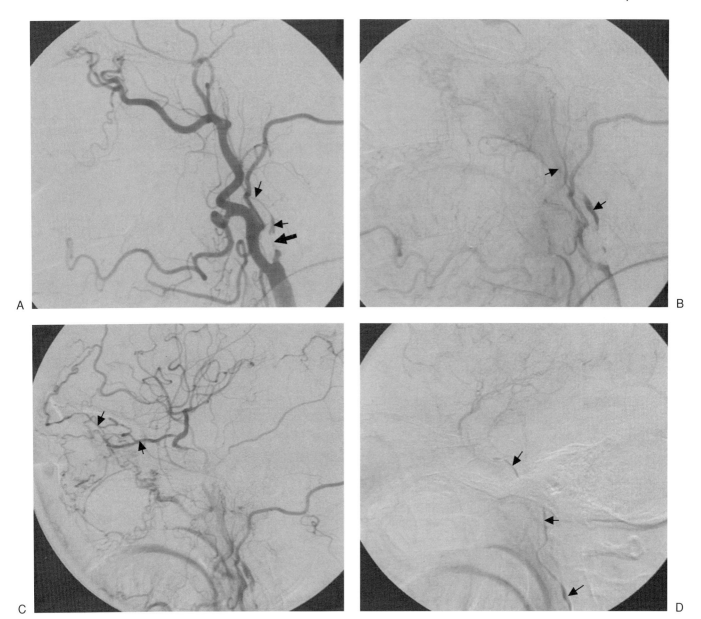

FIG. 16-13. An angiographic string sign (also known as carotid pseudoocclusion) is illustrated. **A:** Left common carotid angiogram, mid-arterial phase, lateral view, discloses a 99% stenosis (*large arrow*) of the proximal internal carotid artery (ICA). A trickle of contrast is seen in the ICA distal to the stenosis (*small arrows*). **B:** Late arterial phase shows contrast in the cervical ICA (*arrows*). **C:** Lateral view of the intracranial circulation obtained in the mid-arterial phase shows that filling of the intracranial ICA is occurring mostly via collaterals from the external carotid artery through the ophthalmic artery (*arrows*). **D:** The early venous phase of the study shows an antegrade trickle of contrast in the cervical and cavernous ICA segments, demonstrating arterial patency (*arrows*).

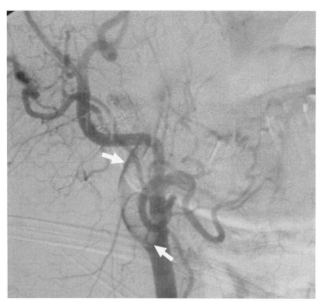

FIG. 16-14. Right common carotid angiogram, arterial phase, oblique view, in this patient with onset of right hemisphere transient ischemic attacks (TIAs) shows an intralumenal filling defect (*white arrows*) in the proximal internal carotid artery. Surgery disclosed an acute intralumenal thrombus loosely attached to a shallow ulcerated plaque.

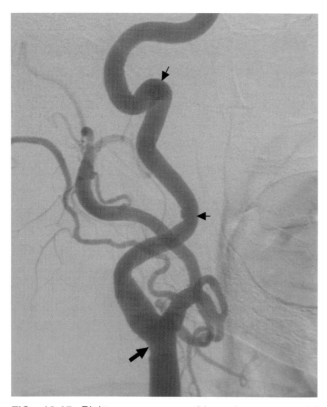

FIG. 16-15. Right common carotid angiogram, arterial phase, oblique view, in a 74-year-old man with a TIA and an irregular pulse. Results of carotid ultrasound were normal. The cervical internal carotid artery is elongated and tortuous (*small arrows*). A very shallow, smooth plaque (*large arrow*) is present at the carotid bifurcation.

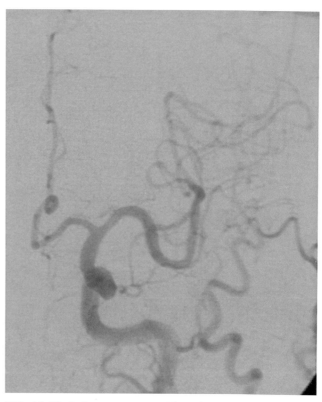

FIG. 16-16. Left common carotid angiogram, arterial phase, AP view, in another case shows ectatic, elongated intracranial vessels. This is normal for the patient's age of 65 years.

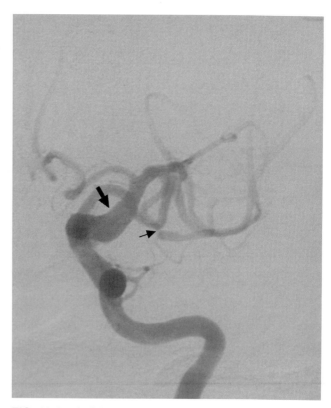

FIG. 16-17. Left internal carotid angiogram, arterial phase, oblique view, shows fusiform dilatation of the supraclinoid internal carotid artery (*large arrow*). Note narrowing of a middle cerebral artery branch (*small arrow*).

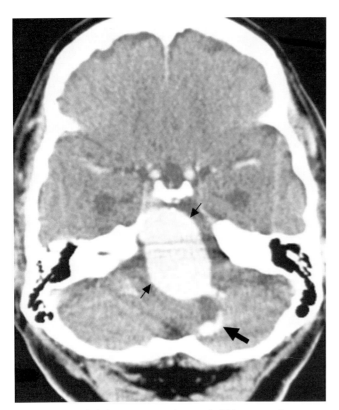

FIG. 16-18. Axial contrast-enhanced CT scan shows an ectatic vertebral artery (*large arrow*) with saccular enlargement of the basilar artery (*small arrows*).

rare lesions are associated with other disease processes. Fibromuscular dysplasia, trauma, spontaneous dissection, and infection have all been reported as causes of extracranial aneurysms (see Chapter 18) (26).

Intracranial aneurysms secondary to ASVD range from small fusiform dilatations of a single vessel to giant dolichoectatic aneurysms that are largely filled with thrombus. The latter are sometimes called *giant serpentine aneurysms* (Fig. 16-19). These aneurysms lack a definable neck. The parent vessel is often circumferentially involved by fusiform aneurysmal dilation or disappears in a large thrombosed mass with distal branches that arise from the aneurysm dome (27).

Vasculitic Atherosclerosis

Atherosclerotic vascular disease is by far the most common cause of intracranial arterial narrowing and occlusion in adults. Diffuse involvement of the cortical vessels may result in an angiographic appearance that is very similar to vasculitis. Atherosclerotic plaques in the medium-sized arteries cause these alternating areas of fusiform stenosis and enlargement. Intracranial ASVD is a dynamic process and lesion progression, particularly in these medium-sized vessels, is common (27a). Both the carotid (Fig. 16-20) and vertebrobasilar (Fig. 16-21) circulations may be affected.

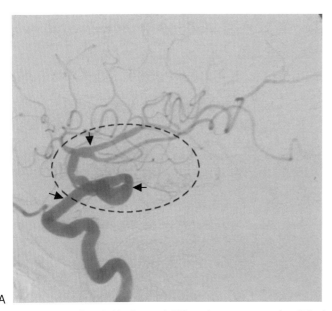

A

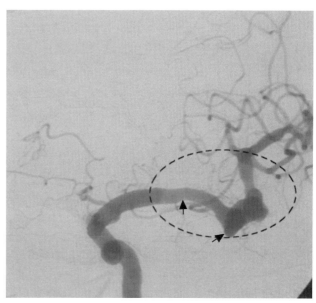

B

FIG. 16-19. Lateral **(A)** and anteroposterior **(B)** views of the left internal carotid angiogram in this 48-year-old man with transient ischemic attacks demonstrate a giant serpentine aneurysm. Note bizarre-appearing elongation and irregularity of the middle cerebral artery (*arrows*). An MR scan and MR angiogram confirmed the presence of a partially thrombosed giant atherosclerotic aneurysm. The approximate diameter of the aneurysm as shown on the MR scan is indicated by the dotted lines.

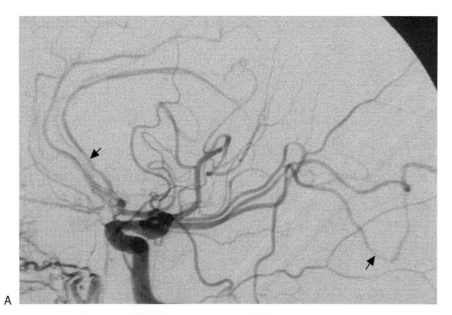

A

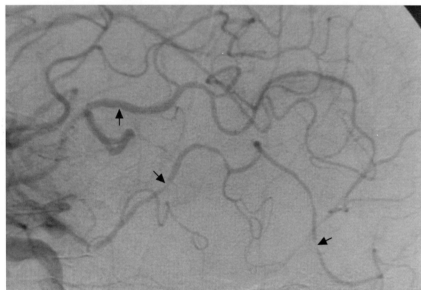

B

FIG. 16-20. Standard lateral (A) and magnified (B) views of a left common carotid angiogram show multifocal irregularities of the distal anterior and middle cerebral arteries (arrows) in this 74-year-old woman with diffuse ASVD. The most common cause of this vasculitislike pattern is atherosclerosis.

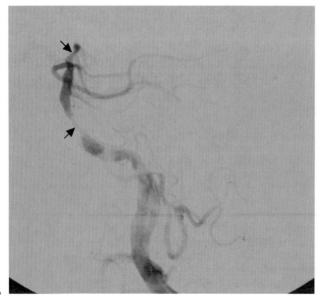

A

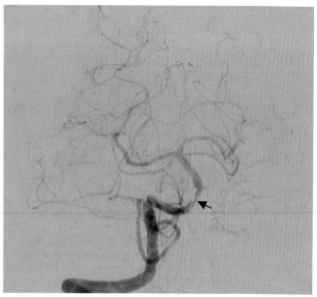

B

FIG. 16-21. Lateral (A) and anteroposterior (B) views of a right vertebral angiogram show multifocal irregularities of the distal basilar artery and its branches (arrows). This patient had diffuse, multisystem atherosclerotic disease.

CAROTID STENOSIS: MEASUREMENT, CLINICAL SIGNIFICANCE, AND TREATMENT OPTIONS

The North American Symptomatic Endarterectomy Trial (NASCET), European Carotid Surgery Trial (ECST), and Asymptomatic Carotid Atherosclerosis Study (ACAS) trial have demonstrated the necessity of determining carotid stenosis accurately (19,28,29). Although noninvasive studies such as CT and MR angiography and ultrasound play an increasing role in evaluating patients with suspected carotid disease, conventional angiography remains the "gold standard" with which these other methods are still compared (13).

Measurement Methods

Most major clinical trials calculate the percentage of stenosis by using diameter reduction at the narrowest site, comparing it with the assumed normal vessel diameter. Each measurement method differs in important ways from the others.

ECST Measurement Method

The minimal residual lumen (MRL) is measured and compared with the subjectively estimated (calculated) normal lumen (NL_c) (Fig. 16-22A). The percentage of stenosis is then calculated as follows:

$$\% \text{ stenosis} = (NL_c - MRL) \div NL_c \times 100$$

NASCET Method

This widely used method is similar to that employed by the ACAS and Veteran's Affairs Carotid Studies Group (VACSG). The maximum area of narrowing is chosen and the minimal residual lumen is measured. The stenosis is then compared with the presumably normal distal lumen (DL) well beyond the bulb, where the vessel walls become parallel (Figs. 16-22B and 16-23) (30). The percentage of stenosis is then calculated as follows:

$$\% \text{ stenosis} = (DL - MRL) \div DL \times 100$$

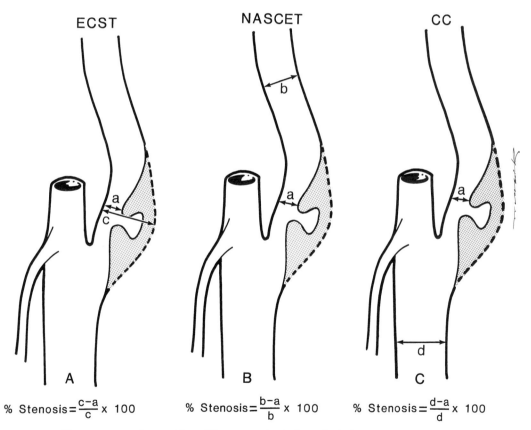

ECST

NASCET

CC

$$\% \text{ Stenosis} = \frac{c-a}{c} \times 100 \qquad \% \text{ Stenosis} = \frac{b-a}{b} \times 100 \qquad \% \text{ Stenosis} = \frac{d-a}{d} \times 100$$

FIG. 16-22. Three commonly used but different methods for calculating carotid stenosis are illustrated and compared. **A:** European Carotid Surgery Trial (ECST) method. **B:** North American Symptomatic Carotid Endarterectomy Trial (NASCET) method. **C:** Common carotid method (also called the carotid stenosis index). a, minimal residual lumen; b, normal ICA lumen (distal to the stenosis, where the walls become parallel); c, estimated (subjectively completed) diameter of the "normal" vessel; d, common carotid diameter.

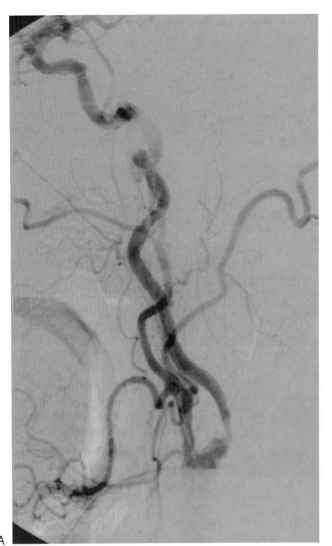

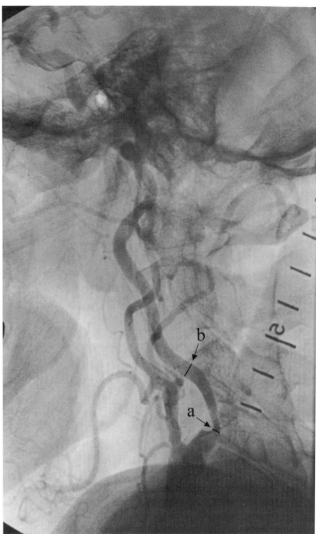

A

B

FIG. 16-23. Manual calculation of carotid stenosis is illustrated in this case. Subtracted **(A)** and unsubtracted **(B)** films of a right common carotid angiogram, arterial phase, lateral view, were performed with centimeter markers to correct for magnification. The 2-mm diameter of the residual lumen at the area of greatest narrowing (*arrow a*) is compared with the 8-mm normal lumen above the constriction (*arrow b*). The stenosis is 75%, a hemodynamically significant lesion by the NASCET criteria.

Common Carotid Method

A third method, called the common carotid artery method or carotid stenosis index (CSI), uses the diameter of the visible disease-free distal common carotid artery (CCA) for comparison. The percentage of stenosis is calculated as follows (Fig. 16-22C) (31):

$$\% \text{ stenosis} = (CCA - MRL) \div CCA \times 100$$

Some investigators feel that the CSI is more reliable, less prone to technical error, and correlates well with duplex and carotid pathology (32).

Other Methodologies

The measurement of stenoses can be automated by using electronic methods. These include digital subtraction angiography with calculated densitometry changes for contrast material at a stenotic site and edge tracing programs that automatically calculate the percentage of stenosis of the vessel in the region of interest (Fig. 16-24) (13).

Comparisons

There are major and clinically important disparities between stenosis calculations using the different mea-

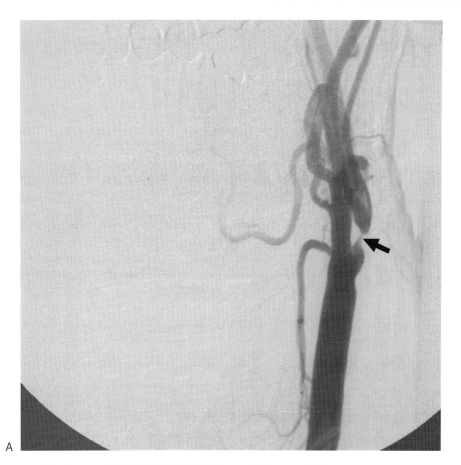

A

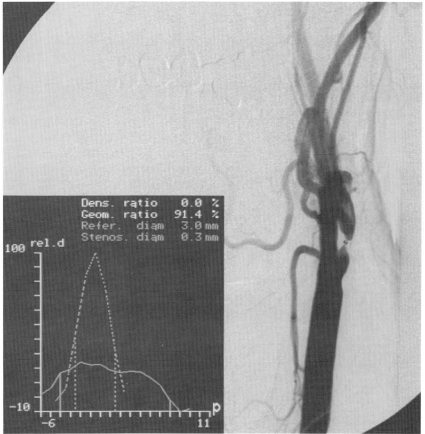

B

FIG. 16-24. Electronic calculation of carotid stenosis is illustrated in this case. **A:** View with the maximum narrowing (*arrow*) of the internal carotid artery (ICA) is selected from multiple projections that were obtained. **B:** Electronic calculation of stenosis and contrast density ratio is performed. The high-grade stenosis is slightly greater than 90%.

surement methods described above (33). This difference is most marked between the ECST and the methods used in other large trials such as NASCET.

European Carotid Surgery Trial calculations usually result in a smaller percentage of stenosis compared with results using the NASCET method. For example, 50% stenosis by ECST standards is approximately equivalent to 70% stenosis calculated using the NASCET method (13,31,34,35). There is also some variability in the published accuracy of noninvasive techniques such as CT angiography as well as difficulty with artifacts induced by factors such as lumen eccentricity (36,36a).

Clinical Significance

Results from some of the multicenter carotid stenosis trials are widely accepted, whereas others are hotly debated.

NASCET

Results from NASCET indicate that surgical intervention is highly beneficial for symptomatic patients with high-grade (more than 70% to 99%) internal carotid artery stenosis (19) (Fig. 16-25). In this selected group, carotid endarterectomy (CEA) results in a 17% absolute risk reduction for any ipsilateral stroke compared with the best medical management (37).

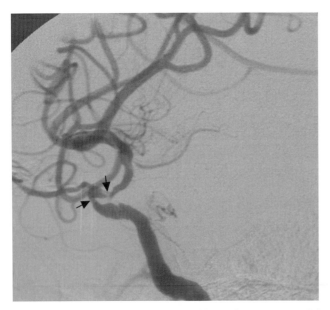

FIG. 16-25. Right common carotid angiogram, arterial phase, lateral view, shows isolated high-grade stenosis of the carotid siphon (*arrows*). Only minimal irregularity of the ICA origin (not shown) was present.

ECST and VACSG/Symptomatic Studies

Equivalent positive benefit for endarterectomy in patients with symptomatic stenosis were reported in these studies despite different methodologies, end points, and formats compared with NASCET (37).

ACAS

The ACAS trial, although criticized on multiple points, concluded that surgery plus best medical management significantly reduces the risk of stroke when compared with best medical management alone in patients with asymptomatic carotid stenoses of 60% or greater (29). Carotid endarterectomy conferred a statistically significant 55% 5-year relative risk reduction for ipsilateral stroke and any perioperative stroke or death and a 5.8% absolute reduction (29,37).

Despite the controversies surrounding this study, its results have significantly affected practice patterns. One study has reported a dramatic increase in the number of carotid endarterectomies performed following release of the ACAS study data (37).

Because angiography and surgery must be performed with less than a 2.3% risk of stroke or death, some surgeons have recommended eliminating conventional angiography in favor of noninvasive testing to improve the risk-benefit ratio for carotid endarterectomy in these patients (38).

Treatment Options and Imaging Implications

Carotid Endarterectomy

Cervical CEA is not effective in patients with siphon stenosis (Fig. 16-25) or in cases where two flow-reducing lesions (so-called tandem stenosis) are present in the same vessel (Fig. 16-26). However, multicenter trials have conclusively demonstrated the effectivenss of CEA in certain selected subpopulations of patients who have cervical carotid occlusive disease (see above). The treatment of asymptomatic patients remains debated and to date the optimal treatment for patients with mild to moderate (30% to 60%) stenosis has not been defined.

In experienced hands, complications from CEA are relatively rare. *Hypertension* affects more than 80% of patients undergoing CEA. Carotid endarterectomy-associated hypertension usually occurs 1 to 2 hours after surgery and can last for 24 hours (39).

In some cases, hypertension leads to cerebral hyperemia and intracerebral hemorrhage, and may be complicated by myocardial infarction. The so-called *hyperperfusion syndrome* typically occurs in hypertensive patients with long-standing high-grade carotid stenosis, poor collateral blood flow, and chronic cerebral vasodilation with impaired vasomotor reactivity. Revascularization in some

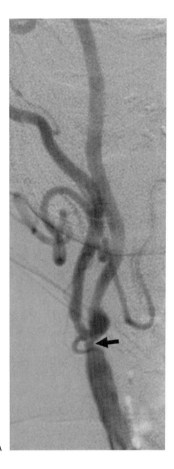
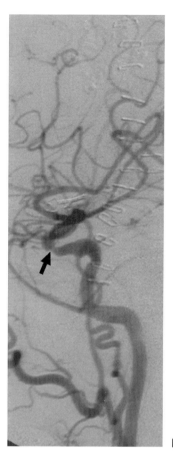

A

B

FIG. 16-26. Tandem carotid stenosis is illustrated in this case. **A:** Right common carotid angiogram, arterial phase, AP view, shows moderate stenosis of the distal common and proximal internal carotid arteries (*arrow*). **B:** Right common carotid angiogram, arterial phase, lateral view of the intracranial circulation shows that a second area of high-grade stenosis is present in the carotid siphon (*arrow*). The flow reduction caused by these two hemodynamically significant lesions is greater than would result from either lesion alone.

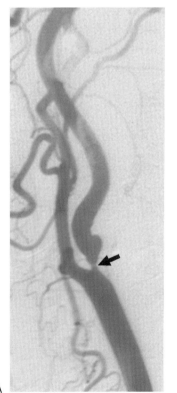
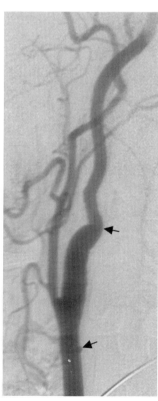

A

B

FIG. 16-27. Pre- **(A)** and post- **(B)** carotid endarterectomy (CEA) common carotid angiograms were performed in this patient with high-grade stenosis of the ICA at its origin (**A**, *arrow*). The post-CEA study shows resolution of the ICA stenosis. The extent of the endarterectomy is indicated (**B**, *arrows*).

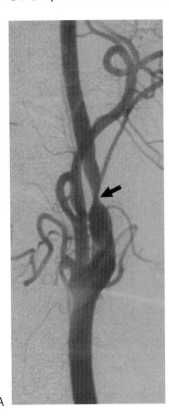
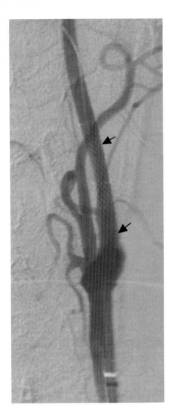

A   B

FIG. 16-28. Pre- (**A**) and post- (**B**) carotid stenting studies were performed in this patient with high-grade ICA stenosis (**A**, *arrow*). The stent (**B**, *arrows*) has enlarged the residual carotid lumen, and the stenosis is no longer present.

of these patients results in perfusion pressure breakthrough and large increases in cerebral blood flow (CBF) with pathological changes similar to hypertensive encephalopathy (39a).

Hypotension in the postoperative period is usually caused by exaggerated discharge from the carotid bulb after plaque removal (39).

Myocardial infarction is the second most common cause of perioperative morbidity and mortality following CEA, affecting 2% to 3% of patients. Myocardial infarction also accounts for up to 50% of late deaths after CEA (39).

Neurologic deficits may be immediate or delayed. Patients with severe, immediate postoperative deficits should be imaged or emergently reexplored to rule out carotid thrombosis (39). Delayed complications include thrombosis and restenosis.

Post-CEA angiograms in patients with uncomplicated endarterectomies normally show mild lumenal enlargement and demonstrate the proximal and distal endarterectomy sites (Fig. 16-27).

Angioplasty and Carotid Stenting

Percutaneous transluminal angioplasty and carotid stenting are both used for the treatment of critical carotid stenosis (more than 70%) secondary to atherosclerosis as well as a spectrum of other vascular occlusive disorders.

Successful endovascular treatment may reduce stenosis with an acceptably low complication rate (Fig. 16-28) (40).

REFERENCES

1. Consigny PM. Pathogenesis of atherosclerosis. *AJR* 1995;164: 553–558.
2. von Ingersleben G, Schmiedl UP, Hatsukami TS, et al. Characterization of atherosclerotic plaques at the carotid bifurcation: correlation of high-resolution MR imaging with histological analysis—preliminary study. *Radiographics* 1997;17:1117–1123.
3. Garcia JH, Ho K-L. Carotid atherosclerosis: definition, pathogenesis, and clinical significance. *Neuroimag Clin North Am* 1996;6:801–810.
4. Kalimo H, Kaste M, Haltia M. Vascular diseases. In: Graham DI, Lantos PL, eds. *Greenfield's neuropathology*, 6th ed. Vol. 1. London: Arnold, 1997:315–396.
5. Winn WB, Schmiedl UP, Reichenbach DD, et al. Detection and characterization of atherosclerotic fibrosis caps with T2-weighted MR. *AJNR* 1998;19:129–134.
6. Imbesi SG, Kerber CH. Why do ulcerated atherosclerotic carotid artery plaques embolize? A flow dynamics study. *AJNR* 1998;19:761–766.
7. Davies PF. Atherosclerosis. Presented at the second basic science course, American Society of Neuroradiology, Chicago, 1990.
8. Osborn AG. Atherosclerosis. In: *Diagnostic neuroradiology*. St. Louis: Mosby, 1994:330–341.
9. Kessler Ch, von Maravic M, Brückmann H, et al. Ultrasound for the assessment of the embolic risk of carotid plaques. *Acta Neurol Scand* 1995;92:231–234.
10. Brant-Zawadzki M. The roles of MR angiography, CT angiography, and sonography in vascular imaging of the head and neck. *AJNR* 1997;18:1820–1825.
11. Huston J, Nichols DA, Luetmer PH, et al. MR angiographic and sonographic indications for endarterectomy. *AJNR* 1998;19:309–315.

12. Manninen HI, Räsänen H, Vanninen RL, et al. Human carotid arteries: correlation of intravascular US with angiographic and histopathologic findings. *Radiology* 1998;206:65–74.

13. Dean BL, Borden N. Conventional angiography. *Neuroimag Clin North Am* 1996;6:843–851.

14. Wolpert SM, Caplan LR. Current role of cerebral angiography in the diagnosis of cerebrovascular disease. *AJR* 1992;159:191–197.

15. Jones EF, Kalman JM, Calafiore P, et al. Proximal aortic atheroma: an independent risk factor for cerebral ischemia. *Stroke* 1995;26: 218–224.

15a. Tenenbaum A, Garniek A, Shemesh J et al. Dual-helical CT for detecting aortic aromas as a source of stroke comparison with transesophageal echocardiography. 1998;208:153–158.

16. Griffiths PD, Worth S, Gholkar A. Incidental intracranial vascular pathology in patients investigated for carotid stenosis [Abstract]. *Neuroradiology* 1995;37:167–168.

17. Sitzer M, Muller W, Siebler M, et al. Plaque ulceration and lumen thrombus are the main sources of cerebral microemboli in high-grade internal carotid artery stenosis. *Stroke* 1995;26:1231–1233.

18. Streifler JY, Eliasziw M, Fox AJ, et al. Angiographic detection of carotid plaque ulceration. *Stroke* 1994;25:1130–1132.

19. North American Symptomatic Carotid Endarterectomy Trial collaborators: beneficial effect of carotid endarterectomy in symptomatic patients with high-grade stenosis. *N Engl J Med* 1991;325:445–453.

20. Berman SS, Devine JJ, Erdoes LS, Hunter GC. Distinguishing carotid artery pseudo-occlusion with color-flow Doppler. *Stroke* 1995;26: 434–438.

21. Ogata J, Masuda J, Yutani C, Yamaguchi T. Mechanisms of cerebral artery thrombosis: a histopathological analysis on eight necropsy cases. *J Neurol Neurosurg Psychiatry* 1994;57:17–21.

22. Bonithon-Kopps C, Touboul PJ, Berr C, et al. Factors of carotid arterial enlargement in a population aged 59–71 years. *Stroke* 1996;27: 654–660.

23. Nakamura K, Saku Y, Torigoe R, et al. Sonographic detection of haemodynamic changes in a case of vertebrobasilar insufficiency. *Neuroradiology* 1998;40:164–166.

24. Passero S, Filosomi G. Posterior circulation infarcts in patients with VBD. *Stroke* 1998;29:653–659.

25. Stehbens WE. Etiology of intracranial berry aneurysms. *J Neurosurg* 1989;70:823–831.

26. Moreau P, Albat B, Thévenet A. Surgical treatment of extracranial internal carotid artery aneurysm. *Ann Vasc Surg* 1994;8:409–416.

27. Anson JA, Lawton MT, Spetzler RF. Characteristics and surgical treatment of dolichoectatic and fusiform aneurysms. *J Neurosurg* 1996;84: 185–193.

27a. Akins PT, Pilgram TK, Cross TD III, Moran CJ: Natural history of stenosis from intracranial atherosclerosis by serial angiography. *Stroke* 1998;29:433–438.

28. European Carotid Surgery Trailists Collaborative Group. MRC European carotid surgery trial: interim results for patients with severe (70–99%) or with mild (0–29%) carotid stenosis. *Lancet* 1991;337: 1235–1243.

29. Executive Committee for ACAS Study. Endarterectomy for asymptomatic carotid artery stenosis. *JAMA* 1995;273:1421–1428.

30. Vainnen R, Manninen H, Koivisto K, et al. Carotid stenosis by digital subtraction angiography: reproducibility of the European Carotid Surgery Trial and the North American Symptomatic Carotid Endarterectomy Trial: Measurement Methods and Visual Interpretation. *AJNR* 1994;15:1635–1641.

31. Rothwell PM, Gibson RJ, Slattery J, et al. Equivalence of measurements of carotid stenosis. *Stroke* 1994;25:2435–2439.

32. Bladin CF, Alexandrov AV, Murphy J, et al. Carotid stenosis index. *Stroke* 1995;26:230–234.

33. Eliasziw M, Smith RF, Singh N, et al. Further comments on the measurement of carotid stenosis from angiograms. *Stroke* 1994;25: 2445–2449.

34. Fox AJ. How to measure carotid stenosis. *Radiology* 1993;186: 316–318.

35. Rothwell PM, Gibson RJ, Slattery J, et al. Prognostic value and reproducibility of measurements of carotid stenosis. *Stroke* 1994;5: 2440–2444.

36. Dix JE, Evans AJ, Kallmes DF, et al. Accuracy and preciser of CT angiography in a model of carotid artery bifurcation stenosis. *AJNR* 1997;18:409–415.

36a. Wise SW, Hopper KD, Ten Have T, Schwartz T. Measuring carotid stenosis using CT angiography: The dilemma of artifactual lumen eccentricity. *AJR* 1998;170:919–923.

37. Huber TS, Wheeler KG, Cuddleback JK, et al. Effect of the asymptomatic carotid endarterectomy in Florida. *Stroke* 1998;29: 1099–1105.

38. Zabramski JM. Asymptomatic carotid stenosis: a neurosurgeon's perspective. *BNI Q* 1996;12:24–25.

39. Holland MC, Spetzler RF. Carotid endarterectomy. *Neuroimag Clin North Am* 1996;6:939–956.

39a. Baker CJ, Mayer SA, Prestigiacomo CJ et al. Diagnosis and monitoring of cerebral hyperfusion after carotid endarterectomy with single photon emission computed tomography: Case report. *Neurosurg* 1998;43:157–161.

40. Urwin RW, Higashida RT, Halbach VV, et al. Endovascular therapy for the carotid artery. *Neuroimag Clin North Am* 1996;4:957–973.

CHAPTER 17

Stroke

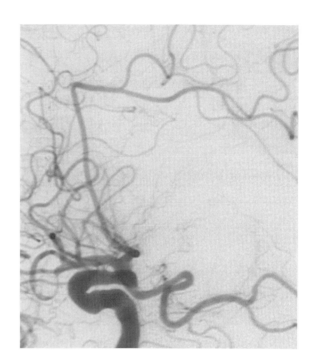

Aggressive stroke therapies focus on timely, accurate diagnosis and preserving "at risk" tissue by rapidly establishing reperfusion (1). That thromboembolic stroke may be amenable to therapy—if rapidly and appropriately instituted—is becoming more widely recognized among the general public through the use of phrases such as "brain attack" and "time is brain."

A complete discussion of noninvasive diagnostic studies and the role of techniques such as diffusion-weighted magnetic resonance (MR) imaging in the new treatment approaches is beyond the scope of this text. However, both conventional angiography and computed tomography (CT) and MR angiography are used to help determine which stroke patients are suitable candidates for emergent thrombolysis.

There are four major types of stroke (Table 17-1). Most are caused by acute occlusion of a cerebral artery (2). This chapter focuses on the angiographic findings that are seen in acute cerebral ischemia. A less common but underdiagnosed type of stroke, sinovenous occlusive disease, is also discussed. The chapter concludes by briefly delineating some common patterns of collateral circulation in the head and neck.

CEREBRAL ISCHEMIA AND INFARCTION

Definitions

Stroke

Stroke is defined as an abrupt onset of focal or global neurologic symptoms caused by ischemia or hemorrhage. By convention, these symptoms must persist for more than 24 hours. If the symptoms resolve within 24 hours, the event is called a *transient ischemic attack* (TIA) (3).

"Stroke" encompasses a heterogenous group of cerebrovascular disorders that ranges from thromboembolic events and aneurysmal subarachnoid hemorrhage to sinovenous occlusions.

Ischemia

"Ischemia" describes the condition in which blood flow decreases to a level at which either temporary or permanent loss of organ function occurs (4). Cerebral ischemia is significantly diminished blood flow to all parts (global ischemia) or selected areas (regional or

TABLE 17-1. *Stroke: etiology and frequency*

Type	Percent
Cerebral ischemia	80–85
Primary intracranial hemorrhage	15
Hypertensive hemorrhage	
Amyloid angiopathy	
Vascular malformation	
Miscellaneous (tumor, drugs, hemorrhagic diathesis)	
Nontraumatic subarachnoid hemorrhage	5
Aneurysm	
Nonaneurysmal SAH	
Cerebral venous thrombosis	1
Sinovenous occlusion	
Isolated cortical vein thrombosis	

focal ischemia) of the brain. The clinical manifestations of cerebral ischemia are predicated on a number of factors, including flow decrement, location, duration, and tissue volume involved (5).

Infarct

An *infarct* is an area of coagulation necrosis that develops as a result of an ischemic event. Severe ischemia, defined as cerebral blood flow (CBF) values below 10 mL/100 g/minute, is the physiologic prerequisite for the development of coagulation necrosis or infarct, although not all ischemic injuries become infarcts (4). *Infarction* is the process by which an infarct develops.

Physiology: Basic Concepts and the Pathogenesis of Stroke

Cerebral Blood Flow Thresholds

Briefly summarized, the crucial events in the pathogenesis of ischemic brain injury are set into motion at critical thresholds of reduced CBF. Reducing CBF to 30% to 35% of normal causes functional suppression (failure of synaptic transmission), whereas greater reductions (to 15% to 20% of normal) cause failure of energy-requiring ion pump mechanisms in the affected brain (6).

There are two physiologically different areas in most acute infarcts: (a) the central *ischemic "core" zone* and (b) a less densely *ischemic "penumbra"* that lies just peripheral to the core zone. The penumbra is metabolically unstable and electrophysiologically dynamic. Cerebral blood flow in the penumbra is approximately 20% to 40% of normal (6). In acute stroke there is a limited period during which the ischemic penumbra has the capacity to recover if perfusion is restored (3).

Time Dependence

There is a curvilinear relationship between the intensity and duration of CBF decrements that correlates with neuronal injury. Near-total CBF reductions (e.g., as in cardiac arrest) may cause neuronal damage within minutes. Longer periods of reduced CBF can be sustained without permanent injury in thromboembolic strokes that retain some collateral circulation (6).

Selective Vulnerability

Sensitivity to ischemic damage varies with different cell types. There is a well-defined *histologic hierarchy of sensitivity* to ischemic damage among the different cell types that constitute the neuropil. Neurons are the most vulnerable. They are followed (in descending order of susceptibility) by astrocytes, oligodendroglia, microglia, and endothelial cells.

There is also a *geographic hierarchy of sensitivity* to ischemic damage among the neurons themselves. Neurons in the CA_1 area of the hippocampus, neocortex layers III, V, and VI, and the neostriatum are the most vulnerable (7).

Collateral Supply

The consequences of cerebral arterial occlusion, regardless of etiology, vary because alterations in cerebral blood flow change with a number of factors. Duration of CBF reduction, location, and available collateral circulation all influence clinical outcome.

Pathology

Gross Pathology

The major gross features of recent *"ischemic infarction"* are blurring of the gray/white matter demarcation, narrowing of the sulci, softening of ischemic tissues as a result of water retention, and displacement of neighboring anatomic structures (i.e., mass effect) (4).

Hemorrhagic infarction occurs when there are numerous petechial hemorrhages in the affected area. Hemorrhagic infarcts are usually confined to the gray matter. In autopsy studies, 18% to 48% of brain arterial infarcts have identifiable hemorrhagic components (3,4). The prevalence of hemorrhage is higher in venous occlusions.

Hemorrhagic transformation occurs when perfusion within ischemic tissue is reestablished. These reperfusion hemorrhages are probably secondary to extravasation from necrotic, leaking blood vessels (3).

Microscopic Pathology

Frank cerebral *infarction* is characterized by irreversible damage to all cells within the infarcted zone. This includes neurons, glia, and endothelial cells. Histologic findings in acute stroke range from coagulative necrosis (in the densely ischemic central focus) to astrocytic swelling (in the penumbral zone).

Imaging

Noninvasive Screening Studies

The decision to consider thrombolytic agents in patients with acute stroke is often based on clinical considerations together with information from noninvasive studies such as CT or MR. Acute stroke subtypes based on evidence of territory distributions are incorrect in 30% to 50% of cases. The concept that stroke mechanisms (e.g., hemodynamic compromise versus embolic disease) can be inferred from scan patterns alone is also incorrect. Because there is such significant variablitity in intracranial arterial territory distributions (see Figs. 6-5, 7-15, 8-16), these patterns are inadequate to determine acute stroke subtype and underlying pathogenesis accurately. This is true regardless of the brain imaging technique applied (7a).

Clinical Considerations

Conventional angiography in the setting of acute stroke is now performed only when primary intracranial hemorrhage with an underlying vascular lesion is suspected or the patient has acute cerebral ischemia and is a potential candidate for thrombolysis.

In patients with ischemic stroke this implies that (a) the patient has presented within the so-called therapeutic window (preferably within 3 or 4 and no longer than 6 hours after ictus) and (b) there is no evidence for hemorrhage on preliminary imaging studies (typically a nonenhanced CT scan). Other important determining factors include the site of arterial occlusion (middle cerebral or basilar artery) and the presence and volume of salvageable brain (e.g., as determined by diffusion-weighted or echo-planar MR imaging) (8).

Conventional Angiographic Findings

The angiographic signs of acute cerebral infarction are summarized in the box below. The most common—and specific—findings are the presence of intravascular thrombus and vessel occlusion.

Intravascular *thrombus* is seen as a filling defect within the lumen of an opacified vessel. The most common sites are the extracranial internal carotid artery (ICA) (see Fig. 16-14) and the middle cerebral artery (MCA) (Fig. 17-1). *Occlusion* is identified as a tapered narrowing (see Fig. 17-5A) or sharp termination of the contrast column, sometimes seen as a meniscal filling defect (Fig. 17-2).

Other angiographic abnormalities observed in acute cerebral infarction are *slow antegrade flow* with prolonged circulation time and delayed "washout" of arterial contrast in the affected area (Fig. 17-1). *"Bare" areas* with a paucity of vessels in nonperfused or slowly perfused brain are seen in some cases (Figs. 17-1D, 17-3A, and 17-6). *Retrograde filling* of patent but proximally obstructed branches from pial collaterals across the vascular watershed zone is also common (Figs. 17-3 to 17-5).

A vascular blush, sometimes called *"luxury perfusion,"* refers to contrast accumulation in ischemic brain parenchyma that is sometimes seen within a few hours to a few days after stroke onset (Figs. 17-4; see also Fig. 18-5D). The pathophysiologic basis of luxury perfusion is

---

Angiographic Signs of Acute Cerebral Ischemia

Common
  Intraluminal thrombus
  Vessel occlusion
  Slow antegrade flow with delayed arterial
    emptying
  Slow retrograde filling through collateral
    vessels
  "Bare" areas (regions of nonperfused or slowly
    perfused brain)
Less common
  Hyperemia (vascular blush or "luxury
    perfusion")
  Arteriovenous shunting with "early draining"
    veins
Uncommon
  Mass effect (rare in hyperacute stroke; very
    common in later stages)

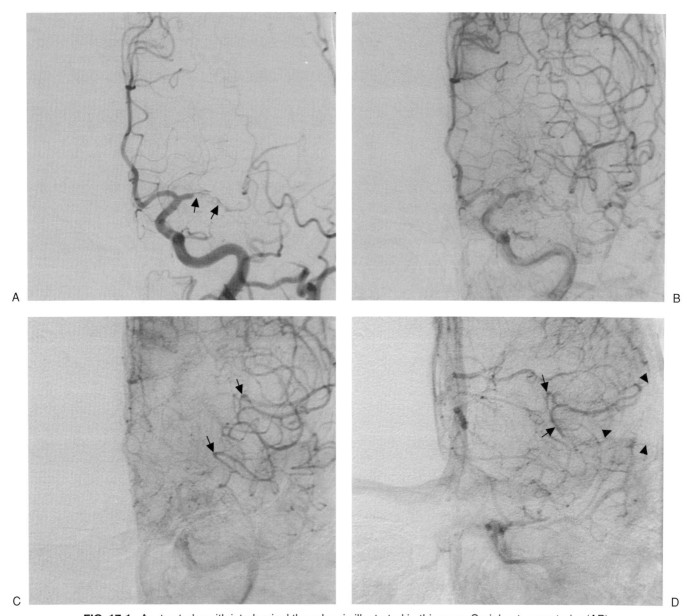

FIG. 17-1. Acute stroke with intraluminal thrombus is illustrated in this case. Serial anteroposterior (AP) views **(A–D)** and lateral **(E–H)** views are shown. **A:** Left common carotid angiogram, early arterial phase, AP view, shows a filling defect (*arrows*) in the horizontal (M1) segment of the middle cerebral artery (MCA). Late arterial **(B)**, capillary **(C)**, and venous phases **(D)** show very slow antegrade flow with contrast stasis in the distal MCA (*arrows*) that persists well into the venous phase of the angiogram. Note the small wedge-shaped bare area of nonperfused parenchyma (**D**, *arrowheads*).

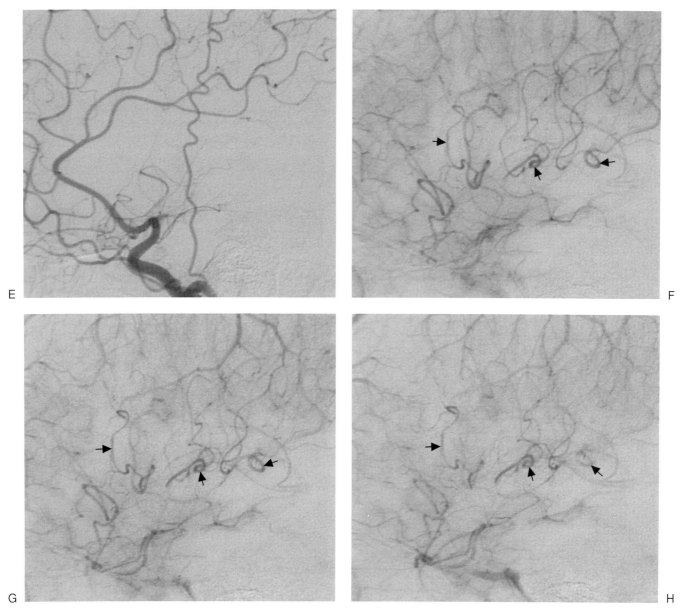

FIG. 17-1. *Continued.* **E–H:** Serial lateral views demonstrate late opacification of the M2 and M3 branches (*arrows*), with some contrast still opacifying these vessels in the early venous phase of the angiogram.

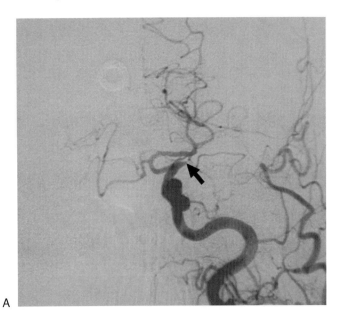

A

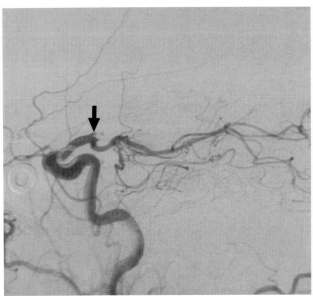

B

FIG. 17-2. Acute stroke with complete embolic occlusion of the supraclinoid internal carotid artery (ICA) is illustrated. Anteroposterior **(A)** and lateral **(B)** views of a left common carotid angiogram show ICA occlusion just distal to the origin of a "fetal" posterior cerebral artery. A meniscus of contrast outlines the clot (*arrows*). There is no filling of the intracranial vessels beyond the thrombus.

incompletely understood. Proposed mechanisms include arteriolar-venular shunting, capillary dilation with shortened circulation time, and increased flow through residual preserved vascular channels (9). In some cases luxury perfusion is accompanied by *arteriovenous shunting* with early appearance of contrast in veins that drain the ischemic focus.

Mass effect in the early stages of acute cerebral ischemia is uncommon but is a major cause of death within the first week after stroke (10).

CT Angiographic Findings

Triphasic helical CT with early arterial, perfusion, and delayed scans after bolus injection of contrast material may be useful for the early diagnosis of acute proximal MCA occlusion and assessment of the ischemic zone. The major signs of acute occlusion are decreased arterial enhancement (early arterial phase), nonenhancing arterial segment (perfusion phase), and asymmetric arterial enhancement (delayed phase) (11).

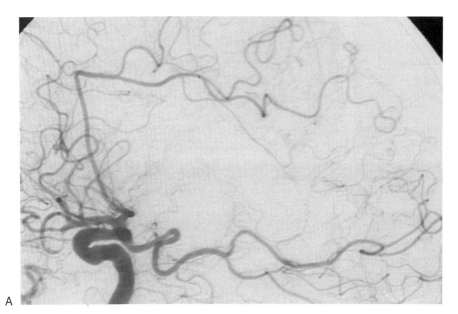

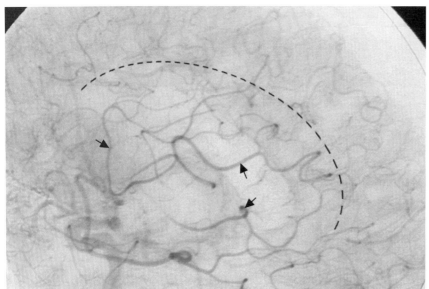

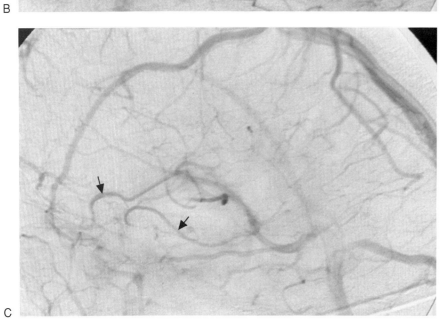

FIG. 17-3. This 78-year-old man with atrial fibrillation experienced acute onset of speech difficulties and right-sided hemiparesis. A left common carotid angiogram was performed prior to thrombolysis. **A:** Early arterial phase, lateral view, shows a large bare area in the middle cerebral artery (MCA) distribution. The anterior (ACA) and posterior (PCA) arteries are opacified normally. **B:** Pial collaterals from the ACA and PCA fill the MCA branches (*arrows*) across the vascular watershed zone (*dotted lines*). Slow retrograde flow in the MCA opacifies some insular branches well into the venous phase of the angiogram (**C**, *arrows*).

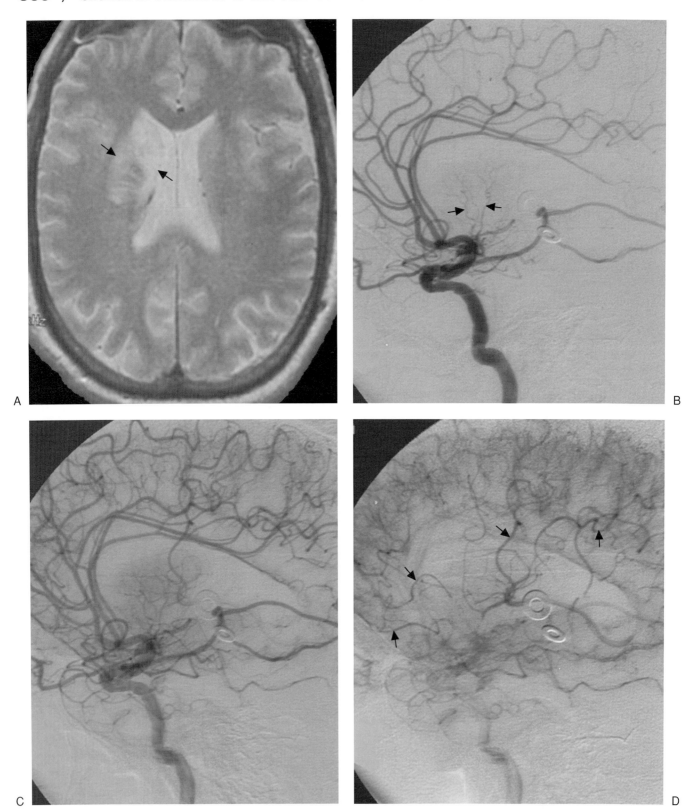

FIG. 17-4. A: Axial T2-weighted MR scan in this patient with a right middle cerebral artery (MCA) occlusion shows increased signal intensity that appears limited to the basal ganglia (*arrows*). **B:** Right internal carotid angiogram, early arterial phase, lateral view, shows a bare area of absent perfusion in the MCA territory. Only the lenticulostriate arteries (*arrows*) are opacified. **C:** Mid-arterial phase shows a dense vascular blush in the region of the basal ganglia. This represents hyperemia, so-called luxury perfusion. **D:** Late arterial phase shows that pial watershed zone collaterals opacify the MCA cortical branches (*arrows*).

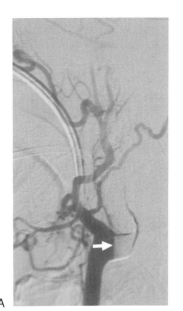
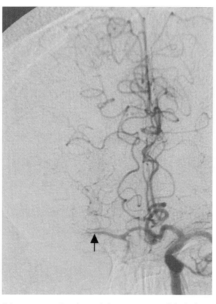
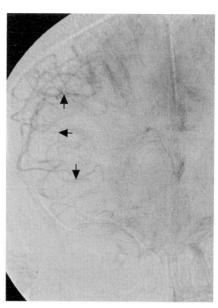

A

B,C

FIG. 17-5. This 52-year-old woman had sudden onset of left hemiparesis. **A:** Right common carotid angiogram, arterial phase, lateral view, shows an acutely thrombosed cervical internal carotid artery (ICA). Note fluid–fluid level between the contrast column and unopacified blood in the dependent portion of the carotid bulb (*arrow*). **B:** Left internal carotid angiogram, arterial phase, AP view, shows that distal embolization from the thrombus has occluded the horizontal middle cerebral artery (*arrow*). **C:** Capillary phase shows that collateral flow (*arrows*) from the anterior carotid artery opacifies over the watershed zone.

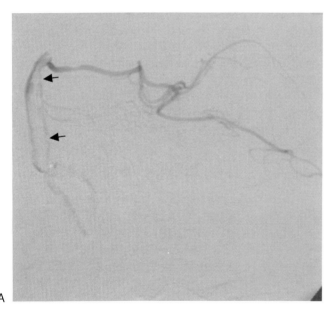
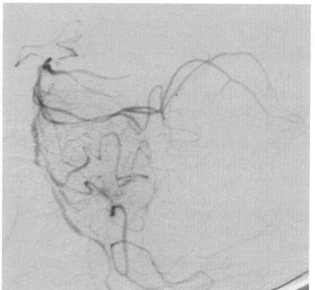

A

B

FIG. 17-6. This 62-year-old woman presented with a 2-week history of flulike symptoms and gradually increasing malaise. She suddenly collapsed and became obtunded. MR scan with MR angiography disclosed a "top of the basilar" syndrome. Angiography was performed prior to intraarterial thrombolysis. **A:** Left vertebral angiogram, late arterial phase, lateral view, shows that extensive clot fills the basilar artery (*arrows*). The only branches that are patent are one superior cerebellar artery and two small pontine perforating arteries. **B:** Improved filling of the posterior circulation branches is seen following thrombolysis.

VENOUS OCCLUSIONS

Cerebral venous thrombosis (CVT) is an underdiagnosed cause of acute neurologic deterioration. Because clinical signs and symptoms are often nonspecific, imaging is critical to the diagnosis of venous occlusion and infarction (7). As one investigator put it recently, "Venous infarction may be more common than is generally thought; half the battle is thinking of it in the first place" (12).

Pathology

Gross Pathology

Cerebral *venous thrombosis* is a multistep process that begins when thrombus forms in a dural sinus. As the clot propagates, it usually first obstructs the sinus and then extends to involve cortical tributaries. Markedly distended veins and adjacent subarachnoid hemorrhages are common (7).

Venous infarction often complicates sinovenous occlusive disease. Venous infarcts tend to become hemorrhagic early in the course of the disease process. In contrast to the petechial cortical hemorrhages that occur with reperfusion in an ischemic infarct, venous infarcts extend widely into the subcortical white matter (3,4). Subarachnoid hemorrhage and gross cerebral edema with descending transtentorial herniation may occur with occlusion of a major dural sinus such as the superior sagittal sinus (SSS).

Microscopic Pathology

Microscopically, the parenchymal lesions that occur secondary to sinovenous occlusions are characterized by large lakes of extravasated plasma, pronounced sponginess in the absence of neuronal necrosis, and periadventitial and parenchymal hemorrhages (3,4).

Etiology

A multitude of different conditions can cause CVT. Both localized and systemic disease processes have been implicated (see box, next column).

Local Predisposing Conditions

Local disease processes such as sinusitis, otitis media and mastoiditis, trauma, and tumor can occlude dural sinuses. In the past, infections were the most common cause of CVT. More recently, less than 10% of venous occlusions had an infectious etiology (3).

Generalized and Systemic Disorders

Congenital coagulation disorders such as protein C, protein S, and antithrombin deficiencies as well as variations in the prothrombin (factor II) gene are associated with an increased risk of deep vein thrombosis and pulmonary embolism (12a).

Cerebral Venous Thrombosis:
Some Reported Predisposing Conditions

Local predisposing conditions
  Sinonasal infection
  Otitis media, mastoiditis
  Trauma
  Tumor (e.g., meningioma, metastasis)
Generalized and systemic disorders
  Dehydration
  Septicemia
  Drugs (e.g., oral contraceptives)
  Pregnancy, puerperium
  Systemic malignancy, paraneoplastic
    syndromes
  Blood dyscrasias
  Lupus anticoagulant, antiphospholipid syndrome
  Hypercoagulable states (protein S, protein C, and
    antithrombin deficiency, Leiden proaccelerin
    allele, etc.)
  Inflammatory bowel disease
  Behçet's disease
  Collagen vascular disease

Acquired predisposing conditions include dehydration, systemic infection, hematologic diseases and hypercoagulable states, drugs (e.g., oral contraceptives), puerperium, pregnancy, systemic malignancy and paraneoplastic syndromes, collagen vascular diseases, antiphospholipid syndrome, inflammatory bowel disease, Behçet's disease, and high-flow vasculopathic changes (13).

No cause for CVT is identified in one fourth of all cases (7).

Clinical Presentation

Numerous factors such as location, degree of venous stasis, rate of occlusion, and availability of collateral veins all influence the clinical and morphologic signs of CVT (14). The symptoms of CVT are often nonspecific, and the diagnosis is frequently elusive. Headache, increased intracranial pressure, vomiting, and lethargy are common. Mild paresis or visual disturbances can occur. More severe complications include seizure, stupor, and coma (15).

Location

In general, the topography of CVT corresponds to one of the major venous drainage territories (see Fig. 11-13). Four general patterns can be identified: (a) A superficial pattern in which a major dural sinus and its adjacent cortical tributaries are occluded; (b) a deep central pattern in which the internal cerebral veins (ICVs) and their tributaries become thrombosed; (c) a deep basal pattern in which the cavernous sinus (CS) is occluded; and (d) isolated cortical venous thrombosis (see box below).

Superficial Pattern of CVT

The *superior sagittal sinus* (SSS) is the most common site, followed by the transverse, sigmoid, and cavernous sinuses. Dural sinus thrombosis is often accompanied by extensive cortical and subcortical hemorrhages in the parenchyma adjacent to the occlusion.

Deep Central Pattern of CVT

Internal cerebral vein (ICV) thrombosis accounts for only 10% of CVT cases (16). The *vein of Galen* and sometimes the *straight sinus* are also thrombosed. Internal cerebral vein thrombosis usually causes bilateral venous infarcts in the basal ganglia and thalami. Adjacent white matter and the upper mid-brain are often affected as well.

Deep Basal Pattern of CVT

Cavernous sinus (CS) thrombosis is now an uncommon form of CVT, representing less than 5% of cases. It

---

is a potentially catastrophic condition associated with a variety of disease processes. The CS is the most common site of septic CVT and usually occurs as a complication of pyogenic sinonasal infections (17).

Contrast-enhanced CT or MR scans typically show filling defects in an expanded CS. Collateral drainage routes through expanded CS tributaries such as the superior ophthalmic vein, inferior petrosal sinus, and sphenoparietal sinus may occur (18). Parenchymal hemorrhage is uncommon in CS thrombosis.

Isolated Cortical Venous Thrombosis

Cortical venous thrombosis in the absence of dural sinus occlusion is a rare but recognized cause of parenchymal hemorrhage. Because positive identification of an isolated thrombosed cortical vein may be difficult, knowledge of associated predisposing conditions is important (see box on page 390) (19).

Imaging

Noninvasive Studies

Cavernous sinus thrombosis is initially diagnosed on noninvasive studies. Nonenhanced CT scans may disclose hyperdense thrombus in the affected dural sinus or cortical vein (cord sign). The cortical and subcortical hemorrhages that often occur early in the course of CVT also can be delineated. Contrast-enhanced CT scans show enhancing dura surrounding intraluminal clot (the so-called empty delta sign). Magnetic radiance with MR venography easily confirms the diagnosis of CVT in almost all cases (16).

Cerebral Angiography: Technical Considerations

Cerebral angiography is now performed almost exclusively as a prelude to thrombolysis and is only occasionally required to establish the diagnosis of CVT itself.

Aortic arch injection with the head filmed in a slightly oblique position is preferred by many angiographers because this technique opacifies all of the craniocerebral vessels as well as the dural sinuses and cortical veins. Inflow of unopacified blood thus cannot be mistaken for clot (20). Alternatively, standard selective carotid and vertebral angiograms can be performed. In either case, it is very important to examine carefully venous phase views obtained late in the angiographic sequence.

Cerebral Angiography: Signs of CVT

A partially thrombosed sinus is characterized by intraluminal filling defects, whereas a completely occluded sinus appears as an empty channel devoid of contrast (Figs. 17-7 and 17-8). The occluded sinus may be surrounded by dilated venous channels contained within the

---

> ## Cerebral Venous Thrombosis: Patterns
>
> **Superficial pattern**
>   Most common type (85%)
>   Dural sinus occlusion (Superior sagittal sinus is most common location)
>   Parenchymal hemorrhage common
> **Deep central pattern**
>   Less common (10%)
>   Internal cerebral vein, vein of Galen, sometimes straight sinus are involved
>   Bilateral infarcts in basal ganglia, thalami, deep white matter
> **Deep basal pattern**
>   Cavernous sinus thrombosis (less than 5%)
>   Sinonasal infection is common (pyogenic, less often fungal)
>   Usually bilateral; unilateral thrombosis occurs but is less common
>   Multiple cranial neuropathies common
>   Parenchymal hemorrhage, infarction rare
> **Isolated cortical pattern**
>   Rare (1%) in the absence of coexisting dural sinus occlusion
>   Focal parenchymal hemorrhage common
>   Anastomotic vein of Labbé, Trolard occlusion may cause large area of hemorrhagic venous infarction
>   Difficult to diagnose; knowledge of predisposing factors, high index of clinical suspicion helpful

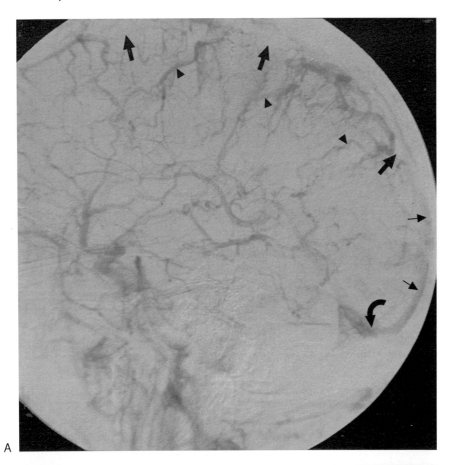

A

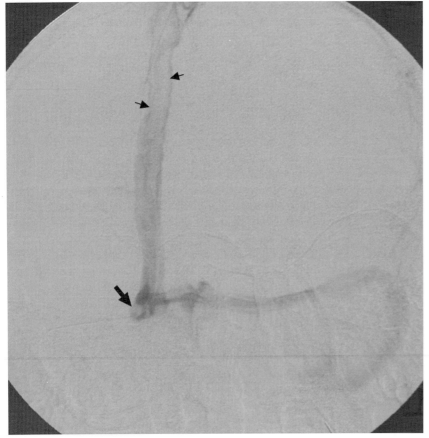

B

FIG. 17-7. A 37-year-old woman began taking oral contraceptives approximately 4 weeks before developing headache and acute left upper extremity paresthesias. An MR scan (not illustrated) showed superior sagittal (SSS) and right transverse (TS) sinus occlusion. She was referred for thrombolysis. **A:** Right internal carotid angiogram, venous phase, lateral view, shows nearly complete SSS thrombosis (*large arrows*). The descending portion of the SSS is partially patent (*small arrows*), but the torcular is filled with clot (*curved arrow*) and the transverse sinus is occluded. Note contrast stasis in numerous tortuous cortical veins (*arrowheads*) providing collateral drainage to the superficial middle cerebral vein and deep subependymal veins. **B:** Retrograde catheterization of the SSS via the right TS shows filling defects in the SSS (*small arrows*) and an occluded right TS (*large arrow*). Thrombolysis was successful. Follow-up MR venogram 1 month later demonstrated patent dural sinuses.

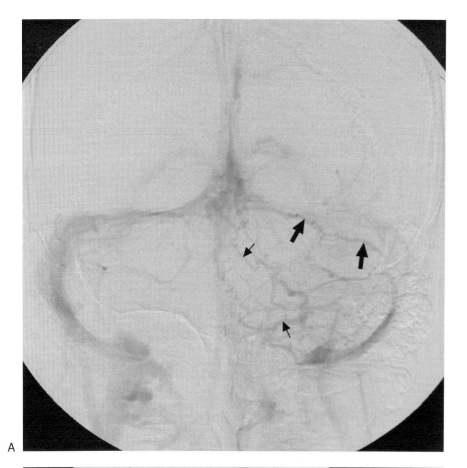

A

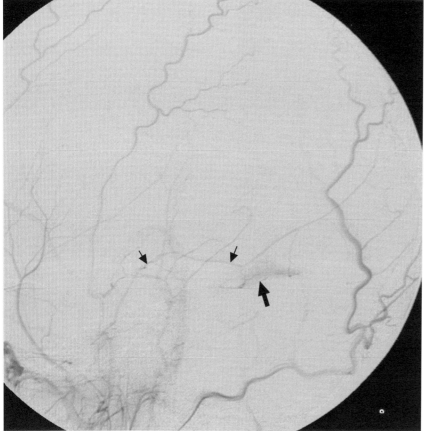

B

FIG. 17-8. This 22-year-old man had a first-time seizure during treatment for extragonadal seminoma. An MR scan (not shown) demonstrated left transverse sinus occlusion with unusually striking leptomeningeal enhancement. **A:** Left vertebral angiogram, arterial phase, anteroposterior view, shows thrombus filling the left transverse sinus (*large arrows*) with numerous tortuous collateral draining veins (*small arrows*). **B:** Left external carotid angiogram, late arterial phase, lateral view, shows that an enlarged posterior meningeal branch (*small arrows*) supplies a small plexus of vessels in the wall of the occluded transverse sinus (*large arrow*). This represents the initial stage in developing an acquired dural arteriovenous fistula (dAVF).

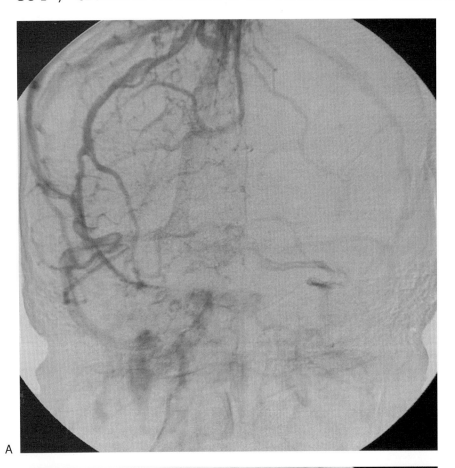

A

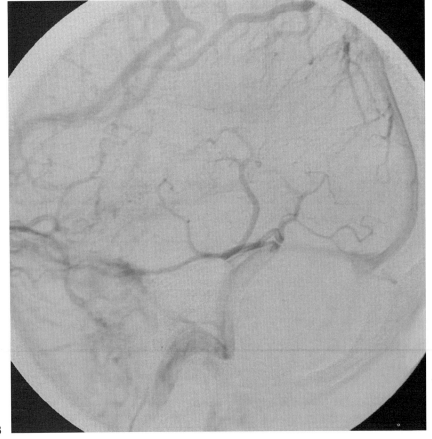

B

FIG. 17-9. Anteroposterior **(A)** and oblique lateral **(B)** venous phase views of a right internal carotid angiogram show that the superior sagittal and transverse sinuses are patent. The internal cerebral vein, vein of Galen, and straight sinus are not visualized. This case demonstrates deep venous thrombosis.

dural leaves. Cortical veins are often seen as prominent, unusually tortuous channels with delayed contrast washout. Enlargement of deep white matter (medullary) and other collateral veins is common in CVT.

Deep central CVT is seen as nonfilling of the ICVs and vein of Galen. Enlarged collateral channels may be present. The straight sinus is often occluded as well (Fig. 17-9). Although outflow from the deep venous system can be substituted in part by choroidal, thalamic, and striate anastomoses with the basal vein (21), deep CVT is always serious and often fatal.

Cerebral angiography is generally unhelpful in diagnosing isolated cortical venous thrombosis and cavernous sinus thrombophlebitis. The CS is visualized in less than half of normal angiograms, and opacification is often suboptimal (17).

Differential Diagnosis

The differential diagnosis of CVT includes intraluminal filling defects caused by *"giant" arachnoid granulations* (Fig. 17-10). Congenital absence or *segmental hypoplasia* may mimic CVT. When interruption of a dural sinus occurs as a congenital variant, parenchymal hemorrhage is absent and the collateral channels usually do not appear congested and tortuous.

COLLATERAL FLOW

Collateral circulation plays a crucial role in the event of cervical or intracranial vascular occlusion (22). Understanding these pathways is also a prerequisite for safe diagnostic angiography as well as neurointerventional procedures. In this section we discuss some of the more important potential anastomoses and their significance in occlusive vascular disorders.

Intracranial Anastomoses

Circle of Willis

The largest and most important potential collateral pathway for cerebral circulation is through the circle of Willis. When anatomically complete, this large anastomotic vascular ring can supply the entire brain from only one of the four major cervical vessels. However, a so-called "complete" circle of Willis occurs in only one fourth of all cases (see Chapter 5). Moreover, some investigators suggest that the circle of Willis is frequently incompetent as a collateral pathway and that arteriographic cross-filling is not a reliable index of vascular sufficiency (23).

Important potential collateral flow patterns through the circle of Willis are from one anterior cerebral artery (ACA) to the other via the anterior communicating artery (ACoA) (Fig. 17-11A and B) and from the poste-

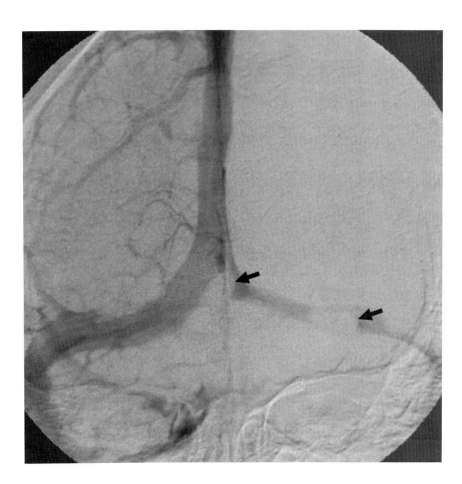

FIG. 17-10. Right common carotid angiogram, venous phase, AP view, demonstrates normal filling defects in the left transverse sinus and torcular herophili (*arrows*). These ovoid, sharply delineated intrasinus masses are normal arachnoid granulations.

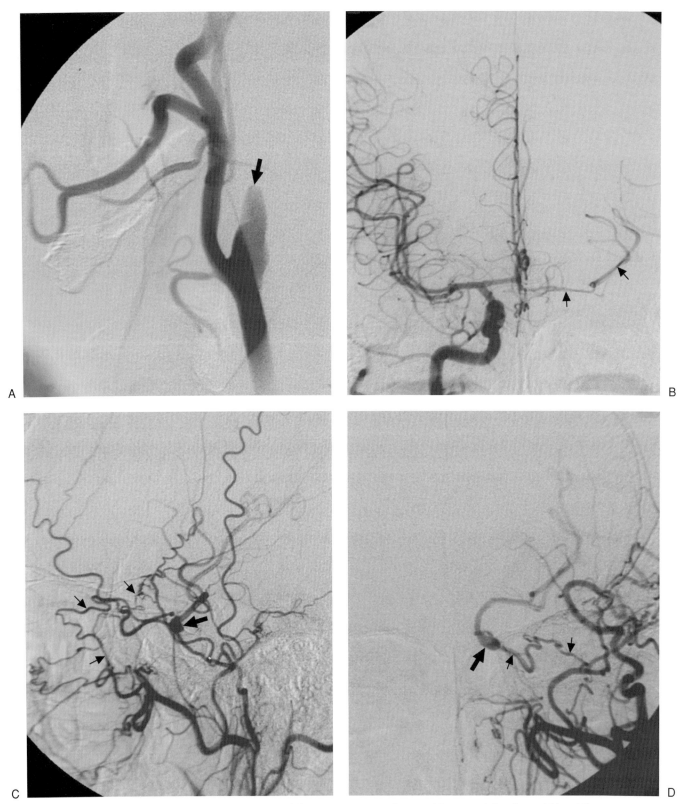

FIG. 17-11. This case illustrates some of the most common forms of intracranial collateral blood flow. **A:** Left common carotid angiogram, arterial phase, lateral view, shows occlusion of the left internal carotid artery (ICA) just beyond the bulb (*arrow*). **B:** Right common carotid angiogram, arterial phase, AP view, shows filling of the left anterior and middle cerebral arteries (*arrows*) via the anterior communicating artery. **C** and **D:** Left common carotid angiogram, late arterial phase, lateral **(C)** and antero-posterior **(D)** views, shows filling of the cavernous ICA (*large arrow*) via collateral flow from the external carotid system (deep maxillary and recurrent meningeal branches) (*small arrows*).

rior (vertebrobasilar) circulation to the anterior circulation via the posterior communicating arteries (PCoAs) (see box below and Fig. 17-12A) (24). A small or absent ipsilateral PCoA has been identified as a risk factor for ischemic cerebral infarction in patients with ICA occlusion (25).

Pial (Leptomeningeal) and Dural Collaterals

Pial collaterals are small but important end-to-end arterial anastomoses that exist across the vascular watershed zone. In the event of intracranial occlusive disorders, they may dilate and provide flow from one branch

---

Collateral Flow Patterns

Intracranial anastomoses
  Circle of Willis
  Pial (leptomeningeal) collaterals
  Transdural collaterals
Extra- to intracranial anastomoses
  External carotid artery (ECA) to ICA
    Maxillary artery
      Middle meningeal artery (MMA), recurrent meningeal to ethmoidal branches of the
        ophthalmic artery (OA)
      MMA to inferolateral trunk (ILT; foramen spinosum)
      Artery of foramen rotundum to ILT
      Accessory meningeal artery to ILT (foramen ovale)
      Anterior, middle deep temporal arteries to OA
    Via vidian artery to petrous ICA (anterior tympanic artery)
    Facial artery
      Angular branch to orbital branches of OA
    Superficial temporal artery (STA)
      Transosseous perforators to anterior falx artery
    Ascending pharyngeal artery
      Superior pharyngeal artery to cavernous ICA (foramen lacerum)
      Rami to cavernous ICA branches
      Inferior tympanic artery to petrous ICA
    Posterior auricular, OA to petrous ICA
      Stylomastoid artery
    Iatrogenic
      STA-MCA bypass graft
  ECA to vertebral artery (VA)
    Occipital artery
      Transosseous perforators
      C1 anastomotic branch (first cervical space)
      C2 anastomotic branch (second cervical space)
    Ascending pharyngeal
      Hypoglossal (odontoid arterial arch)
      Musculospinal branch
  Subclavian artery (SCA) to VA
    Ascending cervical branch
      C3 anastomotic branch
      C4 anastomotic branch
Extracranial anastomoses
  Subclavian steal (VA to basilar artery with flow reversal in contralateral VA to distal SCA)
  Carotid steal (common carotid artery [CCA] occlusion with patent ECA, ICA, and flow reversal
    in ECA)
  Direct vertebral to vertebral (via segmental branches)
  ECA to ECA (via contralateral branches)
  Iatrogenic (SCA to CCA anastomosis, bypass graft)

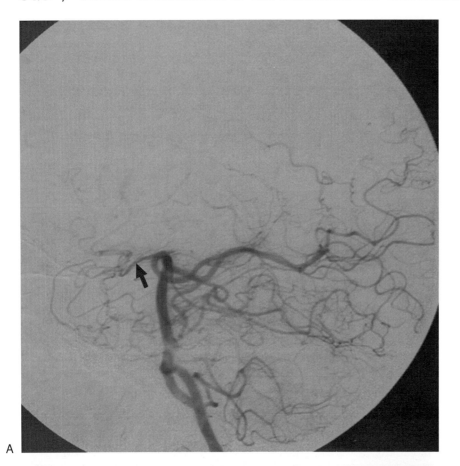

A

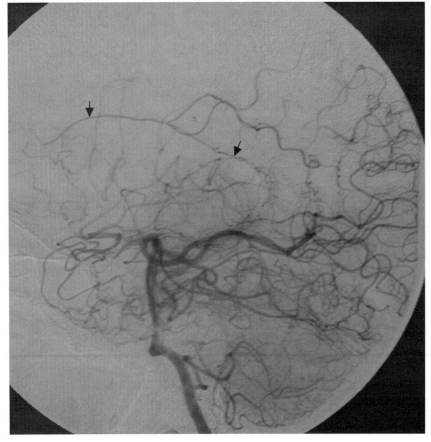

B

FIG. 17-12. Another case illustrates intracranial collateral blood flow. The left cervical internal carotid artery was occluded (not shown). Left vertebral angiogram with early **(A)** and late **(B)** arterial phase films, lateral view, shows collateral filling of the middle cerebral artery via the posterior communicating artery **(A,** *large arrow*). The distal anterior cerebral artery **(B,** *small arrows*) is opacified via splenial and pial branches from the posterior cerebral artery.

to another within the same vascular distribution or from one major cerebral artery to another (Figs. 17-1, 17-3 to 17-5, and 17-12B) (25a).

Dural anastomoses with cortical vessels may develop. These uncommon collaterals are most often seen in the setting of slowly progressive bilateral internal carotid occlusions (26). They may arise from intracranial dural channels or from transosseous perforating branches that originate from the external carotid artery (ECA).

Extra- to Intracranial Anastomoses

External Carotid to Internal Carotid Collaterals

A number of ECA to ICA anastomoses exist normally (see Chapters 2 and 4). In the event of cervical ICA occlusion, they may provide some collateral flow to the intracranial circulation. The most important extracranial source is the *internal maxillary artery* (IMA) (27). The IMA may supply the eye and brain via its extensive ethmoid, ophthalmic, or cavernous anastomoses with the ICA (Figs. 17-11C and D; see also Fig. 16-13) (28,29).

External to internal carotid collaterals also can be created surgically. *Superficial temporal to middle cerebral artery bypass grafts* have been used in selected cases of supraclinoid ICA or MCA occlusive disease (Fig. 17-13).

External Carotid–Vertebral Anastomoses

The muscular branches of the occipital and vertebral arteries provide a rich potential source of collateral blood flow. These suboccipital craniocervical anastomoses can provide flow in either direction (Fig. 17-14; see also Fig. 2-16). Intracranial embolization through these abundant anastomoses, sometimes called the suboccipital carrefour (knot) poses a significant potential risk for neurointerventional procedures (30).

Small but potentially very dangerous anastomoses also exist between the ascending pharyngeal artery, the stylomastoid branch of the occipital artery, and the vertebral artery (VA) (Fig. 17-15; see also Fig. 2-17). Spinal cord and cranial nerve infarction may occur if one of these channels is open and inadvertently embolized during diagnostic or therapeutic procedures.

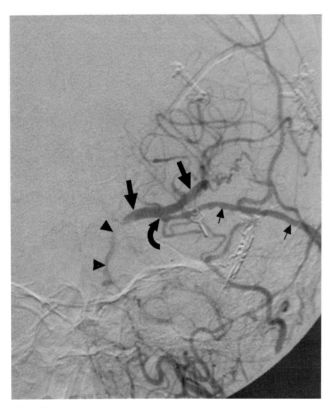

FIG. 17-13. This case demonstrates a surgically created extra- to intracranial source of collateral blood flow. The left common carotid angiogram, mid-arterial phase, AP view, shows an anastomosis (*curved arrow*) between the superficial temporal artery (*small arrows*) and the middle cerebral artery (*large arrows*). The supraclinoid internal carotid artery has a high-grade stenosis (*arrowheads*).

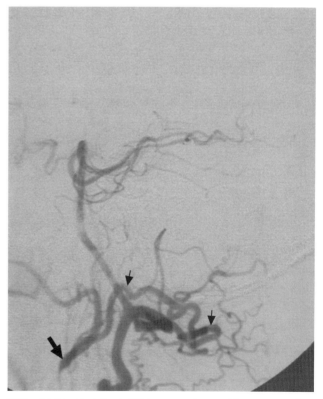

FIG. 17-14. Vertebral (VA)-external carotid artery (ECA) anastomoses are illustrated in this case. The ECA had been ligated previously for epistaxis. The ipsilateral VA fills the ECA (*large arrow*) via collaterals to muscular branches of the occipital artery (*small arrows*). This pattern is sometimes called the suboccipital "carrefour" or "knot."

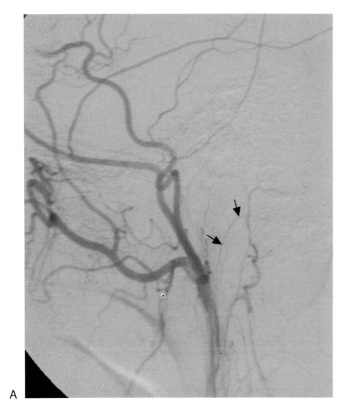

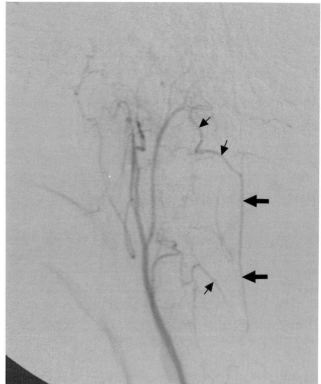

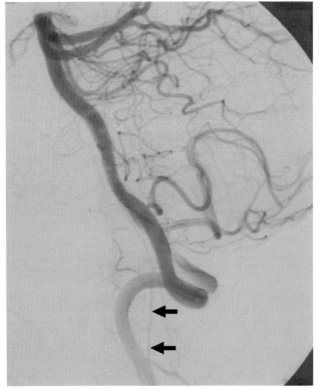

FIG. 17-15. Normal but potentially dangerous external carotid to vertebral anastomoses are illustrated by this case. **A:** Left common carotid angiogram, arterial phase, lateral view, shows the posterior division of the ascending pharyngeal artery (APA) (*arrows*). **B:** Selective APA injection shows filling of the anterior spinal artery (*large arrows*) via collaterals from the APA (*small arrows*). **C:** Left vertebral angiogram, arterial phase, lateral view, again shows the anterior spinal artery (*arrows*).

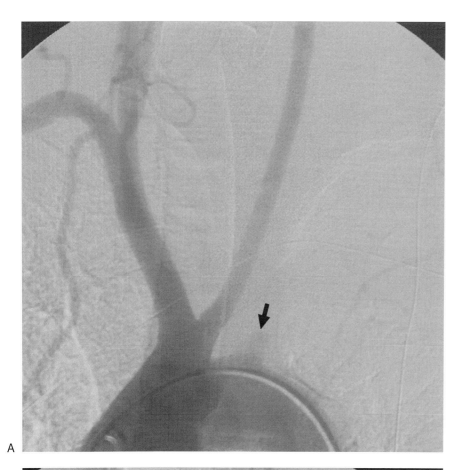

A

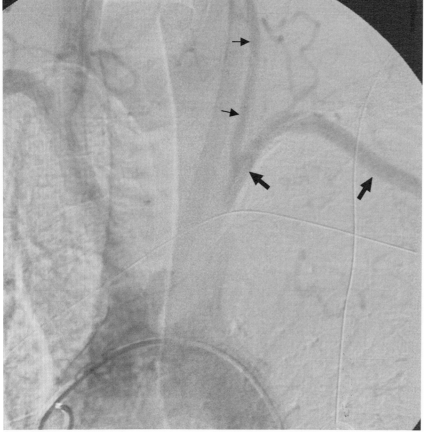

B

FIG. 17-16. Subclavian steal syndrome is illustrated by this case. **A:** Aortic arch angiogram, early arterial phase, left anterior oblique view, shows an occluded left subclavian artery (LSCA) (*arrow*). **B:** Late arterial phase shows filling of the LSCA (*large arrows*) via retrograde flow through the left vertebral artery (VA) (*small arrows*).

(Continued)

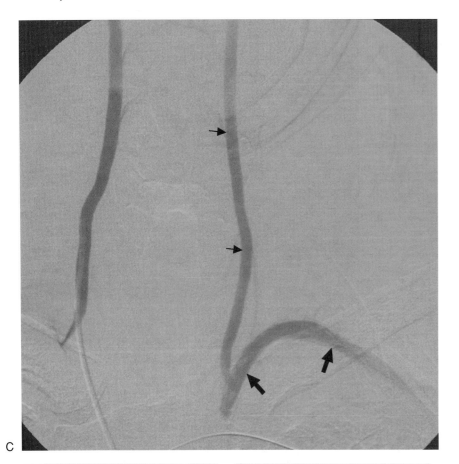

C

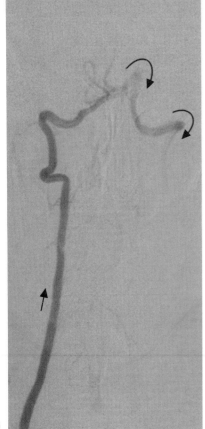

D

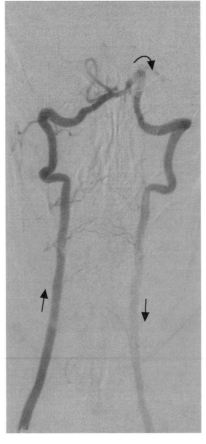

E

FIG. 17-16. *Continued.* **C:** Right vertebral angiogram, arterial phase, AP view, shows opacification of the left VA (*small arrows*) and SCA (*large arrows*) from the right vertebral injection (*curved arrow*). **D** and **E:** The right VA supplies the left VA across the basilar junction. Flow direction is shown by the arrows.

Extracranial Anastomoses

External Carotid Artery

Three major collateral pathways provide extracranial collateral flow to the ECA. These arise from (a) branches of the thyrocervical trunk (from the subclavian artery) that anastomose with the superior thyroid artery; (b) muscular branches from the ipsilateral vertebral artery that anastomose with branches of the occipital artery (the suboccipital carrefour described above); and (c) branches from the contralateral ECA that anastomose with their counterpart vessels (e.g., the ascending pharyngeal, occipital, facial, and temporal arteries) (31).

Vertebral Artery

The extracranial VA may receive collateral flow from the occipital artery as well as the contralateral VA via the posterior fossa. Direct vertebral-to-vertebral anastomoses also occur between muscular and segmental branches.

Steal Syndromes

So-called *subclavian steal* may occur if a subclavian artery is occluded at its origin from the aortic arch. Collateral circulation is recruited from the opposite vertebral artery, crosses the basilar artery junction, and flows down the opposite VA into the subclavian artery. Reversal of flow in the VA is produced when the poststenotic intraluminal pressure in the subclavian artery drops by 10% of the systemic pressure (32).

In classic subclavian steal syndrome, flow is reversed in the affected VA to supply the shoulder and arm distal to the subclavian obstruction (Fig. 17-16). Symptoms are due to ipsilateral arm ischemia and episodic neurologic symptoms from posterior fossa ischemia (steal). Diminished or absent pulse or decreased blood pressure in the affected arm may occur.

Subclavian steal syndrome is relatively uncommon, with a reported incidence that varies between 0.22% and 13.1% (33).

In the uncommon *carotid steal* syndrome the common carotid artery (CCA) is occluded, but the ICA and ECA are both patent beyond the occluded CCA. Flow direction in the ECA is reversed but normal in the ICA distal to the obstruction (30,31).

REFERENCES

1. Brint SU. Acute stroke therapies. *Surg Neurol* 1996;46:446–449.
2. International Stroke Trial Collaborative Group. The International Stroke Trial (IST): a randomised trial of aspirin, subcutaneous heparin, both, or neither among 19,435 patients with acute ischaemic stroke. *Lancet* 1997;349:1569–1581.
3. Kalimo H, Kaste M, Latia M. Vascular diseases. In: Graham DI, Lantos PL, eds. *Greenfield's neuropathology*, 6th ed. London: Arnold, 1997:315–396.
4. Garcia JH, Anderson ML. Circulatory disorders and their effects on the brain. In: Davis RL, Robertson DM, eds. *Textbook of neuropathology*. Baltimore: Williams & Wilkins, 1997:715–822.
5. ter Penning B. Pathophysiology of stoke. *Neuroimag Clin North Am* 1992;2:389–408.
6. Ginsberg MD. The new language of cerebral ischemia. *AJNR* 1997; 18:1435–1445.
7. Osborn AG: Stroke. In: *Diagnostic neuroradiology*. St. Louis: Mosby, 1994:330–398.
7a. Hennerici M, Daffertshofer M, Jakobs L. Failure to identify cerebral infarct mechanisms from topography of vascular territory lesions. *AJNR* 1998;19:1067–1074.
8. Dillon WP. CT techniques for detecting acute stroke and collateral circulation: in search of the holy grail [Editorial]. *AJNR* 1998;19:191–192.
9. Hurst RW. Angiography of nonatherosclerotic occlusive cerebrovascular disease. *Neuroimag Clin North Am* 1996;6:651–678.
10. Kucinski T, Koch C, Gryzska U, et al. The predictive value of early CT and angiography for fatal hemispheric swelling in acute stroke. *AJNR* 1998;19:839–846.
11. Na DG, Byun HS, Lee KH, et al. Acute occlusion of the middle cerebral artery: early evaluation with triphasic helical CT—preliminary results. *Radiology* 1998;207:113–122.
12. Bakaç G, Wardlaw JM. Problems in the diagnosis of intracranial venous infarction. *Neuroradiology* 1997;39:566–570.
12a. Biousse V, Conard J, Brouzes C, et al. Frequency of the 20210G → A mutation in the 3'-untranslated region of the prothrombin gene in 35 cases of cerebral venous thrombosis. *Stroke* 1998;29:1398–1400.
13. Martin PJ, Enevoldson TP. Cerebral venous thrombus. *Postgrad Med J* 1996;72:72–76.
14. Bitzer M, Topka H, Morgalla M, et al. Tumor-related venous obstruction and development of peritumoral brain edema in meningiomas. *Neurosurgery* 1998;42:730–737.
15. Hasso AN, Stringer WA, Brown KD. Cerebral ischemia and infarction. *Neuroimag Clin North Am* 1994;4:733–752.
16. Lafitte F, Boukobza M, Guichard JP, et al. MRI and MRA for diagnosis and follow-up of cerebral venous thrombosis (CVT). *Clin Radiol* 1997;52:672–679.
17. Kriss TC, Kriss VM, Warf B. Cavernous sinus thrombo-phlebitis: case report. *Neurosurgery* 1996;39:385–389.
18. Schuknecht B, Simmen D, Yüksel C, Valavanis A. Tributary venosinus occlusion and septic cavernous sinus thrombosis: CT and MR findings. *AJNR* 1998;19:617–626.
19. Derdeyn CP, Powers WJ. Isolated cortical venous thrombosis and ulcerative colitis. *AJNR* 1998;19:488–490.
20. Elsherbiny SM, Grünewald RA, Powell T. Isolated inferior sagittal sinus thrombosis: a case report. *Neuroradiology* 1997;39:411–413.
21. Andeweg J. The anatomy of collateral venous flow from the brain and its value in aetiological interpretation of intracranial pathology. *Neuroradiology* 1996;38:621–628.
22. Hedera P, Bujdakova J, Traubner P. Effect of collateral few patterns on outcome of carotid occlusion. *Eur Neurol* 1995;35:212–216.
23. AbuRhama AF, Robinson PA, Short Y, et al. Cross-filling of the circle of Willis and carotid stenosis by angiography, duplex ultrasound, and oculopneumoplethysmography. *Am J Surg* 1995;169:308–312.
24. Cassot F, Vergeur V, Bossuet P, et al. Effects of anterior communicating artery diameter on cerebral hemodynamics in internal carotid artery disease. *Circulation* 1995;92:3122–3131.
25. Schomer DF, Marks MP, Steinberg GK, et al. The anatomy of the posterior communicating artery as a risk factor in ischemic cerebral infarction. *N Engl J Med* 1994;330:1565–1570.
25a. Robertson SC, Brown P III, Loftus CM. Effects of etomidate administration on cerebral collateral flow. *Neurosurgery* 1998;43:317–324.
26. Gillilan LA. Potential collateral circulation to the human cerebral cortex. *Neurology* 1974;24:941–948.
27. Helgertner L, Szostek M, Malek AK, Staszkiewicz W. Collateral role of the external carotid artery and its branches in occlusion of the internal carotid artery. *Int Angiol* 1994;13:5–9.
28. García-Mónaco R. Transcranial arterial anastomoses. *Riv Neuroradiol* 1994;7(suppl 4):63–66.
29. Ho WY, TerBrugge KG. The role of angiography in the evaluation of vascular and neoplastic disease in the external carotid artery circulation. *Neuroimag Clin North Am* 1996;6:625–644.
30. Ayad M, Viñuela F, Rubinstein EH. The suboccipital carrefour: cervical and vertebral arterial anastomosis. *AJNR* 1998;19:925–931.
31. Stassi J, Cavanaugh BC, Siegal TL, et al. US case of the day. *Radiographics* 1995;15:1235–1238.
32. Mirfakhraee M, Benzel EC, Guinto FC, et al. Unusual subclavian steal: bidirectional and antegrade blood flow in the vertebral artery. *Neuroradiology* 1995;37:503–511.
33. Morvay Z, Milassin P, Barzó P. Assessment of steal syndromes with colour and pulsed Doppler imaging. *Eur Radiol* 1995;5:359–363.

CHAPTER 18

Trauma

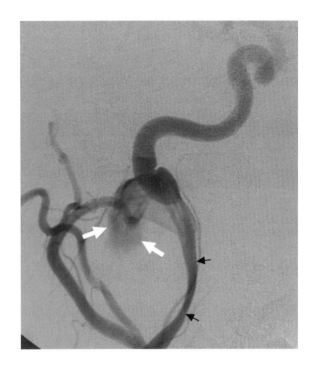

Trauma may injure the cervical and cerebral arteries as well as damage the dural sinuses and cortical veins (see box, next column). These injuries can be direct or indirect, and primary or secondary. They represent a broad, heterogeneous spectrum of abnormalities that ranges from relatively minor local perfusion disturbances to aneurysms, arteriovenous fistulae (AVFs), venous occlusions, and brain death.

Although noninvasive techniques are the primary screening procedures in patients with head and neck trauma, cerebral angiography provides high-resolution detail that may be very helpful in managing some patients with vascular injuries.

The focus of this chapter is on the most important direct manifestations of craniocerebral vascular injury, i.e., arterial dissection, traumatic aneurysms, and arteriovenous fistulae (AVFs). In closing, there is a brief discussion of "brain death." Some secondary effects (such as vascular occlusion induced by cerebral herniation syndromes) have been considered in previous chapters.

ARTERIAL DISSECTION

Pathology and Etiology

Pathology

The underlying pathology of arterial dissection is the same, regardless of whether the dissection is spontaneous (see Chapter 15) or traumatic. Arterial disruption results

---

Vascular Manifestations of Craniocerebral Trauma

Angiographically apparent lesions
    Intimal tear, flap
    Dissection
    Transection
    Vasospasm
    Intraluminal thrombus
    Occlusion
    Pseudoaneurysm
    Arteriovenous fistula
    Dural sinus injury
        Laceration
        Intraluminal thrombus
        Occlusion
        Venous epidural hematoma (EDH)
    Mass effect
    Herniation syndromes
    Global perfusion alterations and brain
        death
Angiographically occult lesions
    Local perfusion disturbances
    Shearing injury
    Cortical contusion
    Focal edema (without significant mass effect)

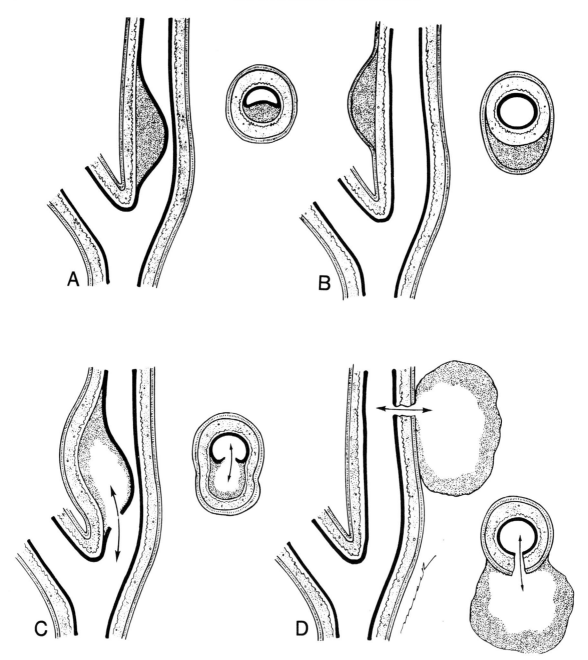

FIG. 18-1. Anatomic diagrams compare carotid artery dissection, dissecting aneurysm, and pseudoaneurysm. Lateral views are shown on the left of each figure; cross-sectional drawings are illustrated on the right. **A:** A typical *subintimal dissection* is shown. The subintimal hematoma is indicated by the heavily dotted area. Subintimal hematomas often compromise the parent vessel lumen. **B:** A *subadventitial dissection* is much less common. The paravascular hematoma is located just under the adventitia, external to the media. The vessel lumen may remain normal in these cases, and conventional angiography can appear unremarkable. Fat-suppressed T1-weighted MR scans are helpful in detecting these unusual paravascular hematomas. **C:** If the intima overlying a typical dissection ruptures, communication between the hematoma and the vessel lumen is established. This creates a true *dissecting aneurysm*. Conventional and CT angiography demonstrate opacification of both the outpouching (false lumen) and the narrowed "true" lumen. **D:** A complete vessel wall laceration may cause a paravascular hematoma to develop. If the hematoma cavitates and communicates with the parent vessel lumen, a *pseudoaneurysm* is created. The pseudoaneurysm is contained only by the organized hematoma wall and the surrounding fascia. (Reprinted with permission from Osborn AG, Tong KT. *Handbook of neuroradiology: skull and brain,* 2nd ed. St. Louis: Mosby, 1996.)

in extravasation of blood into the vessel wall. Dissection occurs as clot extends between the planes of the vessel wall, usually between the intima and media. The most common type is *subintimal dissection* (Fig. 18-1A). Dissection between the media and adventitia, *subadventitial dissection*, is less frequently encountered (Fig. 18-1B) (1).

Etiology

Most traumatic dissections are associated with intimal injury. However, it is unclear whether the initiating lesion

is an intimal tear that allows clot propagation within the vessel wall or a primary intramural hematoma that subsequently ruptures through the intima into the vessel lumen (2).

Traumatic dissections may occur with penetrating, nonpenetrating, or blunt injury. *Penetrating injury* includes gunshot or knife wounds as well as intraoral trauma from sharp objects such as pencils or sticks (2). *Nonpenetrating injury* occurs with spine fracture–subluxation. It also occurs with neck torsion and hyperextension, the so-called "blunt" injuries. *Blunt injuries*, espe-

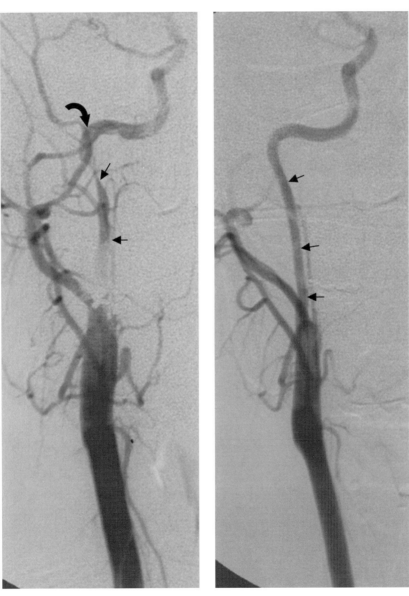

FIG. 18-2. This 26-year-old man sustained blunt neck injury. **A:** Right common carotid angiogram, arterial phase, AP view, shows a carotid dissection with smooth narrowing of the mid- and upper cervical ICA (*straight arrows*). The dissection spares most of the petrous ICA (*curved arrow*). **B:** Follow-up examination 6 months later shows the dissection has healed. The ICA now appears somewhat small (*arrows*).

cially to the carotid artery, are an underdiagnosed cause of cerebral ischemia following trauma (3,4).

Clinical Considerations

Vascular injuries from neck trauma are clinically asymptomatic in 20% to 33% of patients (5). Delayed symptom onset for a few days or even weeks is not uncommon (see Fig. 18-8).

In the case of penetrating injury, clinicians divide the neck into three anatomic zones:

Zone 1 is below the cricoid cartilage.
Zone 2 lies between the level of the cricoid and the mandibular angle.
Zone 3 is above the angle of the mandible.

Color Doppler sonography has been recommended for screening clinically stable patients with zone 2 or zone 3 injuries and no clinical signs of active bleeding (5).

Screening helical computed tomography (CT) is highly sensitive for revealing vascular injuries in all three zones (6). Catheter angiography is often postponed unless there is clinical suspicion or preliminary imaging evidence of injury (2,7).

Location

Carotid dissections may involve either the extra- or intracranial segments. The cervical *internal carotid artery* (ICA) is the most common site of all craniocervical dissections. Cervical ICA dissections usually spare the bulb. Approximately 70% involve both the cervical and petrous segments (2). Intracranial ICA dissections are rare. They typically involve the distal supraclinoid segment and often extend past the terminal ICA bifurcation into the horizontal middle cerebral artery (MCA).

Vertebral artery (VA) dissections are relatively uncommon, accounting for only 20% of cervical vascular injuries (2). The most common site is between the skull base and the upper cervical spine (C1–2 or atlantooccipital). Less commonly, the VA is injured between its origin from the subclavian artery and the C6 foramen transversarium. Mid-cervical VA injuries are generally underrecognized and occur in approximately 5% of patients with fractures that involve the foramina transversaria (7).

Angiographic Findings

Screening angiography in penetrating neck injuries is very sensitive, but findings are negative in up to 92% of stab wounds and in 73% of gunshot wounds (8). Penetrating trauma often causes *dissections*, with or without *intimal tears or flaps.* Dissections have a variable appearance, ranging from circumferential long segment narrow-

ing (Fig. 18-2) to smooth tapered occlusions (Fig. 18-3). *Occlusion without dissection* also occurs but is less common (see Fig. 18-4B).

Complications of traumatic injury include *vasospasm, stenosis, occlusion, intraluminal clots, retrograde thrombosis, dissecting aneurysm,* and *distal embolization* with *cerebral ischemia* or *infarction* (Figs. 18-4 and 18-5).

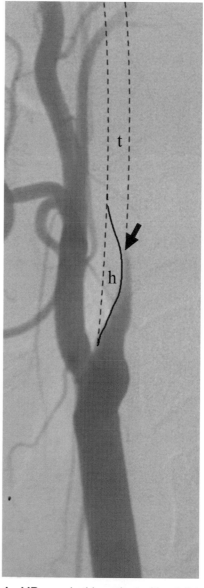

FIG. 18-3. An MR scan in this patient with a left hemisphere stroke 3 days after an auto accident disclosed a subintimal hematoma with distal occlusion of the internal carotid artery (ICA). Left common carotid angiogram, arterial phase, oblique view, shows a traumatic dissection. The true lumen tapers rapidly and terminates in a pointed, blind pouch (*large arrow*). The dotted lines indicate the approximate position of the ICA; the solid line represents the subintimal hematoma (h). The ICA was thrombosed (t) distal to the dissection.

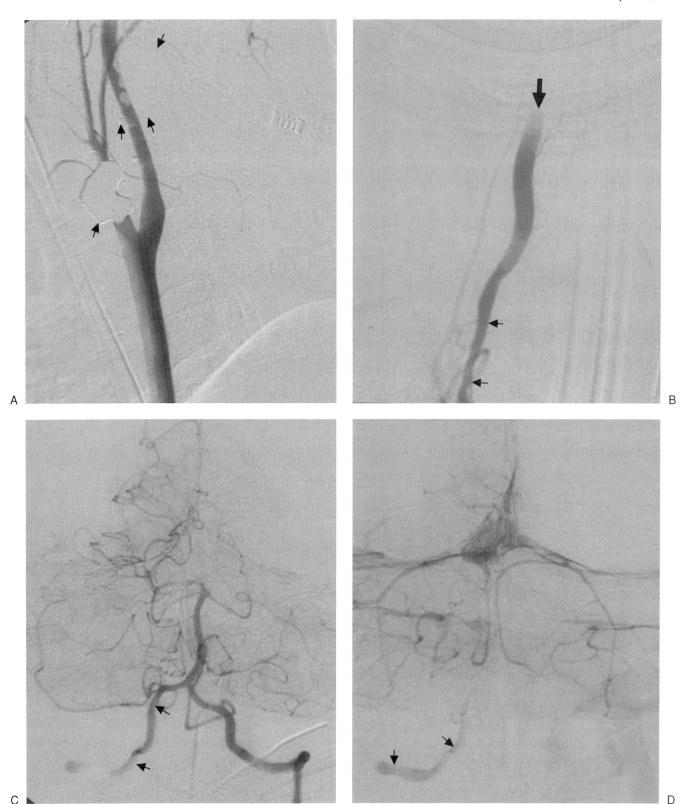

FIG. 18-4. A gunshot wound to the neck prompted this cerebral angiogram. **A:** Right common carotid angiogram, arterial phase, lateral view. Several bullet fragments (*small arrows*) are seen adjacent to the internal carotid artery (ICA). The external carotid branches are stretched and draped around a paravascular hematoma that surrounds the ICA. The ICA appears diminished in caliber, secondary to vasospasm or mass effect from the carotid space hematoma, but is otherwise intact. **B:** Right vertebral angiogram, arterial phase, oblique view, shows that the VA is narrowed proximally (*small arrows*) and terminates abruptly at the upper cervical level (*large arrow*). **C:** Left vertebral angiogram, arterial phase, AP view, shows contrast refluxes across the basilar artery into the distal right VA (*small arrows*). **D:** Venous phase shows persisting contrast stasis in the VA (*arrows*). Surgery disclosed a transected right VA.

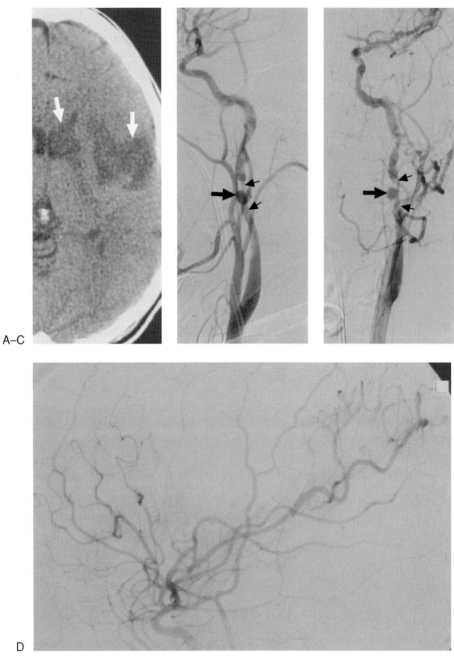

A–C

D

FIG. 18-5. This 38-year-old woman had blunt neck trauma 3 weeks prior to developing acute onset of neurologic symptoms. **A:** Nonenhanced CT (NECT) scan shows a partial left middle cerebral artery infarct (*white arrows*). Lateral **(B)** and anteroposterior **(C)** views of her left common carotid angiogram demonstrate carotid dissection (*small arrows*) with a dissecting aneurysm (large arrows). **D:** Lateral view of the intracranial circulation shows a large wedge-shaped bare area of nonperfused brain. Some luxury perfusion is present, seen as the faint vascular blush surrounding the infarcted area.

TRAUMATIC ANEURYSM

Pathology, Etiology, and Incidence

Pathology

There are several types of traumatic aneurysms. If a dissecting intramural hematoma dilates the parent artery and then ruptures through the intima, continuity with the true vessel lumen is established and a *dissecting aneurysm* is created (Fig. 18-1C).

Rupture of all three arterial layers accompanied by an organized hematoma that then cavitates and communicates with the true vessel lumen results in a *pseudoaneurysm* (Fig. 18-1D). Pseudoaneurysms are surrounded by cavitated clot and fascia; they do not contain normal arterial wall components. If the adventitia is preserved, the result is a rare traumatic *true aneurysm* (9). Most traumatic aneurysms are actually pseudoaneurysms.

Etiology and Incidence

Trauma accounts for less than 1% of all intracranial aneurysms but causes 20% of aneurysms in children (10,11). Traumatic aneurysms occur with both penetrating and blunt injuries as well as closed head injury (3,12).

Presentation and Location

Presentation

Symptoms of traumatic aneurysms vary from an asymptomatic neck mass to sudden rupture with devastating hemorrhage and death. Delayed onset of symptoms is very common.

Location

Extracranial traumatic pseudoaneurysms are usually found in the middle and upper cervical ICA; the VA is an uncommon site. Intracranial lesions occur at several locations, usually within the supratentorial fossae (13). Multiple aneurysms are rare.

The *petrous or cavernous ICA* may be lacerated by basilar skull fractures (see Fig. 12-25). The *distal anterior cerebral artery* is occasionally injured when this vessel is impacted against the falx cerebri. The *posterior cerebral artery* and even the *superior cerebellar artery* can be damaged as they are forced against the tentorium during closed head injury. *Cortical arteries* adjacent to skull fractures or penetrating injuries are a less common site for traumatic pseudoaneurysm.

Angiographic Findings

In general, angiographic findings with traumatic pseudoaneurysms are similar to those seen with true aneurysms (13) (see Chapter 12). Abnormalities in extracranial pseudoaneurysms vary from small saccular lesions (Fig. 18-5B and C) and fusiform dilatations (Fig. 18-6) to collections within huge cavitating hematomas (Fig. 18-7).

Traumatic intracranial aneurysms occur in atypical locations. They are usually found proximal to or beyond the circle of Willis and major arterial bifurcations (Figs. 18-8 and 18-9).

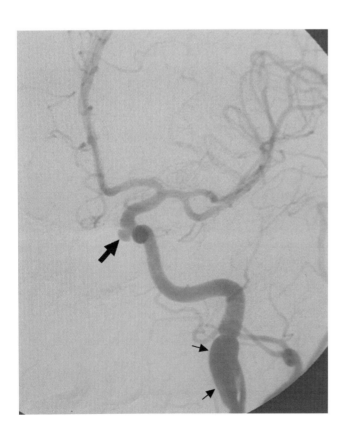

FIG. 18-6. This 33-year-old woman sustained severe head and neck trauma in a motor vehicle accident. A comminuted basilar skull fracture was demonstrated on NECT scans (not shown). Because the fracture involved the carotid canal, an angiogram was obtained. Two traumatic aneurysms are present: a saccular aneurysm of the cavernous internal carotid artery (ICA) (*large arrow*) and a dissecting aneurysm of the cervical ICA just below the exocranial opening of the carotid canal (*small arrows*).

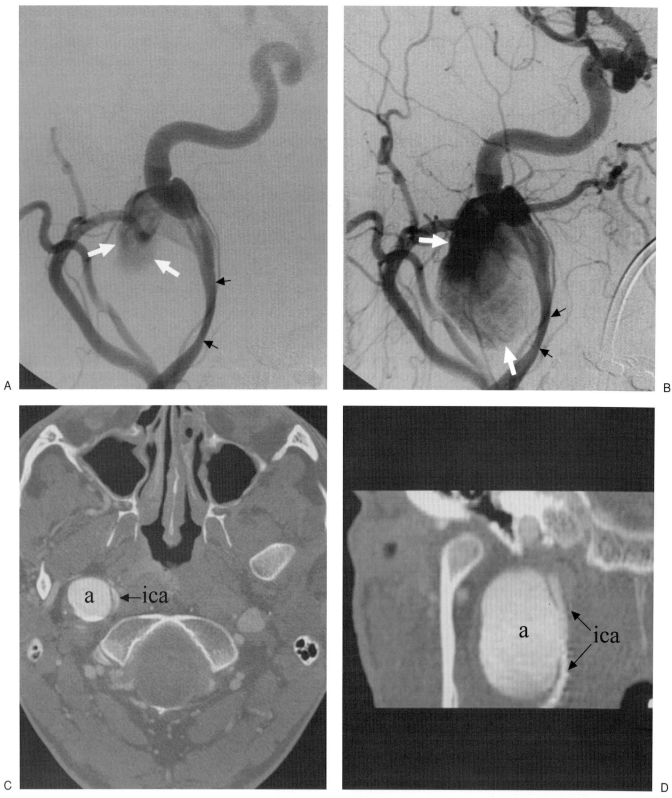

FIG. 18-7. Penetrating neck injury resulted in this large traumatic cervical carotid pseudoaneurysm. Early **(A)** and mid-arterial **(B)** phase films, oblique view, of a right common carotid angiogram show stretching and draping of the internal and external carotid arteries around a large mass. Contrast (*open arrows*) slowly fills the mass. Note severe compression and displacement of the true carotid lumen (*small arrows*). **C:** Axial contrast-enhanced CT scan demonstrates a double lumen sign. The false lumen of the large pseudoaneurysm (a) compresses the true lumen of the parent internal carotid artery (ica**). D:** Coronal reconstruction nicely demonstrates the pseudoaneurysm (a) and the compressed lumen of the internal carotid artery (ica). Surgery confirmed a pseudoaneurysm. The pseudoaneurysm was contained by organized hematoma and adjacent fascia. No normal arterial components were identified in the pseudoaneurysm wall.

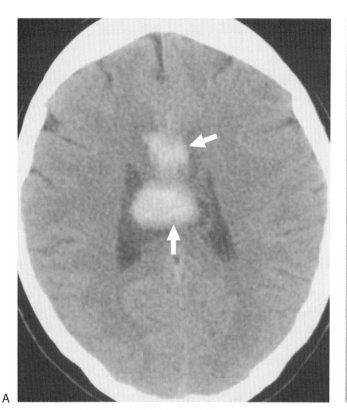
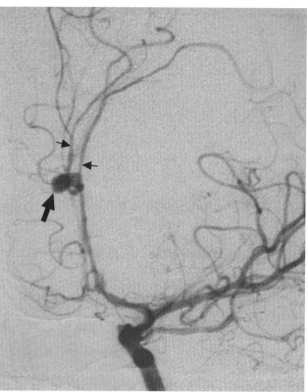

A   B

FIG. 18-8. This 48-year-old woman sustained closed head injury 3 weeks prior to developing an acute hematoma in the corpus callosum and interhemispheric fissure. **A:** Axial NECT scan demonstrates the unusual hematoma (*arrows*). **B:** Left internal carotid angiogram, arterial phase, oblique view, demonstrates a lobulated aneurysm at the distal A2 anterior cerebral artery (ACA) segment (*large arrow*). Note narrowing of both ACAs secondary to vasospasm (*small arrows*). Surgery disclosed a pseudoaneurysm, presumably secondary to ACA impaction against the falx cerebri.

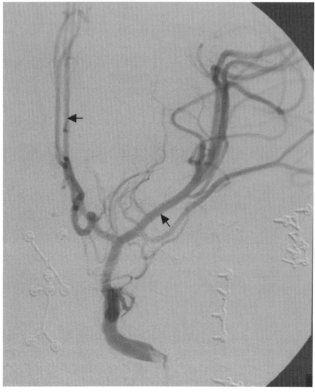
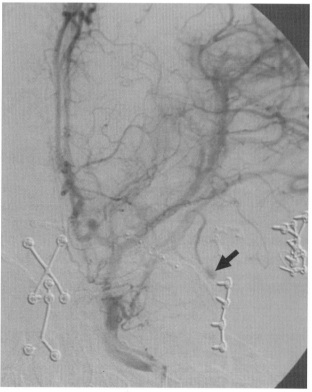

A   B

FIG. 18-9. Early **(A)** and late **(B)** arterial phase films, anteroposterior view, demonstrate a large holotemporal mass effect with elevation of the horizontal middle cerebral artery (MCA) and subfalcine herniation of the anterior cerebral artery (**A**, *arrows*). Surgical evacuation of a large, expanding hematoma did not demonstrate its etiology. Continued bleeding prompted this angiogram, which demonstrated a pseudoaneurysm arising from an anterior temporal MCA branch (**B**, *arrow*).

ARTERIOVENOUS FISTULAE

Carotid-cavernous fistulae (CCFs), dural fistulae involving the meningeal vessels, and extracranial direct AVFs can all occur with craniocerebral trauma. The most common intracranial traumatic vascular injury is carotid-cavernous fistulae.

Carotid-Cavernous Fistula

Definition and Classification

Carotid-cavernous fistulae are abnormal arteriovenous anastomoses between the internal carotid artery (ICA) and the cavernous sinus (CS). These fistulae may be classified by cause (spontaneous or traumatic), by flow velocity (high or low), or by anatomy (direct or indirect arterial supply) (14).

The most common classification is based on arterial supply. Type A CCFs are direct shunts between the ICA and the CS. Types B, C, and D are dural CCFs representing different types of fistulous connections between meningeal branches of the carotid arteries and the cavernous sinus (see Chapter 13). Traumatic CCFs are almost always high-flow, direct shunts between the ICA and the CS (14).

Pathology

Arterial blood in the cavernous ICA and venous blood in the surrounding CS are normally separated only by the carotid wall and a thin endothelium that invests the multiseptated venous spaces of the CS. In the usual traumatic CCF, a direct high-flow communication between the two structures is established.

Etiology

Traumatic direct CCFs usually involve laceration of the cavernous ICA. They may occur with rapid deceleration, direct trauma (e.g., skull fracture or gunshot wound), or thermal injury (transformation of the kinetic energy of a projectile into heat as its velocity is reduced) (15). Direct CCFs also may be caused by rupture of a posttraumatic cavernous ICA aneurysm.

Clinical Presentation

Traumatic CCFs usually occur a few days to a few weeks following injury. In contrast to spontaneous indirect CCFs (in which the patients are usually middle-aged women), most patients with traumatic direct CCFs are men with an average age of 37.5 years (15). Typical presenting symptoms include bruit, pulsating exophthalmus, edema of the preseptal orbital tissues, enlargement, and restriction of motion of the extraocular muscles, and ocular ischemia (7).

Location

Most CCFs occur at the proximal horizontal or posterior vertical portions of the cavernous ICA (2).

Angiography: Technical Considerations

Because most direct CCFs are high-flow lesions, very rapid frame rate or filming is necessary. In some cases the flow is so rapid that the cavernous sinus is immediately opacified and the precise communication site is obscured. In these cases, injection of the vertebral artery with temporary compression of the ipsilateral common carotid artery may slow the flow and successfully demonstrate the fistula site.

Biplane acquisition with relatively high contrast volumes and injection rates is required in most cases. Multiple views may be necessary. Visualization of the entire intracranial vasculature is needed to evaluate collateral blood supply, venous drainage patterns, and vascular steal (2).

Angiography: Imaging Findings

Rapid shunting of blood into a distended cavernous sinus and from the CS into a variety of collateral venous drainage pathways is typical (Fig. 18-10). The most common venous effluence is through the superior and inferior ophthalmic veins. The superior and inferior petrosal sinuses, pterygoid plexus, sylvian veins, and contralateral cavernous sinus are also often involved.

Angiographic findings associated with an increased risk of morbidity and mortality with CCF include presence of an associated pseudoaneurysm, cavernous sinus varices, cortical or deep venous drainage, and obstruction or thrombosis of venous outflow channels (2).

Miscellaneous Traumatic AVFs

Trauma-induced arteriovenous communications can occur in any location where an artery and vein are in close proximity. In actual practice, traumatic fistulae other than CCF are quite uncommon.

Extradural vertebral AVFs can be produced by blunt trauma, penetrating injury, or fracture. Tinnitus and vertigo are the most common presenting symptoms (7). Traumatic vertebral AVFs occur more frequently in the mid- and lower cervical spine, whereas spontaneous fistulae are more common at or above the C2 level (2). Skull fracture with middle meningeal artery laceration usually results in an epidural hematoma (EDH). On rare occasions trauma can cause a *middle meningeal artery AVF* without an accompanying EDH. Traumatic pseudoaneurysms and fistulae involving the *occipital artery* or the *superficial temporal artery* may occur as delayed complications of penetrating scalp injuries.

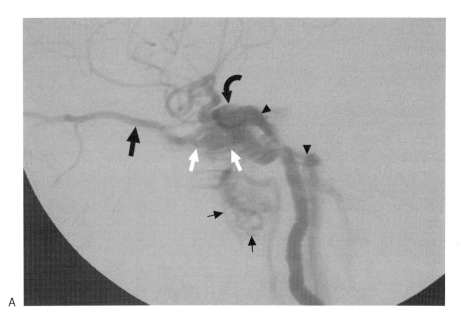

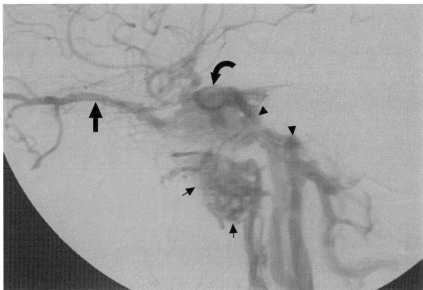

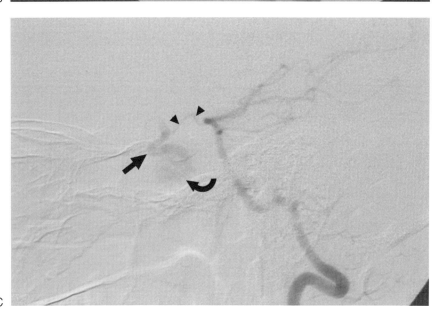

FIG. 18-10. This patient developed proptosis and chemosis 2 weeks after closed head trauma. Early **(A)** and mid-arterial **(B)** phase films, lateral view, of a left internal carotid angiogram demonstrate a high-flow direct carotid-cavernous fistula (*curved arrow*) with rapid opacification of the cavernous sinus (*white arrows*), clival (*arrowheads*), and pterygoid venous plexuses (*small arrows*), and the superior ophthalmic vein (*large arrow*). The precise site of communication between the internal carotid artery (ICA) and cavernous sinus could not be detected. **C:** Left vertebral angiogram, arterial phase, lateral view, performed with temporary compression of the left common carotid artery to slow flow refluxes contrast into the ICA (*large arrow*) via a small posterior communicating artery (*arrowheads*). The arteriovenous fistula site is just below the junction between the vertical and horizontal ICA segments (*curved arrow*), a typical location.

VENOUS OCCLUSIONS

Skull fractures that cross dural sinuses may tear interdural veins or lacerate the sinus itself, resulting in a "venous" EDH. Other complications of dural sinus injury include thrombosis and venous infarction (see Chapter 17). Dural sinus thrombosis (DST) has been described with penetrating and closed head injuries, fractures, disseminated intravascular coagulopathy, and following neurosurgical as well as non-neurosurgical operations. The reported incidence of DST is less than 5% with penetrating trauma and is extremely rare with nonpenetrating (i.e., closed) head injury (16).

BRAIN DEATH

Concept and Definitions

Medical Versus Legal Concepts

The medical definition of brain death is the "irreversible loss of function of the brain, including the brainstem" (17,18). However, the legal definition of brain death and the criteria for establishing its diagnosis vary widely according to country and province, institution, and even patient age. In some countries imaging is mandated to verify absent cerebral blood flow, whereas in others clinical examination and electroencephalographic recordings are sufficient to establish the diagnosis (19).

Clinical Diagnosis

The American Academy of Neurology has analyzed the issue of brain death extensively, refining the clinical criteria for establishing the diagnosis of brain death as well as recommending procedures for testing in patients older than 18 years (17,18).

Imaging

Although conventional angiography has been considered the most valid modality for verifying brain death, other techniques such as nuclear medicine, xenon-enhanced CT, transcranial Doppler ultrasonography, magnetic resonance (MR) imaging with MR angiography, and two-phase spiral CT have all been advocated (19,20).

Angiographic Findings

Computed tomography and conventional angiography demonstrate stagnation and arrest of contrast medium at the level of the internal carotid and vertebral arteries. Enhanced visibility of the superior ophthalmic veins and superficial temporal arteries plus absent opacification of the pericallosal artery, terminal cortical arteries, internal cerebral vein, vein of Galen, and straight sinus are ancillary signs of brain death (Fig. 18-11).

Filling of the superior sagittal sinus occurs on contrast-enhanced CT scans in 50% of brain-dead patients and does not contradict the diagnosis of brain death. Delayed opacification and stagnation of contrast medium in basal arachnoid arterial segments (subarachnoid "stasis filling") also may occur (20).

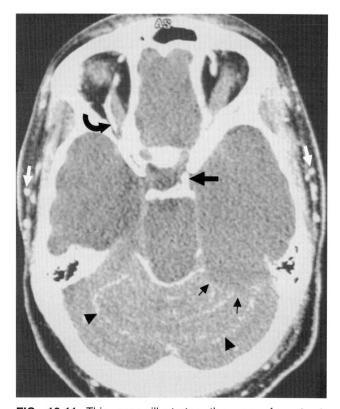

FIG. 18-11. This case illustrates the use of contrast-enhanced helical CT and CT angiography to document brain death. The axial source image obtained during rapid contrast infusion demonstrates markedly edematous temporal lobes with complete obliteration of the gray–white matter interfaces. Severe descending transtentorial herniation is present, demonstrated by displacement of the temporal lobes through the incisura into the posterior fossa (small arrows). No flow is seen in the right internal carotid artery (ICA). The left cavernous ICA is opacified with contrast (large arrow), but there was no intracranial flow. The basilar artery is not opacified. Some posterior fossa enhancement is seen (arrowheads). This represents contrast in basal arachnoid arterial segments, so-called stasis filling, and is not inconsistent with the diagnosis of brain death. Note intense enhancement in the superior ophthalmic veins (curved arrow) and branches of the superficial temporal arteries (white arrows), a common pattern in brain death cases.

REFERENCES

1. Kalimo H, Kaste M, Haltia M. Vascular diseases. In: Graham DI, Lantos PL, eds. *Greenfield's neuropathology*, 6th ed. London: Arnold, 1997:315–396.
2. Gaskill-Shipley MF, Tomsick TA. Angiography in the evaluation of head and neck trauma. *Neuroimag Clin North Am* 1996;6:607–624.
3. Mulloy JP, Flick PA, Gold RE. Blunt carotid injury: a review. *Radiology* 1998;207:571–585.
4. Prall JA, Brega KE, Caldwell DM, Breeze RE. Incidence of unsuspected blunt carotid injury. *Neurosurgery* 1998;42:495–499.
5. Montalvo BM, LeBlang SD, Nuñez DB, et al. Color Doppler sonography in penetrating injuries of the neck. *AJNR* 1996;17:943–951.
6. Nuñez D, Rivas L, McKenny K, et al. Helical CT of traumatic arterial injuries. *AJR* 1998;170:1621–1626.
7. Bula WI, Loes DJ. Trauma to the cerebrovascular system. *Neuroimag Clin North Am* 1994;4:753–772.
8. North CM, Ahmadi J, Segall HD, Zee CS. Penetrating vascular injuries of the face and neck: clinical and angiographic correlation. *AJNR* 1986;7:855–859.
9. Quintana F, Díez C, Guitierrez A, et al. Traumatic aneurysm of the basilar artery. *AJNR* 1996;17:283–285.
10. Buckingham MJ, Crone KR, Ball WS, et al. Traumatic intracranial aneurysms in childhood: two cases and a review of the literature. *Neurosurgery* 1988;22:398–406.
11. Holmes B, Harbaugh RE. Traumatic intracranial aneurysms: a contemporary review. *J Trauma* 1993;35:855–860.
12. Amirjamshidi A, Rahmat H, Abbassioun K. Traumatic aneurysms and arteriovenous fistulas of intracranial vessels associated with penetrating head injuries during war: principles and pitfalls in diagnosis and management. *J Neurosurg* 1996;84:769–780.
13. Meder JF, Gaston A, Merienne L, et al. Traumatic aneurysms of the internal and external carotid arteries. *J Neuroradiol* 1992;19:248–255.
14. Jacobsen BE, Nesbit GM, Ahuma A, Barnwell SL. Traumatic indirect carotid-cavernous fistula: report of two cases. *Neurosurgery* 1996;39:1235–1238.
15. Caldas JGMP, Vale BP, Ramos F Jr, et al. Endovascular treatment of traumatic and spontaneous direct carotid cavernous fistulas. *IJNR* 1998;4:127–131.
16. Kuether TA, O'Neill O, Nesbit GM, Barnwell SL. Endovascular treatment of traumatic dural sinus thrombosis: case report. *Neurosurgery* 1998;42:1163–1167.
17. Quality Standards Subcommittee of the American Academy of Neurology. Practice parameters for determining brain death in adults [Summary Statement]. *Neurology* 1995;45:1012–1014.
18. Wijdicks EFM. Determining brain death in adults. *Neurology* 1995;45:1003–1011.
19. Ishii K, Onuma T, Kinoshita T, et al. Brain death: MR and MR angiography. *AJNR* 1996;17:731–735.
20. Dupas B, Gayet-Delacroix M, Villers D, et al. Diagnosis of brain death using two-phase spiral CT. *AJNR* 1998;19:641–647.

SECTION III

Technical Aspects of Cerebral Angiography

CHAPTER 19

Diagnostic Neuroangiography
Basic Techniques

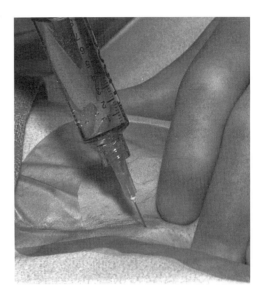

John M. Jacobs

In the current era of increasingly sophisticated noninvasive imaging, angiography is seldom the first study of choice for imaging of the central nervous system. As opposed to the pre–computed tomography (CT) era, when angiography was used to detect intracranial masses and mass effect from a variety of space-occupying processes, angiography today is used to evaluate specific abnormalities of the cerebral vasculature. With advances in technology that include CT, magnetic resonance (MR), Duplex ultrasonography, CT angiography, and MR angiography, in some instances angiography is unnecessary. Clearly, if equivalent information can be obtained by noninvasive means, then catheter angiography is not indicated. But today, as in the past, catheter angiography remains an important tool in the armamentarium for imaging the cerebral vessels.

The purpose of this chapter is to provide the reader with a basic template of the technical aspects of cerebral angiography. Through experience, an accomplished angiographer discovers "tricks" that are safe and effective but are ill advised for the novice angiographer. The goal of angiography is to answer diagnostic questions about the cerebral vasculature in as rapid and safe a fashion as possible to facilitate appropriate therapy.

PREPROCEDURAL ASSESSMENT

Patient Evaluation

It is important whenever possible to visit the patient in advance of the angiogram. The preprocedural evaluation should be used to determine if the angiogram is indeed indicated. Although there are no absolute contraindications to cerebral angiography, it is important to determine if one of the noninvasive techniques mentioned previously could suffice to answer the questions posed. The preprocedural evaluation also should be used to assess the patient's clinical status, past medical history, and history of medications and allergies. Specifically, it is important to note if the patient has ever had prior exposure to contrast media and if a serious adverse reaction occurred.

Laboratory Evaluation

Assessment of pertinent laboratory data should include blood urea nitrogen and creatinine to screen for renal insufficiency or renal failure. Prothrombin time (PT), partial thromboplastin time (PTT), international ratio (INR), and platelet count should be checked to screen for bleeding diathesis. It is important to note if the patient is receiving heparin therapy. We routinely perform angiograms on patients who are fully anticoagulated with heparin but keep adequate doses of protamine sulfate available if reversal of the heparin is necessary. In contrast, we try to avoid angiography in patients anticoagulated with sodium warfarin (Coumadin, Dupont Pharmaceutical) because reversal of this anticoagulant with fresh frozen plasma takes longer. Ideally, if a patient on Coumadin requires angiography and continued anticoagulation is necessary, he or she is hospitalized and converted to heparin prior to the angiogram. If angiography must be performed on patients fully anticoagulated with Coumadin, there are devices available that aid in achieving hemostasis once the catheter is removed (VasoSeal, Bioplex Medical/Datascope Corp., Vaals, The Netherlands).

Patient Education

In addition to educating the radiologist about the patient, the preprocedural evaluation allows the patient to become educated about the procedure and the physician who will perform that procedure. An educated patient is a more cooperative and relaxed patient. The preprocedural evaluation allows the radiologist to develop a rapport with the patient by reviewing what is to be expected during the examination.

The procedure should be explained to the patient in a brief but thorough step-by-step fashion. It is important to review the sensations that the patient may experience when the groin is anesthetized, when the femoral artery is punctured and the catheter manipulated, and when contrast is injected. Forewarning of these events often makes them much more tolerable. It is important to point out to the patient that the angiogram is degraded by motion artifact and that there will be brief episodes when he or she will be positioned a certain way and asked to hold very still or perhaps hold their breath and not swallow. It is useful to describe to the patient your usual commands prior to the injection of contrast and practice this one or two times prior to the placement of a catheter in a vessel. Likewise, it is important that you be consistent in those commands. For example, if you have the patient take a deep breath, exhale, take a half a breath, and hold it on the first injection of a common carotid artery angiogram, the same commands should be used for each additional run. By establishing a standard routine, there will be less need for repeating injections because of miscommunication and patient motion. This results in decreased contrast usage and less catheter time, which relates directly to decreased complications of cerebral angiography.

Informed Consent

The angiographer should outline candidly the hazards and complications that angiography can produce and the likelihood of their occurrence (1). It is important to obtain written informed consent from the patient when-

ever possible prior to performing the procedure. If written consent cannot be obtained from the patient or a responsible family member, it is equally important to document in the patient's medical record that the procedure was an emergency and that an attempt was made to obtain consent. But it is inappropriate when consenting a patient for the procedure that the risks be overemphasized to the extent that a patient is too frightened to have a procedure that is in his or her best interest.

PATIENT PREPARATION

Patient Support and Monitoring

Once in the angiography suite, the patient is appropriately positioned on the table. A reasonable sized (18- to 20-gauge), adequately flowing intravenous line is started that will serve as a means to administer intravenous fluids, sedative, and analgesic medications. Importantly, this intravenous line also serves as a "lifeline" in the event of a life-threatening emergency. In our laboratory, the patient is connected to continuous electrocardiography (ECG), oxygen saturation monitoring, and intermittent automatic blood pressure monitoring equipment (Fig. 19-1). If sedation is given, the patient is provided with low-flow oxygen, usually by nasal cannula or in some instances by ventilatory mask. Ideally, there should be an adequately trained individual, other than the physician performing the procedure, present to monitor the patient's vital signs and clinical status throughout the procedure. It is important to record the data in such a fashion that upward or downward trends can be monitored. It is equally important that all personnel involved in the angiography suite be educated regarding your institution's policies and procedures with respect to conscious sedation.

Filming Technique

If cut film angiography is to be employed, it is best to obtain preliminary films (scout films) prior to beginning the procedure. This will allow for minor adjustments in both filming technique and patient positioning prior to the placement of a catheter in an artery. This is important because complications of angiography are directly related to the length of time a catheter is in an artery. Any measures that can be taken ahead of time to improve the efficiency of the procedure should reduce complication rates.

Tray Set-up

Once the patient has been placed on adequate monitoring devices and the groin prepared, the actual procedure can begin. The angiography tray should be checked for completeness. Several commercially available, disposable angiography tray set-ups are available to order but

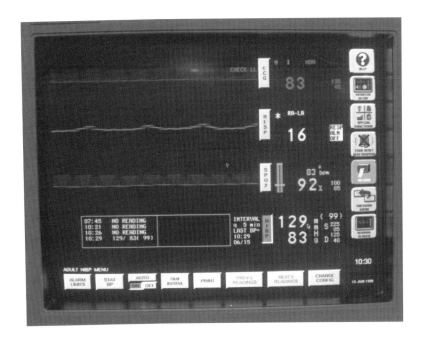

FIG. 19-1. Monitor indicating (from top to bottom) pulse, respiratory rate, oxygen saturation, and blood pressure.

may not include everything needed for a particular case (Fig. 19-2). At our institution, the items frequently used during the procedure are transferred from the tray to a Mayo stand mounted onto the procedural table to facilitate rapid and easy access to supplies such as flush and contrast syringes (Fig. 19-3). Because cerebral angiography is an area of radiology in which simple errors can result in serious injury to the patient or even death, meticulous attention to details is necessary to ensure a safe outcome. As a precaution, the arterial sheath and/or catheter should be flushed with heparinized saline prior to inser-

tion into the body. This will ensure that any debris from the manufacturing process is purged from the lumen of the catheter and will not result in an inadvertent embolus. Additionally, the guide wire should be checked for appropriate fit through both the arterial needle and the catheter.

Catheter and Guide Wire Preparation

Many manufacturers of both catheters and guide wires have introduced versions that are coated with hydrophilic compounds to facilitate smoother transmission of the

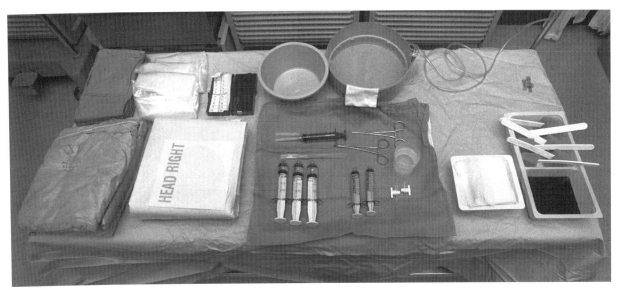

FIG. 19-2. Angiographic tray set-up. Note that lidocaine and contrast syringes are labeled. The types of syringes are also color coded: white, flush; blue, contrast; red, lidocaine. The large bowl has an interior lip to hold wires and catheters in place.

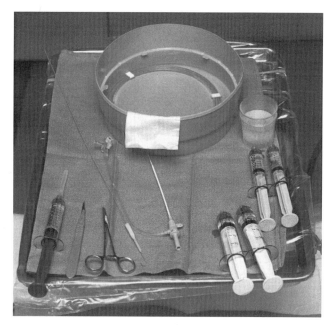

FIG. 19-3. Mayo stand attached to the side of the procedure table to allow frequently used syringes, wires, catheters, and instruments to be easily accessed.

blood. By prewetting the wire or catheter, the material is bound to heparinized saline. Electron micrography of the exterior surface of hydrophilically coated wires, when used properly, has demonstrated less platelet aggregation to these wires than standard Teflon-coated braided wires (2). Although the hydrophilically coated guide wires can be moistened by injecting heparinized saline into an injection port on the circular plastic container or by wiping it with a wet Telfa (Kendall) pad or sponge, it is preferable to actually dip the product into a bowl filled with heparinized saline. The same is true for the hydrophilically coated catheters.

VASCULAR ACCESS

Local Anesthesia

Successful cerebral angiography begins with local anesthesia. Usually a 1% solution of lidocaine is used for local anesthesia at the skin site and for infiltration around the femoral artery. Because of the pH of lidocaine, it can be painful as it is infused. A 20-mL bottle of 1% lidocaine can be buffered with 2 mL of sodium bicarbonate just prior to use to improve patient tolerance.

wire and catheter (Fig. 19-4). These products are in common use in many angiography suites and have some distinct advantages over noncoated catheters and wires because of their reduced friction. However, it is important to thoroughly moisten the exterior surface that is coated before these products are used. In most instances the coating material binds with the first substance that it contacts. As a result, if a dry wire or catheter is inserted into the body, the first substance the material contacts is

Arterial Puncture

The common femoral artery is located just over the medial aspect of the femoral head. In some instances it is worthwhile to spot fluoroscope this location prior to anesthetizing. This is especially true in obese patients, in whom the usual anatomic landmarks are more difficult to discern. The femoral artery should be punctured approx-

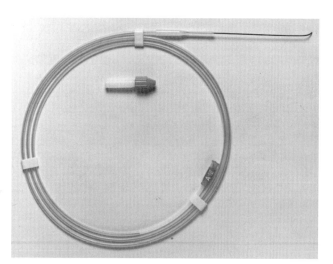

FIG. 19-4. Hydrophilically coated guide wire with distal curve. Note the plastic container with Luer lock hub for flushing the wire with heparinized saline. A torque device is also shown in the center of the figure.

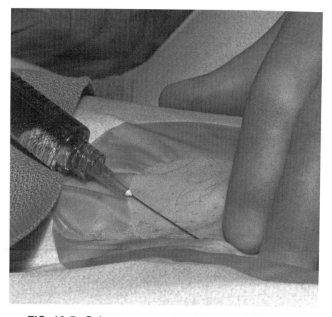

FIG. 19-5. Subcutaneous administration of lidocaine.

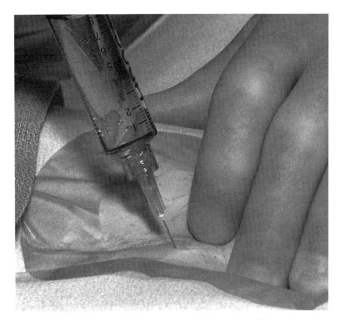

FIG. 19-6. Deep administration of lidocaine. Note that the femoral artery is localized and fixed into position with compression with the left hand.

imately 2 to 3 cm below the level of the inguinal ligament to prevent the development of an intraperitoneal hematoma. The approximate position of the inguinal ligament is a line between the symphysis pubis and the iliac crest. The femoral artery is usually coursing obliquely across the center of this imaginary line that overlies the medial aspect of the femoral head. The femoral artery runs lateral to the femoral vein and medial to the femoral nerve.

Once the location of the femoral artery is ascertained, a 1-cm wheal is raised using a 25-gauge needle on a 10-mL syringe of the lidocaine suspension (Fig. 19-5). The needle is then exchanged for a longer 21-gauge needle. While palpating the femoral artery, the long, thin needle is then used to infiltrate the soft tissues on each side and above the artery (Fig. 19-6). Care should be taken not to puncture the femoral artery or vein at this time, and before injecting the lidocaine suspension, the syringe should be aspirated to be certain that the needle is not intravascular. If the femoral artery or vein is inadvertently punctured with the anesthetizing needle, the needle is simply removed and the vessel is manually compressed until hemostasis is achieved.

Prior to puncturing the femoral artery, a small skin incision is made with a no. 11 blade held flat and parallel to the skin to prevent laceration of a vessel. The sharp side of the blade should be held away from your fingers to prevent personal injury and potential contamination (Fig. 19-7). A hemostat can then be used to bluntly dissect the subcutaneous tissues approximately 1 cm deep. This not only allows for smoother passage of the needle, guide wire, and sheath or catheter, but also helps to prevent the accumulation of a hematoma because it creates a tract between the artery and the skin.

The femoral artery can be fixed into position for the puncture in one of two ways. The artery can be gently compressed and fixed in position using the left hand with the third, fourth, and fifth fingers positioned parallel to the vessel above the skin incision and the index finger positioned just below the skin incision (Fig. 19-8). Alternatively, the index finger and middle finger can be positioned on each side of the vessel just above the skin inci-

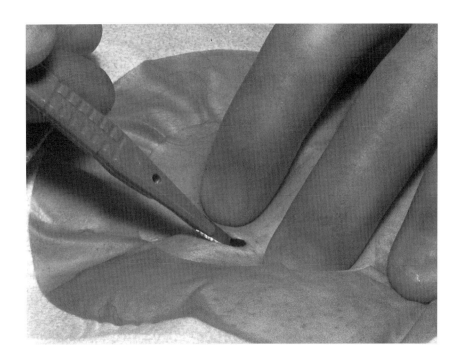

FIG. 19-7. Skin incision. Note that the blade is held with the sharp side facing away from the left hand and in a near horizontal position with the skin surface to prevent injury to the operator and deep penetration and vessel laceration, respectively.

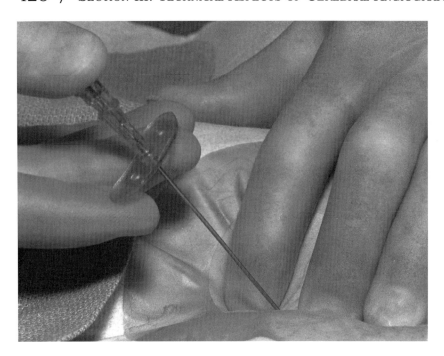

FIG. 19-8. For arterial puncture, the artery is localized with the third and fourth digits above the skin incision and the index finger just below the incision parallel to the course of the femoral artery. The needle is held at approximately a 45 degree incident angle.

sion pointing toward the foot with the femoral artery isolated between the two fingers (Fig. 19-9). When using a styletted needle, the needle is held in the right hand between the index and middle finger with the palm facing upward. The needle is held at a 45-degree angle to the skin. The needle is then gently advanced throughout the incision and subcutaneous tissues with the thumb, which is positioned on the hub. As the tip of the needle approaches the artery, a transmitted pulse can frequently be felt against the operator's thumb. At this point the nee-

dle can be firmly advanced through the artery (Fig. 19-10). The stylet is then removed. If the patient experiences pain during the insertion of the needle, 1 to 2 mL of lidocaine can be infused through the puncture needle at this time to anesthetize the deep tissues and periosteum. Again, it is important to gently aspirate the needle to assure that the tip is not intravascular before infusing more local anesthetic. The needle is then slowly withdrawn until the tip is within the lumen of the artery. When the tip of the needle is cleanly in the lumen of the artery,

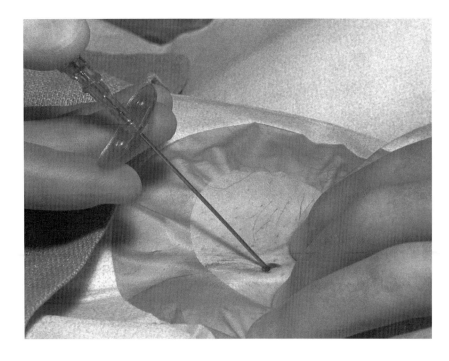

FIG. 19-9. For arterial puncture, the index and third digits of the left hand face caudally and are positioned such that the femoral artery is trapped between them. The needle is held at approximately 45 degrees incident angle.

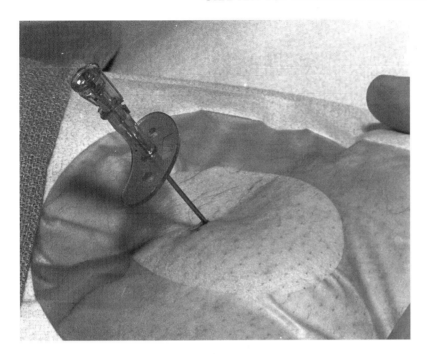

FIG. 19-10. Positioning of the needle after arterial puncture.

vigorous spurting of blood should occur and the guide wire can be introduced (Fig. 19-11). If only a weak blood return is encountered, the needle may be in the femoral vein or against the wall of the artery, or it may even be subintimal. The guide wire should not be introduced until satisfactory arterial flow is achieved. If there is a question about the positioning of the needle, a syringe and exten-

sion tubing filled with water-soluble contrast can be attached to the needle. A small amount of contrast can then be injected under fluoroscopic visualization to check the position of the needle. As a general rule, it is more desirable to remove the needle and compress the artery for 5 to 10 minutes if brisk arterial flow is not achieved than to risk raising an intimal flap in the femoral artery.

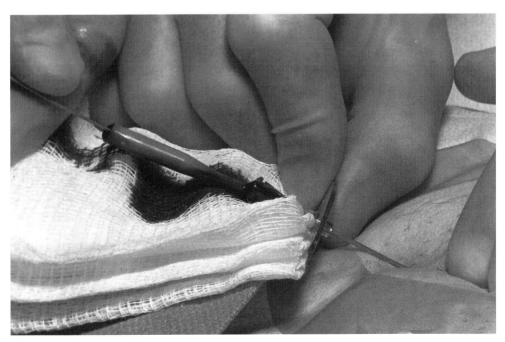

FIG. 19-11. Insertion of the guide wire. Note that there is a brisk, pulsatile back flow of blood, confirming the intraluminal arterial placement of the needle tip. The left hand is used to control the artery while the right is used to control the needle hub. If an assistant is not available, the index finger and thumb of the left hand can be used to secure the needle while the wire is inserted with the right hand.

If a single wall puncture is desired, the needle is held with the right thumb and index finger with the hub exposed to allow blood to return upon entry into the artery. The needle is slowly advanced at a 45-degree angle with the bevel of the needle facing upward. When vigorous arterial blood returns through the needle, the bevel is turned so that it faces dorsally and the guide wire is inserted.

Cannulating the Artery

Once the needle is intraarterial, a guide wire should be inserted through the needle to at least the level of the proximal iliac artery. Many sheaths come with a 3-mm J tip 0.35-inch wire designed to fit the dilator (Fig. 19-12). If a sheath is not used, a 0.35- or 0.38-inch standard wire can be used (3 mm J, Benson, LLT, Rosen, etc.). The wire should advance through the needle in a smooth, unencumbered fashion. Fluoroscopy should be used to visualize the advancement of the wire. If any increase in resistance is felt, this should be investigated prior to advancing the wire further.

Although the author's preference is to use hydrophilically coated wires through the diagnostic catheter, these wires should probably not be used through the needle because the hydrophilic coating can be damaged or stripped off of the wire by manipulation through the needle. Also, there is some belief that the hydrophilically coated wires advance so effortlessly that there may be a greater tendency to inadvertently dissect under iliofemoral plaque. Lastly, when properly hydrated the wire is quite slippery, which can cause inadvertent removal from the femoral artery during attempted place-

ment of the catheter or sheath, resulting in loss of arterial access.

Once the wire is in position, the needle is removed over the wire while firmly gripping the wire with the thumb and index finger of the left hand. The last three fingers can then be used to maintain firm pressure on the femoral artery to prevent bleeding (Fig. 19-13). The guide wire should then be wiped clean of blood to prevent thrombus from being introduced into the catheter. We prefer the use of a Tefla sponge dipped in heparinized saline, but other devices are commercially available that perform just as well.

With the guide wire in position, an appropriately sized arterial dilator is then advanced over the wire into the artery. As the dilator is advanced, a firm rotary motion is invoked to facilitate a smooth entry through the percutaneous tissues and fascia into the vessel (Fig. 19-14). The dilator is then removed in the same fashion as the needle, and the wire is again wiped clean. I prefer to use an arterial sheath that comes with its own dilator and guide wire. Once in position within the artery, the sheath should be secured with sterile strips, a Tegaderm (3M Health Care, St. Paul, MN), or suture.

The arterial sheath allows the angiographer to rapidly exchange catheters with no additional trauma to the artery. A sheath also improves the transmission of torque to the catheter by reducing the friction that would be encountered by the surrounding tissues. Also, there is less trauma to the arteriotomy site from the inward and outward movement of the catheter. The sheath can be connected to a continuous pressurized heparin saline flush for longer cases or can be intermittently flushed by hand for shorter cases (Fig. 19-15). Although the arteriotomy is made

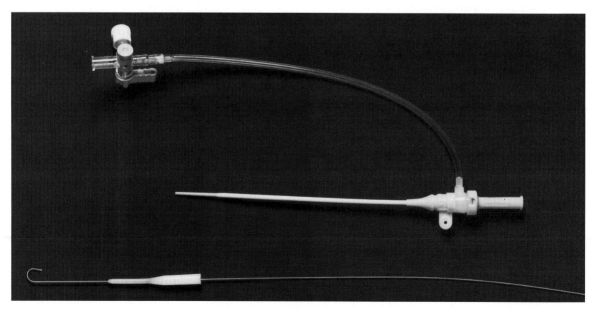

FIG. 19-12. Arterial sheath with dilator and 3-mm J wire with tip straightener.

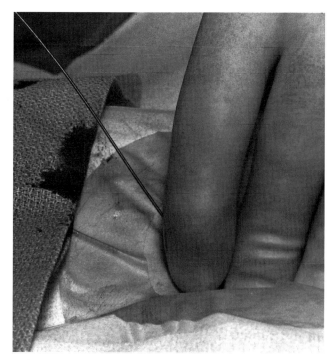

FIG. 19-13. The thumb and index finger of the left hand are used to secure the wire. The third and fourth digits are used to control the artery. The right hand is free to wipe the wire and prepare to insert the sheath.

larger by approximately half a French size when using a sheath, the benefits far outweigh the disadvantages.

For vascular access in infants and children and to make high brachial artery punctures, a micropuncture set (Cook, Inc., Bloomington, IN) is recommended (Fig. 19-

16). This set incorporates a short beveled 22-gauge needle, a modified Cope 0.18-inch introducing wire, and a finely tapered 4 or 5 French dilator and interlocking sheath. Although this system allows for atraumatic access into small arteries, the interlocking sheath is not large enough to accommodate a diagnostic catheter and must be exchanged. Once the dilator and sheath are in position, the dilator and Cope wire are removed. The sheath will accommodate a 0.35-inch standard wire, facilitating exchange for the diagnostic catheter or a standard sheath through which a catheter can be passed.

Safety Tips

Once vascular access is obtained, a quick check should be made to assure that all sharp objects have been removed from the field. I strongly recommend that a standardized place be established for all sharp objects so that no one involved in the procedure inadvertently becomes injured by a contaminated needle or instrument (Fig. 19-17).

Once in the body, a catheter requires frequent flushing. On average, a catheter should be flushed every 90 to 120 seconds, before and after each wire exchange, and just prior to connecting to a power injector and immediately after disconnecting from the power injector. A double flush technique is used. A syringe with 5 to 10 mL of heparinized saline is attached to a stopcock, which in turn is attached to the hub of the catheter. The syringe is gently aspirated with approximately 2 to 3 mL of blood, checking for clot. The first syringe is disconnected and a second clean flush syringe of saline is connected to the end of the catheter. The second syringe is then also aspirated

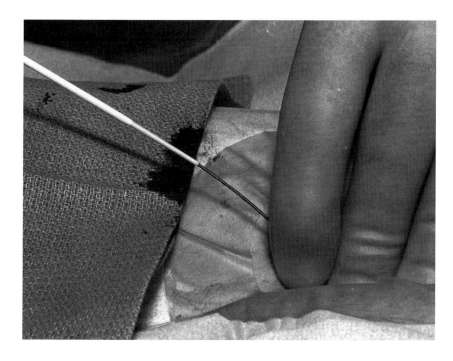

FIG. 19-14. Dilator and sheath being advanced over the wire.

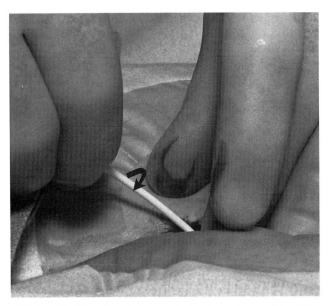

FIG. 19-15. The sheath is inserted using a forward pushing motion with rotation (*curved arrow*) to facilitate smooth access through the tissues and into the artery.

back slightly. The tip of the syringe should be oriented downward so that any bubbles of air will rise toward the plunger and away from the hub of the catheter. It is often helpful to tap the side of the syringe to force any bubbles toward the plunger. The syringe is then injected, flushing

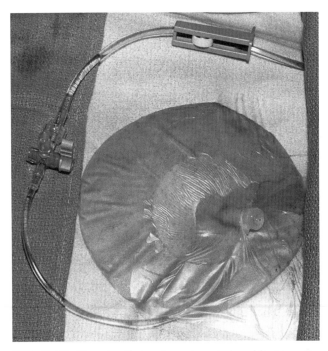

FIG. 19-16. The sheath has been inserted and is now connected to a continuous heparinized flush system and is secured in place with a Tegaderm. Note that the control for the flow rate is within easy reach.

the catheter with a continuous stream of heparinized saline. The stopcock is turned to the off position in mid-injection. This last point, although seemingly trivial, is very important. Turning the stopcock off in mid-injection ensures that heparinized saline has filled the entire length of the catheter, including the tip. If one were to stop injecting prior to turning the stopcock to the off position, there is a chance that blood could backflow into the tip of the catheter, clot, and produce a thromboembolus.

As a syringe, either flush or contrast, is connected to the catheter or stopcock, it is best to allow a meniscus of blood to form by allowing slight backflow into the hub of the catheter. A meniscus is also formed on the tip of the syringe. The two are then brought together in a meniscus-to-meniscus technique. This technique reduces the likelihood of air being trapped between the tip of the syringe and the hub.

After the syringe has been removed from the end of the catheter, the hub should be irrigated. The best technique for doing this is to have a separate syringe filled with heparinized saline with an angiocatheter (approximately 20 gauge) attached to the tip (Fig. 19-18). The tip of the angiocatheter fits very easily into the hub and allows a jet of flush to be injected for irrigating the blood from the hub.

Lastly, after the syringes have been cleaned and refilled with fluid, it is important to ensure that the Luer lock tip of the syringe is clean. A small container filled with flush can be used to dip the tip of the syringe for cleaning.

Similar safety techniques are employed when using an automatic injector. At the onset of the procedure, the injector is filled with contrast. The connecting tubing is attached to the tip of the injector syringe. The injector should be tipped straight up so that all air rises to the top of the injector syringe. The plunger of the injector syringe is then manually advanced until contrast fills the proximalmost aspect of the tubing. The side of the syringe should then be tapped to ensure that no bubbles of air are trapped in the system. The remainder of the tubing is then purged with contrast, producing a closed air-free system. The injector should be prepared prior to establishing vascular access so that time is not wasted once the catheter is in position. Before connecting the injector to the catheter, a test injection of contrast should always be performed to ensure that the position of the tip of the catheter is appropriate.

When connecting the tubing of the injector to the hub of the catheter, the same meniscus-to-meniscus technique previously described should be used. My personal preference is to remove the stopcock from the hub of the catheter prior to connecting the injector tubing, thus eliminating one of the connections that can potentially trap air. However, many angiographers prefer to keep the stopcock on the hub of the catheter and do not feel that it creates a problem. Once the tubing is connected to the

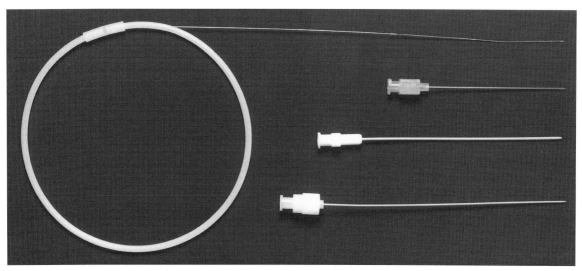

FIG. 19-17. Micropuncture set with long 22-gauge needle, Cope wire, dilator, and sheath. The dilator interlocks with the sheath via a Luer lock adapter.

catheter, the connection site should be gently tapped and visualized to detect whether any air may have become trapped in the system. The injector syringe should be gently aspirated backward until a contrast blood interface is visualized to once again ensure that no air has been introduced during the connection process. The syringe is then gently advanced forward to clear the connecting tubing

and catheter. The automatic injector can now be armed for injection.

To the novice angiographer this may seem like a lot of steps to remember. With experience these safety tips become habit and are performed with little thought. Just remember, stagnant blood clots and clots are the main enemy of the cerebral angiographer.

CATHETERS AND GUIDE WIRE SELECTION

The choice of catheters and guide wires is largely a personal one. Numerous shaped catheters are available that are appropriate for cerebral angiography from a variety of vendors. The list is voluminous and in a constant state of flux as new materials are developed and are incorporated into catheter designs. My philosophy is to become very familiar with a few catheter shapes rather than to mix and match multiple types of catheters. In general, catheters come as simple curve end-hole and complex curve end-hole designs. Several examples of simple and complex curve catheters are illustrated in Figs. 19-19 and 19-20, respectively. As a point of reference, the distal curve of a catheter is referred to as the primary curve, whereas the more proximal curve is referred to as the secondary curve. Simple curve catheters have only a primary curve and do not need to be formed but may not be able to access tortuous vessels. Complex curve catheters have a primary and secondary curve and require reforming of the shape of the distal catheter. Although these catheters greatly facilitate proximal catheterization of tortuous cerebral vessels, the secondary curve may prevent the catheter from

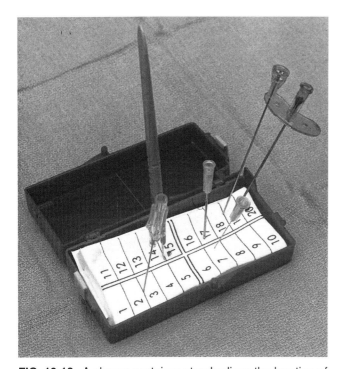

FIG. 19-18. A sharps container standardizes the location of all potentially dangerous needles and instruments.

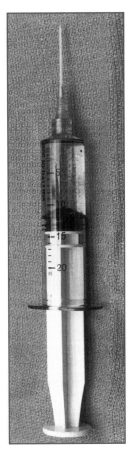

FIG. 19-19. An angiocatheter is attached to a flush syringe and is used to flush the hub of the catheter.

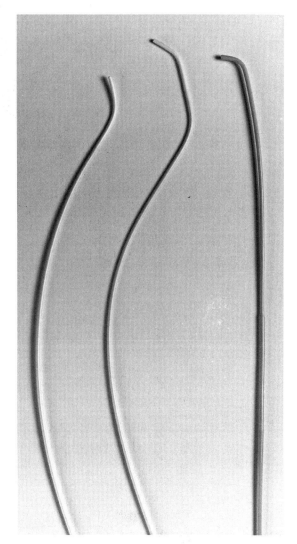

FIG. 19-20. Examples of some simple curve end-hole catheters.

tracking over the wire, making selective and subselective angiography impractical.

If there is a question as to which type of catheter is appropriate for a given patient, a cervicothoracic arch aortogram performed with a multi-hole pigtail catheter is often useful prior to catheter selection.

Simple Curve Catheters

If a simple curve catheter is chosen to perform selective catheterization of the cerebral vessels, the guide wire is advanced over the arch of the aorta into the ascending aorta. The catheter is advanced over the arch, and the guide wire is then removed (Fig. 19-21A). The catheter is then flushed. The tip of the catheter will usually be facing downward toward the aortic valve and must be turned by torque upward so that it faces the origin of the great vessels. The torque applied to a catheter is best transmitted to the end of the catheter if it is simultaneously pulled back as the torque is applied (Fig. 19-21B). Until this concept is learned, the novice angiographer is destined to see the tip of the catheter making 360-degree revolutions

in the aortic arch because torque builds up in the shaft of the catheter and is then suddenly released into the tip.

Once the catheter is oriented in a cephalad direction, it can be pulled back with gentle injections of contrast material until the origin of the desired great vessel is engaged (Fig. 19-21C). Once in the ostium of the desired great vessel, more selective catheterization can be accomplished by reinserting the guide wire and advancing the catheter in a coaxial fashion. The tip of the catheter should not be advanced beyond the end of the guide wire.

If difficulty is encountered, either advancing the guide wire into the common carotid artery or the catheter over the guide wire, there are a few tricks that are useful. When trying to position the guide wire into the common carotid artery, it may become dislodged back into the arch due to proximal tortuosity. If this happens repeatedly,

Complex Curve Catheters

If a complex curve catheter is chosen, it is necessary to reform the curve of the catheter before selecting the cerebral vessels. For the purpose of illustration, the procedure to reform a Simmons II catheter is shown in Fig. 19-22. There are a variety of ways to reform the curve. When using a complex curve catheter, the easiest and perhaps least traumatic means of forming the curve is to use the left subclavian artery. A cervicothoracic arch aortogram will demonstrate the origin of the left subclavian artery. Often the guide wire will engage the left subclavian artery as the catheter and wire are being advanced up the descending aorta. If not, the wire and catheter can be advanced over the arch. The wire is removed and the catheter flushed. Contrast can then be injected through the unformed catheter as it is withdrawn. The ostium of the left subclavian artery can then be engaged in a similar fashion as described above using a simple curve catheter. Once the ostium of the left subclavian artery is engaged, the guide wire can be advanced into the distal subclavian artery (Fig. 19-23A). The catheter is then advanced coaxially over the wire until the secondary curve is just proximal to the origin of the subclavian artery. The wire is then pulled into the catheter to just below the secondary curve (Fig. 19-23B and C). Now by simply advancing and gently rotating the catheter, the system advances into the ascending aorta with the curve formed on the catheter (Fig. 19-23D). Keeping the wire just below the secondary curve of the catheter creates an environment where the shaft of the catheter remains stiff while the curve is more supple. As the catheter is advanced, there is a natural tendency for it to bend at the secondary curve, thus facilitating the formation of the catheter into the desired shape. The hook-shaped loop on the catheter can now be used to engage the great vessels (Fig. 19-23E and F). The left common carotid and innominate arteries also can be used to reform the curve in the catheter if for some reason the subclavian approach is not feasible

If the subclavian artery or other great vessels cannot be accessed to form the catheter, a second approach is to use the ascending aorta (Fig. 19-24). In this instance, the catheter is advanced over the arch. The guide wire is then advanced in such a fashion as to loop back on itself as it slides off of the aortic valve (Fig. 19-24A). The catheter can then be advanced over the wire to form the loop (Fig. 19-24B). Although this technique is a good one to know, it has some distinct disadvantages. If there are calcifications or vegetations on the aortic valve, there is the potential for emboli; if the aorta is very tortuous or the patient is tall, the catheter may not be long enough, and the catheter can flip into the ventricle, producing cardiac arrhythmias. The coronary arteries must also be avoided. But, with careful technique and judicious use of this approach, it is worth having in one's armamentarium.

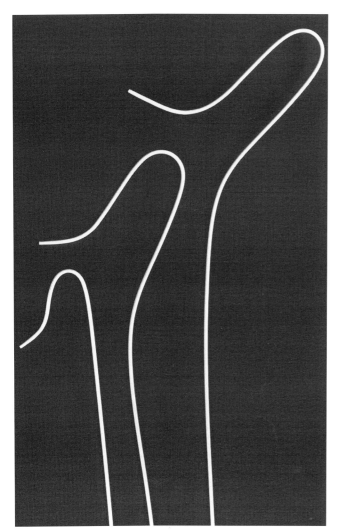

FIG. 19-21. Examples of some complex curve end-hole catheters. Note the varying lengths of the distal segment.

breath holding of the patient in deep inspiration will often elongate and straighten the proximal great vessels, allowing the guide wire to be advanced successfully. An additional maneuver that may prove helpful is to turn the patient's head as far as possible away from the vessel that is to be catheterized. This also can elongate and straighten the vessel.

Once the guide wire is in the desired position, if difficulty is encountered getting the catheter to track over the wire, simultaneously pushing and torquing the catheter may allow the catheter to advance. In addition to the maneuvers described above for positioning the guide wire, having the patient cough intermittently while pushing the catheter may be useful. Each of these maneuvers is an attempt to either straighten a tortuous vessel or reduce the friction coefficient between the guiding wire and the catheter. If these maneuvers fail, then one can resort to using a complex curve catheter.

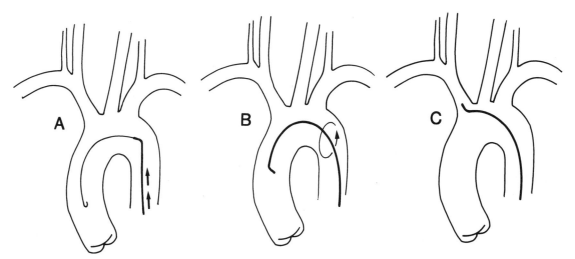

FIG. 19-22. A: To position a simple curve end-hole catheter, the wire is first advanced over the aortic arch followed by the catheter in coaxial fashion (*straight arrows*). **B:** The catheter is usually oriented downward. By torquing the catheter (*curved arrow*) and pulling it back slowly, it can be turned upward toward the ostium of the great vessel. **C:** The catheter can then be pulled back slowly while injecting contrast to engage the vessel.

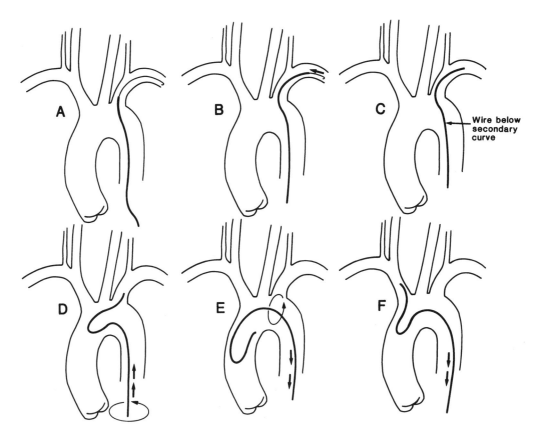

FIG. 19-23. A: To form a loop in a complex curve catheter in the left subclavian artery, the catheter is positioned in the ostium of the artery and the wire is advanced into the distal subclavian artery. **B:** The catheter is advanced over the wire into the subclavian artery and the wire is pulled back (*arrow*) into the catheter. **C:** The wire is pulled back into the catheter until it is just below the secondary curve. **D:** The catheter is then pushed forward (*straight arrows*) with gentle rotation (*curved arrow*) until the loop forms. **E:** The loop is often facing downward, but by simultaneous retraction (*downward arrows*) and torque (*curved arrow*) on the catheter it can be turned upward. **F:** The catheter can now be pulled back (*downward arrow*) while injecting contrast to engage the vessel.

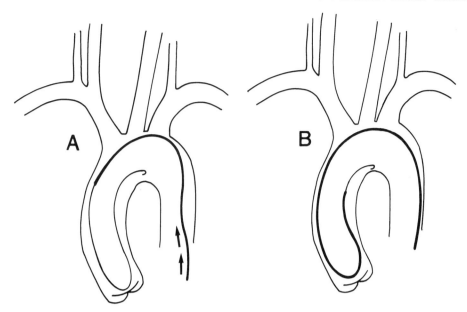

FIG. 19-24. A: To form a loop in a complex curve catheter in the aorta, the wire is advanced until it reflects off of the aortic valve and into the ascending aorta (*arrows*). **B:** The catheter is advanced until the tip follows the wire back up the ascending aorta. The wire is then withdrawn and the loop is formed.

In some instances it is possible to advance the catheter up the iliac artery on the side of puncture, then advance the wire into the opposite iliac artery. The catheter can then be advanced into the contralateral iliac artery until the secondary curve is situated in the distal aorta. The guide wire can then be pulled back into the catheter to just proximal to the secondary curve. The catheter is formed by advancing it into the aorta. In a similar manner, other vessels, such as a renal artery, can be used to form the catheter, but this is a less desirable approach.

When selecting a complex curve catheter for common carotid artery catheterization, the distal tip is available in different lengths. The aortic arch injection should be used to estimate the length between the origin of the innominant artery and the origin of the common carotid artery in selecting the appropriate catheter. The angiographer should become familiar with the specifications of the various catheters used in cerebral angiography.

Once the complex curve has been reformed, it takes on a hooklike appearance. Either the left or right common carotid artery can be selected by simply advancing the catheter over the aortic arch into the opening of the appropriate vessel. The tip of the catheter should be directed cephalad toward the ostium of the vessel. Once the tip engages the origin of the desired great vessel, the catheter is pulled back gently as contrast is injected. To position the catheter tip in the proximal right common carotid artery, the innominate artery is negotiated by slowly pulling back further on the catheter under fluoroscopic visualization while injecting small amounts of contrast until the tip is in position. The injection of con-

trast while positioning the catheter is important because the tip of the catheter can dissect beneath a plaque if caution is not exercised. Positioning of the tip of the catheter also can be accomplished over a guide wire, but the wire will have a tendency to straighten the hook in the catheter and in some instances will cause the shape to be lost completely.

If the left common carotid artery is to be catheterized after the right, the catheter should be advanced until the tip is no longer engaged in the innominate artery. The hook of the catheter is directed downward away from the origin of the great vessels. The catheter can then be pulled back and torqued to point up once the innominate artery origin has been passed.

There are two instances in which the tip of the complex curve catheter must be further altered to effect a successful catheterization of the desired vessel. When the tip of the catheter advances into the proximal right subclavian artery rather than the proximal right common carotid artery and when there is a common origin of the left common carotid artery with the innominate artery, the catheter may have to be formed into a figure of eight or reverse loop (Fig. 19-25). This often occurs when the origin of either the right or left common carotid artery arises along the proximal and medial aspect of the innominate artery (low origin of the right common carotid artery and bovine origin of the left common carotid artery, respectively). If the curve is used in the conventional position, the primary curve is pointing away from the origin of the vessel. Forming a figure-of-eight loop on the catheter redirects the primary curve toward the origin of the vessel.

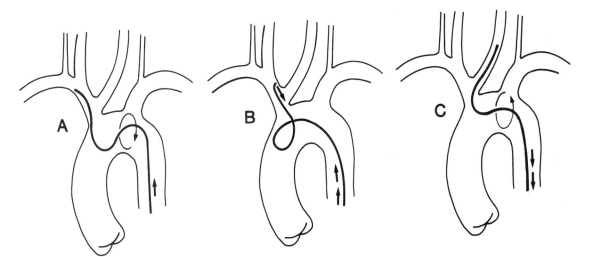

FIG. 19-25. A: To form a figure-of-eight or reverse curve, the catheter is initially positioned into the proximal right subclavian or innominate artery and torque is applied (*curved arrow*) while the catheter is advanced slightly (*upward arrow*). **B:** Once the reverse curve is formed, the tip of the catheter will be oriented medially. By advancing the catheter (*upward arrows*), the tip will engage the vessel (*downward arrow*). **C:** By pulling the catheter back (*downward arrows*) and simultaneously torquing the catheter (*curved arrow*) in the opposite direction that was used to form the loop, the catheter will unfold and engage the more distal aspect of the vessel.

In this instance, the catheter is initially positioned in the innominate or proximal right subclavian artery (Fig. 19-25A). Torque is then applied to the catheter until it rolls over 180 degrees and forms a figure-of-eight appearance (Fig. 19-25B). The primary curve and tip of the catheter is now oriented medially toward the origin of the common carotid artery. As the figure-of-eight curve is formed, the angiographer should remember which direction the catheter was turned to form the figure-of-eight loop. Now that the tip is pointing toward the ostium of the common carotid artery, a small amount of forward advancement of the catheter will allow it to engage the common carotid artery. Once the catheter has engaged the ostium of the common carotid artery, it should be pulled back and simultaneously torqued in the opposite direction in which it was formed to unfold the figure-of-eight loop (Fig. 19-25C). This will firmly seat the catheter into the proximal aspect of the cervical common carotid artery.

These two scenarios are relatively common occurrences in aortic arch anatomy. In such instances, the figure-of-eight loop may be the only means of catheterizing the vessel.

Once the catheter is in position, a test injection of contrast into the common carotid artery under fluoroscopy should be performed. This not only ensures appropriate catheter positioning but also allows visualization of the common carotid artery bifurcation for appropriate centering during angiography.

The advantages of a complex curve catheter are that it can be used more effectively in tortuous vessels and can be used as described above to engage anatomic variations that may be difficult, if not impossible, with a simple curve catheter. The disadvantage of the complex curve catheter is that the very feature that allowed the angiographer into the proximal aspect of the vessel may prevent access into the distal aspect of the vessel. Specifically, although a complex curve catheter may access the proximal common carotid artery or subclavian artery and even allow a guide wire to be advanced into the internal carotid artery (ICA) or vertebral artery, respectively, the catheter may not follow the wire because the secondary curve of the catheter will continually want to reform the loop. If more selective catheterization is necessary, the complex curve catheter can be exchanged over an exchange length guide wire for a simple curve catheter.

Exchanging Catheters

Once access to the proximal aspect of a vessel is achieved, the catheter may not advance over the guide wire despite good positioning of the guide wire tip. This may necessitate exchange of the catheter for a larger-sized or different-shaped catheter or both. Multiple guide wires are available for catheter exchange in lengths ranging from 180 to 300 cm with straight and curved tips. When selecting an exchange length guide wire, the length of the longest catheter to be used and the length of wire to remain in the patient must be added together. Then at least a few additional centimeters are added to the calculation so that the wire can be grasped and controlled and there is some play in the wire within the vessels. The average cerebral catheter is in the range of 90 to 120 cm in length. The average length of wire that must remain in the patient is also in the range of 90 to 120 cm. Therefore, in most adult patients a standard 260-cm exchange length wire is adequate.

The exchange of a catheter is greatly facilitated if two operators are involved. To exchange a catheter, the exchange wire is advanced through the existing catheter to the desired location. Under fluoroscopic visualization, the catheter is gradually and smoothly pulled back as the wire is advanced at the same rate by a second operator. The goal of this maneuver is to remove the catheter without moving the wire tip either forward or backward. Once the catheter tip exits the insertion site, the proximalmost aspect of the exposed wire should be secured with a firm grasp of the thumb and index fingers of the left hand. The wire is wiped clean and the next catheter that has been prepared prior to the attempted exchange is then introduced over the wire. Care should be taken not to advance or withdraw the wire at this point. Once the catheter tip is at the insertion site, the distal aspect of the wire that is now extending out of the hub of the catheter is pinned into position with a firm grasp of the thumb and forefinger. The proximal segment of the wire is released, and the catheter is inserted.

As the catheter is advanced, fluoroscopy of the distal aspect of the wire to include the tip and the aortic arch is recommended. Care should be taken not to dislodge the wire from the great vessel into the aortic arch and not to blindly advance the wire as the catheter is advanced.

Once the catheter has been advanced to the appropriate location, the wire is removed and the catheter is flushed.

Catheter exchanges over a wire are not particularly difficult but are greatly facilitated by communication between operators and close attention to detail, especially with respect to the location of the tip of the guide wire. Usually the most critical points in the exchange of a catheter are the points where the original catheter is pulled below the origin of the great vessel, the point where the catheter tip is removed from the sheath or insertion site, and the point where the second catheter is attempting to engage the great vessel. It is at these times that the guide wire is most likely to migrate.

CONTRAST

Numerous contrast agents are available that are suitable for injection into the cerebral vessels. A list of contrast agents and some of their characteristics are provided in Table 19-1. The two general classes of contrast agents are ionic water-soluble and nonionic water-soluble agents. The nonionic agents are the newest and are described according to the content of organic iodine per milliliter. Ionic contrast agents are described by the weight per volume percentage of iodine-containing salt solution (3). As a general rule, a nonionic contrast agent designated 300 is equivalent in iodine concentration and vessel opacification to an ionic agent designated 60. These two concentrations are the most commonly used in adult cerebral angiography because they offer an excellent ratio between vessel opacification and iodine load.

There remains significant division among angiographers as to whether ionic or nonionic contrast should be the agent of choice for routine cerebral angiography.

TABLE 19-1. *Contrast agents for cerebral angiography*

Product name		Chemical structure	Osmolality (mOsmol/kg water)	Total iodine (mg/mL)	Vendor
Nonionic					
Omnipaque	180	Iohexol	480	180	Winthrop/Nycomed, Princeton, NJ
Omnipaque	240		520	240	
Omnipaque	300		675	300	
Omnipaque	350		844	350	
Isovue	200	Iopamidol	413	200	Squibb/Bracco, Princeton, NJ
Isovue	300		616	300	
Isovue	370		796	375	
Optiray	160	Ioversol	355		Mallinckrodt, St. Louis, MO
Optiray	240		502	240	
Optiray	320		702	320	
Ionic					
Conray	43	Iothalamanate	430	202	Mallinckrodt, St. Louis, MO
Conray	60		1,539	282	
Hypaque	60	Diatrizoate meglumine	1,415	282	Winthrop/Nycomed, Princeton, NJ
Hexabrix		Ioxaglate meglumine	600	320	Mallinkrodt, St. Louis, MO
Angiovist	370	Diatrozoate meglamine	1,405	370	Berlex, Wayne, NJ

Because both agents are safe and adequate for vessel opacification, the major issue dividing the two groups was the cost of the nonionic agents when they were first released. Now that more agents are available on the market, competition and contracts with vendors have driven the cost down, but the cost of the nonionic agents is still higher. There is general agreement that in patients categorized as high risk and in patients undergoing neurointerventional procedures, nonionic agents are preferable. Although there appears to be no significant difference in the rate of neurologic complications when comparing the two types of agents, the nonionic contrast agents appear to have less systemic effects and a lower rate of allergic reactions. In addition, the nonionic agents appear to be better tolerated by the patient in terms of the unpleasant burning sensation that is experienced during injection (4–13).

At our institution, nonionic contrast is routinely used for all patients undergoing cerebral angiography. Anecdotally, many of my patients who have had prior angiograms with ionic contrast have reported significantly less discomfort with nonionic agents. Valid reasoning exists for either choice.

If a patient has had a significant allergic reaction to contrast in the past and cerebral angiography is required, precautionary measures can be taken that may reduce the risk of another reaction. Prior reactions to ionic contrast may not occur with nonionic contrast. Furthermore, the preprocedural treatment of the patient with steroids and antihistamines may play a role in preventing allergic reactions (14).

MECHANICAL AUTOMATIC INJECTORS

There is a jargon that the novice angiographer should learn before using an automatic injector. In general, contrast injections administered via automatic injector are described using the following adjustable criteria: contrast volume per second, total contrast volume and linear rate rise, and PSI (pounds per square inch of pressure). As would be implied, contrast volume per second refers to the volume of contrast that the injector will deliver during each second of the injection, whereas the total volume reflects the amount of contrast that will be injected by the end of the injection interval. By dividing the volume per second by the total volume, one can establish the length of the injection. For example, if the injector is programmed for a common carotid artery angiogram to inject 5 mL/second at a total volume of 10 mL, the injector will deliver 5 mL of contrast in each second of the injection, which will last for 2 seconds. Similarly, if one wanted to decrease the rate per second but prolong the injection yet deliver a similar volume of contrast, the injector could be set at 3 mL contrast per second for a total volume of 9 mL, thus extending the injection time an additional second.

Angiography laboratories vary as to the order in which these numbers are expressed. It is important to understand the jargon in your angiography suite so that everyone involved understands exactly how much contrast is to be injected and at what rate. For the purposes of this text, the rate per second will be expressed first followed by the total volume. For the first example listed above, the instruction would be to set the injector at 5 for 10.

The linear rate rise feature of the injector allows for a linear acceleration of the contrast injection over the first timing interval of the injector. The timing interval on an automatic injector can be set for various time increments. The injector is set for seconds in cerebral angiography. Therefore, a rate rise in cerebral angiography refers to a progressive acceleration of contrast over the first second of the injection. The linear rate rise feature is most useful when a catheter is positioned near the origin of a vessel and a sudden injection of contrast might result in recoil or dislodgement of the catheter from the vessel. Using the previous example, an injection of 5 mL/second for a total of 10 mL with a rate rise of 0.4 seconds would result in the same contrast given over the same time interval, except that the first 5 mL would be injected in a linear accelerating fashion with the desired injection rate being reached 4/10 of a second into the injection rather than from the beginning.

Table 19-2 offers suggested injection rates and volumes depending on the vessel being opacified and type of lesion being studied. With experience, an angiographer learns how to make adjustments in flow rates, total volume, and linear rise to maximize each injection of contrast.

The PSI setting on the injector refers to the maximum pressure that the injector will generate while injecting the contrast. All catheters have specifications that are indicated on the label. These specifications should be followed or it is possible to rupture the catheter. Although

TABLE 19-2. Suggested contrast injection rates and volumes for DSA vs. film

Vessel	Linear rise	Rate (mL/second) DSA	Film	Total volume (mL) DSA	Film
CCA	0–0.2	4–5	5–6	8–10	10–12
ICA	0–0.5	3–4	4–5	6–8	8–10
ECA (proximal) versus hand injection	0–0.5	2–3	3–4	4–6	6–8
ECA (distal) versus hand injection	0–0.5	2–3	3–4	3–4	4–6
ECA (selective branches) versus hand injection	0–0.5	1–2	2–3	2–4	3–5
Vertebral	0–0.5	4–5	5–6	8–10	10–12

DSA, digital subtraction angiography; film, "cut" film.

this should obviously be avoided, catheters are designed to fail in a linear fashion parallel to and near the hub so that if a mistake is made the rupture will most likely occur in a segment of the catheter that is outside of the patient.

ANGIOGRAPHY OF THE CEREBRAL VESSELS IN SPECIFIC DISEASES

In the selective catheterization of cerebral vessels, there is no substitution for experience and common sense. For example, we generally perform selective ICA angiography when evaluating a patient with a suspected intracranial aneurysm. But in an elderly patient with very tortuous and diseased vessels, it may be the better part of valor to settle for less selective angiography of the common carotid artery that will still assess the patient but will put him or her at less risk during the procedure. The following section is designed to point out some basic principles and guidelines in catheterizing the cerebral vessels.

The two most common indications for cerebral angiography at our institution, and probably elsewhere, are cerebrovascular atherosclerosis and the evaluation of intracranial aneurysms. The techniques used for catheterizing cerebral vessels in these two entities are identical to the techniques used for other disease processes. Other chapters in this text have more directly addressed pathophysiology, natural history, and common angiographic appearances, so this section will focus merely on the technical aspects of angiography in specific disease entities.

Cerebrovascular Atherosclerosis

In the evaluation of cerebrovascular atherosclerosis, a cervicothoracic arch aortogram is performed, followed by selective catheterization of both common carotid arteries (see Figs. 16-3 and 16-4). The aortogram is usually performed using a 5 French pigtail catheter, although safe aortography can also be performed using an end-hole catheter. The catheter is advanced under fluoroscopic guidance over a guide wire into the ascending aorta proximal to the origin of the innominate artery. If an end-hole catheter is used, a small test injection should be performed to ensure that the catheter tip is not in a coronary artery or graft.

The arch aortogram gives the angiographer a clear picture of the relationship of the great vessels to one another, the tortuosity of the proximal aspect of the great vessels, and the presence of disease at the origin of the great vessels that may preclude more selective catheterization. Using digital angiography, the usual injection rate is 15 mL/second for 2 seconds, amounting to a total of 30 mL of nonionic 300 contrast. The tube is angled at 30 to 45 degrees left anterior oblique (LAO). Prior to the injection of contrast, fluoroscopy of the catheter while angling the tube will illustrate a view that opens the arch of the aorta.

In rare instances, additional views may be needed, but in our experience the LAO arch view yields an excellent look at the origin of the innominate, left common carotid, and left subclavian arteries (see Fig. 1-11). Additionally, both the ostium and proximal cervical segments of the vertebral arteries can be evaluated from this projection. If necessary, anteroposterior (AP) and right anterior oblique (RAO) or selective injection of the subclavian arteries can be performed to profile the vessel origins (see Figs. 1-12 and 9-5).

Once the aortic arch has been evaluated, the appropriate catheter can be chosen for selective catheterization of the common carotid arteries. As a general rule, if the great vessels are relatively straight or exhibit only mild to moderate tortuosity, one of the many simple curve endhole catheters will suffice. In truth, selective catheterization of the common carotid arteries can be performed with either a simple curve catheter or a complex curve catheter with relative ease if there is minimal tortuosity. My personal bias is to use a simple curve catheter whenever possible because it offers more options in selecting other vessels if the need arises. Specifically, simple curve end-hole catheters are better suited for selective catheterization of internal carotid, external carotid, and vertebral arteries.

The strategy for the catheterization of the common carotid arteries in patients with atherosclerotic disease should be to catheterize and study the symptomatic or diseased vessel first. Usually, the clinical history, duplex ultrasonography, or MR angiogram will give some indication of the suspected site of disease. In the event of a problem that necessitates premature termination of the procedure, the necessary data to implement therapy will have been obtained.

When performing angiography of the common carotid artery, we typically inject contrast at 4 to 5 mL/second for 2 seconds, totaling 8 to 10 mL. Using a biplane digital angiography system, four views of the common carotid artery can be obtained with two injections of contrast. The four views include AP, lateral, 45 degree LAO, and 45 degree RAO (see Fig. 16-5). If a single plane unit is used, an AP, lateral, and ipsilateral oblique view will suffice. Intracranial views are also obtained routinely in AP Caldwell and lateral projections (see Fig. 17-1).

We do not routinely catheterize and inject the vertebrobasilar system if the signs and symptoms of atherosclerotic disease are isolated to the anterior circulation. An exception to this principle is made when symptoms are more likely to be vertebrobasilar in origin. Also, if there is internal carotid artery occlusions it may be necessary to evaluate the vertebrobasilar system to access the collateral circulation to the usual distribution of the occluded vessel.

When it is necessary to catheterize and inject the vertebrobasilar system, the arch aortogram is useful in selecting the larger more dominant vertebral artery. If the two vertebral arteries are about equal in size, the left vertebral artery is usually the easier to catheterize because the relationship of the descending aorta, left subclavian artery, and origin of the left vertebral artery is a relatively straight course compared with the route into the right vertebral artery from the femoral approach.

Cerebral Aneurysm

Two groups of patients are referred for cerebral angiography for evaluation of intracranial aneurysms: patients who present with subarachnoid hemorrhage from rupture of an aneurysm and those who have unruptured aneurysms and present with either mass effect or are incidentally discovered. In both instances the angiographer usually has the benefit of noninvasive imaging tests such as CT, MR, or CT or MR angiography to direct the catheter angiogram toward the pathology.

In the setting of acute subarachnoid hemorrhage, the patient's condition can range in symptoms from mild headache to frank coma. From the time of presentation to the time of operation, there is a very real potential for further decompensation for any number of reasons. More so than for probably any other instance in neuroradiology, it is essential to obtain the necessary information to implement appropriate therapy as quickly and safely as possible.

A noncontrast CT scan of the brain is always obtained prior to the angiogram and in the majority of instances has already been performed before an angiogram is requested. This should be reviewed prior to the start of the procedure to determine, based on the pattern of subarachnoid blood, which vessel territory is most likely to have bled (15,16). The most suspicious vessel should be injected first (see Fig. 12-4). For example, if the majority of the blood is localized to the right sylvian fissure, the right internal carotid artery should be the first vessel injected, even if the catheter practically falls into another artery. In contrast, if the majority of blood is in the posterior fossa and fourth ventricle, the right and left vertebral arteries should both be studied prior to studying the carotid arteries. That way, in the event of sudden decline in the patient's status, the surgeon will have the necessary information to take the patient to the operating room and clip the aneurysm.

If the pattern of subarachnoid blood is diffuse, therefore offering no clue on the CT scan as to the vessel of origin, an organized pattern of study is taken such that all of the intracranial cerebral vessels are seen.

In patients suspected of having a nonruptured aneurysm, there is no significant difference in the angiographic approach to the lesion. The suspicious vessel is injected first, followed by a logical approach to the remainder of the cerebral vasculature. The preprocedural noninvasive imaging, however, is likely to be more variable and to include MR and MR angiography.

Once the aneurysm has been found and well delineated, the remainder of the cerebral vessels also should be studied (see Fig. 12-22). Two or more aneurysms will be present in 15% to 20% of patients (17,18). The additional aneurysms may be treatable through the same exposure at the time of surgery. Also, temporary and sometimes permanent occlusion of the parent artery is necessary to facilitate treatment of the aneurysm. A working knowledge of the collateral circulation to the involved vessel territory can be the difference between a good outcome and a poor outcome. Lastly, in the setting of subarachnoid hemorrhage, vasospasm is usually a delayed complication but in rare instances can be seen acutely (see Fig. 12-27). Visualizing all of the cerebral arteries on initial presentation will not only reveal acute vasospasm but also serve as an important frame of reference for comparison should delayed vasospasm occur.

Compared with the workup for atherosclerotic stenosis, more selective angiography of the cerebral vessels is desirable in the case of an aneurysm evaluation. By selectively catheterizing each ICA, the overlying image of the external carotid artery (ECA) is eliminated and the intracranial vessels are easier to interpret.

Although some angiographers feel more comfortable performing an arch aortogram prior to selecting the great vessels, others may skip this step because it adds little to the evaluation of a patient whose vessels are not difficult to catheterize and increases the contrast load. Whether or not an arch aortogram is performed is to some degree a matter of judgment. For example, a 30-year-old who presents with subarachnoid hemorrhage is unlikely to have an abnormality at the take-off of the great vessels that would preclude selective catheterization, and an arch aortogram is probably unnecessary. In contrast, in a 72-year-old with a long history of poorly controlled hypertension, an arch aortogram may be necessary for mapping purposes as well as to screen for proximal arterial disease.

In general, a simple curve end-hole catheter is preferred for the examination because it is well suited for selective catheterization of the internal carotid and vertebral arteries. Using the guide wire, either the common carotid artery or the subclavian artery is then catheterized. The wire is removed, the catheter is flushed with heparinized saline, and the vessel is injected under fluoroscopic visualization with contrast material. Road mapping with live digital subtraction, if available, is very useful at this point of the procedure to visualize the vessel to be catheterized. If there is no prohibitive disease, such as atherosclerotic stenosis involving the internal carotid or vertebral artery, more selective catheterization is undertaken. The guide wire is reinserted and, using torque to steer the tip, is advanced into the vessel to be catheterized. The catheter is then advanced under fluoroscopy over the wire into the appropriate position. As described previously, the tip of the catheter should not extend beyond the distal aspect of the guide wire.

For internal carotid artery catheterization, the mid-cervical level between C3 and C4 is usually suitable. For the vertebral artery, the catheter can be positioned just distal to the C6 level, where it curves into the foramen transversarium, but proximal to the posterior curve at the C2 level. These two positions, respectively, offer a good location for preventing catheter dislodgement from recoil during injection or reflux of contrast into proximal vessels that you do not intend to opacify. Also, this portion of the respective vessels is generally a straighter segment; therefore, there is less likelihood of the end hole of the catheter becoming occluded by the intima of the vessel wall (side walling). The internal carotid and vertebral arteries are more susceptible to spasm and iatrogenic traumatic injury than are larger vessels; therefore, care should be taken to advance the wire and catheter smoothly and with as little manipulation as possible. Whenever possible, the primary curve of the catheter should be oriented so that it corresponds with the natural curve of the cervical aspect of the vessel. This will help to prevent end-hole occlusion from side walling and spasm.

Once into position, the guide wire should be removed. While removing the guide wire, especially in smaller vessels, it is a good idea to irrigate the hub of the catheter continuously with the syringe affixed with the angiocatheter previously described. If by chance the catheter tip is side walled, a negative pressure will be generated when the wire is removed, which creates a vacuum due to the dead space of the wire and draws air into the catheter. By holding the catheter hub upward and infusing saline flush into the hub as the wire is withdrawn, saline flush rather than air is drawn into the catheter.

If the catheter is side walled, it should be withdrawn slightly and repositioned until backflow into the catheter hub is established. Prior to contrast injection using the automatic injector, a test injection of contrast should be performed to check for spasm at the tip of the catheter, which will also necessitate repositioning, and to check the flow rate within the vessel to establish contrast volume and flow rates.

The goal of cerebral angiography in the evaluation of intracranial aneurysms is to thoroughly study all of the cerebral vessels at the base of the skull and above (19). Because most aneurysms occur at flow dividers or branch points, special attention is directed to the circle of Willis and the other usual locations of aneurysm (see Fig. 12-2). It is insufficient to merely diagnose an aneurysm. For thorough treatment planning, either by neurosurgical clipping or by endovascular means, the anatomy of the aneurysm must be profiled. Specifically, special views should be obtained that lay out the anatomy of the parent artery with the neck and the dome of the aneurysm (see Fig. 12-19). Table 19-3 outlines the usual locations of aneurysms and the views that are most helpful in profiling an aneurysm. Remember, however, that every patient is different and that subtle changes in these views are often necessary to eliminate artifacts or adjust for anatomic variations. Our approach to cerebral angiography in patients suspected of having an aneurysm is to include at a minimum at least one oblique view in addition to the usual AP and lateral projections. In the early phase of learning cerebral angiography for aneurysm evaluation, it is beneficial to go to the operating room and view the intracranial vessels through the operating microscope to better appreciate the neurosurgeon's view of the vessels. This experience is invaluable in getting a three-dimensional sense of the complex relationship of the intracranial cerebral vessels and will better prepare the

TABLE 19-3. Angiographic positions for cerebral aneurysms

Location	Additional views	Percentage of rotation	Angulation (cephalad/caudal)
ACOM	Transorbital oblique	15–30	7 cephalad
	Caldwell's oblique	15–30	7 caudal
MCA	Transorbital oblique	15–30	7 cephalad
	Submentovertex	0	90 to baseline
	Haughton lateral	90	45 cephalad
ICA/PCOM	Tranorbital oblique	15–30	7 cephalad
	Paraorbital oblique	55	7 cephalad
	Haughton lateral	90	45 cephalad
ICA bifurcation	Transorbital oblique	15–30	7 cephalad
	Submentovertex	0	90 to baseline
Basilar tip and VBJ	Towne's oblique	10–30	25–30
	Submentovertex	0	90 to baseline
ICA/ophthalmic	Transorbital oblique	15–30	7 cephalad
	Caldwell's oblique	15–30	7 caudal
Cavernous ICA	Paraorbital oblique	55	7 cephalad
	Haughton lateral	90	45 cephalad
SCA, AICA, PICA	Towne's oblique	10–30	25–30

ACOM, anterior communicating artery; PCOM, posterior communicating artery; VBJ, vertebrobasilar junction; SCA, superior cerebellar artery; AICA, anterior inferior cerebellar artery; PICA, posterior inferior cerebellar artery.

angiographer to choose appropriate angled views to profile the aneurysm.

In order to properly visualize the circle of Willis, additional variations or maneuvers may be necessary. For example, higher injection rates and volumes may be needed to reflux across communicating arteries. To visualize the distal ICA territory under usual circumstances, an injection rate of 4 mL/second for 2 seconds, totaling 8 ml of contrast may be adequate. But to opacify the anterior communicating or posterior communicating artery in the same patient, the contrast injection may need to be increased by 2 to 4 mL to 5 to 6 mL/second, for a total of 10 to 12 mL.

Additionally, cross-compression may be necessary (see Fig. 12-20). To visualize the anterior communicating artery, the carotid artery on the opposite side of the vessel catheterized is manually compressed during the injection. The temporary arrest of flow forces the contrast across the anterior communicating artery. Similarly, the posterior communicating artery can be visualized by manually compressing the carotid artery during a vertebral injection (Huber maneuver). Care should be taken in elderly patients or in patients with diseased cervical vessels not to compress too vigorously. Additionally, during manual compression of the carotid artery, close supervision of the patient's heart rate is important because carotid body stimulation can result in bradycardia.

It is important when evaluating the intracranial circulation for aneurysms that all intradural vessels be visualized. To that end, the circulation in the posterior fossa can sometimes be seen from the injection of only one vertebral artery. If the vertebral artery is injected at a rate of 5 to 6 mL/second for a total volume of 10 to 12 mL of contrast, there is frequently sufficient reflux down the opposite vertebral artery into the high cervical segment such that the posterior inferior cerebellar artery is opacified. This area is one in which clinical judgment and experience play a critical role. Whether or not it is safe to inject the vertebral artery in this fashion or there is sufficient opacification to evaluate the opposite distal vertebral artery and its branches is a matter of judgment. If it is felt for any reason that the opposite vertebral artery is incompletely evaluated, selective catheterization and injection of that vertebral artery is then necessary.

Regardless of the technical expertise and experience of the angiographer, there are times when a vessel simply cannot be catheterized selectively. This usually occurs in the vertebrobasilar circulation but can also occur in the carotid circulation. In such instances, the only option is to inject contrast in a more proximal vessel. Nevertheless, there are ways to augment the pattern of blood flow temporarily to improve opacification of the vessel in need of examination. For example, if a vertebral artery cannot be accessed, the catheter can be positioned in the proximal subclavian artery near the origin of the vertebral artery. A blood pressure cuff can then be placed on the appropriate arm and inflated to just above the patient's known systolic blood pressure. Then, when contrast in injected, it is diverted into the vessel in question. This technique usually requires a slightly longer injection interval and higher volumes, as well as a longer filming sequence to achieve adequate distal vessel opacification.

Arteriovenous Malformations and Fistulae

Most other entities that involve the cerebral vascular system can be evaluated by the techniques outlined for the study of atherosclerosis and aneurysm. But brain arteriovenous malformations (AVMs), dural AVMs or arteriovenous fistulae (AVFs), and carotid cavernous fistulae deserve a few additional technical notes. Although these lesions are different with respect to their etiology, pathophysiology, and natural history, they share a common characteristic: they are high-flow lesions. Because of the high-flow nature of these lesions, the angiographer must alter techniques from the usual routine or the lesion will not be thoroughly evaluated.

Brain Arteriovenous Malformations

When performing cerebral angiography for brain AVMs, it is rare that the diagnosis is not already known from noninvasive imaging. Therefore, the purpose of the angiogram is usually not to establish a diagnosis but to define the best mode of therapy (20). There are three different specialties interested in the outcome of the angiogram, each with different priorities. These include the neurosurgeon with respect to resection, the interventional neuroradiologist with respect to embolization, and the radiation therapist with respect to stereotactic radiosurgery. The cerebral angiographer must understand the aspect of the angiogram that each of these groups is most interested in to appropriately evaluate the patient. The neurosurgeon wishes to know the location of the lesion especially as it relates to eloquent brain tissue, the size of the lesion, the number and distribution of feeding vessels, the venous drainage pattern with respect to the presence or absence of deep venous drainage, and the presence or absence of associated aneurysms on the proximal feeding arteries. All of these factors relate to patient outcome and prognosis if neurosurgical resection is undertaken (21).

The interventional neuroradiologist is also interested in the location of the lesion, the hemodynamics of the lesion and the degree of proximal tortuosity of the feeding vessels because these factors will effect catheter and embolic material selection and the feasibility of embolization. In addition, the presence or absence of so-called intranidal aneurysms and intranidal fistulae is important to the interventionalist because these areas will be targeted first if embolization is undertaken (22).

The radiotherapist is most interested in the size of the AVM and the hemodynamics. Lesions less than 2 to 3 cm in diameter and slower flow lesions respond more favorably than do larger, higher flow lesions (22,23).

Because the angiographer cannot know prior to the study which modality or combination of modalities will be utilized in the treatment of the patient, it is necessary to obtain a sufficient study to satisfy all three groups.

The first question is, which vessels must be studied? The answer to this question lies in a knowledge of the usual arterial supply to a given territory of the brain. For example, a small, centrally located lesion in the basal ganglia may only require the injection of a single ICA. In contrast, a large lesion situated in a watershed territory with a sizable cortical component may require selective study of both ICAs, both external carotid arteries, and the vertebral basilar system to completely evaluate the lesion (see Figs. 13-7 and 13-8). In brain AVMs that occur at the watershed of the anterior cerebral artery (ACA) and middle cerebral artery (MCA), it is often helpful to inject the opposite ICA. There is usually a patent anterior communicating artery that opacifies the involved ACA and isolates its contribution from the MCA contribution. Likewise, in AVMs in the MCA/posterior cerebral artery watershed region, injection of both the anterior and posterior circulation will isolate the contribution from each vessel respectively.

The next question is, how should the vessel be studied? Changes in contrast rate and volume are usually indicated because of the high-flow state and the dilatation of the cerebral vessels. Additionally, faster filming rates are frequently required to understand the hemodynamic characteristics of the lesion. In general, a larger and faster bolus of contrast is required, which needs to be tailored to the expected flow characteristics determined on the initial test injection. Filming should be at a minimum of four frames per second.

Dural AVMs and AVFs

The terms "dural arteriovenous malformation" and "dural arteriovenous fistula" are used interchangeably. Because there is not a discrete nidus as in brain AVMs the term "dural arteriovenous fistula" is probably more precise. Furthermore, a dural fistula involving the cavernous sinus is sometimes referred to as an indirect carotid cavernous fistula.

Dural AVFs are high-flow communications between the arteries that supply the dura and the dural sinuses and/or veins. The arterial supply to a dural AVF will depend on the area of dura involved. A review of the arterial supply to the dura in various locations is beyond the scope of this chapter but is reviewed comprehensively in other texts (24–26). Suffice it to say that the approach to the angiographic evaluation of a dural fistula is to selectively catheterize and inject all vessels that could potentially be involved in supplying a given territory (see Fig. 13-21). Selective and sometimes subselective injection of each branch vessel of the ECA that could potentially supply the lesion is indicated. Additionally, dural branches of the ICA and vertebral artery also should be evaluated when indicated (see Fig. 13-20).

When catheterizing the branch vessels of the ECA, roadmapping and live digital subtraction fluoroscopy can be very useful. Catheterizing branch vessels of the ECA requires the use of a simple curve end-hole catheter. The same over-the-wire technique previously described for catheterizing the ICA can be used to engage various branch vessels of the ECA. Sometimes, however, it is easier to simply guide the catheter by torque control without the use of a guide wire. In the past the thought of advancing a catheter without the use of a guide wire was considered by some to be heresy. But in the current era with smaller caliber, tapered tip catheters, it is safe and feasible in selected instances. It is important to inject contrast as the catheter is being advanced or turned so that it can be guided visually into the proper position without producing injury or spasm in the vessel.

Although dural AVFs are high-flow lesions, they often consist of multiple small vessels that coalesce at the site of the fistula. Therefore, when selective and subselective catheterization is performed, small amounts of contrast can usually be injected through the catheter by hand rather than requiring the use of an automatic power injector. On average, normal branch vessels of the ECA when selectively catheterized can be adequately opacified with 3 to 5 mL of contrast. Depending on the degree of dilatation and flow characteristics, ECA branch vessels supplying dural AVFs can usually be opacified by mild to moderate increases in contrast volume.

When interpreting the angiogram of a dural fistula, the venous drainage pattern is very important because this aspect of the lesion will determine natural history and prognosis. Most dural fistulae drain into a large dural sinus. This type of fistula, although often symptomatic, is at low risk to the patient for hemorrhage. In contrast, the more rare dural fistula that drains into cortical brain veins or has associated venous aneurysms is at higher risk for hemorrhage (see Figs. 13-22 and 13-23) (24,25).

Direct Fistulae

Direct fistulae may be posttraumatic, such as in the case of a carotid cavernous sinus fistula (CCF) following a base of skull fracture, or can be congenital, as in the case of a vein of Galen fistula. Although the pathophysiology of these lesions is quite different, the hemodynamic characteristics are similar. Flow in the lesion is usually extremely high, making it more difficult to identify the site of the fistulous connection between the arterial system and the venous system (see Fig. 18-10). This requires much higher contrast rates and volumes in a range that would usually be unthinkable. For example, in the instance of a CCF, it is not unusual to inject 10 mL/second for a total of 10 mL into the internal carotid artery. The important aspect of the contrast injection in the evaluation of a fistula is to produce a compact bolus that will identify the defect in the vessel. To that end, very rapid filming is also required. Although four frames per second may be adequate in some instances, it may be necessary to increase frame rates even higher. By using rapid frame rates for filming and a compact, high-volume bolus of contrast, the odds are improved in finding the defect or hole in the artery on one or more of the frames before the venous system fills with contrast. The location and number of fistulous communications has therapeutic implications, especially if embolization is the treatment of choice.

With extremely high flow fistulae it is useful to also evaluate the collateral circulation to the territory involved. This has both therapeutic and diagnostic implications. During treatment of a fistula it may become necessary to sacrifice the artery. A knowledge of the collateral circulation to the involved vascular territory becomes essential in that setting. Also, if the site of the fistula cannot be detected by injection of the involved artery because flow into the venous system is too rapid, it can sometimes be better seen with retrograde flow from a collateral pathway. For example, if the hole in the ICA involved with a CCF cannot be clearly identified when the ICA is injected due to very high flow, it may be better seen with an ipsilateral carotid compression maneuver during a vertebral injection (Huber maneuver; see Fig. 18-10C).

SUMMARY

It is fortunate for patients that CT, MR, and MR angiography have replaced the need for cerebral angiography in many settings. It is unfortunate for people in training, however, because the experience that used to be gained during residency and fellowship has been reduced. At the same time, the need for more detailed evaluation to answer specific questions in a given patient has increased because there are more treatment options available to patients with vascular lesions. Specifically, in the past treatment decisions were based mainly on whether to operate or not operate. Now the decisions are more complex because the additional options of endovascular therapy and radiation therapy and medical management have significantly advanced.

In this chapter, guidelines and techniques for performing most cerebral angiograms were discussed. As was stated earlier, there is no substitution for experience and good judgment. Although the guidelines presented work in the majority of instances, they may not be appropriate in all instances. The angiographer must learn to adapt standard techniques to specific situations to arrive at a safe means of obtaining the necessary information to implement appropriate therapy.

In order to fulfill that mission, a thorough understanding of cerebral vascular anatomy, pathophysiology, and disease processes and their treatments is necessary. With respect to the technical aspects of cerebral angiography, one must remain adaptable. Techniques that were considered bad practice or unsafe in the past may be perfectly acceptable today because of advances in catheter material, contrast, and so forth. Rather than using the perspective of correct versus incorrect technique, it may be best to consider techniques from the perspective of safe versus unsafe.

REFERENCES

1. Skalpe IO, Lundervold A, Tjostad K. Complications of cerebral angiography. Comparing metrizamide (Amipaque) and meglumine metrizoate (Isopaque Cerebral). *Neuroradiology* 1980;19:67–71.
2. Pinto RS, Robbins E, Seidenwurm D. Thrombogenicity of Teflon versus copolymer-coated guidewires: evaluation with scanning electron microscopy. *AJNR* 1989;10:407–410.
3. Morris P. *Practical neuroangiography.* Baltimore, MD: Williams & Wilkins, 1997.
4. Bird CR, Drayer BP, Velaj R, et al. Safety of contrast media in cerebral angiography: iopamidol vs. methylglucamine iothalamate. *AJNR* 1984; 5:801–803.
5. Bryan RN, Miller SL, Roehm JO, Weatherall PT. Neuroangiography with iohexal. *AJNR* 1983;4:344–346.
6. Pelz D, Fox AJ, Vinuela F. Clinical trials of iohexol vs. Conray 60 for cerebral angiography. *AJNR* 1984;5:565–568.
7. Kido DK, Potts DG, Bryan RN, et al. Iohexol in cerebral angiography: multicenter clinical trial. *Invest Radiol* 1985;20(suppl 1):55–57.
8. Lovencic M, Jakovac I, Klanfar Z. Iohexol versus meglumine-Ca-metrizoate in cerebral angiography: a randomized double-blind crossover study. *Acta Radiol Suppl (Stockh)* 1986;369:521–523.
9. Pelz DM, Fox AJ, Vinuela F, Lylyk P. A comparison of iopamidol and iohexol in cerebral angiography. *AJNR* 1988;9:1163–1166.
10. Wolf GL, Arenson RL, Cross AP. A prospective trial of ionic vs. nonionic contrast agents in routine clinical practice: comparison of adverse effects. *AJR* 1989;152:939–944.
11. Katayama H, Yamaguchi K, Kozuka T, Takashima T, Seez P, Matsuura K. Adverse reactions to ionic and nonionic contrast media. *Radiology* 1990;175:621–628.
12. Latchaw RE. The use of nonionic contrast agents in neuroangiography. A review of the literature and recommendations for clinical use. *Invest Radiol* 1993;28(suppl 5):55–59.
13. Velaj R, Drayer B, Albright R, Fram E. Comparative neurotoxicity of angiographic contrast media. *Neurology* 1985;35:1290–1298.
14. *The manual on iodinated contrast media.* Reston, VA: American College of Radiology, 1991.
15. Brismar J. Computer tomography as the primary radiologic procedure in acute subarachnoid hemorrhage. *Acta Radiol [Diagn] (Stockh)* 1979; 20:849–864.
16. Davis KR, New PFJ, Ojemann RG, et al. Computed tomographic evaluation of hemorrhage secondary to intracranial aneurysm. *AJR* 1976;127:143–153.
17. Bjorkesten G, Halonen V. Incidence of intracranial vascular lesions in patients with subarachnoid hemorrhage investigated by four-vessel angiography. *J Neurosurg* 1965;23:29–32.
18. Osborn AG. *Introduction to cerebral angiography.* Philadelphia, PA: Harper & Row, 1980.
19. Lin JP, Kricheff II. Angiographic investigation of cerebral aneurysms. Technical aspects. *Radiology* 1972:105;69–76.
20. Jacobs JM. Angiography in intracranial hemorrhage. *Neuroimag Clin North Am* 1992;2:89–106.
21. Spetzler RF, Martin NA. A proposed grading system for arteriovenous malformations. *J Neurosurg* 1986 Oct;65:476–483.
22. Marks MP, Lane B, Steinberg G, Chang P. Vascular characteristics of

intracranial arteriovenous malformations which correlate with symptoms of hemorrhage and steal. *Neuroradiology* 1991;33(suppl): 184–186.

23. Lunsford LD, Konziolka D, Flickinger JC, et al. Stereotactic radiosurgery for arteriovenous malformations of the brain. *J Neurosurg* 1991;75:512–524.

24. Djindjian R, Merland JJ, Theron J. *Super-selective arteriography of the external carotid artery.* Berlin: Springer-Verlag, 1978.

25. Lasjaunias P, Berenstein A. *Surgical neuroangiography. 1. Functional anatomy of craniofacial arteries.* Berlin: Springer-Verlag, 1986.

26. Kupersmith MJ. *Neurovascular neuro-ophthalmology.* Berlin: Springer-Verlag, 1993.

Subject Index

Note: Blood vessels are indexed under their names, e.g., Carotid artery(ies); Cerebral vein(s). Letters after page numbers indicate the following: f, illustrations; t, tables; b, boxes.

Vasculopathy, intracranial (*contd.*)
  congenital, 350–351, 352f–353f
  differential diagnosis of, 357, 357f
  imaging appearance of, 351, 354,
      354f
  primary angiitis, 354
  secondary angiitis, 354–355, 355f
  secondary vasculitis, 355–356,
      356f
  systemic vasculitis, 354
  terminology of, 351
Vasoconstriction, in subarachnoid
      hemorrhage, 259
Vasospasm
  in aneurysm rupture, 256, 256f, 269f
  catheter-induced, 342, 344f, 345f
  in subarachnoid hemorrhage, vs.
      vasculitis, 357, 357f
Vein(s). *See specific artery names, e.g.,*
      Cerebral veins
Vein of Galen
  anatomy of, 202f, 220f, 225–226, 225f,
      226f, 235f
  aneurysmal malformation of, 290,
      290f–292f, 292
  angiography of, 208f, 229, 230f, 231f,
      236f
  development of, 217, 219
  malformations of, 214, 215f, 278f
  thrombosis of, 391, 394f, 395
  vascular territories of, 227f
Vein of Labbé
  anatomy of, 202f, 219, 219f–222f
  angiography of, 200f, 222, 222f
  vascular territories of, 227f
Vein of Trolard
  anatomy of, 202f, 219, 219f–221f
  angiography of, 208f, 209f, 222
Venous angioma (developmental venous
      anomaly), 294–295, 295f–297f
Venous malformations, 278f, 293–298
  arterialized, 287
  cavernous, 278f, 293, 295–296, 298,
      299f
  cutaneous, 310
  developmental venous anomaly,
      294–295, 295f–297f
  varices, 295, 298f
Venous occlusions

stroke in, 390–391, 390b, 392f–395f,
      395
  traumatic, 416, 416f
Venous outflow channels, of arteriovenous
      malformations, 279, 280f
Ventral aortae, 4t, 8f, 9f, 32f, 33
Ventricular branches, of posterior cerebral
      artery, 156, 157f
Ventricular vein, inferior, anatomy of,
      225f, 226f
Vermian arteries, anatomy of, 176f, 178f,
      182f, 189f, 190
Vermian veins
  inferior
    anatomy of, 235, 235f, 237f
    displacement of, in tonsillar
        herniation, 325f
  superior, anatomy of, 233, 234f–236f,
      235
Vertebral artery(ies), 173–184
  anastomoses of, 403
    with external carotid artery, 399,
        399f, 400f
    with pharyngeal artery, 38–39
    in subclavian steal, 401f–402f, 403
  anatomy of, 13f, 14f
    angiographic, 178f–182f, 180
    gross, 173–174, 174b, 175f, 176f
  aneurysms of, 184
  angiography of, 178f–182f, 180
    in aneurysm, 441, 441t, 442
  anomalies of, 174b, 184, 184f, 185f
  arteriovenous fistulae of, traumatic, 414
  atherosclerosis of
    angiography of, 363f
    ectasia in, 371f
    vasculitis in, 372f
  branches of, 174b
    cervical, 174–176
    intracranial, 176–177, 177f, 178f, 180
    meningeal, 176, 176f
  development of, 4t, 5, 7f–11f, 173, 174b
  displacement of, in tumors, 333f
  dissection of, 346
    traumatic, 408, 409f
  duplicate origin of, 184, 184f
  extraosseous segment of, 174, 175f
  extraspinal segment of, 174, 175f, 181f
  fenestration of, 184, 185f

foraminal segment of, 174, 175f, 181f
  intradural segment of, 174, 175f
  left
    anatomy of, 28f, 29, 29f, 177f
    angiography of, 182f, 183f
    branches of, 182f
    origin of, 16, 19f, 28f, 29, 29f
  origin of, 12f, 178f, 179f, 180
    anomalous, 184
    left, 28f, 29, 29f
  relationships of, 174, 174b
  right
    anatomy of, 27, 28f, 36f, 177f
    angiography of, 184f
    hypoplasia of, 19f
  segments of, 173–174, 175f
  termination in, posterior inferior
      cerebellar artery, 180, 183f
  variants of, 174b, 180, 183f, 184f
Vertebral column, aortic arch relationship
      to, 12
Vertebral veins
  anatomy of, 196f
  development of, 218f
Vertebral venous plexus
  anatomy of, 197–198
  angiography of, 198f, 199f
Vertebrobasilar dolichoectasia, ectasia of,
      366
Vertebrobasilar system. *See also* Basilar
      artery; Cerebral artery(ies),
      posterior; Vertebral artery(ies)
  angiographic technique for, in
      atherosclerosis, 439–440
  dissections in, 346
Vesalius, foramen of, 49
Vidian artery (artery of the pterygoid
      canal)
  anastomoses of, 86f
  anatomy of, 49, 52f, 72f, 73, 75f
  enlargement of, juvenile nasopharyngeal
      angiofibroma, 334, 335f
Virchow-Robin space, anatomy of, 201f
von Hippel-Lindau syndrome,
      hemangioblastoma in, 329

W
Watershed zone, 118f, 131, 149, 168
Willis, circle of. *See* Circle of Willis